Idyll Arbor's
Therapy
Dictionary

Idyll Arbor's

Therapy Dictionary

Second Edition

Idyll Arbor, Inc.

PO Box 720, Ravensdale, WA 98051 (425) 432-3231

Idyll Arbor, Inc. Editor: Thomas M. Blaschko

To the best of our knowledge, the information and recommendations of this book reflect currently accepted practice. Nevertheless, they cannot be considered absolute and universal. Guidelines suggested by federal law are subject to change as the laws and interpretations do. Recommendations for a particular client must be considered in light of the client's needs and condition. The editors, authors, and publisher disclaim responsibly for any adverse effects resulting directly or indirectly from the suggested management practices, from any undetected errors, or from the reader's misunderstanding of the text.

The first edition of this dictionary was titled *Idyll Arbor's Glossary for Therapists*.

Library of Congress Cataloging-in-Publication Data
Idyll Arbor's therapy dictionary / authors, joan burlingame ... [et al.] ; editor-in-chief, joan burlingame; contributing
  editors, Thomas M. Blaschko, Thomas K. Skalko.-- 2nd ed.
    p. cm.
  Previously published under the title: Idyll Arbor's glossary for therapists.
  Includes bibliographical references.
  ISBN 1-882883-46-2
   1.   Medical rehabilitation--Dictionaries. 2. Therapeutics--Dictionaries. 3. Medical care--Dictionaries. I. Title:
Therapy dictionary. II. burlingame, joan. III. burlingame, joan. IV. Blaschko, Thomas M. V. Idyll Arbor's
glossary for therapists.

RM930.B87 2001
617'.03'03--dc21

                         2001024759

ISBN 1-882883-46-2

Staff

Editor in Chief
joan burlingame, CTRS, HTR, ABDA

Contributing Editors
Thomas M. Blaschko, MA
Thomas K. Skalko, PhD, TRS/CTRS

Authors
joan burlingame, CTRS, ABDA, HTR
Anne Battiste, CTRS
Thomas M. Blaschko, MA
Susan Brennen
Mary Ann Devine, CTRS
Maria Jimenez
Carmen V. Russoniello, EdD, CTRS
Ann Nathan
Laree Shanda, CTRS
Thomas K. Skalko, PhD, TRS/CTRS

The difference between the right word
and the almost right word
is the difference between
lightning and the lightning bug.

— Mark Twain

Contents

How to Use This Dictionary

The terms in this dictionary are defined with an emphasis toward providing the type of information a therapist needs. In this way the **Therapy Dictionary** is different from a medical dictionary. While it provides the basic medical definition for most words, it does not stop there. Many of the definitions also include implications for functional ability and therapy intervention. Words in a definition, which are italicized, are defined elsewhere in the dictionary.

We also recognize that, while this **Dictionary** contains thousands of words, there are many more to define. Individuals are invited to submit their own sets of definitions for consideration for the next edition. Individuals who submit groups of their own definitions that are used in the next edition will be recognized as contributors to the **Dictionary.**

Notes on Definitions from Federal Government Documents

Quite often the Federal Government of the United States defines terms in ways that are different from those normally used. At other times, because the term being defined is tied very closely with a federal regulation that the therapist is expected to follow, it is important to know exactly, word for word, what the government's definition is. For that purpose, specific federal definitions used in this book are basically word for word as they can be found in official government publications. To let the reader know when the exact government definition has been used, we have placed an abbreviation in front of the definition. This abbreviation can be used with the key below to determine which government publication the quote came from.

ADA — Americans with Disabilities Act. **Americans with Disabilities Act Handbook**. 1991. Equal Employment Opportunity Commission and the US Department of Justice. United States Printing Office Publication #EEOC-BK-19.

CDC — From the CDC **Glossary of Medical and Scientific Terms Related to CFS** from Centers for Disease Control and Prevention web site (9/14/00)

FB — **Understanding Estimates of the Impact of Health Reform on the Federal Budget**, 1994. Office of Technology Assessment, Congress of the United States of America Publication #OTA-BP-H-132.

HCFA/Questions — Answers to HCFA Frequently Asked Questions HCFA web site 9/18/00

HCO — **Bringing Health Care Online: The Role of Information Technologies**. 1995. Office of Technology Assessment. Congress of the United States of America Publication #OTA-ITC-624.

HHS — definition supplied by the Health and Human Services Department through their web sites.

HHS/NMDP — The National Marrow Donor Program, from their web site.

OBRA — **State Operations Manual for the Nursing Home Reform Provisions of the Omnibus Budget Reconciliation Act of 1987**, updated in 1992 and 1995.

RAPs — **Resident Assessment Protocols**, part of the MDS. (Part of the OBRA legislation).

Note about the DSM-IV

Reference is made to the **DSM-IV** throughout this book. The **DSM-IV** is the **Diagnostic and Statistical Manual of Mental Disorders, Fourth Edition** published by the American Psychiatric Association (1994). The **DSM-IV** is the official guide for behaviors and characteristics associated with recognized psychiatric (mental) disorders. When the term **DSM-IV** is used, the authors are usually indicating that the behaviors and/or characteristics are part of the "official" diagnostic criteria.

A

AA See *Alcoholics Anonymous*.

AAHPERD See *American Alliance for Health, Physical Education, Recreation, and Dance*.

abasement a term coined by Henry Murray used to describe an individual's belief that s/he should surrender to the will of another to make up for imagined or real flaws or shortcomings in himself/herself.

abasia a Greek term literally meaning a negative ability to step. Abasia is the inability to walk due to a variety of causes. There are five primary types of abasia: 1. abasia ataxia, which is due to a defect in coordination causing difficulty in movement, 2. choreic abasia, which is due to chorea of the legs, 3. paralytic abasia, which is due to a paralysis of the leg muscles, 4. paroxysmal trepidant abasia, which is due to the leg muscles stiffening spastically upon attempting to stand, and 5. trembling abasia, which is an inability to walk due to severe trembling of the leg muscles. Also called "astasia." See *chorea movements*.

abbreviated standard survey a survey conducted in response to a complaint, a change of facility ownership, management, or director of nursing services. (OBRA) The abbreviated standard survey does not cover all of the aspects covered in the standard survey, but rather concentrates on the particular areas of concern or concerns. For example, an abbreviated standard survey may be conducted to substantiate a complaint. The survey team can expand the abbreviated standard survey to cover additional areas or decide to conduct a standard survey if, during an abbreviated standard survey, they find evidence that warrants a more extensive review. See *partial extended survey*.

abbreviation expansion a type of "shorthand" typing for entering information into the computer. A *macro* program (a short computer program) tells the computer to recognize a specific string of letters or symbols as a longer entry. An example is the use of "control-c" to copy a piece of text in Microsoft Word instead of clicking "edit" then selecting "copy." This system can save the user time and effort and is especially helpful for people with disabilities who have trouble with data entry and typing.

abdominal belts See *back belts*.

abduction the process of moving a body part away from midline. In the case of the digits (the fingers or toes), abduction refers to the process of moving the digit away from the axis of the limb. Most activities require some degree of abduction. These include walking (abduction of lower limbs, arms), cooking (abduction of arms in mixing), and reading (abducting the arms when turning pages). Contrast with *adduction*.

ABE See *adult basic education*.

aberration deviation from what is considered "*normal*." This term is used in both psychiatric settings and medical settings. It may apply to a patient's behavior, to a biological structure, to the results of a test, or to an outcome of a procedure.

ability grouping the process of dividing individuals into groups based on similar, shared abilities.

ability testing the measurement of an individual's performance in specific domains (e.g., cognitive, physical, or psychomotor) through the use of *standardized testing tools*. Ability testing measures the individual's functional ability at that one moment in time. Disease process (such as sundowning in Alzheimer's disease) or environmental conditions (such as taking the test in a hot, stuffy classroom) may cause significant variations to occur in the individual's performance from one time to the next. The tester should not modify the individual's score on the ability test to "make up for" the disease process or environmental conditions. However, the tester should note on the summary of the individual's test results any process or condition which may have impacted the individual's performance. When accommodation is required, the type of accommodation should be written along with the test results. Any type of accommodation may change the testing tool's *validity*, *reliability*, and meaning of scores.

abnormal different from what is normally expected; outside standard measurements. In psychiatry, "abnormal" historically meant that a behavior was outside the statistically described "normal" behavior and therefore implied that the behavior was undesirable. This definition causes conflict when one tries to be culturally sensitive. It would be considered abnormal in the United States for a woman to be treated as subservient to her husband. However, in many fundamental religions, that would be considered the norm. Homosexuality would, statistically, be considered abnormal. However, many cities and some states have laws making it illegal to discriminate against individuals based on their sexual preference. The Americans with Disabilities Act is a civil rights law that makes it illegal to discriminate against individuals because their physical or psychological abilities are outside "the norm." Abnormal, when referring to lab tests, ability to ambulate, etc., is still used (appropriately) in health care. See *Denver Developmental Screening Tool*.

above elbow amputation an amputation of the arm between the shoulder and elbow joints. Functional ability is improved through the use of a six-unit prosthesis:
1. specially constructed socket to provide maximal axial loading
2. cable and figure eight harness
3. internal locking elbow
4. forearm lift assist
5. wrist unit
6. terminal device

Above elbow amputation is abbreviated "AE."

above knee amputation above knee refers to an amputation of the leg above the knee joint but below the hip joint. Functional ability is improved through the use of a five-unit prosthesis:
1. quadrilateral socket (made of either wood or plastic)
2. pelvic band
3. control belt
4. mechanical knee joint
5. prosthetic foot

The purpose of the socket is to help distribute the weight through the ischial tuberosity to the hip joint. Some patients are fitted with a suction socket instead of a quadrilateral socket, pelvic band, and control belt. An above knee amputation is abbreviated "AKA."

abrasion the unusual or abnormal process of wearing away tissue, body structure, or other body substance. Individuals who have impaired sensation in their legs have an increased risk of receiving abrasions of skin tissue as they bump against hard objects. *Bruxism* is the habitual abrasion of the teeth, which wears down the structure of the teeth.

abscess a collection of pus, resulting from an infection, which is contained in a capsule formed by surrounding healthy cells. The site appears inflamed with signs of redness, swelling, pain, and warmth. An abscess is healed when the pus escapes either through natural breaking of the cell walls or through medical intervention. Care must be taken that the escaping infectious material does not enter the blood stream, infect other parts of the body, or spread to other people. There are over 100 types of abscesses.

absence the momentary loss of mental attention for which the individual has no memory. This is a common aspect of some types of *epilepsy*.

absent sensation lack of awareness of contact. See *sensation*.

absolute score interpretation the use of an individual's (or group's) score on a standardized test to infer a specific level of capability. An example would be IQ testing. While an IQ test may have fewer than 150 questions, scores greater than 130 would infer cognitive "giftedness" and the likelihood that above average performance could be expected on additional, similar questions. For a test to be used for absolute score interpretation, the testing tool must be able to predict performance over a broad area through the use of representative questions or skills. Many standardized testing tools measure performance but cannot state with reasonable certainty that if an individual performs well on the test, then the individual holds the necessary performance skills inferred by the test to successfully repeat that performance outside of the controlled test-taking environment.

abstinence the refraining from indulging in an activity (usually referring to sexual intercourse), food, or other substance. "Abstinence syndrome" is used to refer to the wide range of physiological complications that arise when someone goes "cold turkey" and experiences a quick withdrawal from a drug to which s/he is addicted.

abstract reasoning the ability to look at a situation, picture a variety of actions to take, understand the implications for possible actions, analyze the choices, and then come to a conclusion or decision. See *dementia, executive function*.

abulia a severe, pathological reduction in the ability to initiate activity, develop new ideas, or make decisions as well as the demonstration of indifference to the consequences of one's actions (or inactions).

abuse the misuse of a person, an object, or a drug. By law, therapists are required to report suspected cases of abuse of a child or a person who considered not able to independently take care of himself/herself. While there are many precipitating factors to child abuse, some of the key risk factors identified as increasing a child's chances of being an abuse victim (or abusability) are excessive crying, physical disability, and prematurity. See *confidentiality, consumer rights, drug abuse, mental abuse, neglect, ombudsman, physical abuse, Protection and Advocacy for the Mentally Ill Act of 1986*.

abuse (Medicare) (HCFA/Questions) actions that are inconsistent with accepted, sound medical, business, or fiscal practices. Abuse directly or indirectly results in an unnecessary cost to the program through improper payments. The real difference between fraud and abuse is the person's intent. Both have the same impact: they steal valuable resources from the Medicare Trust Fund that would otherwise be used to provide care to Medicare beneficiaries. Complaints about fraud committed against Medicare frequently take a long time to resolve. All Medicare contractors (the intermediaries and carriers that contract with HCFA to process Medicare claims) have Medicare Fraud Units in place to detect, deter, and prevent fraud and abuse. In addition to the other workload that these units have, they receive and respond to a large number of complaints. Some of these complaints involve fraud and abuse while others are simple misunderstandings. The Fraud Unit staff must treat each complaint seriously. This means that they meticulously investigate each case. Investigations may involve a number of steps including sending surveys to a random sample of beneficiaries, speaking to beneficiaries on the phone, obtaining medical records from providers, conducting on-site audits, and writing a report on the investigation. After the Fraud Unit has completed its investigation, the case is often referred to federal law enforcement and then on to the US Attorney for criminal or civil prosecution. Obviously, this process takes a considerable amount of time. Fraud Units refer the results of their investigations to the US Department of Health and Human Services Office of the Inspector General (OIG). The OIG's Office of Investigations then prepares the case for referral to the Department of Justice for criminal and/or civil prosecution. A person who is found guilty of committing Medicare fraud faces a host of different criminal, civil, and administrative sanction penalties including:

- Civil penalties of $5,000 to $10,000 per false claim and treble damages under the False Claims Act
- Criminal fines and/or imprisonment of up to 10 years if convicted of the crime of Health Care Fraud as provided in the Health Insurance Portability and Accountability Act of 1996 or, for violations of the Medicare/Medicaid Anti-Kickback Statute, imprisonment of up to five years and/or a criminal fine of up to $25,000

Administrative sanctions including up to a $10,000 civil monetary penalty per line item on a false claim, assessments of up to treble the amount falsely claimed, and/or exclusion from participation in Medicare and state health care programs. In addition to the penalties outlined above, those who commit health care fraud can also be tried for mail and wire

fraud. The consequences have never been as great in US history as they are today. See *fraud (Medicare)*.

academic ability the ability to perform the tasks expected by one's school. Academic ability is not the same as intelligence quotient (IQ) but is frequently related.

acathexis the lack of felt and/or demonstrated emotional response to a person, event, or information that would normally cause a significant response.

acceleration 1. an increase in frequency of a behavior or other observable event (e.g. quickening of pulse rate or respiration). 2. a change in speed.

acceleration factors (in head injuries) the type of brain damage typically found in the injuries due to force. The movement of the brain against the skull (an acceleration injury) causes more neurological damage to the brain than the result of the same force crushing the stationary skull. In fact, an acceleration injury to the head causes significantly more damage to the brain than a crushing blow twenty times as intense. (Ylvisaker, 1985, p. 5)

acceptable daily intake (ADI) (HHS) the amount of chemical that, if ingested daily over a lifetime, appears to be without appreciable effect.

acceptable plan of correction a term used by the United States government for a plan of action(s) to correct Medicare and/or Medicaid deficiencies found during a survey. This plan, written by the facility, indicates the corrections to be made, the steps to make the corrections, and the time period needed to make the correction. The plan of correction is considered to be "acceptable" if the corrections and their time lines are approved by the authority (state or federal survey team) that is responsible for determining a facility's compliance. See *effective date of participation, plan of correction*.

acceptance See *social acceptance*.

access aisle (ADA) an accessible pedestrian space between *elements*, such as parking spaces, seating, and desks, that provides clearances appropriate for use of the elements.

accessibility 1. the degree to which a building, a program, or a position is open to individuals with disabilities; the ability of a site or object to be reached and used by individuals. The *Americans With Disabilities Act* in the United States is a major piece of legislation that outlines the specific measurements for accessibility designs and accommodations. 2. in case management, the availability of services for members of managed care systems. If there are no appointments available in a timely manner, if the phone line is always busy, or if other problems impede the patient's ability to reach and see the professional, the system has poor accessibility. Standards for this accessibility are set by the National Committee for Quality Assurance (NCQA) for the Accreditation of Managed Care Organizations. See *customer service.*

accessible 1. practically defined, a site, building, or facility (or a portion of one of these) is accessible to a patient if the patient can engage in normal uses. 2. (ADA) legally defined, a site, building, or facility, (or a portion of one of these) is accessible if it complies with the ADA Accessibility Guidelines.

accessible element (ADA) an element specified by the ADA regulations (for example, telephone, controls, and the like).

accessible route (ADA) a continuous unobstructed path connecting all accessible elements and spaces of a building or facility. Interior accessible routes may include corridors, floors, ramps, elevators, lifts, and clear floor space at fixtures. Exterior accessible routes may include parking access aisles, curb ramps, crosswalks at vehicular ways, walks, ramps, and lifts.

accessible space (ADA) space that complies with the ADA regulations.

ACCH See *Association for the Care of Children's Health.*

accident See *adolescent injuries, back injury, brain injury, childhood injuries, falls.*

accident and health insurance an insurance policy or entitlement program which pays (in part or whole) for treatment and other benefits in the case of disease, accidental injury, or accidental death.

accident prevention program a written plan to prevent workplace injury and illness. Federal laws in the United States require that an employer provides the employees with a safe place to work. Most states implement this expectation through the requirement of a formal, written accident prevention program. These programs have three components: 1. the written accident prevention program, 2. the formation and maintenance of a safety committee, and 3. the actual employee training programs and equipment purchases which are required to implement the program. The Occupational Safety and Health Act (federal law) requires survey teams to evaluate employer's compliance through unannounced survey visits. By far, the most common OSHA citation is the lack of a written accident prevention program. See *environment of care.*

accommodation changing to adjust to outside circumstances or to the environment as in: 1. the individual's or the environment's ability to adjust to a needed or desired change. Piaget felt that as an individual matures, s/he is able to accommodate the

way that s/he perceives the world to fit a changing understanding of reality, *assimilation;* 2. buildings going through structural changes to accommodate those with different physical needs; 3. an individual's eye lens changing shape to focus on objects at various distances; 4. social groups going through changes (compromise, conciliation, arbitration, or surrender) as a result of two or more cultural groups coming into contact with each other. See *equilibration, Kolb's experiential learning theory.*

accountability being responsible for the consequences of an action or decision. In quality assurance programs, individuals who are responsible for the quality assurance goal are said to have the "accountability."

accreditation referring to the formal certification by a group of recognized authorities that one's work, schooling, program, or facility has met or exceeded minimum standards of quality. Accreditation is a voluntary process. Some of the recognized accrediting bodies in health care are the *Joint Commission on Accreditation of Healthcare Organizations* (JCAHO) and *CARF: the Rehabilitation Accreditation Commission.*

accredited hospital hospitals that are approved by either the Joint Commission on Accreditation of Healthcare Organizations or the American Osteopathic Association (AOA). These hospitals are "deemed" to meet the Medicare conditions of participation. See *deemed status.*

accredited standards committee (HCO) a committee chartered by ANSI to work on standards in a particular area of commerce. For example, ASC X12 is the committee working on standards for the insurance industry, including health.

acculturation the process by which children learn the expectations, responsibilities, and norms of their culture. This acquisition of expected patterns of behavior takes place over an extended period of time and often has its periods of trials and tribulations. An example would be the child who is two years old (the "terrible twos") who goes through a period usually lasting about six months when s/he is making a serious, subconscious attempt to learn just how far s/he can push the cultural expectations. This term is also used to refer to the adult who has entered a different cultural group and is learning how to function within that group's expectations. Acculturation is an important process which helps ensure the individual's acceptance into his/her social group and community. Individuals who live in institutions for a long period of time tend to become less able to fit into the community as a whole. The skills and behaviors that help one survive inside an institution (acculturation to institutional skills and behaviors) tend to be skills and behaviors that help separate (alienate) one from the community as a whole.

Acesulfame K (acesulfame potassium) (HHS) a low-calorie sweetener approved for use in the United States in 1988. It is an organic salt consisting of carbon, nitrogen, oxygen, hydrogen, sulphur, and potassium atoms. It is 200 times sweeter than sucrose, has a synergistic sweetening effect with other sweeteners, has a stable shelf life, and is heat stable. It is excreted through the human digestive system unchanged, and is therefore non-caloric.

acetylsalicylic acid aspirin. While aspirin is an over-the-counter medication, which is primarily used to treat minor aches and pains and prevent heart attacks, it does have potential negative side effects. Adverse reactions include nausea and dyspepsia and increased thirst. The prolonged use of aspirin may lead to a persistent iron deficiency anemia.

achievement test a test designed to measure an individual's current knowledge base. Some of the better-known achievement tests are the Academic Instructional Measurement System (AIMS), Woodcock-Johnson Psycho-educational Battery, and the Kaufman Test of Educational Achievement.

achondroplasia a hereditary disorder which causes inadequate cartilage formation at the end of the long bones and the skull. This results in premature ossification. This disorder causes the most common type of dwarfism, which presents with a normal-sized trunk but other features (e.g., head, limbs) smaller than normal.

acid a "street term" commonly used to refer to the illegal drug lysergic acid diethylamide (LSD).

ACLD See *Learning Disabilities Association of America.*

acousticophobia the irrational fear of sounds.

acoustics pertaining to the physical aspects of sound: just one aspect of auditory perception. See *auditory.*

acquired immune deficiency syndrome (AIDS) the advanced stage of HIV infection. AIDS is caused by a virus that damages the immune system, leaving the body vulnerable to attack from certain infections and cancers that are not a threat to healthy people. The AIDS virus is carried in the blood and in some body secretions; it is most commonly transmitted by sexual contact or by contact with infected blood — for example, by sharing needles used for injecting drugs. See *blood/body fluids precautions, HIV.*

acrocephalia a birth defect where the child's head is abnormally pointed. Originating from the Greek words "acro" which means extremity or topmost and "cephalic" which means head or brain.

acrophobia the irrational fear of heights.

acting out 1. an undesirable explosion of anger, aggression, and/or other anti-social behaviors as one expresses his/her feelings through actions instead of words or "talking things out." 2. a neutral or positive connotation of someone being able to express previously held in feelings in a somewhat controlled manner (e.g., using drama). When a patient is said to be acting out using the first meaning, it usually implies that some type of intervention is needed. The expression of anger in and of itself is not therapeutic. The ability to learn how to resolve and cope with the source of anger, as in the second meaning, is therapeutic. See *anger management, medical play.*

action tremor an involuntary tremor which is evidenced by oscillating and rhythmic movements of the outstretched upper limb during activity. See *tremor.*

action verbs verbs that state an action being taken. Action verbs are used in procedure statements or patient objectives. See *procedures.*

active the act of initiating and sustaining involvement in an activity or social interaction. Opposite of passive. Because active is such a general term it is frequently is used as an adjective to describe some action which is being done actively, e.g., active treatment, active participation. Referring to medications, "active" refers to the ingredients in the medication that cause a change to occur.

active listening a technique of listening in which the listener carefully listens to the other person's communication then restates what the other person said to ensure that the listener understood. Active listening involves a non-judgmental attitude when reiterating what the speaker said. See *listening skills.*

active movement voluntarily done movement through the patient's use of his/her own muscles. See *movement.*

active stretching patient-initiated movement designed to increase *range of motion* in affected soft tissue and joints. This is usually carried out in physical therapy using a prescribed exercise program or in therapeutic activity programs using a prescribed set of activities designed to achieve the desired outcome.

active surveillance See *surveillance.*

active treatment for inpatient psychiatric services The United States Government defines "Active Treatment" for patients receiving inpatient psychiatric services as a professionally developed and physician supervised individual plan of care designed to achieve the individual's discharge from the inpatient status at the earliest possible time and which meets the special staff and medical records requirements necessary to carry out a program of treatment for mentally ill persons as prescribed in regulations at 42 CFR 482.61 and 482.62.

active treatment in intermediate care facilities for the mentally retarded The United States government defines "active treatment" in ICF-MRs as the aggressive, consistent implementation of a program of specialized and generic training, treatment, health services, and related services directed toward the acquisition of the behaviors necessary for the individual to function with as much self-determination and independence as possible; and the prevention or deceleration of regression or loss of current optimal functional status (42 CFR 483.440). Active treatment is an overall combined program of learning and health care for individuals who are mentally retarded or have other significant developmental disabilities and who are receiving Medicaid funding. Active treatment is considered to be a continuum, starting with a comprehensive assessment by the interdisciplinary team, followed by a team meeting with the client to determine the learning and health care goals over the next 12 months, the implementation of the program, the monitoring of the effectiveness of the program, and lastly, the (re)assessment when the program no longer seems to meet the client's needs. Active treatment does not assume that the client will always progress, but rather, that the program is helping the client maximize his/her potential, even if s/he has a deteriorating condition. Training in leisure skill development (including the skills needed to have an enjoyable retirement) is a vital aspect of the law.

activities of daily living (ADL) skills that are required on a day-to-day basis. In the broader sense, all health care professionals use treatment interventions to help the patient overcome difficulties in performing ADLs. Basic activities of daily living are usually grouped into seven categories: 1. bathing, 2. dressing, 3. toilet hygiene, 4. grooming, 5. feeding/eating, 6. functional mobility, and 7. functional communication (American Occupational Therapy Association, 1989). ADL skills of dressing, hand function, and vocational skills are frequently the treatment domain of Occupational Therapy. However, in practice, all members of the interdisciplinary team work toward the patient's increased independence in ADLs. (RAPs) Personal mastery of ADLs and mobility are as crucial to human existence in the nursing home as they are in the community. The nursing home is unique only in that most patients require help with self-care functions. ADL dependence can lead to intense personal distress — invalidism, isolation, diminished self-worth, and a loss of

control over one's destiny. As inactivity increases, complications such as *pressure sores, falls, contractures,* and muscle wasting can be expected. It is important for the staff to be able to set positive and realistic goals, weighing the advantages of independence against risks to safety and self-identity. In promoting independence, staff must be willing to accept a reasonable degree of risk and active patient participation in setting treatment objectives. Rehabilitative goals of several types can be considered:

- To restore function to maximum self-sufficiency in the area indicated;
- To replace hands-on assistance with a program of task segmentation and verbal cueing;
- To restore abilities to a level that allows the patient to function with fewer supports;
- To shorten the time required for providing assistance;
- To expand the amount of space in which self-sufficiency can be practiced;
- To avoid or delay additional loss of independence; and
- To support the patient who is certain to decline in order to lessen the likelihood of complications (e.g., pressure sores and contractures).

See *adult daycare centers, advanced activities of daily living, decision making, developmental coordination disorder, mania, mental retardation, significant change.*

activity movement, action, behavior, thought process, progression, development, wakefulness, physiological functions, etc.

activity analysis the objective analysis of the components required to complete an activity. This analysis includes a description and sequence of the physical actions, cognitive actions, social knowledge, and physical equipment required to complete a specific activity. Also referred to as task analysis. The easiest way to break any activity into tasks is to do the activity yourself, slowly. As you make each movement, ask yourself four questions: 1. What did I have to know to make this move? (cognitive) 2. What set of muscles did I need to use and/or coordinate? (physical) 3. How and with whom did I need to interact? (social) 4. How did it make me feel? (emotional). (Cunninghis, 1995)

activity intolerance a patient has an activity intolerance when s/he has insufficient physiological or psychological energy to endure or complete a required task. Some of the measurable/observable characteristics include the patient's verbal report of fatigue, weakness, or inability to stay in the activity; an abnormal heart rate or blood pressure in response to activity; discomfort upon exertion; or an abnormal change in the patient's heartbeat (e.g., arrhythmias).

activity professional an individual hired by a long-term care facility to provide free-time activities to maintain and/or enhance a resident's life as well as to provide specific activity interventions to decrease the negative impact of illness, injury, and institutionalization. The majority of activity professionals work in long-term care facilities. In the United States the federal legislation that regulates long-term care facilities is called *OBRA*. The qualification for an activity professional is defined as someone "who is a qualified therapeutic recreation specialist or an activities professional who is licensed or registered, if applicable, by the state in which practicing; and is eligible for certification as a therapeutic recreation specialist; as an activities professional by a recognized accrediting body on or after October 1, 1990; or has two years experience in a social or recreation program within the last five years, one of which was full-time in a patient activities program in a health care setting; or is a qualified occupational therapist or occupational therapy assistant; or has completed a training course approved by the state." (Tag #256 — OBRA).

activity therapy therapeutic services of professionals who use activities as the modality for their therapy. This term is most frequently used in psychiatric facilities when occupational therapy, recreational therapy, and other disciplines such as music, art, dance, and horticultural therapy are combined into one department.

ACTS advanced communications and technology satellite.

actus reus a legal term which means "voluntary conduct." To commit a criminal act an offender must demonstrate two components: the volitional intent to cause harm (actus reus) and the existence of evil intent in doing so (*mens rea*). If the offender is not mentally able to form an evil intent at the time of the crime, the defendant may be found not guilty by reason of insanity. Compare to *competency to stand criminal trial*. See *forensic psychiatry, insanity defense*.

acuity 1. the ability to distinguish fine detail; usually used to describe how well (or poorly) something functions, e.g., visual acuity (how well someone can see) or auditory acuity (how well someone can hear). 2. an indication of how compromised an individual's or group's health is. A high acuity amongst one's patients means that many of them are very ill or medically unstable.

acupuncture a type of medical treatment developed by Eastern medicine. The effects are produced by inserting long needles into critical points in the body and then either twirling the needle or applying an electrical current through the needle to points indicated by ancient charts. In Western medicine, this is most often used for anesthesia.

acute relating to disease, the abrupt onset phase; usually short and relatively severe. Compare with *chronic*. See *acute stage*.

acute lymphoblastic leukemia (ALL) (HHS/-NMDP) a rapidly progressive malignant disorder involving the production of immature white blood cells, which results in the replacement of normal bone marrow with blast cells. Also called acute lymphocytic leukemia. Appears most commonly in children, but can occur in adults. See *leukemia.*

acute myelogenous leukemia (AML) (HHS/-NMDP) a malignant disorder involving the white cells that results in the excessive accumulation of myeloid blast cells in both the bone marrow and the bloodstream. AML occurs in all ages and is the more common acute leukemia in adults. AML affects a different type of white cells than those affected by ALL. See *leukemia.*

acute non-lymphocytic leukemia (ANLL) (HHS/-NMDP) terminology for acute leukemias that are not lymphocytic. See *acute myelogenous leukemia, leukemia.*

acute stage the first of two or more phases of an illness or disease. This stage is usually somewhat severe and short in duration. The acute stage of tissue and bone damage usually involves a decrease in activity caused by pain without exertion, inflammation, immobilization (both voluntary and as treatment), and the sedating effects of pain medications. See s*ubacute stage, chronic stage.*

ADA See *Americans with Disabilities Act.*

adaptability the ability of an individual to adjust to changes in the environment; to successfully change to enhance one's ability to fit into a specific situation. Adaptability may include changes in muscle strength or cardiovascular fitness to meet physical challenges, the ability to learn new information, or the ability to adjust the way one thinks about a situation.

adaptation 1. the ability of an individual's nervous system to adjust to stimulation. If there is a prolonged increase in stimulation (e.g., the pressure of eye glasses on the bridge of the nose), the nerves in the body will respond by reacting less to the stimuli. The reverse is also true. With prolonged decreased stimuli received by the nerves, an increase in sensitivity is experienced (e.g., being able to see better in the dark after ten or twenty minutes of dark adaptation). 2. in a more general sense, an individual's ability to respond to changing stimuli in the environment. A college student who grew up in a quiet house will eventually be able to ignore the noise in the dorm and fall asleep. See *intelligence.*

adaptive activities activities that are modified to meet the needs and abilities of the people engaging in those activities.

adaptive aquatics techniques placing the emphasis on swimming skills modified or adapted to accommodate individual abilities. Skills include pool entry and exit, swimming skill development, and should also encompass community referral.

adaptive behavior the manner in which the individual modifies his/her behavior to better fit into the environment. See *acculturation, adaptation, ineffective individual coping, maladaptive.*

Adaptive Behavior Scale — Residential and Community: 2nd Edition (ABS-RC:2) The ABS-RC:2 is usually administered by a psychologist to identify the patient's strengths and weaknesses in coping with the social demands of his/her environment. The scale is divided into two parts. Part One focuses on personal independence and is designed to evaluate coping skills considered important in daily living. Part Two is concerned with social behavior and includes eight domains related to the manifestation of personality and behavior disorders. This assessment has moderate reliability (.80+) and is best supported with findings from assessments administered by the therapist relating to community integration and leisure competency.

adaptive functioning an individual's ability to successfully integrate with his/her peers and community. While the individual's measured IQ does play a part in his/her ability to adapt to social, work, and other activities of day-to-day living, it is not the sole determining factor. An individual's economic, educational, or vocational situation may also play a significant role in his/her ability to adaptively change to meet challenges. While an individual's IQ measurement will most likely remain stable over his/her life span, the individual's adaptive functioning level is amenable to change through training and life experiences. The trend in health care is for the professional to measure the individual's level of adaptive functioning by comparing his/her level to a chronological age. An individual may have the cognitive ability of a 3 year old (related to IQ) but be able to adaptively function with the social ability of a 7 year old given appropriate training. As the therapist reviews the assessment reports from other professionals, s/he may want to note if the professional is referring to an adaptive functioning level or

an IQ equivalent level. This is a key element for safety, an example being that it requires the neurological/cognitive level of 7 years to anticipate the actual speed of an oncoming car to cross the road safely. An individual who is cognitively 3 and yet is able to demonstrate an adaptive ability to socially function at age 7 may not be able to safely cross the road alone. See *intelligence quotient, mental retardation.*

adaptive physical education the modification of a physical education program to allow the activity and educational components of the program to match the physical, social, emotional, and cognitive skills of the individual(s) enrolled in the program.

adaptive recreation the modification of a leisure education program and/or activity to allow the individual(s) enrolled to participate. The rules, equipment, environment, or tasks of the activity may be modified to match the physical, social, emotional, and cognitive skills of the individual(s) participating.

adaptive skills skills that the individual has learned which allow him/her to balance his/her needs with the demands and needs of those around him/her. The ability to modify one's behavior or methods to accomplish a task. See *mental retardation.*

adaptive switches controls used to operate equipment needed by the patient. All switches perform the same basic job: they either turn something off or turn something on. Adaptive switches are usually either a single switch (controlling just one action — like a light switch on or off) or a dual (multiple) switch (controlling more than one action — like a stereo which has one button for the tape player and another button for the radio). Adaptive switches come in two modes: "momentary contact" which is activated only while the switch is being used (like a door bell) or "normally open" which remains on until turned off by the user (like a nursing call light). Switches are used to help a patient control communication devices, objects in the environment, etc.

ADD no longer an official diagnosis. See *attention deficit hyperactivity disorder.*

addiction an out-of-date term referring to the physiological or psychological over-dependence on a drug or behavior. Because the term "addiction" has been so overused in pop psychology (e.g., addictive love, chocolate addiction) the World Health Organization has suggested that the term "dependence" be used in place of the term "addiction" when referring to dependence on drugs. The **DSM-IV** refers to addiction as *substance-related disorders.* See *compulsion.*

Addison's disease an endocrine disorder that generally occurs when 90% or more of the adrenal gland is destroyed. The most common cause of this destruction is an autoimmune system failure. Some of the primary symptoms of Addison's disease are a bronze coloration of the skin and gastrointestinal disorders (including nausea, vomiting, anorexia, and chronic diarrhea). The patient will likely also complain about weakness and fatigue. Weight loss is common. Because of the underlying symptoms associated with Addison's disease, patients experience a variety of functional changes. Cardiovascular abnormalities associated with Addison's disease include light-headedness upon standing up quickly (hypotension), irregular pulse, and decreased ability to tolerate stressful situations (e.g., colds, family fights). In addition to lowered tolerance for activity due to fatigue and nausea/vomiting, patients with Addison's disease are at an increased risk of dehydration. Physician's orders should be obtained prior to allowing the patient to participate in physical activity. Patients with Addison's disease are at risk for hypoglycemia and a sudden, significant change in physical activity might cause the patient to go into crisis. Patients with Addison's disease experience times of medical crisis related to the disease. At these times the therapist should monitor the patient's vital signs carefully, looking for symptoms of shock, hypotension, depletion of body fluids, and impaired consciousness. See *adrenal gland.*

addition (ADA) an expansion, extension, or increase in the gross floor area of a building or facility.

additives (to food) (HHS) any natural or synthetic material, other than the basic raw ingredients, used in the production of a food item to enhance the final product; any substance that may affect the characteristics of any food, including those used in the production, processing, treatment, packaging, transportation, or storage of food.

adduction the process of moving a body part toward midline. In the case of the digits (fingers and toes) adduction refers to the process of moving the digit toward the axis of the limb. Contrast with *abduction.*

ADHD See *attention-deficit hyperactivity disorder.*

adhesions collagen fibers that adhere to surrounding anatomical structures and cause a reduction in the normal elasticity and movement of those structures. Adhesions are frequently a complication of surgery, trauma, or immobilization.

adjudication in Medicare and Medicaid, the cycle of processing a claim submitted to the private company which processes claims for the government. See *fiscal intermediary.*

adjunctive therapy a term from the 1970's and before which grouped therapy and other services as being separate and secondary (less important) to medicine or nursing. Occupational therapy, recreational therapy, and social services were frequently considered adjunctive therapies.

adjusted historical payment base (AHPB) the average amount paid by Medicare within each geographical region for specific services that were provided.

adjustment 1. the patient's ability to modify his/her behavior, feelings, or actions to improve function and well-being, 2. the manipulation of a patient's spine and joints by a chiropractor, and 3. the modifications made to a patient's bill as a result of preferred provider status of the health care professional. See *identity.*

ADL See *activities of daily living.*

administrative authority (ADA) a governmental agency that adopts or enforces regulations and guidelines for the design, construction, or alteration of buildings and facilities.

administrative data (HCO) data used in the administration of public programs or agencies or private businesses. In health care, examples of administrative data are hospital discharge abstracts, health insurance claims, and enrollment records. Compare with *clinical data.*

administrative law judge (ALJ) one of a group of specifically designated individuals from the Office of Hearing and Appeals, Social Security Administration, responsible for conducting evidentiary hearings under the Medicare and Medicaid administrative appeals process. Typically an administrative law judge is involved in health care (Medicare and Medicaid) when a facility is legally contesting the results of a survey. See *appeals council review.*

administrative simplification (HCO) efforts to reduce the cost and complexity of health care through increased standardization and automation of health care providers' and insurers' administrative activities.

admission/discharge record (HCO) a synopsis of a patient record containing basic identifying and financial information about a patient, along with clinical information, including the admitting *diagnosis* and final diagnosis and a summary of procedures performed. Also known as a discharge abstract.

admissions See *psychiatric admissions.*

adolescence a stage of human development. While the recognized age of onset of adolescence varies from facility to facility, it is generally considered to be the onset of puberty (around 11 to 13 years of age) until around 18 years of age. This is a critical stage of development where the individual learns to function independently of his/her family and rely more upon himself/herself and peers.

adolescent injuries (CDC) At least one adolescent (10-19 years old) dies of an injury every hour of every day; about 15,000 die each year. Injuries kill more adolescents than all diseases combined. For every injury death, there are about 41 injury hospitalizations and 1100 cases treated in emergency departments. Unintentional injury accounts for around 60% of adolescent injury deaths, while violence (homicide and suicide) accounts for the remaining 40%. In general, males are more likely than females to die of any type of injury. The most pronounced differences between sexes in injury death rates occur within the older adolescent group (15-19 years). In this group, males are about 2.5 times more likely to die of an unintentional injury and 5 times more likely to die of homicide or suicide. The gender difference is most pronounced in drowning, where males are 10.6 times more likely to die than females of the same age. Among adolescents 15-19 years old, one in every four deaths is caused by a firearm. For this age group, the risk of dying from a firearm injury has increased by 77% since 1985. The largest proportion of adolescent injuries is due to motor vehicle crashes. Adolescents are far less likely to use seat belts than any other age. Adolescents are especially vulnerable to fatal crashes at night; they do 20% of their driving at night, but they have more than 50% of their fatalities at night. When adolescents drive after drinking alcohol, they are more likely than adults to be in a crash, even when drinking less alcohol than adults. Adolescents also cause a disproportionate number of deaths among non-adolescent drivers, passengers, and pedestrians. Alcohol is involved in about 35% of adolescent (15-20 years) driver fatalities. Alcohol is involved in about 40% of all adolescent drownings. See *head injury.*

ADP See *alternative disposition plan.*

adrenal gland a gland located on the superior aspect of the kidney. The adrenal gland is made up of two primary sections, each secreting different sets of *hormones.* The inner portion, the adrenal medulla, secretes epinephrine (adrenaline), norepinephrine (noradrenaline), and dopamine. The outer aspect of the adrenal gland, the adrenal cortex, produces glucocorticoids (cortisol, cortisone, corticosterone), mineralocorticoids (aldosterone), androgens (ketosteroid), estrogens (estradiol), and progesterone. The adrenal gland is part of the *endocrine system.*

adrenalin a hormone that is usually referred to now as epinephrine. See *epinephrine.*

adult basic education Congress passed two laws in the 1960's to make getting a high school education easier for individuals who dropped out of school before they graduated. In 1964 the Economic Opportunity Act was passed which described the content of adult basic education to include elementary education, social skills, and community responsibility. In 1969 the Adult Education Act was passed to provide basic education for adults who had dropped out of high school.

adult daycare centers day treatment centers for adults who require some supervision and structured activity to be able to remain at home instead of a health care facility. These centers usually provide help in activities of daily living, cognitive and sensory stimulation, friendship, and nutritional support. While each center may have a few professionally trained health care workers, most of the staff are para-professionals or support staff. The need for more options in adult daycare centers has increased greatly since the 1980's as many households have both adults working outside of the home (who therefore cannot take care of aging parents), because long-term care facilities are very expensive, and because people realize that an aging parent's quality of life is usually improved by living at home instead of in a long-term care facility. Compare with *day treatment program.* See *Medicaid.*

adulthood a level in human development that follows adolescence. Adulthood is generally considered to begin around the age of 18. Some theories end adulthood at death, others end adulthood at "old age."

advanced activities of daily living (AADLs) Advanced activities of daily living may be grouped into seven categories: 1. basic environmental *community safety skills,* 2. community *mobility skills,* 3. *consumer skills,* 4. community *resource identification,* 5. advanced *dressing skills,* 6. *time management skills,* and 7. *social interaction skills.* These advanced skills are frequently the treatment domain of recreational therapy while the basic ADLs frequently are covered by the occupational therapist. See *activities of daily living.*

advance directive a legal document that describes what a person wants to have happen if they are incapacitated and unable to make decisions about health care for themselves. Depending on state laws, it may 1. outline what the patient's wishes are concerning his/her desire for extra-ordinary measures (CPR, life support equipment, etc.) to be used in case of a life-threatening event (serving as a "Living Will"); 2. also extend to cover routine life-support measures such as feeding and hydration; or 3. be used as a Durable Power of Attorney for Health Care to assign the right to make decisions concerning health care to another person when the patient is no longer able to make decisions. By federal law, each patient being admitted to a hospital is to be offered an advanced directive to be signed and placed in his/her chart. See *terminal care*.

Advanced Technology Program (HCO) a Commerce Department program that funds cooperative development and validation of enabling technologies, including computer and information technologies.

adverse actions procedures applied by the Health Care Financing Administration (HCFA) or the Medicaid state agency, when a provider or supplier is found not to meet one or more of the *conditions of participation* for coverage. See *due process, intermediate sanction*, *nonrenewal*, *termination*.

advocacy the act of working to make changes for the benefit of someone else or a group which one does not necessarily belong to.

aerobic activities with paced movements that:

1. allow the heart and circulatory system to keep up with oxygen needs of the body,

2. use a continuous amount of energy for muscle contraction, and

3. maintain a heartbeat faster than resting rate for a minimum of 10 minutes.

When leading *exercise* activities for patients with heart conditions, the professional should delay arm exercises until after both the warm up exercises and aerobic activities of the lower extremity (e.g., walking, leg raises). This delay will lower the chance of having the patient experience *angina* episodes (chest pain), *dysrhythmias* (uneven heartbeat), muscle soreness, and fatigue (Karam, 1989, p. 8). The safest aerobic schedule for most patients is 10-20 minutes of exercise three or four times a week. Individuals who exercise over 30 minutes at a time and/or five or more days a week do not significantly increase their aerobic ability and significantly increase the risk of orthopedic injury (Karam, 1989, pp. 16, 17). When using aerobic activities with patients with *diabetes* the biggest challenge is to balance the exercise with diet modifications, especially in Type I diabetes mellitus. This balance is the responsibility of the physician and the dietitian. The professional should also limit the aerobic activity to less than 40 minutes, even with a patient who has a balanced program (Karam, 1989, p. 63).

AFB isolation an isolation procedure for patients with currently active pulmonary tuberculosis who have a positive sputum smear or a chest X-ray appearance that strongly suggests current (active) tuberculosis. The isolation procedure includes: 1. masks are indicated only when patient is coughing and does not reliably cover mouth, 2. gowns are indicated only if needed to prevent gross contamination of clothing, 3. gloves are not indicated, 4. hands must be washed after touching the patient or potentially contaminated articles and before taking care of another patient, 5. articles should be discarded, cleaned, or sent for decontamination and reprocessing. The sign for AFB isolation is always gray. See *isolation*.

AFDC See *Aid to Families with Dependent Children*.

affect a person's *emotions*. Historically, affect is considered to be one of the three elements of mental functioning (along with cognition and volition). Affect is the outward expression of a person's feelings, tone, or mood, which can be observed. (Affect and emotion are commonly used interchangeably.) Because it is such a general term it is almost always used with a qualifier. Some of the qualifiers that go along with affect are shown in the adjacent column. The **DSM-IV** lists five specific affect disturbances:

Qualifiers for Affect

absent	animated
apathetic	appropriate
belligerent	bland
blunted	broad
calm	cheerful
constricted	contained
controlled	dazed
deep	despondent
detached	dispassionate
eager	energetic
euphoric	expressionless
exuberant	flat
generalized	inappropriate
inexpressive	integrated
intense	joyous
labile	low intensity
low key	motivated
muted	normal range
overwhelmed	passive appearing
pervasive	puzzled
remote	responsive
restricted	restricted in range
self-effacing	serious
shallow	smiling
subdued	sullen
supple	unattached
unchanging	uncomplaining
uninvolved	unresponsive
unspontaneous	unvarying
vacant stare	

1. *blunted* (significant reduction in the intensity of emotional expression)
2. *flat* (absence or near absence of any signs of affective expression)
3. *inappropriate* (discordance between affect expression and the content of speech or ideation)
4. *labile* (abnormal variability in affect with repeated, rapid, and abrupt shifts in affective expression)
5. *restricted or constricted* (mild reduction in the range and intensity of emotional expression) (p. 763)

See *Global Assessment of Functioning Scale, schizophrenia.*

affective related to a person's emotions or *affect.*

affective disorder a term found in the **DSM-III** (1987) to refer to mood disorders, but which was dropped in the **DSM-IV** (1994) edition of the terminology and diagnostic book. See *bipolar disorder, mood.*

afferent referring to the process of transmitting nerve impulses from the sensory neurons to the central nervous system. Compare to *efferent.*

affiliations relationships that offer a supportive environment usually with those who share common beliefs and goals. More formally, an affiliation may refer to a professional group to which one belongs.

affordances (HCO) behaviors and actions that are allowed or enabled by a specific technology.

aftercare the services provided to a patient after discharge from a treatment center. The purpose of an aftercare program is to facilitate the smooth integration back into the community after surgery or other intervention. As more managed care programs institute a continuum of care from inpatient through home health this term will likely become obsolete. See *continuity of care.*

age a term usually referring to chronological age (length of time since the person was born). It may also refer to developmental age (the age that most individuals are when they can perform a specific set of skills), psychological age (the emotional and social skill level that an individual has achieved), and mental age (the measurement of a person's intellectual development as compared to his/her peers).

age appropriate appropriate for a given age. Age appropriate is often used to imply that an individual with cognitive limitations should engage in activities appropriate for his/her chronological *age* instead of activities appropriate for his/her cognitive age and/or appropriate for his/her interests. This topic tends to be a heated one with strong supporters on both sides. In reality, it may be more appropriate and pleasurable for an adult with profound mental retar-

dation to play with bubbles or beach balls. However, the social stigma that goes along with those activities may result in significant barriers to normalization and integration into the community. Professionals who work with individuals who tend to select "age *in*appropriate" activities may be able to help the individual the most by being able to identify the aspects of the age inappropriate activity that the individual enjoys the most and then find an "age appropriate" activity that shares most of those same aspects. See *medical play.*

ageism an assumption (prejudice) that one age is preferable to another. Older individuals frequently experience age discrimination because people assume that they are less capable because of their age.

age of onset the individual's chronological age at the time an illness or disease was noted. The same cause may result in different diagnoses depending on the age of onset. For example, if an individual sustains a head injury at age three from a motor vehicle accident, s/he would be considered to be developmentally disabled. If an individual sustains a head injury at age twenty-two, the diagnosis is traumatic brain injury. The three year old does not get re-classified as s/he reaches adulthood; the diagnosis remains. Since the disabilities due to developmental disability and due to head trauma may be so different, the trend is increasingly to use the diagnosis which best describes the situation. In this example, traumatic brain injury would usually be used. Other diagnostic groups also have age of onset requirements. For example, the diagnosis of autism is only used if the symptoms and diagnosis come before the age of three.

aggression generally, the forceful and hostile actions taken by a person. This action usually originates from three causes (Reber, 1985): 1. fear or frustration; 2. a desire to produce fear or flight in others; or 3. a tendency to push forward one's own ideas or interests. A fourth cause would be organic — related to a neurological damage of impulse control from such diagnoses as traumatic brain injury (TBI) or *lead poisoning.* See *Freud.*

aggressive behavior hostile behavior toward another individual or the environment. Patients may demonstrate aggressive behavior as a means of getting attention or because they lack coping strategies. Impulse control and anger management are important skills for patients learning to demonstrate strong, angry feelings in socially acceptable ways. See *assault cycle, violence in the workplace.*

agitation the appearance that a patient is anxious because s/he is demonstrating motor restlessness. Motor activity may be uninfluenced by external stimuli.

One therapy goal may be to determine if cues or triggers that proceeded agitation can be identified. Measurement of the typical duration, intensity, and frequency of the agitation episode may help determine the effect of intervention on reducing the agitation. Agitation is frequently due to neurological damage or due to a side effect of medication. See *alcohol dependence, bipolar disorder, delirium tremens, mania, metabolic disorders, mood state, physical restraint, psychomotor agitation.*

agnosia the diminished ability to know familiar persons or objects caused by cerebral trauma. It may affect any of the five senses: auditory, gustatory, olfactory, tactile, and visual.

agonist muscle(s) that are contracting to move a body part against the force of another muscle (the *antagonist*).

agoraphobia the most common type of phobia, agoraphobia is the fear of open spaces in which escape may be difficult or embarrassing. The **DSM-IV** does not consider agoraphobia as a true diagnosis: it can only be used as a qualifying descriptor of another disorder, usually *Panic Disorder.*

Agreement (1864) Under section 1864 of the Social Security Act (the Act) HCFA contracts with the states to perform various survey and certification functions with respect to providers and suppliers participating in Medicare. Under this Agreement (1864), states consent to perform survey and certification functions, while the Secretary consents to pay the states for reasonable costs related to the performance of these functions. (Under section 1902 of the Act the states must utilize the same state agency to perform survey and certification functions for Medicaid). See *entitlement programs.*

AHCPR Agency for Health Care Policy and Research.

AHTA See *American Horticultural Therapy Association.*

AIDS acquired immune deficiency syndrome. See *acquired immune deficiency syndrome, blood/body fluids precautions, HIV/AIDS.*

AIDS-related complex See *AIDS-wasting syndrome.*

AIDS-wasting syndrome a grouping together of signs and symptoms into a syndrome associated with AIDS. The signs and symptoms include weight loss, fever, malaise, lethargy, oral thrush, and the immunological problems common with the AIDS virus. AIDS-wasting syndrome is a more current term for AIDS-related complex.

Aid to Families with Dependent Children (AFDC) a federal and state cash assistance program for families who meet their state's Medicaid eligibility guidelines. See *entitlement programs.*

air carrier access rules In 1986 the United States Government passed the Air Carrier Access Act of 1986, which was further updated in the Americans with Disabilities Act of 1990. This Act required the Department of Transportation (DOT) to develop regulations that ensure that individuals with disabilities are treated without discrimination in a way consistent with the safe carriage of all passengers.

air fluidized bed commercially known as a "Clinitron" or a "FluidAir," these beds are used with patients who are at severe risk for *pressure sores* and oozing of body fluids. The mattress is usually filled with silicone pebbles suspended inside the mattress by a constant flow of air. Implications for treatment include a potential increased risk for loss of *range of motion* as these beds have few positioning options, increased risk of sensory deprivation as the flowing air and machinery associated with the bed produces a "white" noise making it difficult to hear other sounds and increased sense of social isolation as patients placed on air fluidized beds seldom are transferred off the beds (due to their medical condition), are visually impaired due to the massiveness of the bed (the sides of the bed are above the patient's side vision) and due to the white noise. See *bed.*

AITN Arizona-International Telemedicine Network.

akathisia motor restlessness ranging from a feeling of inner disquiet, often localized in the muscles, to inability to sit still or lie quietly; a side effect of some antipsychotic drugs.

akinesia 1. diminished or absence of voluntary motion. 2. paralysis of a muscle.

alanine aminotransferase (a. transaminase; ALT) (HHS) enzymes that facilitate the conversion of one amino acid into another, thus helping to maintain a balanced supply of amino acid building blocks for protein synthesis. Elevated alanine aminotransferase levels provide a useful indicator for liver disorders.

albinism a type of inherited pigment disorder that is characterized by a lack of normal levels of melanin in the skin. While the term "albino" is used as if the pigment disorder was just a single disorder, it actually represents at least thirteen different types of pigment disorders. Individuals with these pigment disorders are often referred to as "albinos."

albino See *albinism.*

albumin (HHS) a type of protein widely distributed in the tissues and fluids of plants and animals. It is the single most abundant protein in blood. Albumin acts as a carrier for numerous substances.

alcohol abuse A person is considered to be abusing alcohol if s/he meets the criteria for *substance abuse.* A person does not need to be dependent on alcohol to be an abuser of alcohol. If his/her use of alcohol causes problems at home, school, or work and/or if the person engages in behavior that is dangerous (driving while intoxicated) or anti-social (physically violent when drunk or unable to participate in family activities due to a hang over), the person is abusing alcohol.

alcohol amnestic disorder a dated term used in the **DSM-III** but now referred to as "alcohol-induced persisting dementia." See *alcohol-induced disorders.*

alcohol consumption patterns Over 100 million Americans use alcohol with an estimated 10-13% experiencing significant problems as a result of drinking (Institute of Medicine, 1989). The consumption of alcohol is closely associated with normal leisure activities. Individuals perceive that alcohol will have three effects on their leisure: 1. help disengagement from responsibility and tension, 2. increase self-assurance and acceptance, and 3. increase ability to be involved in the leisure activity (Carruthers 1993). The perceived benefits of leisure and alcohol consumption are very close in many people's minds. People expect consumption to increase the quality of their leisure. Individuals who come to rely on alcohol as a vital component of being able to enjoy leisure activities have moved from potentially healthy leisure lifestyles to an unhealthy one. It is when the individual crosses the line from enjoying alcohol during leisure to having it as an important component of leisure that a pathological change has occurred.

alcohol dependence A person is considered to be dependent on alcohol if s/he meets the criteria for *substance dependence.* Another clinical manifestation of alcohol dependence for those who have a history of prolonged, heavy intake, is the development of withdrawal symptoms 12 hours after significantly reducing the normal amount of intake. Not all patients develop withdrawal symptoms; some experience severe complications. For those who experience withdrawal symptoms, the symptoms may be so unpleasant that they will tolerate the negative consequences of alcohol use just to avoid the withdrawal period. Therapists who see patients in a community setting should be aware that while most patients demonstrate withdrawal symptoms within 12 hours of reduced intake, some may not experience the first significant signs of withdrawal until two days later. The **DSM-IV** lists the symptoms of withdrawal as at least two of the following: autonomic hyperactivity (e.g., sweating or pulse rate greater than 100); increased hand tremor; insomnia; nausea or vomiting; transient visual, tactile, or auditory hal-

lucinations or illusions; psychomotor agitation; anxiety; and grand mal seizures. For most patients these symptoms peak the second day but may persist for three to four more days. Some symptoms (anxiety, insomnia, and autonomic dysfunction) may persist up to six months after acute withdrawal. See *neuropathy.*

alcoholic halluncinosis a dated term used in the **DSM-III.** The condition is now referred to as an "alcohol-induced psychotic disorder, with hallucinations." See *alcohol-induced disorders.*

alcoholic paralysis See *neuropathy.*

Alcoholics Anonymous (AA) Alcoholics Anonymous is a voluntary, worldwide fellowship of men and women from all walks of life who meet together to attain and maintain sobriety. The only requirement for membership is a desire to stop drinking. There are no dues or fees for AA membership. Anonymity is the spiritual foundation of AA. It disciplines the Fellowship to govern itself by principles rather than personalities. AA considers itself a society of peers. The organization strives to make

The Twelve Steps of Alcoholics Anonymous

1. We admitted we were powerless over alcohol — that our lives had become unmanageable.
2. Came to believe that a Power greater than ourselves could restore us to sanity.
3. Made a decision to turn our will and our lives over to the care of God as we understood Him.
4. Made a searching and fearless moral inventory of ourselves.
5. Admitted to God, to ourselves and to another human being the exact nature of our wrongs.
6. Were entirely ready to have God remove all these defects of character.
7. Humbly asked Him to remove our shortcomings.
8. Made a list of all persons we had harmed and became willing to make amends to them all.
9. Made direct amends to such people whenever possible, except when to do so would injure them or others.
10. Continued to take personal inventory and, when we were wrong, promptly admitted it.
11. Sought through prayer and meditation to improve our conscious contact with God, as we understood Him, praying only for knowledge of His will for us and the power to carry that out.
12. Having had a spiritual awakening as the result of these steps, we tried to carry this message to alcoholics and to practice these principles in all our affairs.

known its program of recovery, not individuals who participate in the program. Anonymity in the public media is assurance to all AA members, especially to newcomers, that their AA membership will not be disclosed. AA was started in 1935 by a New York stockbroker and an Ohio surgeon (both now deceased), who had been "hopeless" drunks. They founded AA to help others who suffered from the disease of alcoholism and to stay sober themselves. The twelve steps of the Alcoholics Anonymous program are shown on the previous page. (Material provided by Alcoholics Anonymous.)

alcohol idiosyncratic intoxication a dated term used in the **DSM-III,** which is no longer used as a diagnostic term. It was felt that there was not enough supporting evidence in the literature to consider this a specific diagnosis.

alcohol-induced disorders disorders which originate in the overuse/abuse of alcohol. Alcohol is part of most cultures in the world, working as a brain depressant. All cultures who use alcohol experience morbidity as a result. In the United States approximately 90% of the adult population has used alcohol with a substantial percentage (60% of males, 30% of females) using alcohol in a pathological manner at least once (e.g., driving after drinking, missing work or school due to hangovers) (American Psychiatric Association, 1994). The **DSM-IV** recognizes eleven alcohol-induced disorders shown in the table on the next page. See *aversion therapy, cirrhosis.*

alcohol intoxication a medical diagnosis which indicates that the patient has recently ingested alcohol, has clinically significant behavioral or psychological changes which are maladaptive in nature, and has at least one of the following signs: "slurred speech, incoordination, unsteady gait, nystagmus, impairment in attention or memory, and a stupor or coma." (**DSM-IV,** p. 197)

alcoholism the combined social and physiological symptoms that go along with *alcohol dependence* and/or *alcohol abuse.*

alcohol-related disorders disorders in one of two groups: alcohol use disorders and alcohol-induced disorders. alcohol use disorders include two diagnoses: alcohol dependence and alcohol abuse. alcohol-induced disorders has thirteen diagnoses: alcohol intoxication, alcohol withdrawal, alcohol intoxication delirium, alcohol withdrawal delirium, alcohol-induced persisting dementia, alcohol-induced persisting amnesiac disorder, alcohol-induced psychotic disorder with delusions, alcohol-induced psychotic disorder with hallucinations, alcohol-induced mood disorder, alcohol-induced anxiety disorder, alcohol-induced sexual dysfunction, alcohol-induced sleep

disorder, and alcohol-related disorder not otherwise specified. See *alcohol-induced disorders, alcohol use disorders, comorbidity, dual diagnosis, substance abuse.*

alcohol use disorders alcohol-related disorders found in the **DSM-IV,** which includes two diagnoses: *alcohol dependence* and *alcohol abuse.* The World Health Organization's test for alcohol use disorder is shown on the second following page. See *substance abuse, substance dependence.*

alcohol with dementia a dated term referring to dementia inducted by prolonged alcohol abuse. The current diagnostic term is "alcohol-inducted persisting dementia." See *alcohol-induced disorders.*

alcohol withdrawal a medical diagnosis with four general criteria: 1. The patient has stopped (or greatly reduced) his/her alcohol intake after prolonged and heavy usage; 2. at least two of the following occur within a few hours to a few days of stopping (or greatly reducing) alcohol intake: "a. autonomic hyperactivity (e.g., sweating or pulse rate greater than 100), b. increased hand tremor, c. insomnia, d. nausea or vomiting, e. transient visual, tactile, or auditory hallucinations or illusions, f. psychomotor agitation, g. anxiety, and h. grand mal seizures; 3. The symptoms from #2 are significant enough to cause distress, and 4. The symptoms are not explained by other medical diagnoses" (American Psychiatric Association, 1994, pp. 198-199). Therapists find that the length of stay on most in-patient units is very short. The amount of time for treatment intervention is shortened even more when the patient is going through alcohol withdrawal, as s/he will likely not be physically or cognitively able to tolerate activity for the first few days of withdrawal.

alexithymia an inability to consciously experience or to communicate feelings. This mood disorder is one of the possible symptoms of mental illness and is a common feature of *post-traumatic stress disorder.* After prolonged and painful abuse, such as that experienced by prisoners tortured during ethnic cleansing activities or children sexually abused through childhood, alexithymia may be more of a massive regression than a true dissociative disorder.

algolagnia a psychiatric disorder in which an individual derives pleasure, usually of a sexual nature, through inflecting pain, abuse, or humiliation upon himself/herself (passive algolagnia or *masochism*) or upon another individual (active algolagnia or *sadism*) who may or may not be a consenting participant in the activity. When the individual engages in both active and passive algolagnia, it is called *sadomasochism.*

Table of Alcohol-Induced Disorders

Disorder	Description
Alcohol Intoxication	Negative behavioral changes (inappropriate sexual behaviors, aggressive behaviors, *mood* swings, impaired judgment) and impaired physical function (slurred speech, impairment in coordination, impaired gait, *nystagmus*, impaired cognitive and *memory* skills, possible stupor or coma) that occurs during or shortly after ingesting alcohol.
Alcohol Withdrawal	The cessation or reduction in the heavy and prolonged use of alcohol which produces the following symptoms: autonomic hyperactivity, nausea or vomiting, hand tremors, insomnia, hallucinations or illusions, anxiety, psychomotor agitation, and possibly grand mal seizures. The symptoms are significant enough to cause a measurable change in *functional ability* and must be related to either alcohol intoxication or alcohol withdrawal. The symptoms usually peak by the second day and tend to diminish by the fifth day.
Alcohol Intoxication Delirium	Fluctuating impairment of consciousness (decreased ability to demonstrate skills associated with *attention span*), impairment of cognition (decreased perception skills, decreased short and long-term *memory* capabilities, language impairment) that develop over a period of hours to days and can be tied to the use of alcohol.
Alcohol Withdrawal Delirium	Fluctuating impairment of consciousness (decreased ability to demonstrate skills associated with *attention span*), impairment of cognition (decreased perception skills, decreased short and long-term *memory* capabilities, language impairment) that developed shortly after or during alcohol withdrawal.
Persisting Dementia	Memory impairment, deterioration of language function (aphasia, apraxia, and/or agnosia), impairment of *executive function* significant enough to impair ability to function in the community traced to a prolonged and substantial abuse of alcohol. The symptoms are slow to develop and persist even after the use of alcohol has stopped. The deficits are usually permanent.
Persisting Amnestic	Impairment in either short-term *memory* (ability to learn new information) or long-term memory (ability to access information previously encoded in the brain) significant enough to impair the person's ability to function in the community. This impairment is separate from alcohol-induced delirium or dementia and lasts longer than the usual duration of alcohol intoxication or withdrawal. There must be evidence that the impairment is tied to the long-term use of alcohol.
Psychotic Disorder with Delusions	Delusional beliefs or *hallucinations* evident for at least one day to one month tied to the prolonged use of alcohol. Onset may be linked to alcohol intoxication or to withdrawal.
Mood Disorder	A noticeable change in *mood* that is prominent and persistent. This mood change is either characterized by a decreased interest in life (*anhedonia*) or feelings that are elevated, expansive, or irritable. This change in mood is significant enough to cause a measurable change in *functional ability* and must be related to either alcohol intoxication or alcohol withdrawal.
Anxiety Disorder	Symptoms of *anxiety* (panic attacks, obsessive or compulsive behavior, or significant worry predominates thinking) that are significant enough to cause a measurable change in *functional ability* and must be related to either alcohol intoxication or alcohol withdrawal.
Sexual Dysfunction	Symptoms of sexual dysfunction (impaired desire, arousal, orgasm) along with the person experiencing distress and interpersonal difficulty which is significant enough to cause a measurable change in *functional ability* and must be related to either alcohol intoxication or alcohol withdrawal.
Sleep Disorder	A disturbance in the individual's sleep which is severe enough to require medical attention and is significant enough to cause a measurable change in *functional ability* and must be related to either alcohol intoxication or alcohol withdrawal.

Alcohol Use Disorder Inventory Test

Should You Worry? No questionnaire can tell you for sure if you're a problem drinker. But many alcohol-abuse experts use the following test. (Source: Alcohol Use Disorder Inventory Test, World Health Organization, 1987)

	0	1	2	3	4	Total
1. How often do you have a drink containing alcohol? (one drink is a beer, glass of wine, or mixed drink)	Never	Monthly or less	2-4 times a month	2-3 times a week	4 or more times a week	
2. How many drinks containing alcohol do you have on a typical day when you are drinking?	1 or 2	3 or 4	5 or 6	7 to 9	10 or more	
3. How often do you have six or more drinks on one occasion?	Never	Less than monthly	Monthly	Weekly	Daily or almost daily	
4. How often during the past year have you been unable to stop drinking once you started?	Never	Less than monthly	Monthly	Weekly	Daily or almost daily	
5. How often during the past year have you failed to do what was normally expected of you because of drinking?	Never	Less than monthly	Monthly	Weekly	Daily or almost daily	
6. How often during the past year have you needed a drink in the morning to get going after a heavy drinking session?	Never	Less than monthly	Monthly	Weekly	Daily or almost daily	
7. How often during the past year have you had a feeling of guilt or remorse after drinking?	Never	Less than monthly	Monthly	Weekly	Daily or almost daily	
8. How often during the past year have you been unable to remember what happened the night before because of drinking?	Never	Less than monthly	Monthly	Weekly	Daily or almost daily	
9. Have you or someone else been injured as a result of your drinking?	No		Yes, but not in the past year.		Yes. During the past year.	
10. Has a relative, friend, doctor, or other health worker been concerned about your drinking or suggested you cut down?	No		Yes, but not in the past year		Yes. During the past year.	
Scoring: A total score of 8-15 may indicate a problem with alcohol use. You may want to ask your physician about cutting down or becoming abstinent. A total score of 16 or more suggests a more serious problem. You should contact your physician or an alcohol-treatment program for help.						**Total**

17

algophobia an irrational fear of pain for oneself or for others. Not an official **DSM-IV** diagnosis.

alienation feeling of being separate or different from others, to not fit in, or to feel not wanted. In the theory of *existentialism*, alienation implies a separation from part of one's self, usually due to an extreme desire to conform to the wishes of others and not being "true to one's self."

alimentation to provide an individual with nourishment, usually referring to the delivery of nourishment through a tube. See *feeding tubes*.

alkaline phosphatase (HHS) a group of enzymes that belong to the class known as hydrolases. They are thought to play an important role in the transport of sugars and phosphates in the intestine, bone, kidney, and placenta. Elevated serum levels of alkaline phosphatase activity may indicate liver disease.

allele (HHS/NMDP) alternate forms of a gene. Some genes, like the ones that control expression of HLA antigens, have many alternate forms. In HLA, each allele specifies a specific tissue type.

allergen (in food) (HHS) the part of a food (a protein) that stimulates the immune system of food-allergic individuals. A single food can contain multiple food allergens. Carbohydrates or fats are not allergens.

allergy a hypersensivity to elements (allergens) in the environment. An allergic reaction is the body's response to allergens entering the body and combining with immunoglobulin E (IgE). IgE then attaches itself to specific cells that release histamines. These, in turn, cause the surrounding blood vessels to dilate resulting in a loss of fluid from the vessels. The resulting body reaction to this process produces runny noses, sneezing, rashes, and hives. Treatment includes changing the environment to reduce exposure, immunotherapy (allergy shots), and other medications. See *diet — prescribed*.

allergy (to food) (HHS) any adverse reaction to an otherwise harmless food or food component (a protein) that involves the body's immune system. To avoid confusion with other types of adverse reactions to foods, it is important to use the terms "food allergy" or "food hypersensitivity" only when the immune system is involved in causing the reaction.

allogeneic bone marrow transplant (HHS/NMDP) transplant of bone marrow cells from a family member (other than an identical twin) or from an unrelated individual.

allograft a graft that is not matched genetically but which does come from the same species. Also known as an allogenic graft. This kind of graft is a temporary graft.

alloplastic maneuver making a change to the external environment; causing change or movement to things other than oneself.

allowed coverage the actual dollar amount that will be paid by the insurance carrier for services and equipment provided as outlined by the insurance policy or entitlement program. This is not the same as the amount billed. See *assignment (Medicare)*.

alogia a poverty in thinking that is inferred from deficits in speech which might include a lack of frequency of speech, a lack of content of speech, a blocking of speech, or an increased response time when answering.

ALS See *amyotrophic lateral sclerosis*.

alteration (ADA) a change to a building or facility made by, on behalf of, or for the use of a public accommodation or commercial facility that affects or could affect the usability of the building or facility or part thereof. Alterations include, but are not limited to, remodeling, renovation, rehabilitation, reconstruction, historic restoration, changes, or rearrangement of the structural parts or elements, and changes or rearrangement in the planned configuration of walls and full-height partitions. Normal maintenance, re-roofing, painting, or wallpapering or changes to mechanical and electrical systems are not alterations unless they affect the usability of the building or facility.

altered body image a change in the way that a patient perceives his/her own body image. The patient may actually have a change in his/her body function or structure or it may be a perceived change in his/her body function or structure.

alternating air bed See *static air bed, bed*.

alternative disposition plan the "second choice" option for placement and services after *discharge* if the original disposition plan does not work out. See *discharge plan, discharge summary*.

Alzheimer's disease named after Alois Alzheimer, a German neurologist. This disease is a kind of organic mental disorder that leads to a general loss of cognitive ability. The loss can be observed as a loss in long-term memory, judgment, abstract thinking, and changes in personality. To meet diagnostic criteria for Alzheimer's Type dementia the patient must have developed significant multiple cognitive deficits which reduce independent functioning. The cognitive loss must be significant and impair the patient's ability to learn new information or to recall information learned previously. The cognitive loss must include at least one of the following cognitive disturbances: "*aphasia* (language disturbance), *apraxia* (impaired ability to carry out motor activities despite intact motor function), *agnosia* (failure to recognize or identify objects despite intact sensory function), and disturbance in *executive function* (i.e., planning, organizing, sequencing, abstracting)." (**DSM-IV** p. 142) Alzheimer's disease is difficult to separate from other dementias. The physician must rule out dementias caused by nervous system conditions such as cerebrovascular disease and brain tumors as well as systemic conditions such as hypothyroidism, vitamin B12 deficiency, HIV infection, or other Axis I disorders such as schizophrenia. The length of time that a person lives after developing the first signs of Alzheimer's disease is usually 5 to 10 years. See *visual function.*

AMA 1. against medical advice (stopping treatment or changing treatment against the physician's advice). See *elopement.* 2. American Medical Association.

amaurosis partial or total blindness, from a cause besides injury to the eye itself.

ambi a prefix meaning "both."

amblyopia a loss of visual function not caused by refractive errors or by an organic disease. In layman's terms, this disorder is frequently called "lazy eye" and is typically the result of a congenital defect or of a traumatic accident. Other possible causes are poisons like lead or quinine.

ambulatory able to walk. This usually refers to the patient's ability to walk functionally to the places s/he needs to get to on a daily basis, whether using a walker, cane, braces, or no assistive devices. Lewis (1989) lists seven neurological changes that occur with age which decrease an individual's ability to ambulate safely. They are 1. decreased proprioception of toes, 2. increased sway, 3. increased reaction time, 4. decreased sense of vibration at the ankles, 5. decreased number of neurons, 6. decreased cerebral blood flow, and 7. increased cerebrovascular resistance. See *falls, four-point gait, locomotion, physical restraint.*

ambulatory status a patient's ambulatory status refers to the patient's current functional level when walking or moving about.

ambulatory surgical center (ASC) a health care facility that operates exclusively for the purpose of providing surgical services to patients not requiring hospitalization and that meets the conditions for coverage at 42 CFR Part 416, Subpart B.

amelia refers to the absence of one or more limbs from birth; a congenital defect.

American Alliance for Health, Physical Education, Recreation, and Dance (AAHPERD) a professional organization that is involved in the transmission of knowledge related to physical education, recreation, and dance. The address is 1900 Association Drive, Reston, VA 22091, www.aahperd.org, 800-

213-7193.

American Art Therapy Association the professional organization that represents art therapists. 1202 Allanson Rd., Mundelein, IL 60060, 847-949-6064.

American Association for Music Therapy See *American Music Therapy Association.*

American Health Security Act of 1993 (H.R.1200/S.491) (FB) a health reform proposal sponsored by Rep. Jim McDermott and Sen. Paul Wellstone in the 103rd Congress that would have established a single-payer national health insurance program, federally mandated and administered by the states. This program would have replaced private health insurance and public program coverage with comprehensive health and long-term care benefits. A national board would have established a national health budget to be distributed among the states, based on the national average, per-capita cost of covered services, adjusted for differences among the states in costs and the health status of their populations. This Act did not pass.

American Horticultural Therapy Association (AHTA) the professional organization which represents horticultural therapists. The address is 9090 York St., Denver, CO 80206, www.ahta.org, 303-331-3862.

American Music Therapy Association (AMTA) the national professional organization for music therapists. The American Music Therapy Association was formed when the American Association for Music Therapy and the National Association for Music Therapy merged in 1997. The new association's address is 8455 Colesville Rd., Suite 1000, Silver Spring, MD 20910, www.musictherapy.org, 301-589-3300.

American Occupational Therapy Association (AOTA) the national professional organization for occupational therapists and occupational therapy assistants. The organization's address is 4720 Montgomery Lane, PO Box 31220, Bethesda, MD 20824-1220, www.aota.org.

American Occupational Therapy Certification Board (AOTCB) the group that oversees the credentialing of occupational therapists and occupation\al therapy assistants. American Occupational Therapy Certification Board, 800 South Frederick Avenue, Suite 200, Gaithersburg, MD 20877, 301-990-7979, www.nbcot.org. See *Joint Commission.*

American Physical Therapy Association (APTA) the national professional organization for physical therapists. The address is 1111 North Fairfax Street, Alexandria, VA 22314, www.apta.org, 800-999-2782.

American Recreation Society (ARS) the name given to the first formal organization of hospital-based recreators. The organization was formed in 1949. It then joined other groups to become a section under the National Recreation and Park Association. In 1985 a large group of hospital-based therapists separated again from the National Recreation and Park Association to become the *American Therapeutic Recreation Association.* See *National Association of Recreation Therapists.*

American Sign Language (ASL) the use of gestures, finger manipulation, and finger spelling to communicate in English. Also called Ameslan.

American Speech, Language and Hearing Association (ASHA) the national professional organization for audiologists and speech-language pathologists. The address is 10801 Rockville Pike, Rockville, MD 20852, www.asha.org, 800-638-8255.

Americans with Disabilities Act 1990 a United States federal civil rights law. This law has five sections, called "Titles." Title I covers equal employment opportunities for individuals with disabilities. Title II covers nondiscrimination on the basis of disability in the receipt and use of state and local government services. Title III covers nondiscrimination on the basis of disability by public accommodations and in commercial facilities. Title IV covers telecommunications relay services for individuals who have a hearing impairment or a speech impairment. Title V covers miscellaneous provisions including construction, (lack of) state immunity, prohibition against retaliation and coercion, regulations by the Architectural and Transportation Barriers Compliance Board, attorney's fees, technical assistance, federal wilderness areas, coverage of Congress and the agencies of the legislative branch, illegal use of drugs, definitions, amendments to the Rehabilitation Act, and alternative means of dispute resolution. The ADA opens up many opportunities to individuals with disabilities as it helps break down architectural and attitudinal barriers. See the ADA Table of Contents on the following page. See *consumer rights, employer, inclusive recreation.*

American Therapeutic Recreation Association (ATRA) one of the two professional organizations for recreational therapists in the United States. ATRA's office is 1414 Prince St., Suite 204, Alexandria, VA 22314, www.atra-tr.org, 703-683-9420. See *National Therapeutic Recreation Society.*

Ameslan See *American Sign Language.*

AMI acute myocardial infarction.

amino acids (HHS) the building blocks of proteins. Chemically, amino acids are organic compounds containing an amino (NH_2) group and a carboxyl (COOH) group. Amino acids are classified as essential, nonessential, and conditionally essential. If body synthesis is inadequate to meet metabolic need, an amino acid is classified as essential and must be supplied as part of the diet. Essential amino acids include leucine, isoleucine, valine, tryptophan, phenylalanine, methionine, threonine, lysine, histidine, and possibly arginine. Nonessential amino acids can be synthesized by the body in adequate amounts, and include alanine, aspartic acid, asparagine, glutamic acid, glutamine, glycine, proline, and serine. Conditionally essential amino acids become essential under certain clinical conditions.

amnesia an inability to recall past events. Some types of amnesia include post-traumatic amnesia (due to trauma to the brain), anterograde amnesia (an inability to recall events after the onset of amnesia with memory intact for events of long ago), and retrograde (an inability to recall events which happened prior to the onset of amnesia).

amniocentesis a test in which fluid is withdrawn from the amniotic sac around a fetus to test for metabolic and chromosomal aberrations.

ampere the amount of electrical current passed through a resistance of 1 ohm by an electrical potential of 1 volt; the International System of Units unit of electrical current, equal to a constant current that would produce a force of 2×10^{-7} newton per meter of length when maintained in two straight, parallel conductors of infinite length and negligible circular cross section, placed one meter apart in a vacuum.

amphetamine a drug that stimulates the central nervous system.

amputation the removal of a part of the body including cutting through the bone. An amputation is usually the last choice of a medical team. However, injury due to trauma or burns, infection, malignancy, or a loss of the circulatory system may dictate the need for an amputation. Occasionally a nonviable limb is amputated to allow the fitting and use of a prosthetic limb to increase function. See *disarticulation, residual limb.*

amputee an individual who has had an amputation.

amylase (HHS) an enzyme that breaks down complex carbohydrates such as starch.

amyotrophic lateral sclerosis (ALS) also known as Lou Gehrig disease, ALS is a degenerative disease of the lower motor neurons and pyramidal tracts. This degeneration causes the individual to experience progressive motor weakness and spastic conditions of his/her limbs. The disease progresses through muscular atrophy, fibrillary twitching, and eventual involvement of the nuclei in the medulla. Death results within two to five years.

ADA SECTION 1. SHORT TITLE; TABLE OF CONTENTS

Short Title: This Act may be cited as the "Americans with Disabilities Act of 1990"

ADA TITLE I EMPLOYMENT

ADA TITLE II PUBLIC SERVICES

Subtitle: A Prohibition Against Discrimination and Other Generally Applicable Provisions

Subtitle: Actions Applicable to Public Transportation Provided by Public Entities Considered Discriminatory

Part I: Public Transportation Other Than by Aircraft or Certain Rail Operations

Part II: Public Transportation by Intercity and Commuter Rail

TITLE III PUBLIC ACCOMMODATIONS AND SERVICES OPERATED BY PRIVATE ENTITIES

TITLE IV TELECOMMUNICATIONS

TITLE V MISCELLANEOUS PROVISIONS

anaclitic depression depression in infants that is caused by sudden separation from the mother figure. It can lead to severe problems, including death if the mother figure is not replaced in one to three months.

anaerobic activities activities of short duration that deplete energy stores in the body by using oxygen faster than the heart and lungs can replace it.

analincuts the penetration of a man's penis into the rectum of another person, male or female. This activity has a high risk of exposure to HIV. Some of the "slang" for analincuts includes: cornholing, dog-fashion, and stern job.

analingus contact with the anus by another person's mouth. Some "slang" terms for analingus include: kiss ass, rimming, and bite-the-brown. This activity is associated with a high risk of contracting HIV.

anal intercourse See *analincuts*.

anal stage a term used in psychoanalytic theory to indicate a second step in development. This step is usually associated with an individual's taking pleasure in learning to control his/her bowel movements. Most individuals tend to move through this phase between the ages of 1½ to 3 years.

analysis of covariance (ANCOVA) a series of statistical procedures that help researchers determine if the differences between two or more sets of observations are due to chance or due to differences in the situation.

analysis of variance (ANOVA) a method for statistically analyzing data that makes simultaneous comparisons between two or more means. The ANOVA process provides the researcher with a series of values called "F values." These F values can be statistically tested to determine if there is a significant relationship between any of the experimental variables.

anaphylactic shock (HHS) an allergic reaction marked by contraction of smooth muscle and dilation of blood vessels. If not checked rapidly by an injection of epinephrine, the reaction can be fatal.

anastomosis the surgical connection between tubular structures inside the human body. Literally meaning "to provide a mouth," an anastomosis is created to allow flow from one structure to the other (fecal matter in the intestines, blood in the arteries as with by-pass surgery). Tubular structures include blood vessels and the intestines.

andragogy the study of how adults learn. Malcolm Knowles (1978, 1984) theorized that since adults don't learn the same way as children, the educational techniques used with adults should be different from what is typically seen in schools. Adults learn differently for four primary reasons: 1. They are more self-directed than children, 2. They come to the learning environment with significantly more real-world experience, 3. They identify learning closely with their social and occupational role(s) in life, so learning has an important place in their lives, and 4. They usually have an immediate application for the learning that is taking place, unlike children who are not sure where they will use the information. See *Brookfield's principles, learning disabilities, pedagogy, teaching*.

androgen any of the male sex hormones which are responsible for the development of masculine traits. A small amount of this hormone is also produced by the ovaries in females.

androphobia irrational fear of men.

anemia (including sickle cell anemia) Anemia refers to a variety of conditions, all of which have either an inadequate number of red blood cells (RBCs) or hemoglobin (which carries oxygen throughout the body). Cause: The subnormal amount of oxygen carrying cells is either caused by: 1. the body's inability to produce a normal amount of RBCs or hemoglobin (due to iron deficient diet, lead poisoning, kidney disease, chronic infection, B12 deficiency, bone marrow damage from irradiation, etc.) or 2. the RBCs are destroyed faster than the body can replace them (immune diseases, sickle cell disease, certain toxic substances, certain drugs, etc.). Impact on functional ability: The condition of anemia places a child at risk for developing at a slower pace than his/her peers. A child with anemia tends to have a suboptimal level of energy and alertness. Anemia due to sickle cell disease has additional concerns because of the patient's increased susceptibility to serious infections. A patient with a sickle cell crisis (event) also experiences extreme pain associated with the death of cells in the part of the body affected and his/her awareness of the environment is further reduced by the side effects of the medications which address the crisis. Lead in the blood interferes with the RBCs ability to bind with iron. Patients who live in older building with lead soldered water pipes or patients with *pica* are at increased risk for lead ingestion. Since lead is not shed by the body, but accumulates over the patient's life span, ongoing monitoring may be required. One of the groups at the greatest risk for anemia includes individuals with a developmental disability who also have difficulty with chewing and swallowing. Issues related to activity with anemia are listed on the next page. See *aplastic anemia, bone marrow transplant.*

anencephaly a genetic defect which results in the brain and spinal cord failing to develop during pregnancy.

anergia 1. the patient's apparent lack of energy or desire to engage in any activity that requires effort

Issues Related to Activity with Anemia

Concern	Intervention
iron deficient diet	Promote the desire for and the knowledge of how to prepare or to select when eating out: meat, fish, poultry, iron-fortified, enriched breads, dried beans, peanut butter, dark green vegetables, and dried fruit.
high risk activities	Certain activities and environmental conditions induce a crisis, especially in patients with sickle cell disease. Education on the reasonable/safe selection of activities is extremely important.
anemia due to medical treatment	Anemia due to radiation, blood loss during surgery, medications, etc., would indicate the need for an activity program that is varied (balanced) but requires reduced energy levels. Extra care needs to be taken with infection control and sterilization techniques, especially with bone marrow transplant.

beyond passivity. 2. a deficit in the immune system, usually caused by an advanced disease, which prevents the body from fighting off foreign substances.

aneurysm the dilation or bulging out of the wall of an artery or vein. It may rupture and cause a spontaneous hemorrhage.

anger management specific training in techniques to control one's anger. This training usually includes identification of triggers, re-assessment of values (is it *really* important enough to get angry about?), relaxation techniques, and coping techniques. See *conflict, coping skills training, relaxation techniques.*

angina the feeling of pain in the chest and perception of difficulty in breathing (due to pain) as a result of the heart's reaction to overexertion or excitement. For individuals with *angina pectoris* (occasional lack of blood flow to the heart) such an event is very frightening, as the patient has the feeling of impending death. See *aerobic, atherosclerosis.*

angular movement movement that changes the angle of two bones joined together by a common joint. See *movement.*

anhedonia the apparent lack of ability to derive pleasure from life; to not be able to appreciate the pleasures that most people enjoy. Anhedonia is a primary feature of *depression.* See *alcohol-induced*

disorder, dysthymia, mood. Compare to *hypoactivity.*

animal facilitated therapy the use of animals (interaction with and care of) as a modality to help patients move toward wellness and wholeness. Certain patients find animals less threatening than people, helping remove some barriers to treatment. The therapist will need to be cautious in the use of animals, as some patients dislike or are frightened by them. Each state and province has specific regulations concerning the presence of animals in health care facilities. Check your local regulations to ensure that you have addressed all of the requirements. See *chlamydial infection, Lyme disease, zoomatology.*

animism the belief that inanimate objects are alive. Depending on one's culture, animism may be an indication of mental illness.

ankle and foot The ankle and foot have three primary functions: To provide a means of mobility including being able to provide a rigid structure to push the body forward and a flexible structure to absorb the shock of foot contact with hard surfaces, to provide a means of stability on even and uneven surfaces and to provide a means to bear weight using a limited amount of energy. See *Chopart amputation.*

ankylosis the abnormal immobility of a joint as a re-

Terms Related to Ankylosis

Term	Description
bony ankylosis	the abnormal fusion of bones at a joint — considered to be true ankylosis
extracapsular ankylosis	an immobility of the joint due to a structure exterior to the joint — frequently the direct result of a surgically implanted piece of bone
false ankylosis	an immobility of the joint which is not caused by an abnormal union of the joint and bones around the joint
fibrous ankylosis	an immobility of the joint as a direct result of the formation of fibrous bands around the joint causing restriction
intracapsular ankylosis	an immobility caused by an unnatural rigidity of the joint structure itself
ligamentous ankylosis	an immobility of the joint as a direct result of rigidity of the ligaments around the joint
spurious ankylosis	another term for false ankylosis

sult of a buildup of fibrous tissue or bony tissue forming a bridge across the joint. See the terms related to ankylosis below. Contrast with *contracture.*

anniversary reaction a strong emotional response which occurs near or on the anniversary date of a previously experienced traumatic event. This reaction generally tends to be depressive in nature.

annual care conference (OBRA) Long-term care facilities are seeing fewer and fewer patients who are living in the facility for over 12 months. For those who do, the federal law in the United States (OBRA) requires that the interdisciplinary team conduct a re-assessment of the patient's needs, then meet as a group with the patient (and family) to outline a general course of treatment for the next year. This annual care conference is in addition to the quarterly and other care conferences that have taken place.

anomaly a characteristic that is significantly different from the norm. Anomaly does not necessarily have a negative connotation; it is just a statement that something is different. Birth defects would be considered to be anomalies.

anorexia nervosa a type of psychological eating disorder where the individual is unable or unwilling to maintain a minimally normal body weight. Individuals (usually female) with anorexia nervosa have a severely distorted perception of what their body looks like and are extremely afraid of gaining weight. One of the diagnostic criteria for anorexia nervosa is that the individual is less than 85% of what is considered a normal body weight for his/her age and height and yet still considers his/her weight to be a "problem" (i.e., being too fat). In females the diagnosis requires the absence of at least three consecutive menstrual cycles that would normally be expected to occur. For a variety of reasons, including their lack of accurate perception about their own self-image, individuals with anorexia nervosa tend to be poor historians. Therapists should take this tendency into account when they are interviewing the patient. In addition, many individuals with anorexia nervosa have secondary symptoms of depressed *mood,* social withdrawal, *irritability,* insomnia, and diminished interest in sex (**DSM-IV**), which adds significant complexity to the development of a suitable treatment intervention. See *body image, childhood psychiatric disorders.*

ANOVA See *analysis of variance.*

anoxia oxygen deficiency. After just a short time (three minutes) of anoxia the human body will start experiencing reduced functioning and death of cells. See *secondary brain injury.*

ANSI American National Standards Institute.

Antabuse a medication (disulfiram) that causes a very unpleasant physical reaction whenever the patient drinks alcohol, even in small amounts. The reactions include "flushing, throbbing in head and neck, throbbing headaches, respiratory difficulty, nausea, copious vomiting, sweating, thirst, chest pain, palpitations, dyspnea, hyperventilation, tachycardia, hypotension, syncope, marked uneasiness, weakness, vertigo, blurred vision, and confusion." (**Facts and Comparisons,** 1995, p. 3084) Because of these extremely unpleasant effects of mixing alcohol with Antabuse, the medication tends to be a good tool in helping some individuals avoid alcohol. Patients take one dose a day for months to years until they are socially and behaviorally able to abstain from alcohol without the Antabuse.

antagonist 1. a muscle that has the opposite action of its opposing muscle. 2. an individual who tends to function in an oppositional manner; a person who takes the opposite point of view. Compare *agonist.*

antecedent an event or action that takes place prior to a behavior or movement that influences that behavior or movement. The therapist should always be watching for patterns of antecedents, especially when working with patients with cognitive disorders like traumatic brain injuries. Many behavioral outbursts are triggered by an event or action just prior to the outburst. Startle responses in individuals with cerebral palsy can often be traced to an antecedent event.

anterior referring to the front of the body or organ or indicating a location toward the head.

anterograde moving forward.

anterograde amnesia See *amnesia.*

antianxiety medications See *anxiolytic.*

antibiotic a chemical that destroys targeted bacteria or other cells without excessive harm to the individual taking the antibiotic. Many antibiotics cause individuals to develop a sensitivity to the sun (*photosensitivity*) as a side effect of the antibiotic. This photosensitivity lasts while the individual is taking the medication and adequate precautions should be taken during that period of time.

antibiotic resistance (CDC) Antibiotic resistance occurs when bacteria that cause infection are not killed by the antibiotics taken to stop the infection. The bacteria survive and continue to multiply causing more harm. Widespread use of antibiotics promotes the spread of antibiotic resistance. The Centers for Disease Control and Prevention (CDC) estimates that about 100 million courses of antibiotics are provided by office-based doctors each year. Approximately half of those are unnecessary, being prescribed for colds, coughs, and other viral infections. Smart use of antibiotics is the key to decreasing, or even reversing, the spread of resistance. Although the solution to the problem of antibiotic resistance is complex, we do know that when communities have decreased antibiotic use, they also have decreased resistance. CDC recommends that everyone only use antibiotics when they are necessary. It is important to understand that, although they are very useful drugs, antibiotics are not useful for a viral infection such as a cold, cough, or flu. This understanding will help you work with your doctor to decide what treatment is best for your illness.

Facts about Antibiotics and Antibiotic Resistance (CDC)

- In 1928, Alexander Fleming, a Scottish scientist discovered the first antibiotic.
- Antibiotics became widely available in the 1940's.
- In 1954, two million pounds of antibiotics were produced in the United States.
- Today the figure exceeds 50 million pounds.
- Antibiotics work by either killing bacteria (bactericidal) or by inhibiting growth (bacteriostatic).
- Humans consume 235 million doses of antibiotics annually. It is estimated that 20%-50% of that use is unnecessary.

antibody immunoglobulin; protein produced by the immune system of humans and higher animals in response to the presence of a specific *antigen*. There are five major classes of antibodies: IgG, IgA, IgM, IgE, and IgD. The IgE class is involved in hypersensitivity reactions. The others can neutralize the effects of toxins or lyse cell membranes.

antidepressant (CDC) pharmaceutical agents used to treat clinical depression.

antigen a particle in the body that is identified by the immune system as being foreign. The presence of an antigen usually causes the body to react, initiating an immune response. Certain viruses, like HIV, cause the body to react, but the body is not able to develop an immune response. In bone marrow transplants, this immune response is graft-versus-host disease or rejection.

anti-inflammatory (CDC) agents that reduce inflammation without directly antagonizing the agent that caused it.

antimicrobial resistance (CDC) Antimicrobial resistance can develop in any type of microbe (germ). Microbes can develop resistance to specific medicines. A common misconception is that a person's body becomes resistant to specific drugs. However, it is microbes, not people, that become resistant to the drugs. Drug resistance happens when microbes develop ways to survive the use of medicines meant to kill or weaken them. If a microbe is resistant to many drugs, treating the infections it causes can become difficult or even impossible. Someone with an infection that is resistant to a certain medicine can pass that resistant infection to another person. In this way, a hard-to-treat illness can be spread from person to person. In some cases, the illness can lead to serious disability or even death.

antinuclear antibody (HHS) anti-self antibodies directed against the DNA. It is one indicator for the autoimmune disorder systemic lupus erythematosus (SLE).

antioxidant (HHS) Antioxidants protect key cell components by neutralizing the damaging effects of "free radicals," natural byproducts of cell metabolism. Free radicals form when oxygen is metabolized, or burned, by the body. They travel through cells, disrupting the structure of other molecules, causing cellular damage. Such cell damage is believed to contribute to aging and various health problems.

antipsychotics medications that are used to reduce the symptoms of psychoses. Also referred to as neuroleptics.

antisense (HHS) a piece of DNA that produces the mirror image, or antisense messenger RNA, that is exactly opposite in sequence to one that directs the cells to produce a specific protein. Since the antisense RNA binds tightly to its image, it prevents the protein from being made.

antisocial behaviors which violate the rights of others and are against customs, standards, and moral principles of the society in which the individual lives. Antisocial behavior does not necessarily indicate mental illness. See *antisocial personality disorder, comorbidity, conduct disorder.*

antisocial personality disorder a psychiatric disorder that usually presents itself during childhood and adolescence and endures through adulthood. The key features of this disorder are deceit and manipulation used in a manner which shows little regard for others or things. To be formally diagnosed as having an antisocial personality disorder the individual must be 18 years of age. However, many of these individuals have been diagnosed as having a *conduct disorder* as a youth. One of the criteria for this diagnosis is that the individual has demonstrated a persistent disregard for socially acceptable norms of behavior in at least one of the fol-

Anxiolytic Medications

Drug	Principle Side Effects
Benzodiazepines alprazolam (Xanax) chlordiazepoxide (Librium) clorazepate (Tranxene) diazepam (Valium) halazepam (Paxipam) lorazepam (Ativan) oxazepam (Serax) prazepam (Centrax) temazepam (Restoril)	Side effects are not usually considered significant enough to discontinue medication. Noted drowsiness, ataxia, and confusion may be seen in patients who are older or who are physically impaired. May change behaviors (sometimes problematic) with hypoactivity, irritability, and some memory impairment possible. (Note: encourage patients not to crush or chew sustained release formulas of Valium, as this changes the rate of delivery of the medication.)
Non benzodiazepines buspirone (BuSpar) hydroxyzine HCL (Atarax) hydroxyzine pamoate (Vistaril)	Side effects include dream disturbances, dizziness, light-headedness, and nausea. May cause enough drowsiness that extra caution is needed during activities that require greater attention to detail. May also cause abnormal movements (e.g., motor restlessness, involuntary repetitive movements of the face or neck muscles).

lowing categories: aggression to people and animals, destruction of property, deceitfulness or theft, or serious violation of rules. Impulsivity, irritability, and aggressiveness along with frequent job and living situation changes are features of this diagnosis. People with antisocial personality disorder tend to ignore the feelings of others, and frequently blame the victims, saying that any harm was deserved and/or asked for. See *dual diagnosis, dyssocial behavior.*

antitoxin a substance which helps neutralize specific toxins produced by bacteria.

anxiety the most common psychological disorders. Anxiety is the psychological and physical response to an exaggerated, imagined danger or imagined pending discomfort. In response to this imagined or over-emphasized threat, the patient may experience an increased heart rate, a change in breathing rate, sweating, fatigue, weakness, choking, nausea or abdominal distress, numbness, dizziness or unsteadiness, hot flashes or chills, and/or trembling. While anxiety is seldom so severe that it makes a normally functional patient non-functional, it can interfere with the patient's ability to integrate into his/her community. Bourne (1995) stresses that successful intervention to reduce anxiety must include three elements: 1. reduction of physiological reactivity,

2. elimination of avoidance behaviors, and 3. a change in subjective interpretations (or "self-talk") that perpetuate a state of apprehension and worry (p. 2). See *alcohol-induced disorders, anxiolytic, biofeedback, breathing, bruxism, catharsis, comorbidity, displacement, coping skills training, deconditioning, defense mechanism, desensitization, meditation, Minnesota Multiphasic Personality Inventory, mood state, panic attack, progressive relaxation, refuting irrational ideas, stress.*

anxiolytic medications that cause a reduction in the patient's high level of anxiety. The therapist should be familiar with the side effects of the specific anxiolytic medication the patient is receiving, as restrictions in activity may be indicated. See the table of medications above.

aortic stenosis a narrowing of the aortic valve. The aortic valve helps control the movement of oxygen-enriched blood from the left ventricle to the aorta. See *congenital heart disease.*

APA American Psychiatric Association, American Psychological Association.

Apgar Test a test developed to measure the relative health of an infant at birth. The treatment team measures the infant's Apgar score at one minute and five minutes after birth and continues to measure the infant's Apgar score until the infant's condition

Apgar Test Scoring Criteria

Function	Zero Points	One Point	Two Points
Heart Rate	Absent	Slow (< 100 beats/min.)	> 100 beats per minute
Respiratory Effort	Absent	Slow or irregular	Good: crying lustily
Muscle Tone	Limp	Some flexion of extremities	Active motion; well flexed
Reflex Irritability	No response	Grimace	Cough or sneeze; vigorous cry
Color	Blue or pale	Body pink; extremities blue	Completely pink

stabilizes. A score of 7 to 10 indicates that the infant is adjusting well to extrauterine life; a score of 4 to 6 indicates that the infant is experiencing moderate difficulty adjusting to extrauterine life and a score of 0 to 3 indicates that the infant is experiencing significant difficulty adjusting to extrauterine life. See the scoring criteria below. See *Family APGAR Scale.*

aphasia the loss or decrease in the ability to speak, understand, read, or write. Compare to *apraxia.* See *fluent aphasia, cerebral vascular accident, nonfluent aphasia, paraphasia.*

apheresis (HHS/NMDP) a process by which particular blood components, such as platelets, plasma, or white blood cells, are obtained for transfusion. The procedure is somewhat more time consuming than routine blood donation and involves separation of whole blood into its component parts. Platelet transfusions are used to prevent and control bleeding in transplant patients.

aplastic anemia the failure of the bone marrow to produce white blood cells, red blood cells, and platelets, which causes an increased risk of infection and bleeding. The functional symptoms of aplastic anemia develop over time, making it difficult for the patient to identify just when s/he started feeling weaker, fatiguing quicker, experiencing an increased shortness of breath, and headaches. Without treatment aplastic anemia eventually develops into tachycardia and congestive heart failure. See *anemia.*

apnea cessation of breathing.

apparatus equipment, especially mobility or speech equipment including wheelchairs, crutches, etc.

appeal process (Medicaid) an evidentiary hearing by the state before the effective date of the denial, termination, or nonrenewal or within 120 days after the effective date of the adverse action initiated by the state. (An informal reconsideration must be provided prior to the adverse action if the state elects to provide a full evidentiary hearing after the effective date of the adverse action.)

appeal process (Medicaid look behind) Under federal look behind authority, if termination is based on deficiencies that pose an immediate and serious threat to patient health and safety, an *administrative law judge* (ALJ) hearing is available after the effective date of termination. If the deficiencies do not pose an immediate and serious threat, an ALJ hearing is provided before the effective date of termination and the provider agreement is continued pending the outcome of the hearing, if requested. In either case, if the provider is dissatisfied with the decision of the ALJ, the provider may request appeals

council review and may further appeal to the United States District Court.

appeal process (Medicare suppliers) the process that provides for reconsideration following an initial determination or revised initial determination by the Regional Office of HCFA. If the supplier is dissatisfied with this decision, the supplier may request an *administrative law judge* (ALJ) hearing and if the supplier is dissatisfied with the ALJ decision the supplier may request appeals council review of the ALJ decision. If the supplier is still dissatisfied with the decision of the appeals council, it may appeal to the United States District Court.

appeals council review When the state or federal survey team cites a facility for significantly failing to meet regulations and the facility disagrees with the findings, the facility may appeal. This appeal is part of a facility's right to due process under the law. The appeals council review is the final step in the administrative phase of due process for providers/suppliers who are dissatisfied with the results of the *administrative law judge* hearing. A request for appeals council review must be filed within 60 days following the administrative law judge decision. See *appeal process (Medicare suppliers).*

appeals mechanism all of the regulatory and voluntary health care accreditation organizations have specifically outlined processes (mechanisms) for a facility which feels that the survey finding(s) are incorrect.

appendicular the limbs of the body; to be distinguished from the trunk of the body.

applied relaxation a type of relaxation technique. Applied relaxation is actually a progressive program using six specific techniques to produce immediate relaxation in less than thirty seconds for individuals who have mastered the technique. Developed in the 1980's by L. G. Öst, this technique is especially helpful for patients with phobias and panic attacks. The six stages of applied relaxation training are *progressive relaxation*, release-only relaxation, cue-controlled relaxation, differential relaxation, rapid relaxation, and applied relaxation. With practice twice daily (15 minutes each) each stage will take between one and two weeks to master. See *relaxation techniques.*

appropriateness the degree to which the health care that was received was correct. The key elements of appropriateness are shown in the table at the top of the next page. See *concurrent review, gatekeeper, practice guidelines, quality assessment.*

appropriations the funds approved by a governmental body to pay for services or supplies.

approval For Medicare, a function performed by the

Elements of Appropriateness of Treatment/Services Received

Element	Description
clearly indicated	• assessment of need based on standardized testing tools or on clinical impression • matching diagnosis • meets standards of practice
adequate in quantity	• service and treatment provided frequently enough to cause measurable gain and chance of carryover of gain
setting best suited for both patient and type of service/treatment delivered	• choice takes into account best location/equipment to produce the greatest gain with the least amount of resources • choice of setting takes into account the socioeconomic and insurance coverage of patient
not excessive in nature	• treatment team has known indicators/benchmarks as to when further treatment and services will provide only diminishing returns

HCFA Regional Offices based on the state agency's certification recommendation.

apraxia the inability to carry out purposeful, voluntary movements without presence of muscle weakness, paralysis, or impaired sensations. This can be found in physical activities and in speech. Contrast with *aphasia.* See *ideational apraxia, ideomotor apraxia.*

APTA See *American Physical Therapy Association.*

aptitude referring to an individual's ability to demonstrate a skill or other observable trait. When the professional uses the term "aptitude" in describing a patient's abilities, s/he is indicating that there is a high likelihood that the patient will be able to repeat his/her performance at the level indicated.

aptitude test a test that is designed to predict how well an individual will achieve, independent of his/her current knowledge base.

aquatic therapy a clinical specialty, sometimes referred to as a treatment modality. Aquatic therapy entails a purposeful progression of skills focusing on psychosocial, cognitive, leisure and motor performance utilizing the properties of water to enhance the benefits of the experience. See *mask/snorkel/fin, personal safety (aquatics), proprioceptive neuromuscular facilitation.*

aquatic therapy evaluation evaluation of performance within a water environment. Water performance differs significantly, but directly relates to land-based performance. Land-based evaluations provide information but cannot replace a water-based assessment, which must take hydrophysics into account.

ARC See *Association for Retarded Citizens.*

architectural barriers physical restraints on mobility or usage due to the design of the physical building or structure. Some types of architectural barriers are regulated by state and federal law. See *consumer rights, Americans with Disabilities Act.*

Architectural Barriers Act of 1968 federal law requiring that buildings and facilities be designed and constructed to be accessible to and usable by individuals with disabilities. It also requires that when major changes are made in a building, the issue of architectural barriers in that building must be addressed and corrected. The significant limitation to this law, which the ADA has corrected, was that this law only applied to buildings that received federal funds, although many local building departments included the specifications in their local building codes. See *consumer rights, Americans with Disabilities Act.*

architecture (of databases) In health care settings, the architecture of a database is the model or blueprint used to guide developers as they develop a system to handle the desired information, including what information is to be entered, how it is to be entered, how it is to be utilized, and the types of output configurations. The architecture of a database takes into consideration the software, hardware, and peripherals needed to provide the desired capabilities of the database.

Arden syntax (HCO) a computer language for encoding and sharing medical knowledge in discrete modules.

area of rescue assistance (ADA) an area, which has direct access to an exit, where people who are unable to use stairs may remain temporarily in safety to await further instructions or assistance during emergency evacuation.

arrhythmia an uneven or unusual beat in the rhythm of the heart.

arteriosclerosis a disorder characterized by thickening, calcification, and loss of elasticity of the blood vessels that is a common problem among the elderly, especially elderly who have diabetes. Blood supply is reduced most often in the lower extremities and the cerebrum. See *atherosclerosis*, a type of arteriosclerosis.

arteriosclerotic vascular disease the blood flow to the extremities decreases over time due to a narrowing and fibrosis of the medium to large arteries. This disease is most commonly seen in patients who are elderly or have a long history of diabetes mellitus. Some of the clinical signs include: 1. decreased skin temperature in extremities, 2. chalky white coloring of skin and/or blanching of the skin in the affected limbs, 3. decreased hair growth over affected area, 4. increased susceptibility to skin ulceration, and 5. pain. This disease is commonly referred to as "hardening of the arteries." The patient may experience a decreased tolerance to temperature extremes leading to discomfort during certain activities. The pain experienced by the patient may fall into two separate categories: pain upon exertion (*intermittent claudication*) and pain during periods of inactivity.

arthogenic gait a gait noted by the elevation of one hip and the swinging out of the leg (instead of a straight through swing). This gait is often caused by a deformity or stiffness of either the hip or the knee.

arthritis a potentially disabling disability which causes inflammation of a joint or joints. While not always degenerative in nature, arthritis affects 50% of people over the age of 65% and 75% of people over the age of 80 (Rodman, McEwen, and Wallace, 1973). The symptoms of arthritis that may interfere with a patient's level of activity include pain, swelling, stiffness, and weakness. There are many different types of arthritis. See *bed rest, chronic inflammation, degenerative joint disease.*

arthrodesis fusion of bony surfaces. At times the limitations on a patient's activity level caused by chronic joint pain or chronic joint instability require the fusing of bony surfaces. These limitations are so severe that the loss of range of motion due to the fusion is secondary to the pain or instability. The internal fusion is usually done using plates, pins, or by bone grafts. A patient who has undergone arthrodesis may need significant re-education for the use of movement and balance during activities. Not only is it likely that the premorbid movement pattern was abnormal due to pain and/or instability, but the post-morbid movement pattern will also be different due to a loss of normal range of motion. Re-education of movement patterns and balance may be required, as well as the potential need for adapted equipment.

arthrogryposis a birth defect that causes prenatal contractures, compressed joints, and often, joints developed at abnormal angles. Caused by either neuromuscular problems in the fetus or by uteral problems (too little amniotic fluid or a misshapen uterus), this disorder is treated by exercises and when needed, surgery and casting. The most involved form of arthrogryposis is called arthrogryposis multiplex congenita (abbreviated AMC). Lesser forms of this disorder, estimated to occur at the rate of approximately 500 new cases each year in the United States (Goldenson, et al, 1978), include bilateral clubfoot. Many of the children born with arthrogryposis have normal cognitive abilities. Individuals who have developed arthrogryposis due to a birth defect are found to have changes in their motor neurons prenatally. This limitation of motor neurons may impact an individual's strength later on in life.

arthroplasty the surgical reconstruction of a joint required because of trauma or *ankylosis* or to reduce excessive motion of the joint. A variety of materials may be used in this reconstruction including silicone, metal, or other types of implants.

articular sensation awareness of the contact and movement of joints. See *sensation.*

articulation disorder a deficit in the ability to control the movement of facial muscles, mouth muscles, and breathing to produce understandable speech.

artifact a flaw in a research experiment; often discovered when different tests of the same hypothesis produce conflicting results.

artificial airway a surgically placed alternative passage for air to reach the lungs. The two most common types of artificial airways are the endotracheal tube and the *tracheostomy*. Between 20% and 40% of patients with *burns* treated at burn centers have a secondary complication from an associated respiratory insult requiring an artificial airway (DiGregorio, 1984). See *endotracheal airway.*

artificial neural network (HCO) a linked network of simple software-based processors, analogous to a biological neural network, that can be trained as an ensemble to respond consistently to a set of input stimuli.

art therapy a human service profession that utilizes art media, images, the creative arts process, and patient/client responses to the created products as reflections of an individual's development, abilities, personality, interests, concerns, and conflicts. Art therapy practice is based on knowledge of human developmental and psychological theories, which are implemented in the full spectrum of models of assessment and treatment including educational, psychodynamic, cognitive, transpersonal, and other therapeutic means of reconciling emotional conflicts, fostering self-awareness, developing social skills, managing behavior, solving problems, reducing anxiety, aiding reality orientation, and increasing self-esteem. Art therapy is an effective treatment of the developmentally, medically, educationally, socially, or psychologically impaired; and is practiced in mental health, rehabilitation, medical, educational, and forensic institutions. Populations of all ages, races, and ethnic backgrounds are served by art therapists in individual, couples, family, and group therapy formats. Educational, professional, and ethical standards for art therapists are regulated by the American Art Therapy Association. The Art Therapy Credentials Boards, Inc. (ATCB), an independent organization, grants postgraduate registration (ATR) after reviewing documentation of completion of graduate education and postgraduate supervised experience. The Registered Art Therapist who successfully completes the written examination administered by the ATCB is qualified as Board Certified (ATR-BC), a credential requiring maintenance through continuing education credits. (Reprinted with permission from the American Art Therapy Association, Inc. All rights reserved, ©1995.) For more information contact the American Art Therapy Association, Inc. at 847-949-6064.

ASA abbreviation for *acetylsalicylic acid.*

ASC See *accredited standards committee, ambula-*

The Assault Cycle

Cycle Phase	Characteristics of the Phase	Staff Response
Phase One **Perceived Loss**	The first stage of the assault cycle is when a potentially violent person receives information which signals a loss or a threat of loss to that person.	
Phase Two **Escalation**	The therapist may be able to observe specific warning signs which include: staring, flushed face, rapid breathing, tense or anxious posture, pacing, regularly shifting body positions, challenging staff's authority, shouting, using profanity, or making sexual comments.	• Listen to the person express his/her feelings and frustrations. Within reason, try not to rush the person. Being a good listener may defuse the situation. • Show respect and sympathize with the person's feelings while trying not to intimidate or be intimidated.
Phase Three **Attack**	The person who is feeling the loss releases his/her built up stress. This may be limited to yelling and verbal abuse but may also include violence against people and things.	• Staff should call security or police. • Get support and help from other staff; a *show of force* may interrupt the violence the perpetrator is exhibiting. • If you are physically or verbally threatened, place your body in an assertive stance: standing up straight, feet hip's distance apart looking the perpetrator in the eyes. • Keep the perpetrator at arms length and try to position yourself near an exit.
Phase Four **Recovery and Post-Crisis**	Phase four has two parts. During the recovery phase the perpetrator has released most of his/her stress and feelings of anger so presents with a more relaxed physical stance. Risk of returning to the attack phase is still high. During the post-crisis phase the perpetrator may become withdrawn, showing signs of depression. S/he may also verbalize regret for his/her actions.	• Staff may still feel symptoms of severe stress and possibly physical injury 30 minutes or more after the assault. Take appropriate steps to receive immediate care as needed. • Get away from both the area of the assault and the perpetrator to calm down. Talk about what happened with a counselor or supportive co-worker. This emotional support is different than the debriefing a supervisor will need to complete to write an incident report. • Common symptoms of being involved in a crisis situation include self-blame, professional self-doubt, emotional disturbances, anger, irritability, feelings of helplessness, distancing yourself from others, body tension, soreness of injury, difficulty sleeping, and loss of self-control.

tory surgical center.

ASHA See *American Speech, Language, and Hearing Association.*

ASIA Impairment Scale (AIS) American Spinal Injury Association Impairment Scale. See *spinal cord injury.*

aspartame (HHS) a low-calorie sweetener used in a variety of foods and beverages and as a tabletop sweetener. It is about 200 times sweeter than sugar. Aspartame is made by joining two protein components, aspartic acid and phenylalanine.

asphyxia the decrease of oxygen and increase of carbon dioxide in the blood due to insufficient breathing or insufficient oxygen in the air. Brain, heart, and other tissue damage happen relatively quickly and may lead to death.

aspirin See *acetylsalicylic acid.*

aspirin hypersensitivity triad a syndrome that combines *asthma*, *nasal polyposis*, and aspirin intolerance. Individuals with aspirin hypersensitivity triad tend to have recurring nasal congestion, aspirin intolerance (rash, runny nose, and severe asthma attacks), and nasal polyposis. Symptom relief (decreasing the chronic runny nose through medications, decreased presence of polyps through surgery and decreased severity through *avoidance therapy*) allows greater comfort during activity. Working and playing in environments which are smoke free with little to no air pollution enhances symptom reduction.

assault cycle Violence in the workplace is becoming more and more of a problem for health care workers. By being able to recognize the four phases of the assault cycle shown on the previous page, staff will be better prepared to reduce the impact of violence in the workplace (Coastal Health Train, 1996).

assembly area (ADA) a room or space accommodating a group of individuals for recreational, educational, political, social, or amusement purposes or for the consumption of food and drink.

Assembly areas have specific accessibility requirements under the *Americans with Disabilities Act.*

assertiveness a communication skill which is a prerequisite for healthy survival in one's community. Assertiveness is the ability to: 1. identify that some force in the environment is pressuring for a change in behavior (environmental awareness), 2. identify that you do not want to change or are willing to offer a compromise in the pressured change (self-awareness), and 3. communicate (verbally and/or nonverbally) your position to the force in the environment (interpersonal skill). The ability to demonstrate appropriate assertiveness is an advanced social skill.

assertiveness training the teaching and enhancement of skills required for appropriate assertiveness in a variety of situations. These techniques allow the individual to stand up for his/her rights and at the same time recognize (and honor) the rights of others. Assertiveness is a learned behavior. The individual first learns to identify three different types of interpersonal styles: aggressive behavior, passive behavior, and assertive behavior. Time is taken to identify which interpersonal style is being used in different situations throughout the day. The patient also keeps a log of the type of his/her interpersonal response and how comfortable s/he was with that behavior. Using the log and memory of past interactions, the individual identifies sensitive topics, problematic interpersonal relationships, and uncomfortable situations. The next step is to plan specific actions, behaviors, and conversations for the next time the interaction takes place. This step involves the appropriate use of assertive body language, learning to listen, being able to arrive at a workable compromise, and avoiding manipulation. Davis, et al (1995) suggests using the LADDER approach. An example of the LADDER approach is shown below. See *assertiveness.*

assessment the process of placing a value on some-

LADDER Approach to Assertiveness Training

Look At	I'm not sure why my co-worker can't carry her own share of the load when it comes to cleaning and ordering supplies.
Arrange	I will ask her to meet with me on Tuesday so that we can talk about it.
Define	I figure that there are two hours of clean up and ordering each week in the splinting room and another hour in the durable equipment room. Right now I am doing all of the durable equipment each week and the splinting room every other week while she is doing only the splinting room every other week.
Describe	I feel uncomfortable doing most of the drudgery work. I feel like she is implying that she is the better therapist and that is why she sees more patients and cleans and orders less. I want to know how this assignment was scheduled originally and if it still needs to be this way.
Express	I'd like to talk with you about how the cleaning and ordering duties are divided up as I'd like to change some of the division of work.
Reinforce	I want to work with you on this because I think that together we can reach a fair arrangement.

thing through *measurement* and quantification. Assessment is not the same thing as an evaluation. See *clinical privileging, communication, concrete thinking, diagnosis, discharge summary, evaluation, functional assessment, instrument, intake assessment, Joint Commission, multiaxial system, partial extended survey, preadmission review, predictor, psychiatric rehabilitation, quality assessment, resident assessment instrument, resident assessment protocols, social history, therapy process.*

assignment (Medicare) an agreement with a physician and/or treatment team to accept the *allowed coverage* as a payment in full and not to charge the patient for any remaining balance due.

assimilation to incorporate an object, element, or idea into something else. This term has a very broad meaning that has a more narrow definition depending on the context. In sociology, assimilation usually refers to the mixing of two (or more) cultural groups that have different cultural beliefs into a new, single group that shares one set of common beliefs. In physiology, assimilation usually refers to the body's absorption of food, converting it into protoplasm for use by the body. Numerous well-known theorists in psychology have defined assimilation to fit into their theoretical base as shown in the table below. See *accommodation, equilibration.*

assisted living a residential setting where adults who are not related to one another receive assistance with some activities of daily living and other personal care. These centers provide 24-hour supervision and assistance designed to accommodate each resident's changing needs. Services offered include housekeeping, some health-related services, and activities geared toward keeping the resident as independent as possible and decreasing the need for nursing home services. The environment of assisted living centers is designed to promote each resident's autonomy, privacy, and independence.

associated features secondary diagnoses caused by the severity of the primary diagnosis. Most often associated features appear with individuals with IQs measured between 35-55 (moderate range). The earlier the age of onset of a severe disability, the greater the possibility of one or more associated features to appear. An earlier version of the **Diagnostic and Statistical Manual of Mental Disorders (DSM-III-R**, p. 35) provided the professional with a list of typical associated features.

- Deficits in cognitive ability that may show up in academic ability, *judgment, pathfinding* skills, etc.
- Deficits in body posture and motor ability that may show up in expression of feelings (excessive response), walking on tiptoe, unusual body postures, and poor coordination that cannot be explained neurologically.
- Deficits in reaction to sensory input which may show up in hyper- or hypo-sensitivity to hot, cold, pain, noise, or smells which cannot be explained neurologically.
- Abnormal eating and/or sleeping patterns that may show up as an extreme limitation in foods liked, frequent periods of wakefulness during the night, or unusual fluid intake patterns.
- Deficits in moods and emotions which may

Theories on Assimilation in Psychology

Type	Description
Herbart	Applied to his theory on how people acquire knowledge — Herbart felt that the only way for individuals to assimilate new information into previously assimilated information (called apperceptive mass) was for the individual to see clear connection(s) between the new information and the previously learned information (recognition, identification, and/or comprehension).
Jung	Applied to the process of adaptation — Jung used the term assimilation to describe the process individuals go through to change the environment, memory of events, or ideas to meet their current situation and need.
Piaget	Applied to his theory of human development — Piaget's theory that individuals function by having a general concept of how things are and should be. As individuals mature, they need to accommodate new ideas when events do not fit into their previously held concepts. The process of accommodation to the development of a new conceptual framework is done through assimilation.
Thorndike	Applied to animal behavior — Thorndike believed that animals would be able to assimilate (cope with) a new situation if they had a previously learned behavior which worked in a similar situation and could generalize the behavior to produce moderate success in the new situation.
Wulf	Applied to his theory of memory — Wulf believed that novel objects, ideas, or events had to be integrated into a person's current cognitive structure before s/he would be able to incorporate it into memory.

show up as laughing or crying at inappropriate times, by being fearful or self-assured in inappropriate situations, by the lack of any demonstrated emotion, etc.

- *Self-injurious behavior* (SIB) which may show up as an action that the individual takes to harm himself/herself, including picking at skin, hitting his/her chin, cheek, or forehead or hitting his/her head against the wall or other hard object. Pain does not stop the individual from the self-injurious behavior.

associated movement movement of body parts which normally would move together, e.g., the eyes. See *movement*.

Association for Children with Learning Disabilities See *Learning Disabilities Association of America*.

Association for the Care of Children's Health (ACCH) a membership organization representing different disciplines and families who promote "humanizing health care for children and families" within the health care arena. ACCH's address is 19 Mantua Rd., Mt. Royal, NJ 08061, 609-224-1742, www.acch.org. See *Child Life Council*.

Association of Retarded Citizens (The ARC) an organization formed by the parents of individuals with mental retardation. The primary purpose of The ARC is to promote a better understanding of mental retardation through education and research. The organization now prefers to be called its new name, "The Arc," to drop the stigma associated with retardation.

astasia See *abasia*.

astereognosis a sensory/cognitive loss of the ability to determine what an object is through touch alone.

asthma a chronic disorder which produces episodic, reversible airway obstruction. This obstruction may be caused by bronchospasms, an increase in the mucous secretion, and/or an increase in mucosal edema. It is most often caused by allergic reactions to an environmental irritant, a specific type of food,

or stress. Approximately 10 million Americans (3% - 4% of the population) have asthma. Asthma attacks with severe wheezing, cyanosis, confusion, and lethargy signal a life-threatening situation. See *autogenics, biofeedback, bronchospasm. chronic obstructive pulmonary disease, cyanosis, lethargy.*

ASTM American Society for Testing and Materials.

asymmetrical lack of symmetry. When comparing the same part on both sides of the body, the observer notices that they are not the same; an implication that they should be symmetrical. A lack of symmetry may be an indication of a clinical condition.

asymmetric encryption (HCO) an encryption scheme in which information intended for an individual is encoded with his/her well-known, public encryption key, but may only be decoded with his/her private key (generated from a guarded password).

asymptomatic without symptoms. When used in health care settings, it means that an individual has been shown to have a disease or disability through lab tests or other clinical tests but is not exhibiting observable, behavioral symptoms. A person who is *HIV* positive may be asymptomatic (not showing the symptoms associated with AIDS) but still be infected with the virus. See *latent infection.*

asynchronous transfer mode (HCO) a fast networking protocol based on small, uniform packets. Asynchronous transfer mode communications are suitable for continuous transfer of large amounts of data, including video streams.

ataxia a lack of the ability to coordinate one's functions. Ataxia is most often associated with gait, but does apply to other domains. See chart below. See *ataxic gait, cerebral palsy, Frenkel's movement.*

ataxic gait gait characterized by an unsteady, wide gait and has two different forms:

1. Spinal ataxia is caused by a disruption of sensory pathways in the central nervous system. This gait is frequently seen in patients with either tabes dorsalis, *multiple sclerosis*, or other

Domain Specific Ataxia

Domain	Definition
Cognitive	A lack of agreement between a person's emotional state and his/her situation. While cognitive *apraxia* usually refers to a severe, chronic discrepancy in behavior — an example of a mental ataxia response would be laughing when one is nervous and emotionally uncomfortable.
Motor	The inability to coordinate the motor function of one's muscles.
Sensory	Due to a dysfunction in an individual's sensory neural pathways (esp. the conduction of *proprioception* information), an individual is not able to fully function within his/her environment.
Speech	Speech that is void of tonation, inflection, and varied pace. Almost robot like.
Static	Due to a loss of the ability to coordinate functions (motor and/or sensory), a person is not able to maintain a normal standing position.

disease processes that affect the central nervous system. The ataxic gait tends to become worse when the patient closes his/her eyes. In addition to the broad-based gait, spinal ataxia is also identified by "double tapping" when the heel comes down first followed by the toes making a double slapping sound (Rothstein, et al., 1991, p. 727).

2. Cerebellar ataxia is caused by lesions in the *cerebellum*. Cerebellar ataxia is characterized by an inability to walk in a straight line but does not worsen when the patient's eyes are closed.

This type of gait limits the patient's ability to participate in mainstream activities like basketball, soccer, and football. While activities like hiking and swimming may need some modification, these should be a realistic option to all but the most involved patients.

atherosclerosis a disorder in which too much cholesterol builds up in the blood and accumulates in the walls of the blood vessels, generally affecting the large vessels coming from the heart. Atheromatous lesions are leading causes of cardiac disorders including *angina* pectoris and *myocardial infarction*.

athetoid movement movement that is marked by slow, continuous, writhing movements, especially in the hands. See *cerebral palsy, movement*.

athetosis See *cerebral palsy*.

ATM See *asynchronous transfer mode*.

ATP See *advanced technology program*.

ATRA See *American Therapeutic Recreation Association*.

atresia the abnormal closure of an opening or pathway due to a congenital defect or due to a pathological event.

atrial septal defect a hole between the atrial chambers that allows a portion of the oxygen-enriched blood to leak back into the oxygen-depleted blood in the right atrium. This leakage causes an abnormal enlargement in both the right atrium and right ventricle. The pulmonary artery is also enlarged. This enlargement (in addition to the hole) decreases the pumping efficiency of the heart. See *congenital heart disease*.

atrioventricular canal multiple defects of the heart, including: 1. a hole in the wall between the two ventricles, 2. a hole in the wall between the two atria, and 3. inefficient valves going between the atria and their corresponding ventricles; relatively common in individuals with *Down syndrome*.

atrophy a decrease (or wasting away) in the size and function of a body part due to inactivity, disease, decrease in the blood supply, or disability. See *bed rest*.

attending behavior individual's tendency to perceptually prioritize one event, object, or other stimuli at any one moment in time. All other stimuli are consciously or subconsciously selected out and ignored. Attending behavior refers to the observable/measurable actions associated with this perceptual prioritizing. Individuals who have studied the art of concentration a long time (as in karate) tend to have strong attending behaviors. Individuals who have attention deficit hyperactivity disorder (ADHD) tend to have weak attending behaviors. See *attention deficit hyperactivity disorder, attention span, attention deficit, General Recreation Screening Tool*.

attending physician the physician who is ultimately responsible for the type and quality of care received by the patient. A title for the physician in charge of the medical treatment team at a teaching university or hospital. The attending physician is the lead physician on the treatment team which includes the "fellow" (post-residency position), "resident" (post-medical school internship), and "medical student" (still in medical school).

attention deficit the inability to attend to a task or a thought due to a lack of: 1. duration of attention, 2. appropriate selectivity of attention, 3. appropriate filtering of attention, and/or 4. ability to maintain attention. See *attending behavior, attention deficit, disruptive behavior disorders*.

attention deficit disorder no longer an official diagnosis. See *attention deficit hyperactivity disorder*.

attention deficit hyperactivity disorder (ADHD) a category of diagnoses found in the **DSM-IV**. ADHD has three types: primarily *attention deficit* (attention deficit hyperactivity disorder, predominately inattention type), primarily *hyperactivity* (attention deficit hyperactivity disorder, predominately hyperactivity type), or both attention deficit and hyperactivity (attention deficit hyperactivity disorder, combined type). In all three cases the behaviors must be age-inappropriate, evident for a duration of at least six months and must be severe enough to negatively impact function at school, home, and/or work. Some of the behaviors must have been present before the person was seven years old. To qualify for this diagnosis, the person must demonstrate at least six of the symptoms. For predominately inattention they must demonstrate six or more symptoms in inattention and fewer than six in hyperactivity. For predominately hyperactivity they must demonstrate six or more symptoms in hyperactivity and fewer than six in inattention. For combined type they must demonstrate at least six in both inattention and hyperactivity. Inattention has nine possible symptoms: 1. often fails to give close attention to details or makes careless mistakes in schoolwork, work, or other activities, 2. often has difficulty sustaining attention in tasks or play activities, 3. often does not seem to listen when spoken to directly, 4. often does not follow through on instructions and fails to finish schoolwork, chores, or duties in the workplace (not due to oppositional behavior or failure to understand instructions), 5. often has difficulties organizing tasks and activities, 6. often avoids, dislikes, or is reluctant to engage in tasks that require sustained mental effort (such as schoolwork or homework), 7. often loses things necessary for tasks or activities (e.g., school assignments, pencils, books, or tools), 8. is often easily distracted by extraneous stimuli, and 9. is often forgetful in daily activities. Hyperactivity includes *impulsivity* and has nine possible symptoms: 1. often fidgets with hands or feet or squirms in seat, 2. often leaves seat in classroom or in other situations in which remaining seated is expected, 3. often runs about or climbs excessively in situations in which it is inappropriate (in adolescents or adults, may be limited to subjective feelings of restlessness), 4. often has difficulty playing or engaging in leisure activities quietly, 5. is often "on the go" or often acts as if "driven by a motor," 6. often talks excessively (impulsivity), 7. often blurts out answers to questions before the questions have been completed, 8. often has difficulty awaiting turn, and 9. often interrupts or intrudes on others (e.g., butts into conversations or games). See *biofeedback, comorbidity, self-injurious behavior.*

attention seeking behaviors that are exhibited by an individual with the conscious or unconscious intention of receiving attention from another individual. This attention may be either positive or negative. Attention seeking behaviors that are usually successful tend to become ingrained in the individual's behavior. Many individuals seen by the therapist may be used to receiving negative attention and in the stressful environment of treatment, these behavior may accelerate. When this happens, it is best for the entire treatment team to decide the best way to address these behaviors to cause their extinction. Consistency of response from the treatment team is vital. Lack of consistency allows the behavior to be retained and allows the patient a chance to play (manipulate) one staff against another. The team may take a passive approach (everyone ignore the behavior) or an active approach using a behavior modification program. A key therapy concept to remember is that the behavior that is identified for extinction has been a functional behavior in the patient's life. It has solved a need. Upon discharge the

patient will likely regress to the old attention seeking behavior unless the staff has helped the patient replace the less desirable behavior with a positive behavior that will work in the patient's home environment. See *extinction, behavior modification program.*

attention span the measured duration of the individual's ability to pay attention to a specific stimuli. Operationally, the patient demonstrates attention by focusing on a selected, relevant stimulus, ignoring other distractions in the environment. The patient who has a good attention span is able to demonstrate goal-directed perception. Developmentally, the length of time an individual is able to attend to a stimulus increases with age. Aspects of attention span include: 1. attention to task (culturally appropriate eye contact plus body language which displays interest), 2. motor quietness (motor activity fairly restricted to that which is required to attend to primary stimuli), 3. cognitive focus (attention to primary stimuli), and 4. ability to ignore interruptions and impulsive thoughts. See *cognitive deficits, delirium, distractibility.*

attention to detail the ability to observe, to know the appropriate next step in sequence, and to maintain focus so tasks are completed in a thorough manner.

attention to task the ability to focus on each phase of a task, to anticipate the next step in the sequence and to complete each step of the task appropriately.

attribution based persuasion the use of an individual's own belief in his/her own ability to convince him/her to believe in something. The individual must believe that something can be accomplished or endured because of his/her own internal strength and belief in self. Individuals tend to take pride in accomplishments that they feel are attributable to their own capabilities. If individuals view their performance as being dependent on someone else's (or the environment's) actions, they are less likely to be intrinsically motivated and satisfied and less likely to be persuaded. Therapists can use attribution based persuasion by setting up experiential situations in which the patient is shown/recognizes his/her own strengths and, because of this knowledge, is willing, able, and persuaded to do something.

attribution theory a sociological theory heavily influenced by Heider and Gestalt therapy. This theory sets a framework to explain how/why people develop attitudes toward others based on inferred thoughts and actions. This inference involves three steps: 1. an individual observes the actions of someone else, 2. the individual then tries to figure out the other person's reason for acting in such a manner

Attribution Theory, Example 1

observation	possible reason	motivation
sees man cutting grass	grass is over 5" long	man does not like untidy lawns

Attribution Theory, Example 2

observation	possible reason	motivation
sees woman smile at him (he opened the post office door for her)	she likes me	she wants to go to bed with me (when smile really just equaled a "thank-you")

(and settles on a reason), and 3. the individual then takes his/her thought process a step further by inferring what motivated the individual to take the action. See example 1 at the top of the page. Quite frequently therapists will work with individuals who act in a socially unexpected or socially unacceptable manner. It may be that the patient has an impaired skill level in one or more of the three steps of the attribution theory. By observing the patient and asking how s/he arrived at the perceived motivation the therapist may be able to pinpoint the area(s) of strength and weakness. A coping strategy may be able to be developed. See example 2 above. The patient is a 18-year-old male with a traumatic brain injury, Rancho Los Amigos level of 6 with socially inappropriate, sexually charged behavior toward females.

attrition the wearing away or progressive deterioration of a body part or skill.

atypical the object or characteristic being discussed is different from what is considered normal or expected. In scientific terms, atypical refers to a characteristic that is at least two *standard deviations* from the mean. In health care, atypical is used to describe a manifestation of a disease or illness that has many of the required attributes but which significantly deviates in one way or another from the norm.

audiometrist an individual who is professionally trained to used an audiometer to measure the qualitative and quantitative values of an individual's hearing. See *hearing impairment.*

audit a review of documents for *quality assurance, utilization review,* or to otherwise determine if standards were met. In health care an audit usually refers to the review of the medical chart and related documents.

audition the sense of hearing including the properties of sound and the organs involved in hearing. The field is concerned with a variety of aspects including: acoustics (the physical properties of sound), hearing (the coordinated use of body organs to receive sound), aural (referring to the physical components of the human ear), and otic (referring to the

nerve cells which receive and help process the sounds). See *hearing impairment.*

auditory pertaining to *audition.*

augmentative communication the use of tools or techniques to allow communication with another person when the individual's ability to communicate is impaired. See *communication board, augmentative communication device.*

augmentative communication device any system, other than the individual's own voice, used to communicate with other individuals. The system may be as simple as a board with a few pictures on it or as sophisticated as a computer-driven system that produces both a written message and computer generated speech. Other therapists may want to assist the speech therapist in determining which augmentative communication device to prescribe for an individual. A device that generates speech may be nice, but if the individual enjoys spending time in the library or at movies and needs to indicate the need to use the restroom, everyone in the room will hear the message. The therapist may also want to help the team anticipate the individual's potential sequence of devices needed. Seldom does the same augmentative communication device work for an individual throughout his/her life span.

aura a sensory-based, subjective experience which may precede a seizure or migraine headache by a few seconds to a few hours.

authenticator (HCO) a device that provides an internally stored or calculated response to verify a user's identity when logging onto a computer. Only authorized users are likely to both know a unique piece of information (the password) and be in possession of a unique piece of equipment (the authenticator).

authorization of services the approval for funding for health care services by the fiscal intermediary or insurance company.

autism a developmental disorder characterized by abnormal or impaired development in social interaction and communication and limited areas of interest. While many developmental disorders produce autistic-like symptoms, to be accurately diagnosed as having autism, the patient must have a qualitative impairment in social interactions; qualitative impairments in communication; and restricted repetitive and stereotyped patterns of behavior, interests, and activities (**DSM-IV**). Cause: Autism, which occurs approximately once in every 2000 live births, is thought to be a type of brain dysfunction. This dysfunction is not identifiable on either a CAT scan or an MRI but is thought to be incurred prenatally. Impact on functional ability: Individuals with autism require extensive intervention to develop rudimentary communication skills and to develop the ability to perform the basic tasks of daily living. Due to the nature of the disorder, the therapist will probably achieve greater success with the individual if s/he concentrates on developing solid skills in just 2 or 3 activities rather than trying to have the individual learn 10 or more activities. (Remember, one of the diagnostic criterion is an extremely limited ability to engage in or tolerate a wide range of activities.) Individuals who are less impaired by autism may eventually tolerate a greater range of activities. See the chart at the bottom of the page for implications for therapy. See *idiopathic, pervasive developmental disorder, self-injurious behavior.*

auto-cosmic play a developmental level where a child's play is centered on his/her body. This is one of the earliest developmental levels in humans.

autogeneic actions and thoughts produced within one's body; self-producing.

autogenics a relaxation technique first suggested by Oskar Vogt in the 1800's and developed further by Johannes H. Schultz in the 1930's. The basic technique involves the patient obtaining a trance-like state through the use of verbal statements such as "my arm is warm." (Schultz discovered that visualizing different body temperatures or body weights can induce a hypnotic state when combined with purposeful reduction of attention to outside stimuli.) Mastery usually requires five to eight 90-second practices a day for ten or so months. Autogenics has been found helpful for patients with *asthma, constipation, ulcers*, high *blood pressure*, irregular heartbeat, and headaches. Autogenics is contraindicated for pre-adolescents or patients with severe cognitive or psychological disorders. See *relaxation techniques.*

autogenous graft a graft taken from the patient's own body. This kind of graft is a permanent type of graft. Therapy activity with the patient must not compromise the grafts ability to "take." Frequently the graft site must be immobilized to reduce trauma and movement. Spillage of paints, juices, and such must be avoided to decrease the risk of infection.

autoimmune disease (HHS) disorders in which the body mounts a destructive immune response against its own tissues.

autologous bone marrow transplant (HHS/NMDP) a transplant procedure where a portion of the patient's marrow is removed, stored, and then returned to the body after the patient receives high doses of chemotherapy and/or radiation therapy.

automated data collection (HCO) direct transfer of physiological data from monitoring instruments to a bedside display system or a computer-based patient record.

Autism, Implications for Therapists

Concern	Intervention
communication skills	Treatment interventions that help teach basic communication and social skills are usually indicated, keep communication concrete and extremely functional.
limited range of activities	Treatment should include introduction and training in one activity at a time, using reinforcement techniques enjoyed by the patient. If possible, build up a repertoire of activities in different domains (cardiovascular activity, creative activity, social activity).
behavior modification	Concrete rewards (toys, food, etc.) tend to be understood better than social rewards (verbal praise, time with peers, etc.). The therapist should continue to use verbal praise during treatment, but do not use verbal praise as the sole reward. Time-outs are usually contraindicated because they tend to be rewarding to the individual.
cognitive ability	An individual with autism may have the capability for reaching a normal IQ if the brain dysfunction (which limits the intake of information in an organized manner) can be overcome. Patience from the therapist mixed with repetitious, rewarding activity will frequently produce a positive outcome.
seizure activity	While few children with autism have *seizures*, up to 25% of the adults with autism develop seizures. The therapist should observe the patient's activity closely to note the onset of any seizure activity.

automated guideway transit (AGT) (ADA) a fixed guideway transportation system that operates with automated (driverless) individual vehicles or multi-car trains. Service may be on a fixed schedule or in response to passenger activated call buttons. Such systems using small, slow moving vehicles, often operated in airports and amusement parks, are sometimes called "people movers." These vehicles must comply with the ADA accessibility standards. The ADA accessibility guidelines for automated guideway transit may be found in the **Automated Guideway Transit Vehicles and Systems Technical Assistance Manual** (US Architectural and Transportation Barriers Compliance Board).

automatic cancellation clause (Medicare and Medicaid) a time-limited agreement may contain an automatic cancellation clause. The clause provides that if corrections of deficiencies are not made by the 60th day following the last date by which all corrections are to have been made or if substantial effort and progress have not been achieved and an acceptable revised *plan of correction* submitted, the agreement for funding will be automatically canceled on that 60th day.

automatic door (ADA) a door equipped with a power-operated mechanism and controls that open and close the door automatically upon receipt of a momentary actuating signal. The switch that begins the automatic cycle may be a photoelectric device, floor mat, or manual switch. See *power-assisted door*.

automatic movement movement caused by the patient's own muscles, but not a voluntary movement, e.g. blinking of eyes. See *movement*.

autonomic dysreflexia a serious medical problem that can occur in individuals with a *spinal cord injury* above the 7th thoracic level. Autonomic dysreflexia can be caused by many type of noxious stimuli below the level of the spinal cord injury and its symptoms may be mild or severe. Severe autonomic dysreflexia is a medical emergency, which, if not properly treated, can result in a cerebrovascular hemorrhage (stroke) and possibly death. Severe autonomic dysreflexia, if not addressed immediately on a community integration outing, can lead to the death of a patient before the therapist can return to the hospital with the patient. Common stimuli that cause autonomic dysreflexia include full or spastic bladders, a full rectum, tight or irritating clothing, a fracture, or another undiscovered, painful stimulus. See *catheterization*.

autonomic hyperactivity the excessive activity of the autonomic system, may be induced by a reduction in the pathological use of alcohol or other sub-stances. Symptoms include sweating or a *pulse* rate above 100, which is not caused by physical activity. See *alcohol dependence*.

autonomic nervous system one aspect of the nervous system which is responsible for the involuntary vital functions including the action of the cardiac muscle, smooth muscles, and glands. The autonomic nervous system has two divisions: the *sympathetic nervous system* and the *parasympathetic nervous system*. The sympathetic nervous system activates the heart to increase the heart rate, causes blood vessels to constrict, and raises *blood pressure*. The parasympathetic nervous system activates to slow down the heart rate; causes the coordinated, rhythmic, and sequential contraction of the smooth muscles of the digestive tract (to digest food), ureters (to urinate), and bile duct (to move bile); and relaxes sphincter muscles.

autonomy making decisions for oneself; deciding which activity to engage in and possessing the functional skills to be able to complete the activity. Patients who are dependent on others for their care, even if for a short time, experience a great loss of autonomy. This loss frequently causes a situational *depression*. Health care workers can make a big difference in the patient's perceived loss of autonomy and subsequent development of situational depression by allowing the patient as many real choices as possible. Remember — the patient is the consumer of health care services and, as such, has the legal right to make the choices in almost all situations. Compare with *dependency*. See *consumer rights for individuals with disability*.

autoplastic 1. referring to the use of tissue and other material from a person's body to replace missing tissue or other material someplace else on the person's body. An example would be the use of a bone graft to strengthen a broken bone. 2. referring to self-produced change or movement; a change that is made internally instead of as a result of outside forces.

autopsy the postmortem examination to evaluate the cause of death and/or to identify pathological events.

auxiliary aides and services (ADA) At times a facility is required to provide auxiliary aides or services for individuals who are disabled because of a hearing or vision impairments. Legally this is defined as qualified *interpreters*, note takers, transcription services, written materials, telephone headset amplifiers, assistive listening devices, assistive listening systems, telephones compatible with hearing aids, closed caption decoders, open and closed captioning, telecommunications devices for individuals who are deaf (TDDs), video text displays, or other effective methods of making aurally delivered materials available to individuals with *hearing impairments*. Qualified readers, taped tests, audio recorders, Braille materials, large print materials, or other effective methods of making visually delivered materials available must be provided to individuals with *visual impairments*.

availability in reference to *managed care* systems, the extent to which services of the correct type and quality are accessible to its members.

average adjusted per capita cost (AAPCC) the government's estimate of what Medicare has paid (on average) for a *fee-for-service* charge, adjusted by county for the beneficiary's age, sex, and program entitlement.

aversion therapy a type of *behavior modification* that relies on the use of painful or unpleasant responses to stop undesired behavior. The use of disulfiram (*Antabuse*) with individuals who are alcoholics is an example of aversion therapy. Generally, the use of aversion therapy requires prior approval from the patient, approval from a human rights committee, and must be written into the treatment plan. It is recommended that less averse interventions be tried first.

aversive the demonstration of feelings and actions which indicate a strong reaction of dislike, repulsion, or displeasure in response to an object or action in the environment.

avoidance therapy a type of health care intervention in which the patient improves his/her health status by avoiding exposure to irritants and allergens. Avoidance therapy is normally used in conjunction with other treatments. An example of avoidance therapy would be getting rid of the cat you are allergic to.

axial referring to the trunk of the body versus the limbs.

axilla the armpit; hollow area below the shoulder between the upper arm and the chest.

axillary crutch also known as the underarm crutch. This is the most common type of crutch used. The crutch has a foam or rubber pad placed on top of the body of the crutch which forms a modified upside down triangle. In the middle of this triangle is a cross bar which the patient grasps with his/her hand. The crutch then tapers down to a single shaft, which is capped with a rubber cap to decrease slipping. These crutches are adjusted at the cross bar (for appropriate distance from the armpit/foam pad at the top of the crutch) and at the point where the modified triangle is connected to the single shaft. Properly fitted axillary crutches should allow a two-inch space between the armpit and the rubber pad as the patient stands in the "crutch stance." See *crutch*.

axillary lymph nodes (HHS) lymphoid organs located near the shoulder joint.

axis 1. the imaginary line, which if drawn through the human body, would extend midline from the head, down through the torso, and end between the ankles. 2. in psychiatry, see *multiaxial system*.

B

Bacillus thuringiensis See *Bt*.

back belts a support device buckled around one's waist that is intended to provide increased protection from *back injury*. However, there has been much discussion as to whether back belts actually prevent injury. (CDC) In recent years, there has been a dramatic increase in the number of workers who rely on back belts to prevent injury during lifting. Back belts, also called "back supports" or "abdominal belts," are currently worn by workers in numerous industries, including grocery store clerks, airline baggage handlers, and warehouse workers. As their use has risen, National Institute for Occupational Safety and Health (NIOSH) has increasingly been asked for advice on back belt selection. In response to these inquiries, the Institute decided to address a more fundamental question. Rather than ask, "Which belt will best protect workers?" NIOSH researchers began with the question, "Do back belts protect workers?" Employers relying on back belts to prevent injury should be aware of the lack of scientific evidence supporting their use. After a review of the scientific literature, NIOSH has concluded that, because of limitations of the studies that have analyzed workplace use of back belts, the results cannot be used to either support or refute the effectiveness of back belts in injury reduction. Although back belts are being bought and sold under the premise that they reduce the risk of back injury, there is insufficient scientific evidence that they actually deliver what is promised. The Institute, therefore, does not recommend the use of back belts to prevent injuries among workers who have never been injured. If you or your workers are wearing back belts as protective equipment against back injury, you should be aware of the lack of scientific evidence supporting their use. NIOSH systematically reviewed published peer-reviewed scientific literature on back belts to determine if they actually reduce the risk of back injury. Because there were few studies on the association between workplace use of back belts and injuries, NIOSH also reviewed studies of the relationship between back belt use and forces exerted on the spine during manual lifting. In other words, much of the existing research is based on theories of what causes back injury, rather than on the actual rates of workplace injury with and without back belt use. For a detailed technical report on the studies NIOSH reviewed, call 1-800-35-NIOSH to request "Workplace Use of Back Belts: Review and Recommendations" (Publication No. 94-122).

backbone 1. vertebral column. 2. (HCO) a high-capacity communications channel that carries data accumulated from smaller branches of a computer or telecommunications network.

back injury (CDC) Back injuries account for nearly 20% of all injuries and illnesses in the workplace and cost the nation an estimated $20 to $50 billion per year. The National Institute for Occupational Safety and Health (NIOSH) believes that the most effective way to prevent back injury is to implement an ergonomics program that focuses on redesigning the work environment and work tasks to reduce the hazards of lifting. However, in response to the increasing human and economic costs of back injury, companies have implemented numerous other measures, either in conjunction with or in place of sound ergonomics programs. For instance, there has been a dramatic increase in the use of industrial *back belts*. The decision to wear a back belt is a personal choice; however, NIOSH believes that workers and employers should have the best available information to make that decision. Companies should not rely on back belts as a "cure all" for back injury, but should begin to undertake prevention measures that reduce the risks of lifting tasks.

back support See *back belts*.

baclofen a medication primarily used for patients with multiple sclerosis and spinal cord injuries that inhibits monosynaptic and polysynaptic reflexes at the spinal cord level. It is used primarily as a means to reduce *spasticity*. Baclofen may cause drowsiness, dizziness, and *fatigue*. While on community integration outings the patient should avoid substances that depress the central nervous system (like alcohol). Not known to cause sun sensitivity.

Bad Ragaz aquatic therapy technique developed in Bad Ragaz, Switzerland, which utilizes the properties of water, allowing for normal anatomical and physiological functions of joints and muscles. For practical purposes, this method applies the theories of *proprioceptive neuromuscular facilitation* using the resistance created by the body's movement through water.

balance 1. an instrument for weighing. 2. a mental

or emotional state that allows for dealing with the world effectively. 3. the ability to maintain a posture. There are four primary systems involved in postural stability. These systems are the visual, vestibular, proprioceptive, and musculoskeletal systems. See the table below. Normal changes related to growth, development, and aging all impact each system differently and at different times of the individual's life. The therapist will want to be aware of how each system contributes to balance and to anticipate changes that may occur due to aging and/or the disease process. See *cocontraction, dynamic balance, equilibrium, homeostasis, kinesthetic, Parkinsonian gait, static balance.*

balance bill/extra bill the amount over the allowed coverage still due to be paid. The fee in excess of what is covered by the individual's insurance.

bandwidth (HCO) the amount of information an electronic connection can carry per unit of time, usually expressed in bits per second.

barbiturate drugs which are highly addictive and which depress the central nervous system. Phenobarbital and Pentothal are two different kinds of barbiturates.

baroreceptor sensitivity the baroreceptor nerve detects pressure applied to body parts. An individual with a baroreceptor sensitivity has hypersensitivity (over sensitivity) to touch and pressure. As a person ages s/he may experience a natural loss of baroreceptor sensitivity. See *hypersensation.*

barriers to recreation See *constraints on leisure.*

baseline 1. the measurement of a patient's functional status prior to the introduction of treatment. The CERT - Psych/R, the TRAA, or the grip strength test

Body Sensory Systems that Affect Balance

System	Discussion
visual system	The visual system provides the brain and the central nervous system with external, static references (such as furniture or floors). The brain uses this information to determine where the person is (and where it wants to be) in relationship to the external, static references. As people age, their eyes do not function as well. They have a harder time adjusting to changes in the intensity of light and greater difficulty with depth perception. Not only does visual acuity decrease (ability to see things clearly), but the eyes also lose sensitivity to contrast and color. A patient experiencing any of these changes may find it harder to maintain functional and safe postural stability.
vestibular system	The vestibular system provides the patient with information about the position of his/her head relative to the rest of his/her body as well as information about acceleration and deceleration. Studying this system's functions related to postural balance has been difficult because the input from this system is so reliant on additional input from the visual and proprioceptive systems (Poole, 1991). However, the therapist should consider the potential increased chance of falls during activity in individuals who have an impairment in the vestibular system. This is especially true if there is also loss of function in the two other closely related systems (visual and proprioception).
proprioceptive system	The proprioceptive system (receptors in the muscles, tendons, and joints) provides the patient with information about the position of his/her body including the sensation of movement. Poor proprioceptive feedback may allow the patient to misjudge where his/her body is in relationship to the environment and/or gravity and increases the likelihood of a loss of balance.
musculoskeletal systems	The musculoskeletal system provides the structure and form to the body. As a person ages there is a general decrease in the muscles' strength and speed of contraction. This decrease in strength and timing of muscle contractions increase "sway" as an individual ages. (Postural sway is the musculoskeletal system's miscoordinated corrective reaction to feedback from the visual, vestibular, and proprioceptive systems indicating that the body is not properly aligned.) Increased sway produces a greater risk of falling. Also, because of changes in the musculoskeletal system, peoples' gait changes as they get older. Men tend to develop a wider, shorter gait and women tend to develop a narrower, shorter gait. Velocity, height of foot pickup, and arm swing all decrease while irregular gait step increases. These changes increase the risk of falls. The greatest number of falls related to musculoskeletal system decline is found with patients with medium velocities (50-60% of normal) (Brummel-Smith, 1990). Lastly, many individuals who are older have developed disorders that impact musculoskeletal function such as strokes and Parkinson's disease.

are examples of measurements that may be used as a baseline. 2. (FB) the state of a system before any proposed policy change or reform in federal health care. It is a benchmark for measuring the effects of proposed policy changes. It can refer to the expenditures, the demographic compositions, or the underlying macroeconomic factors that are generally used as the input parameters in estimating the effects of reform.

basic water safety skills See *functional aquatic activities*.

bathing the process of washing. (OBRA) A patient is considered to be independent in bathing if s/he is able to clean his/her body (excluding back and shampooing hair). This includes a full-body bath/shower and/or a sponge bath. In the United States a patient is technically independent in bathing even if s/he requires "set-up" assistance. Many facilities routinely provide "set-up" assistance to all patients, such as drawing water for a tub bath or laying out bathing materials. If this is the case and the patient requires no other assistance, for survey purposes, this patient is still considered to be independ-

ent in bathing. If a patient is to be discharged to home or participates in an aquatics program, the staff may need to evaluate whether the patient is actually able to complete the set-up himself/herself.

B cell abbreviation for B lymphocyte — the primary cell involved in the human immune response.

Beck Depression Inventory a quick testing tool that helps the professional determine the degree of clinical depression. The Beck Depression Inventory, frequently called the Beck Depression Scale, was originally published in 1961 and modified in 1979. The Inventory contains 21 items, which have four statements each. The patient is instructed to select the truest statement for each item. The questions are written to measure the following (listed in order of occurrence on the Inventory): *mood*, pessimism, sense of failure, lack of satisfaction, guilt feelings, sense of self-punishment, self-hate, self-accusations, self-punitive wishes, crying spells, *irritability*, social withdrawal, indecisiveness, *body image*, work inhibition, sleep disturbance, fatigability, loss of appetite, weight loss, somatic preoccupation, and loss of *libido*. The first question is given below to show

Specialized Hospital Beds

Type	Description	Implications for Treatment
Air Fluidized Bed	Commercially known as a *Clinitron* or a *FluidAir*, these beds are used with patients who are at severe risk for *pressure sores* and oozing of body fluid. The mattress is usually filled with silicone pebbles suspended inside the mattress by a constant flow of air.	• increased risk for loss of *range of motion* because these beds have few positioning options • increased risk of sensory *deprivation* because the flowing air and machinery associated with the bed produce a "white" noise making it difficult to hear other sounds • increased sense of social isolation because patients placed on air fluidized beds are seldom transferred off the beds (due to their medical condition), are visually impaired due to the massiveness of the bed (the sides of the bed are above the patient's side vision) and are unable to hear due to the white noise (see above)
Circular Bed	Commercially known as a *CircOlectric*, these beds are welded to a circular frame, which allows a patient, to be turned 360° while lying flat on his/her back. These beds actually have two mattresses with the patient placed between the two. The two mattresses are jointed at the foot of the bed and open like a clamshell, allowing more space around the patient's head. These beds are usually used with patients with extensive trauma, especially with trauma to the upper torso and head.	• increased risk of isolation due to the massiveness of the bed • increased risk for loss of *range of motion* because it is difficult to conduct range of motion exercises around the framework of the bed • at times it may be difficult to establish and maintain eye contact with the patient when s/he is positioned with his/her face down and when the head is lower than the feet

Specialized Hospital Beds, Continued

Type	Description	Implications for Treatment
Foam Mattress or Gel Cushion	Commercially known as *Egg Crate, Geo-Matt, Spencegel Pad*, these mattresses are used for patients who have intact skin or a lower grade (stage one or a small area stage two) pressure sore. They provide a slightly more therapeutic surface for skin at risk than regular mattresses. They are often placed over an existing mattress.	• when placed over existing mattress, may increase risk of *fall* (patient not used to mattress height) or decrease bed *mobility* (patient may need firm surface to move in bed)
Low-Air Loss Bed	Commercially known as *KinAir, FLEXICAIR,* and *Mediscus*, these beds are made up of multiple independently inflated air sacs that allow an equal distribution of pressure over the body regardless of the position. These beds are used with patients who have *pressure sores* or are at a high risk of developing pressure sores.	• decreased ability to transfer self out of bed • equipment and activities which have sharp points are contraindicated because they may result in a punctured air sac
Oscillating Support Bed	Commercially known as *Roto-Rest, Tilt and Turn,* and *Paragon 9000*, these beds "rock" the patient in a 124° arc from side to side, oscillating continuously like an oscillating fan would. This movement relieves pressure on any one part of the body. The patient is "wedged" into position in the bed with foam wedges and supports. This bed is used with patients who are at high risk of developing *pneumonia* due to bed rest or at risk for developing *pressure sores*.	• increased risk for lost range of motion • increased risk for isolation due to visual blockage (wedges blocking view) and due to noise of machinery (and due to the wedges covering the ears) • hard to conduct conversation with patient as bed moves
Static Air, Alternating Air or Water Mattress	Commercially known as *TENDER Cloud, Soft-Care, Pulsair,* and *Lotus*, these beds have compartments for air or water which either allow the gradual movement between cells or mechanically force the movement between cells (like a wave action), to reduce pressure on the skin.	• decreased ability to transfer self out of bed • equipment and activities which have sharp points are contraindicated because they may result in a punctured air sac • increased risk for sweating due to plastic covers on the mattresses

the types of choices the patient is able to make.

1. I do not feel sad.
   I feel sad.
   I am sad all the time and can't snap out of it.
   I am so sad or unhappy that I can't stand it.

bed Many patients require the use of specialized hospital beds to reduce or prevent further injury and disability. See the table on the previous page and the top of this page for a list of the types of beds. See *falls, gatching, support surface.*

bedfast (OBRA) in the United States, a technical term referring to a patient who is in a bed or recliner 22 hours or more per day for the past seven days. The patient may have bathroom privileges and still be considered bedfast.

bedrate the amount paid by the insurance company or government for the patient's basic care, such as nursing and dietary services. Bedrates are preset daily amounts determined by the typical cost of care within the region. Many of the services provided by the facility are included in the bedrate and may not be billed separately. Most of the services provided by activity professionals in nursing homes or therapists on psychiatric units are covered under bedrates.

bed rest an activity status order usually determined by the patient's physician. Bed rest should be avoided or shortened whenever possible because of the severe physiological and psychological side effects. When a patient has physician ordered bed rest, the professional should try to offset some of the negative aspects through the use of activity. Prior to engaging the patient in activity, the professional needs to know the specific reasons why the patient is on bed rest and to obtain clearance for specific activities and movement. See below for interventions during bed rest. See *bedfast, deconditioning.*

bedsore a descriptive but somewhat antiquated term referring to injury to the skin and other body tissues that results from being in bed. A bedsore can be caused by a prolonged period of pressure on one part of the body or by a sheering force during movement in the bed. See *pressure sore.*

bedwetting See *enuresis.*

behavior the observable actions that an individual demonstrates during any type of activity. See behavior topics below, *extinction.*

behavioral lability a patient's inability to regulate his/her *moods* and behaviors due to cognitive deficits. The patient may fluctuate between being confused/oriented, overly emotional/flat affect, emotional and behavioral outburst/calm, sexually inappropriate behavior/socially and sexually appropriate, failure to recognize behavior as inappropriate/able to recognize inappropriateness of behavior.

Indicated Interventions During Bed Rest

Function Affected	Activity Interventions Indicated
Psychological Effects	
Decreased Sensory Stimulation	Activities to help maintain central brain processing skills, e.g., pattern tracing activities, radio or other auditory stimulation (including emphasizing the need for the patient to wear his/her hearing aid during bed rest), reading, and other activities to stimulate color discrimination, object familiarity, and social interaction.
Altered Body/Self-Image	Activities that reinforce the skills the patient has and can use during bed rest. Activities that reinforce who the patient is (e.g., parent, worker, hobbyist).
Altered Sensation of Time	Provision of calendar, clock, television, radio. Social interaction that deals with what the day and time are as well as what is happening in the community/world in general.
Increased Dependence	Ensure that all interactions with the patient, whether they are treatment oriented or just social in nature, allow the patient real choices that make a difference in his/her life. See *dependency.*
Musculoskeletal Function	
Muscular Atrophy	Activities that promote the frequent, repetitive use of many muscle groups. *Atrophy* of the muscle will be slowed only if the patient uses the muscle with adequate frequency and duration to promote strength and good circulation. Use appropriate precautions with patients who have *arthritis.*
Joint Stiffness	Activities that promote *range of motion* (passive, assisted, or active depending on the patient's orders).
Cardiovascular Function	
Edema	Activities that promote the gentle movement of swollen areas. Proper positioning with frequent positioning changes during activity to facilitate good circulation. See *edema.*
Respiratory Function	
Slower, Shallower Respiration	Activities that encourage the patient to take deep breaths; coughing as needed to bring up secretions from the lungs. Activities that promote the patient's turning from side to side in the bed to help with lung drainage.
Gastrointestinal Function	
Constipation	Since bed rest promotes *constipation* and fecal impaction, activities that promote sitting/bending at the waist, as well as leg movements to exercise the torso and muscles around the abdomen area. Adequate fluids and proper diet (snacks during activity) to promote a healthy level of fluid intake and nitrogen balance.
Skin Integrity	
Pressure Sores	Activities that promote frequent and proper positioning for each patient depending on his/her needs and skin tolerance.

behavioral medicine the development and integration of biobehavioral and biomedical scientific knowledge and techniques relevant to health and illness and the application of this knowledge and these techniques to prediction, prevention, diagnosis, treatment, and rehabilitation. The five functional categories proposed by the National Institutes of Health are 1. biobehavioral mechanisms (processes through which behavior, health, and illness interact); 2. identification and distribution of psychosocial risk and protective factors (factors that lead to or safeguard against illness or substance abuse); 3. development, maintenance, and change of health-related behaviors resulting from a disease or treatment; 4. behaviors resulting from a disease or treatment; and 5. behavioral and social interventions to prevent and treat illness or to promote health. (Blumenthal, 1994, p. 45)

behavioral model a model of therapeutic intervention that feels that most maladaptive behaviors can be controlled or modified through modification of the patient's behavior. Undesirable behaviors are thought to be modified without having to change the entire personality or behavior patterns of the individual. This model is different than the medical model, which feels that many maladaptive behaviors can be explained through body functions and corrected with medications or other interventions that emphasize the work of the health care professional with a more passive role for the patient. See *medical model.*

behavioral objective an objective that can be measured by observing behavior. See *objective.*

Behavioral Risk Factor Surveillance System (BRFSS) a nationwide survey used to measure behaviors that increase risk of *morbidity* and *mortality.* (CDC) By the early 1980's, scientific research clearly showed that personal health behaviors played a major role in premature morbidity and mortality. Although national estimates of health risk behaviors among US adult populations had been periodically obtained through surveys conducted by the National Center for Health Statistics (NCHS), these data were not available on a state-specific basis. This deficiency was viewed as critical for state health agencies that have the primary role of targeting resources to reduce behavioral risks and their consequent illnesses. National data may not be appropriate for any given state; however, state and local agency participation was critical to achieve national health goals. About the same time as personal health behaviors received wider recognition in relation to chronic disease morbidity and mortality, telephone surveys emerged as an acceptable method for determining

the prevalence of many health risk behaviors among populations. In addition to their cost advantages, telephone surveys were especially desirable at the state and local level, where the necessary expertise and resources for conducting area probability sampling for in-person household interviews were not likely to be available. As a result, surveys were developed and conducted to monitor state-level prevalence of the major behavioral risks among adults associated with premature morbidity and mortality. The basic philosophy was to collect data on actual behaviors, rather than on attitudes or knowledge, that would be especially useful for planning, initiating, supporting, and evaluating health promotion and disease prevention programs. To determine feasibility of behavioral surveillance, initial point-in-time state surveys were conducted in 29 states from 1981-1983. In 1984, The Centers for Disease Control and Prevention (CDC) established the Behavioral Risk Factor Surveillance System (BRFSS), and 15 states participated in monthly data collection. Although the BRFSS was designed to collect state-level data, a number of states from the outset stratified their samples to allow them to estimate prevalence for regions within their respective states. CDC developed standard core questionnaires for states to use to provide data that could be compared across states. The BRFSS, administered and supported by the Division of Adult and Community Health, National Center for Chronic Disease Prevention and Health Promotion, CDC, is an on-going data collection program. By 1994, all states, the District of Columbia, and three territories were participating in the BRFSS.

behavioral therapy a philosophy that states that the undesired behaviors exhibited by an individual can be modified without directly addressing the underlying pathology. An example would be the use of a behavioral modification program to reduce *self-injurious behavior* without directly addressing the underlying mental retardation.

behavior modification program (BMP) a planned, systematic way of interacting with a patient and structuring the patient's environment to produce a desired change in the patient's behavior. There are many different types of BMPs that work. The two key elements are to select an age-appropriate method and then to consistently implement the program. See *autism (chart), aversion therapy, cueing, operant conditioning.*

behavior problem (RAPs) Between 60% and 70% of patients in a typical nursing facility exhibit emotional, social, and/or behavioral disorders; about 40% have purely behavioral problems (e.g., wandering, verbal abuse, physically aggressive and/or socially inappropriate behaviors). Patients with behavior problems also frequently have other related problems. Over 80% of those who have behavior problems will have some type of cognitive deficit; about 75% will have *mood* and/or relationship problems. Problem behaviors are often seen as a source of danger and distress to the patients themselves and sometimes to other patients and staff. Nursing facilities often find such patients difficult to cope with and physicians often seem unaware of the wide range of available treatment and management options. As a result, overuse of *physical restraints* or *psychotropic drugs* is too common. About one-half of patients who exhibit "problem" behaviors will be physically restrained and about one-half will receive psychoactive medications — antipsychotics (neuroleptics), antianxiety agents, and to a lesser extent, antidepressants. These interventions, however, have potentially serious, negative side effects and many nurses in nursing facilities report being uncomfortable using only physical restraints and/or psychotropics to manage patients with behavior problems. As a result, there is an increasing trend toward using other interventions and treatment in addressing problem behaviors such as *behavior modification programs* and environmental alterations. See *extrinsic, intrinsic, maintenance program.*

below elbow amputation an amputation between the wrist and the elbow. Function is greatly enhanced with a prosthesis similar to the one used for the *wrist disarticulation* amputation. Movement for activities that require pronation, supination, and flexion are usually retained unless the amputation is close to the elbow. In an amputation close to the elbow a Hepp-Kuhn Socket or a Munster Socket is used in addition to the figure 8 harness, flexible elbow hinges, wrist unit, and terminal device. When either socket is used, the patient will most likely experience limited forearm flexion, requiring some adaptation of activities or positioning. Cosmetically the patient may be concerned about the extensiveness of the prosthetic device.

below knee amputation an amputation located between the knee and the ankle. Functional ability is increased by a three unit prosthesis: 1. soft or hard socket condylar cuff suspension, 2. patellar tendon-bearing prosthesis, and 3. prosthetic foot. A variety of options are available in the patellar tendon-bearing prosthesis.

benchmark the industry-wide, best performance in any given area (e.g., treatment protocols) within a specific group (e.g., traumatic brain injury). A treatment *protocol* that consistently has the best out-

comes for the most functional gain (performance) with patient with a Rancho Los Amigos level of 4-5 at admission would be the *benchmark* for that area. *Quality assurance* programs that want to measure the quality of their treatment protocols with patients with a Rancho Los Amigos level of 4-5 would use the benchmark protocol as a comparison. When benchmarking a protocol, the professional defines the *outcomes* in measurable terms, determines how well the protocol achieves those outcomes, and applies the information learned to improve the program. See *performance goals.*

beneficiary an individual who is entitled to receive Medicare services. Also a term used by health care insurance companies to indicate that an individual is entitled to receive the benefits of a health insurance policy.

bias (HHS) Bias occurs when problems in study design lead to effects that are not related to the variables being studied. An example is selection bias, which occurs when study subjects are chosen in a way that can misleadingly increase or decrease the strength of an association. Choosing experimental and control group subjects from different populations would result in a selection bias.

bile duct (HHS) tubular structures responsible for conducting bile (a substance that aids in digestion) from the liver to the intestine.

biliary calculi See *gallstone.*

biliary obstruction (HHS) blockage or clogging of a bile duct.

bilirubin (HHS) a red pigment formed from hemoglobin during normal and abnormal destruction of red blood cells in the body.

biofeedback a technique of training the individual to be aware of unconscious or involuntary physiological actions of the body to allow him/her to control or modify the body's response to stimuli. Alyce and Elmer Green of the Menninger Foundation first developed biofeedback techniques in the 1960's. Biofeedback generally implies the use of instruments to become more aware of exactly how the body is being affected by stress (obtaining an exact measurement) and then using a variety of *relaxation techniques* to measurably change the body functions which are sub-optimal (obtaining change). In other words, if the patient experiences a rapid heartbeat and fast, shallow breathing during stress, the patient might use biofeedback techniques to slow his/her heartbeat and slow and deepen his/her breathing. The "measurement" would be a monitor to keep track of the pulse and breathing rate. The patient would be "hooked up" to this monitor and observe the rate changes as s/he practiced different relaxa-

Characteristics of Bipolar Disorders

Disorder	Description
Mania	Characterized by excitement, euphoria, expansive or irritable mood, *hyperactivity*, *pressured speech*, flight of ideas, decreased need for sleep, *distractibility*, and impaired *judgment*. *Delusions* consistent with elation and grandiosity may be present.
Depressed	Characterized by lowered *mood*, slowed thinking, decreased movement or *agitation*, loss of interest, guilt, lowered self-esteem, sleep disturbance, and decreased appetite.
Mixed	Characterized by the co-existence of mania and depressive symptoms.

tion techniques to obtain change. Biofeedback is used to reduce or resolve a large group of disorders including: "tension headache, migraine headache, hypertension, insomnia, spastic colon, muscle spasms, anxiety, phobic reactions, asthma, stuttering, teeth grinding (*bruxism*), *epilepsy*, *attention deficit hyperactivity disorder*, tinnitus, chronic pain, *panic attacks*, some tics and tremors, gastrointestinal disorders, decreased blood glucose levels, stress incontinence, painful intercourse, painful menstrual cramps, and increased vaginal muscle tone (Davis, Robbins-Eshelman & McKay, 1995, p. 118)." It is important to note that there are many applications for biofeedback other than treatment. Some other uses include training for optimal performance, product testing, physiological profiling (stress evaluations), and fun (games controlled by physiological responses). Some of the specific machines and types of biofeedback training include electromyogram (EMG) training, thermograph (temperature) training, galvanic skin response (GSR) training, electroencephalogram (EEG) training, and heart rate training. See *multidisciplinary pain center*.

biometric identifier (HCO) a retinal pattern, fingerprint, or other anatomical feature that can be used by a computer program (along with appropriate interface equipment) to positively identify a user.

biopesticide (HHS) any material of natural origin used in pest control derived from living organisms, such as bacteria, plant cells, or animal cells.

biotechnology (HHS) The simplest definition of biotechnology is "applied biology." The application of biological knowledge and techniques to develop products. It may be further defined as the use of living organisms to make a product or run a process. By this definition, the classic techniques used for plant and animal breeding, fermentation, and enzyme purification would be considered biotechnology. Some people use the term only to refer to newer tools of genetic science. In this context, biotechnology may be defined as the use of biotechnical methods to modify the genetic materials of living cells so they will produce new substances or perform new functions. Examples include recombinant

DNA technology, in which a copy of a piece of DNA containing one or a few genes is transferred between organisms or "recombined" within an organism.

bipolar disorder a major *affective disorder* in which there are episodes of both *mania* and *depression*; formerly called manic depressive psychosis, circular, or mixed type. Bipolar disorder may be subdivided into manic, depressed, or mixed types on the basis of currently presenting symptoms. Patients who have a bipolar disorder tend to have a high rate (10% - 15%) of completed *suicide*. For patients who are experiencing a severe manic episode, caution should be taken, as they tend to have a higher incidence of violent behavior (child or spousal abuse or other assaultive or physically destructive behavior). If a patient experiences his/her first bipolar episode after the age of 40, the cause may be secondary to a medical problem or to *substance abuse*. Bipolar I disorder refers to *mood* swings that are manic in nature. Bipolar II disorder refers to mood swings that are *hypomanic* (less severe than mania) in nature. See the chart at the top of the page for characteristics of bipolar disorders. See *medically complex*.

bladder cancers Most bladder cancers (90%) are transitional cell carcinomas. Most frequently seen in patients over 50 years. Treatment includes surgery, radiation, and/or chemotherapy. Functional ability may be limited due to bladder spasms, pain, radiation bowel damage, ureteric obstruction, or bladder hemorrhage.

blank (HHS/NMDP) Individuals have the ability to express two HLA antigens within each category of antigens (one set being inherited from each biological parent). When an individual has apparently inherited the same antigen type from both parents, the HLA typing of that individual is designated by the shared HLA antigen followed by a "blank" (-).

blast cells (HHS/NMDP) blood cells still in an immature stage of cellular development before appearance of the definitive characteristics of the cell.

blast crisis (HHS/NMDP) the stage of chronic myelogenous leukemia (CML) in which large quantities of immature cells are produced by the bone marrow.

This stage of CML is far less responsive to treatment than the chronic or stable phase.

blastogenesis the induction of cell division after exposure to an antigen or mitogen. Blastogenesis is thought to provide an in vitro model of the lymphocyte proliferative response to challenge by an infectious agent.

blind experiment (single or double) (HHS) In a single blind experiment, the subjects do not know whether they are receiving an experimental treatment or a placebo. In a *double blind experiment*, neither the researchers nor the participants are aware of which subjects receive the treatment until after the study is completed.

blood alcohol level the percentage of alcohol in the blood. European countries have had alcohol limits since the 1930's and 1940's with the United States adding its own laws after WWII by enacting a federal definition of "intoxication." President Clinton signed a federal drunk driving law on October 23, 2000, lowering the blood alcohol limit for drunkenness to 0.08%. At the time President Clinton signed the law, 31 states had a blood alcohol limit of 0.10%. States that don't lower their blood alcohol limit to 0.08% by 2007 will lose federal highway funds.

blood/body fluids precautions an isolation procedure for patients who have *AIDS*; arthropod-borne viral fevers; *hepatitis* B or C; malaria, rat-bite fever, syphilis, and other selected diseases. The isolation procedures include: 1. masks are not indicated, 2. gowns are indicated if soiling with blood or body fluids is likely, 3. gloves are indicated for touching blood or body fluids, 4. hands must be washed after touching the patient or potentially contaminated articles and before taking care of another patient, 5. articles contaminated with infective material should be discarded or bagged and labeled before being sent for decontamination and reprocessing, 6. care should be taken to avoid needle-stick injuries; used needles should not be recapped or bent;

they should be placed in a prominently labeled, puncture-resistance container designated specifically for such disposal, and 7. blood spills should be cleaned up promptly with a solution of 5.25% sodium hypochlorite diluted 1:10 with water. The sign for blood/body fluids precautions is always pink.

blood-borne pathogens infectious material, including the *HIV/AIDS* virus and *hepatitis* virus, which are transmitted through contact with infected body fluids. See *exposure control plan, occupational exposure*.

blood pressure a measurement of the volume and of pressure of the blood on the walls of the arteries. Blood pressure is one of the four elements of *vital signs*. Recorded as a fraction, the top measurement, systolic, measures the strength exerted by the heart when it is pumping. The lower number, the diastolic, measures the pressure exerted on the arteries when the heart is resting. The equipment used to measure blood pressure is called a blood pressure cuff, which is used with a sphygmomanometer and stethoscope. All therapists need to know how to take a patient's blood pressure, as blood pressure is an indicator of health. Activity may be contraindicated if the patient arrives at therapy with a questionable blood pressure (either high or low). With certain patients, the physician may request a blood pressure to be taken during activity as a precaution. There are no physiologically observable signs of high blood pressure. The therapist will not be able to guess a patient's blood pressure without measuring it with a blood pressure cuff. See the table of common factors that influence blood pressure at the bottom of the page. See *autogenics, coarctation of the aorta, hypertension, metabolic disorders, sympathetic nervous system*.

B lymphocytes the primary cells of the humoral immune system; derived from bone marrow; lymphocytes that produce immunoglobulin.

body image the sum total of an individual's image of his/her body and who s/he is involving both conscious and subconscious awareness. A severely dis-

Common Factors That Influence Blood Pressure

Factor	Description
Position of Patient	A patient who is lying down will have a lower blood pressure than the same patient sitting up. Blood pressure may go up when the patient's legs are crossed.
Activity	Exertion during activity may raise a patient's blood pressure (more so in patients who are out of shape). If the patient's blood pressure is near the maximum suggested by the physician prior to activity, activity may be contraindicated.
Ingested Substance	Coffee, tobacco, and some medications may raise the patient's blood pressure.
Time of Day	Blood pressure tends to be lowest upon waking and higher mid afternoon to evening.
Gender	Women tend to have slightly lower blood pressures than men of the same age.
Pain and Emotions	Both pain and strong emotional experiences raise a patient's blood pressure.

torted or inappropriate body image is a clinical condition affecting many individuals with neurotic disorders. See *anorexia nervosa, Beck Depression Inventory, bulimia nervosa.*

body language a complex non-verbal system, often influenced by one's culture, of communicating one's feelings and emotions through the stance and movement of one's body. See *interpersonal skills.*

body of knowledge the sum of the information a profession embraces as being pertinent to the practice of the profession. For therapists the scope of this body of knowledge would include professional standards of practice, normal and abnormal physiological process, human development, the body of knowledge directly related to the provisions of services (e.g., splinting techniques, leisure counseling), and management theory and technique. Body of knowledge is different from expertise, which is the ability to translate the body of knowledge into action. See *scope of practice.*

body scheme the automatic, alternating tensing and relaxing of an individual's muscles to be able to maintain a desired body position.

bolus tube feeding When the patient is not able to eat normally, one option is to use a *feeding tube.* A bolus tube feeding consists of a large amount (250 to 400 ml) of liquid of nourishment, which is placed into the patient's stomach over the period of a few minutes. This feeding is repeated four to six times a day and allows for the freer movement of the patient, as the patient can clamp the end of the tube and move about after the feeding. Patients who are unconscious or who take a long time to digest the food are at greater risk of vomiting and aspiration.

bone length the length of a specific bone; more specifically, the amount of bone left after an amputation. This length is usually measured from the medial tibial plateau down to the bone end for patients with below knee amputations or from the ischial tuberosity or the greater trochanter down to the bone end for patients with above the knee amputations. The therapist may want to consider the length of the stump (and the stability provided by prosthesis due to the length) prior to introducing the patient to new activities that require physical skill.

bone marrow (HHS/NMDP) a substance with the consistency of thick blood found in the body's hollow bones, such as legs, arms, and hips. It produces platelets, red blood cells, and white blood cells, the main agents of the body's immune system. Bone marrow for transplant is invariably harvested from the pelvis.

bone marrow transplant a treatment that eradicates the patient's bone marrow and then implants new,

healthier bone marrow. The patient's bone marrow is destroyed over a seven-day period using radiation and chemotherapy. The replacement bone marrow is introduced into the body just as a blood transfusion would be, with approximately one quart of the new bone marrow being dripped into the patient's bloodstream using a catheter. The new bone marrow may be autologous (the patient's own bone marrow which had been removed, frozen, and stored) or from a donor (usually a compatible sibling or unrelated donor). Bone marrow transplants are used to treat many different type of *leukemia*, aplastic *anemia*, and some immune deficiency diseases. Bone marrow produces two different kinds of blood cells, red and white, as well as platelets. Some patients who have gone through bone marrow transplants develop *graft-versus-host disease* (GVH).

boredom the absence of desired arousal and interest. The lack of pleasurable stimulation (boredom) is a relatively new concept. Peters (1975) states that it was not until ten years after the birth of the industrial revolution that the concept of boredom was found in the literature. And even then, little reference to the concept of boredom was found in literature until the late 1960's. Work to define what boredom actually was did not gain popular attention until the 1990's. The concept of "boredom" also is not a singular notion. An individual may be interested in one or two aspects of his/her life, but may find that other aspects are unbearably void of interest. Ragheb and Merydith (1995) studied the construct of boredom and found four major components of free time boredom: physical involvement (the individual has enough physical movement to satisfy him/her), mental involvement (the individual has enough to think about and finds these thoughts emotionally satisfying), meaningfulness (the individual has a focus or purpose during his/her free time), and speed of time (the individual has enough purposeful and satisfying activity to fill his/her time). Boredom is a common complaint. Not only does the therapist hear the complaint from his/her patients but also from staff. Many therapists have had an order for treatment based on the patient's complaint of boredom. But not all "boredom" needs to be addressed nor does it mean that the patient's boredom can be solved through activity. Ragheb and Merydith (1995, p.1) state that "boredom is a pathological event if ill health or a loss of freedom (e.g., incarceration) is a direct result of the patient's lack of desired arousal or interest in his/her environment. Some patients will report that their life has always been boring. While this attitude may not be a desired one, boredom in and of itself is not always a condition that requires direct intervention at the time of admission to health care services. Intervention may be indicated if the therapist determines that the patient's pre-admission boredom is one of the events that led to the current admission or which is reducing the patient's optimal recovery." Patients who have led a very active life may find that they are bored while confined to the hospital. Such boredom does not necessarily call for therapeutic intervention. The therapist needs to determine the causes of the patient's boredom and to use clinical judgment about how important resolving the boredom will be to the patient's overall recovery. Also, the physiological symptoms of boredom are similar to the physiological symptoms of *over-stimulation*. Prior to involving the "bored" patient in activities, the therapist should first rule out emotional and physical "shut down" due to over-stimulation. See *Free Time Boredom Measurement, leisure.*

Borrelia (CDC) a genus of bacteria with numerous species that cause disease in humans. The diseases associated with these organisms are typically relapsing fevers frequently transmitted to humans through bites by ticks or lice. Animals are usually the reservoirs for the bacteria.

botulism (CDC) a rare but serious paralytic illness caused by a nerve toxin that is produced by the bacterium Clostridium botulinum. There are three main kinds of botulism. Food-borne botulism is caused by eating foods that contain the botulism toxin. Wound botulism is caused by toxin produced from a wound infected with Clostridium botulinum. Infant botulism is caused by consuming the spores of the botulinum bacteria, which then grow in the intestines and release toxin. All forms of botulism can be fatal and are considered medical emergencies. Food-borne botulism can be especially dangerous because many people can be poisoned by eating a contaminated food. Clostridium botulinum is the name of a group of bacteria commonly found in soil. These rod-shaped organisms grow best in low oxygen conditions. The bacteria form spores that allow them to survive in a dormant state until exposed to conditions that can support their growth. There are seven types of botulism toxin designated by the letters A through G; only types A, B, E, and F cause illness in humans. In the United States an average of 110 cases of botulism are reported each year. Of these, approximately 25% are food-borne, 72% are infant botulism, and the rest are wound botulism. Outbreaks of food-borne botulism involving two or more persons occur most years and are usually caused by eating contaminated home-canned foods. The number of cases of food-borne and infant botu-

lism has changed little in recent years, but wound botulism has increased because of the use of black-tar heroin, especially in California. The classic symptoms of botulism include double vision, blurred vision, drooping eyelids, slurred speech, difficulty swallowing, dry mouth, and muscle weakness. Infants with botulism appear lethargic, feed poorly, are constipated, and have a weak cry and poor muscle tone. These are all symptoms of the muscle paralysis caused by the bacterial toxin. If untreated, these symptoms may progress to cause paralysis of the arms, legs, trunk, and respiratory muscles. In food-borne botulism, symptoms generally begin 18 to 36 hours after eating a contaminated food, but they can occur as early as six hours or as late as ten days. Physicians may consider the diagnosis if the patient's history and physical examination suggest botulism. However, these clues are usually not enough to allow a diagnosis of botulism. Other diseases such as *Guillain-Barré* syndrome, stroke, and myasthenia gravis can appear similar to botulism, and special tests may be needed to exclude these other conditions. These tests may include a brain scan, spinal fluid examination, nerve conduction test (electromyography or EMG), and a Tensilon test for myasthenia gravis. The most direct way to confirm the diagnosis is to demonstrate the botulinum toxin in the patient's serum or stool by injecting serum or stool into mice and looking for signs of botulism. The bacteria can also be isolated from the stool of persons with food-borne and infant botulism. These tests can be performed at some state health department laboratories and at CDC. The respiratory failure and paralysis that occur with severe botulism may require a patient to be on a breathing machine (ventilator) for weeks, plus intensive medical and nursing care. After several weeks, the paralysis slowly improves. If diagnosed early, food-borne and wound botulism can be treated with an antitoxin that blocks the action of toxin circulating in the blood. This can prevent patients from worsening, but recovery still takes many weeks. Physicians may try to remove contaminated food still in the gut by inducing vomiting or by using enemas. Wounds should be treated, usually surgically, to remove the source of the toxin-producing bacteria. Good supportive care in a hospital is the mainstay of therapy for all forms of botulism. Currently, antitoxin is not routinely given for treatment of infant botulism. Botulism can result in death due to respiratory failure. However, in the past 50 years the proportion of patients with botulism who die has fallen from about 50% to 8%. A patient with severe botulism may require a breathing machine as well as intensive medical and nursing care for several months. Patients who survive an episode of botulism poisoning may have fatigue and shortness of breath for years and long-term therapy may be needed to aid recovery.

bovine spongiform encephalopathy (BSE) (HHS) also known as "mad cow disease." It is a rare, chronic, degenerative disease affecting the brain and central nervous system of cattle. Cattle with BSE lose their coordination, develop abnormal posture, and experience changes in behavior. Clinical symptoms take 4-5 years to develop, followed by death in a period of several weeks to months unless the affected animal is destroyed sooner.

bowel and bladder disorders a bowel or bladder disorder implies that the patient has lost or has abnormal function related to voiding urine or feces. The most common disorders the therapist will see are urinary *incontinence*, *constipation*, and *ostomy*. While these disorders in and of themselves do not produce functional ability deficits, the care associated with these disorders may cause a patient to experience life differently than his/her peers.

Brady dyskinesia an abnormal slowness of *movement*; a sluggishness of a patient's physical or cognitive response.

brain cancers Unless metastases, cancers are usually from glial cells (gliomas) as neuron cells cannot divide. Brain tumors are the second most common cancer in children. The peak age for astrocytomas is 50 to 60 years of age. Treatment includes surgery, radiation, and/or chemotherapy. Functional ability may be impaired by headaches, vomiting, focal brain damage to specific areas of the brain (e.g., motor function, speech), and impaired *executive function*.

brain plasticity the brain's ability to adjust to a physiological insult (e.g., *traumatic brain injury*) by developing the ability to manage a specific function in a part of the brain which usually is responsible for other functions. It is thought that the younger the patient is at the time of the insult, the greater the potential for relearning due to a greater brain plasticity.

brain-skull differential during an acceleration or deceleration of the body, the skull tends to accelerate or decelerate with a faster reaction time than the brain. It is because of this differential that a person sustains coup and contrecoup lesions during a traumatic brain injury. See *coup, contrecoup, lesions*.

brainstem one of three parts of the brain, along with the *cerebellum* and the *cerebrum*; made up of the medulla oblongata, the pons, and the mesencephalon. The brainstem joins the spinal cord with the brain and controls breathing, heartbeat, and involuntary functions. It is also responsible for coordination of motor movement, senses, and reflexes. The brainstem is near the back, lower part of the brain. See *decerebrate rigidity*.

BRAT diet a diet prescribed for children who have been fed intravenously and need to move slowly back to eating solids. BRAT stands for bananas, rice cereal, applesauce, and toast.

breast cancer the second leading cause of death among women in the United States. Signs of breast cancer include persistent lumps, nipple discharge or bleeding, and skin dimpling. Most breast cancers that are detected early are found through the use of mammograms. Treatment includes surgery, radiation, and chemotherapy.

breathing a *relaxation technique* that involves purposeful, slow, rhythmic breathing to increase the amount of oxygen being taken into the body and to exhale carbon dioxide. The patient inhales through the nose with relatively large, deep breaths and exhales through the mouth. The breathing should be deep enough to involve the diaphragm and not just the chest. Poor breathing patterns are evident in disorders such as *anxiety*, *panic attacks*, and *depression* as well as with medical disorders such as headaches and muscle tension. Mastery of this technique can happen within minutes but measurable changes usually require a month or more of regular practice. See *escharotomy*.

breathlessness the inability to take in enough oxygen to satisfy body function needs. Goldenson, et al (1978) reported on the **Standard Classification of Grading Breathlessness** as it relates to activity. This classification system is helpful when charting a patient's respiratory status during activities. See the table on the next page. See *chronic obstructive pulmonary disease, dyspnea, emphysema*.

brief combination techniques a relaxation strategy that combines techniques to best suite the patient's needs. By combining techniques based on the patient's individualized situation, the patient benefits from the synergistic effect of techniques so a progressive, deeper relaxation may be achieved. Many patients find that by combining a couple of brief techniques they are able to become very relaxed even during the short time period covered by a typical coffee break. Mastery usually takes a few weeks of daily practice, especially if the patient has not used relaxation techniques before. Brief combination techniques work well for patients with "flight or fight" symptoms, job related *stress* or stress-induced physiologic disorders. See *relaxation techniques*.

Brief Leisure Rating Scale (BLRS) 25-item assess-

Standard Classification of Grading Breathlessness

Grade	Description
1	Can keep pace walking with person of same age and body build without breathlessness on level ground, but not on hills or stairs.
2	Can walk a mile at own pace without dyspnea (shortness of breath), but cannot keep pace with a normally fit person on level ground.
3	Becomes breathless after walking about 100 yards (92 meters) or for a few minutes on level ground.
4	Becomes breathless while dressing or talking.

ment developed to measure the evaluator's perception of the patient's degree of learned *helplessness*. Originally designed by Ellis and Niles to be used as a means to measure a patient's perceived helplessness in leisure, this assessment has had little formal testing and does not have a manual. The BLRS has a solid foundation behind it because of the skill of the authors and the work that they put into its development. However, before it is used as an instrument for determining treatment, it needs further testing and, possibly, revision.

bronchitis an infection or inflammation of the bronchial tubes or air passages of the lungs. Bronchitis is a common disorder that starts when the lining of the bronchial wall becomes thick and heavy with mucus. This further increases the patient's susceptibility to *infection* or increased irritation from environmental irritants (e.g., pollution, cigarette smoke). Symptoms associated with bronchitis include coughing and the production of phlegm and may last for one to two months (or longer). See *chronic obstructive pulmonary disease.*

bronchopulmonary dysplasia (BPD) a chronic lung disorder found in children and youth who have respiratory distress syndrome and/or who use a *ventilator* to breathe. Illness or trauma at birth (e.g., meconium aspiration) may damage the lungs so that some type of assisted breathing is required. This assisted breathing may be oxygen-enriched air and/or the use of a respirator. Both a higher percentage of oxygen or the forced expansion of the lungs, while necessary to maintain life, damage lung tissue. While many of the children with BPD gradually improve (20% do not survive the first year), there are many secondary problems associated with BPD that the therapist must be aware of. Because of the forced air or oxygen-enriched air, the child will be more susceptible to normal childhood illnesses. This susceptibility often leads to increased episodes of otitis media (ear infections), which may lead to some hearing loss. The patient's increased susceptibility to infection and potential hearing loss makes normal socialization or even the use of standard daycare difficult. In addition, the child usually has an air

tube connected to a stoma in the trachea or near the child's nose, which is connected to a tank or a respirator at the other end. This severely limits the child's ability to move around, get physical exercise, and explore his/her world, leading to a type of sensory *deprivation*. A child with BPD is placed on many medications. These medications (along with limited exercise and often with associated feeding problems) cause fragile bones that break easily. The stress of having a chronically ill child in the home and the financial burden of the required medical services also impacts the child's feeling of security. All of these problems, which are secondary to the BPD, are very significant and call for the services of the therapist. One of the most important aspects of the therapist's job is to ensure that the child experiences a balance of activities to help decrease the chance of developmental delays. See *developmental disability.*

bronchospasm abnormal narrowing and obstruction of the airway due to contractions of the smooth muscle of the bronchi. Acute bronchospasms can be a medical emergency. Relief of the bronchospasm is important to help avoid having to take drastic measures. Patients who have a history of acute bronchospasms should always carry bronchodilator medications (which dilate the bronchi and reduce the spasm). Individuals who have a history of *asthma* have learned through experience that vigorous physical activity leads to bronchospasms. One of the therapist's jobs is to evaluate the patient's degree of avoidance of physical activity and provide any necessary education. Moderate physical activity promotes health and provides opportunities to be with peers. See *chronic obstructive pulmonary disease.*

Brookfield's principles one of the primary authors on how adults learn, Stephen Brookfield (1986) outlined six principles to be used when teaching adults (*andragogy*). The six key ways that adults approach learning differently than children are 1. adults tend to be in class voluntarily, 2. adults tend to approach each other with mutual respect, 3. adults tend to want to take responsibility for their own learning, actively collaborating with the instructor, 4. adults tend to view learning as a dynamic, ongoing process that is a key element related to the quality of their life or job (also known as "praxis"), 5. adults learn best when they are in a setting that promotes a supportive, critical reflection of their work, and 6. adults tend to work best when the learning environment is set up to empower their desire to be self-directed.

bruxism rhythmic or spasmodic grinding of the teeth and other nonfunctional mandible movement. This involuntary habitual grinding is usually seen only during sleep. However, individuals with moderate to severe mental retardation may experience bruxism during waking hours. Bruxism is thought to be caused by an individual's repression of anger, fear, *anxiety*, or other, similarly stressful feelings related to the perceived inability to control one's environment. See *biofeedback, stress.*

Bt (Bacillus thuringiensis) (HHS) one of the most common microorganisms used in biologically-based pesticides. Several of the proteins produced by Bt, principally in the coating the bacteria forms around itself, are lethal to individual species of insects. By using Bt in pesticide formulations, target insects can be controlled using an environmentally benign, biologically-based agent. Bt-based insecticides have been widely used by home gardeners for many years as well as on farms.

budget the written document that shows how much money (and other resources) will be used during a specific time period (usually a year). A department's operating budget usually provides an overview of where the department will get money (revenue) and where the money will be spent (allocation, expenses). Income for therapy services usually comes from four sources: *roomrate* (managed care systems, Medicaid/Medicare and private insurance), direct billing (third party *reimbursement*), donations, and earned income (from arts and crafts sales, etc.).

Buerger's disease See *thromboangiitis obliterans.*

building (ADA) any structure used and intended for supporting or sheltering any use or occupancy.

bulbous referring to the rounding off of a limb at the point of amputation. Different than a *fish mouth amputation* or a *guillotine amputation.*

bulimia nervosa a psychological eating disorder which is evidenced by an individual's binge eating at least two times a week for a minimum of three months. Individuals usually experience feelings of a lack of control during these episodes. The age of onset for bulimia nervosa is early adolescence through early adulthood and occurs most often in females. Bulimia nervosa is usually not fatal, as the individuals are usually near normal weight but do show signs of *depression* and poor *body image.* There are

two forms of the condition, purging and non-purging. The first type regularly engages in purging through self-induced vomiting or the excessive use of laxatives or diuretics. The non-purging type controls weight through strict dieting, fasting, or excessive exercise. See *anorexia nervosa, childhood psychiatric disorders.*

burn tissue damage resulting from four primary causes: 1. open flame, 2. scald, 3. chemicals, and 4. electricity. The degree of injury is measured using two elements: the degree of the burn and the percentage of the body involved. The degrees of severity of a burn are listed in the charts on the next page. In addition to the degree of burns, three other factors influence recovery:

1. the extent of the total body surface area (TBSA) burned (listed in percentages)
2. the patient's ability to withstand pain and treatment
3. pre-existing conditions like cardiovascular disease (causes increased pulmonary edema), renal disease (due to burn-associated renal failure), respiratory disease (decreased tolerance to respiratory challenges), or metabolic disease (poor wound healing and increased susceptibility to infection).

To help fight hypovolemic shock (too little fluid) an intravenous line (IV) and urinary *catheter* are placed and electrolyte-fortified fluids are pumped into the patient. The lack of fluids is caused by intravenous fluid loss. The capillaries become more permeable, causing excess fluid loss and edema (as well as the loss of electrolytes). This permeability happens in both the involved (burned) and the healthy parts of the body, especially in patients with total body surface area burns of 30% or more (Zane, 1984, p. 18). A significant long-term side effect of severe burns is the loss of surface capillary function and the loss of the sweat glands. With a decreased ability to shed the excess intravascular fluid (sweat) around the injured sites, *edema* (swelling) occurs. This intravascular fluid tends to be protein enriched. Protein enriched fluids encourage the production of collagen fibers. *Collagen* fibers reduce the ability of the muscles and tendons to stretch. With decreased activity the collagen fibers thicken and adhere to the surrounding structures, causing an internal loss of *range of motion* (ROM). Since ROM will likely be reduced already due to external fibrosis scarring, it is vital for the patient to participate in a variety of activities which promote ROM. Moderate activity is the key to encourage increased circulation and decrease collagen development. The therapist is challenged to find an appropriate mix of activities that

Degrees of Severity of Burns

Degree	Description
First	An injury to the superficial layer of the skin (like a sunburn).
Second	An injury that extends beyond the superficial layers of the skin into the dermis. This burn is associated with blistering and pain. Except in the cases of excessively deep second-degree burns, skin grafts are not required. Functional ability to participate in activities is challenged by the *fibrosis, contractures,* and joint stiffness that remain after the burned area has healed. Extensive, deep second-degree burns are associated with a high death rate.
Third	An injury that extends through all layers of the skin. Due to the damage to the epidermis and the dermis, self-healing does not occur. Skin grafts are used to replace the skin functions lost. The best grafts tend to be the ones from the patient's own uninjured skin (*autogenous graft*). Due to the significance of loss to the body, a full thickness graft is used to replace a full thickness loss. The therapist should not expect a return to premorbid functional ability and can expect a significant cosmetic disfigurement. Third-degree burns are also called full thickness burns.
Fourth	An injury that extends into the underlying tendon and bone. This degree of burn is also referred to as a "char injury." Any char injury which involves tendons should be noted on the therapist's assessment, as ranging of damaged tendons is contraindicated.

Seven Classifications of Burns, American Burn Association (DiGregorio, 1984, p.2)

Class	Description
Class 1	second-degree burns of 25% or greater total body surface area in adults or 20% in children
Class 2	third-degree burns of 10% or greater total body surface area
Class 3	burns involving specialized areas: that is burns of the hands, feet, face, eyes, ears, or perineum.
Class 4	burns complicated by inhalation injury
Class 5	burns complicated by fractures or other major trauma
Class 6	high voltage electrical burns
Class 7	burns occurring in poor risk groups, such as patients with significant preexisting medical problems, head injuries, cerebral vascular accidents, or psychiatric disabilities

the patient enjoys, that activates all involved structures and is reasonable given the patient's personal and community resources. See *cardiovascular endurance, debridement, artificial airway, eschar, escharotomy, Foley catheter, Jobst.*

bus (ADA) any of several types of self-propelled vehicles, other than an over the road bus, generally rubber tired, intended for use on city streets, highways, and busways, including but not limited to minibuses, forty and thirty foot transit buses, articulated buses, double-decked buses, and electric powered trolley buses, used to provide designated or specific public transportation services. Self-propelled, rubber tire vehicles designed to look like antique or vintage trolleys or streetcars are considered buses. The ADA accessibility guidelines for buses may be found in the **Buses, Vans, and Systems Technical Assistance Manual** (US Architectural and Transportation Barriers Compliance Board).

business plan a plan which outlines where the business intends to be (financially, scope of product, and market position) within a stated period of time. Creating the business plan starts with a defined set of goals and objectives for the business. These are then developed into performance standards for each component of the stated goals and objectives. A time estimate and cost estimate are then determined for each of the components, placing each component in a logical sequence. Next, management needs to determine the types and amount of training required for each staff person or team to allow the business to achieve the goals and objectives. This determination would also include the cost and time required as well as the types and amount of training. To help implement the business plan, policies and procedures should be written which will help guide each staff person and the teams to achieve the goals and objectives in the manner envisioned. Actual performance along the way should be measured against the previously developed performance criteria and *quality assurance* measures should be implemented to improve the process as it goes along.

Bus Utilization Skills Assessment a functional assessment that measures a patient's skill level associated with riding public transportation, including street safety, personal safety, social skills, money skills, and reading a bus schedule. By burlingame, 1989.

C

cadaver graft a graft that is taken from a donor soon after the donor is declared dead. This is a temporary until an *autogenous graft* can be used or until the body is able to heal itself adequately.

cafeteria plan (FB) a type of health care benefit plan provided by employers that allows all participating employees to choose among two or more benefits consisting of cash and qualified benefits (e.g., health insurance and life insurance). Under section 125 of the Internal Revenue Code, employers may contribute flexible benefit credits that employees can allocate toward the purchase of health benefits. Employers may also set up salary conversion mechanisms that allow employees to pay for health insurance premiums with pretax income. Employers may also provide *flexible spending accounts* allowing employees to contribute pretax funds for health care expenditures.

caffeine (HHS) a naturally occurring substance found in the leaves, seeds, or fruits of over 63 plant species worldwide; part of a group of compounds known as methylxanthines. The most commonly known sources of caffeine are coffee and cocoa beans, cola nuts, and tea leaves. Caffeine is a pharmacologically active substance and, depending on the dose, can be a mild central nervous system stimulant. Caffeine does not accumulate in the body over the course of time and is normally excreted within several hours of consumption.

calicivirus (CDC) (also Norwalk-like virus) an extremely common cause of food-borne illness, though it is rarely diagnosed, because the laboratory test is not widely available. It causes an acute gastrointestinal illness, usually with more vomiting than diarrhea, that resolves within two days. Unlike many food-borne pathogens that have animal reservoirs, it is believed that Norwalk-like viruses spread primarily from one infected person to another. Infected kitchen workers can contaminate a salad or sandwich as they prepare it, if they have the virus on their hands. Infected fishermen have contaminated oysters as they harvested them. See *food-borne disease*.

calorie (HHS) the amount of energy required to raise the temperature of one milliliter of water at a standard initial temperature by one degree centigrade.

Campylobacter (CDC) a bacterial pathogen that causes fever, diarrhea, and abdominal cramps. It is the most commonly identified bacterial cause of diarrheal illness in the world. These bacteria live in the intestines of healthy birds, and most raw poultry meat has Campylobacter on it. Eating undercooked chicken, or other food that has been contaminated with juices dripping from raw chicken, is the most frequent source of this infection. See *food-borne disease*.

Canadian crutch crutch with a vertical metal cuff for the patient's lower arms (about 1 - 2 inches below the elbow) and a handle for the hand to allow weight bearing. Also known as the Lofstrand crutch. See *crutch*.

cancer a group of over 200 different types of disease, one of the most common causes of death in the United States. Over 500,000 deaths a year result from cancer, slightly less than the number of deaths due to cardiovascular disease. Cancer is a term applied to cells that grow larger, divide quicker, and are unable to carry out their normal function. These cells have the ability to separate from each other, move through the body to a new location and then establish a new site of abnormal growth called a *metastasis*. The incidence of cancer increases significantly with age. See *physician data query, remission*.

cancer staging and grading the international scale used to determine the severity of the cancer is called the TNM staging system. TNM stands for <u>t</u>umor size, <u>n</u>odal involvement, and <u>m</u>etastatic progress. TNM is used with most cancers with the notable exception of Hodgkin's disease and lymphomas. Another way to describe the degree of involvement is to grade the cancer by measuring the degrees of difference between the normal cell type that the cancer developed from and the cancerous cell.

Candida albicans (CDC) a common saprophyte (an organism that lives on dead organic matter) of the digestive tract and female urogenital tract. It does not ordinarily cause disease, but may do so following a disruption of bacterial flora of the body, or in patients with depressed immune systems.

capital expenditure an expenditure of money for the purchase or replacement of a room, a building, large, expensive pieces of equipment, and/or the development or expansion of services.

capitated a fiscal management technique used by insurance companies (as well as Medicare and

Medicaid) which states that the payer will pay up to a specific dollar amount for the patient's care. If the facility exceeds that ceiling, the facility cannot expect to receive payment for the excess billing above the capitation amount. Only in special situations is the provider allowed to bill the patient for the excess amount. On the other hand, if a facility is able to deliver the services for less than the capitated amount, the facility is allowed to pocket the extra, unused amount. See *independent practice association, managed care.*

CAPS-free diet a prescribed diet which calls for no caffeine, alcohol, pepper, or spicy foods.

carbohydrate (HHS) organic compounds that consist of carbon, hydrogen, and oxygen. They vary from simple sugars containing from three to seven carbon atoms to very complex polymers. Only the hexoses (sugars with six carbon atoms) and pentoses (sugars with five carbon atoms) and their polymers play important roles in nutrition. Carbohydrates in food provide four calories per gram. Plants manufacture and store carbohydrates as their chief source of energy. The glucose synthesized in the leaves of plants is used as the basis for more complex forms of carbohydrates. Classification of carbohydrates relates to their structural core of simple sugars (saccharides). Principal monosaccharides that occur in food are glucose and fructose. Three common disaccharides are sucrose, maltose, and lactose. Polysaccharides of interest in nutrition include starch, dextrin, glycogen, and cellulose.

cardiorespiratory endurance the ability of both the heart and lungs to move oxygen to muscle groups efficiently enough to allow normal activity with reasonable endurance over a period of time. May be increased with the systematic use of activities that stress the heart and other muscle tissues, usually at least three times a week and without causing undue fatigue. Cardiorespiratory endurance can be significantly hindered when the patient has second and third-degree *burns* or skin breakdowns to the anterior trunk area. After consultation with the physician, the professional may want to encourage daily involvement in activities that involve diaphragmatic breathing. Fun activities that involve blowing around balloons suspended from overhead or a game of air hockey using a Ping-Pong ball on a table are good places to begin.

care conference the meeting where a patient's status is discussed. During this meeting the patient's needs and strengths are outlined or updated, priorities for intervention and service agreed upon and specific *outcomes* with anticipated dates are determined. The individuals attending the care conference may in-

clude the patient and his/her family, nursing, therapies (recreation, occupational, physical, speech — as needed by the patient), activity professional, dietitian, physician, and social services director. The length of time spent on each patient depends on the severity/complexity of the patient's needs. The frequency of conferences (daily, weekly, monthly, quarterly) and whether the patient and/or family members are present may vary. A care conference may last for as little as 5 minutes or as long as 90 minutes for each patient. The shorter care conferences, which typically take place on the unit, are called "rounds." When presenting information on a patient during a care conference, the staff need to provide the other team members with information in a clear, concise, and condensed manner. Present enough information to get the information across, no more. (The information presented should be found in the *progress notes* prior to the meeting.) The other members of the team will let you know when they need more information or further clarification. A typical format for presentation might be 1. presentation of specific problem/need, 2. short summary of reasons why there is a need/problem, and 3. what action the professional and/or patient will need to take. See *rounds.*

care domains the twelve categories used in the *quality indicator* process in nursing homes throughout the United States. The twelve domains are 1. *accidents*, 2. behavioral and emotional patterns, 3. clinical management, 4. cognitive functioning, 5. elimination and continence, 6. *infection control*, 7. nutrition and eating, 8. physical functioning, 9. *psychotropic* drug use, 10. *quality of life*, 11. sensory function and communication, and 12. skin care. Within the twelve domains are 30 quality indicators.

care mapping See *critical pathway.*

care plan written document that outlines how the staff are going to address the patient's measured (assessed) needs. This plan is usually interdisciplinary with stated needs/concerns, goals and specific objectives, interventions, and services to be delivered to meet the goals, and the anticipated date of completion for each objective. The needs/concerns are frequently prioritized and state which staff or disciplines are responsible for monitoring the patient's status. Many facilities are using *critical pathways* in place of care plans. A sample care plan is shown on the next page. See *dementia, resident assessment protocol, resident care plan.*

caretaker/caregiver in a broad sense, anyone involved in the delivery of a patient's health care. It is usually applied to individuals (community workers,

Example of Using a Care Plan Within Treatment

Assess-ment	Observa-tion	**_Subjective Data_** "I don't know how to ride the bus to the day treatment center." **_Objective Data_** Patient scored 21/30 on the **CIP**/City Bus Module 4E Pretest Patient scored 10/19 on the **CIP**/City Bus Module 4E Field Trial				
	Clinical Impression	Deficit related to use of public transportation, which places the patient at a high risk for isolation and at a high risk to fail to complete required treatment. Also, this deficit increases stresses within the family, as mom is required to take time off work to drive patient home from the day center. Specific deficits related to obtaining scheduling and route information, choosing routes, and identifying the bus stop where he needs to get off the bus.				
Sample	**Problem #7**	Lack of transportation options/skills.				
Item from Care Plan	**Needs/ Concerns**	**Goal**	**Objective**	**Tx Plan/Intervention**	**Date**	**Staff**
	Potential for isolation and lack of access to health care services due to lack of transporta-tion.	Independ-ent use of city bus	Pt will be able to board bus at his home bus stop and suc-cessfully ride the bus to and from day tx center with no cues except for those found by him in the memory book.	Therapist will construct memory book for patient to use from home to day tx cen-ter and back. Therapist will help patient fill out application for discounted bus pass. Therapist will accom-pany/instruct pt in use of bus 3x week until objective met. Alternative transportation options will be arranged in case of emergency, bad weather, etc.	3/25/01 3/27/01 4/2/01 4/5/01	Speech RT RT MSW
Progress Notes	3/28/01 8:30	Therapist reviewed use of pass with patient. Patient able to role-play presenting pass to the driver when boarding the bus.				
	3/28/01 14:30	Therapist reviewed use of memory book system with patient. Patient was able to re-peat back the basics of the system to the therapist with 75% accuracy after third run through on the unit.				
	4/2/01 15:15	**S:** Patient stated "Now I get it. Won't my mom be happy now that she doesn't have to drive me every day through rush hour traffic!" **O:** Patient readministered the **CIP**/City Bus Module 4E Pretest and scored 27/30 and on the **CIP**/City Bus Module 4E Field Trial scored 17/19. Patient should be able to use the city bus to and from home independently with the use of his memory book.				

paraprofessionals, and/or nurses aides) who provide these services in the community setting. See _Denver Developmental Screening Tool._

CARF: the Rehabilitation Accreditation Commission a private (non-government) accrediting agency which promotes the provision of quality care to pa-tients who have disabilities and others in need of re-habilitation. As of 1996 CARF divided the types of programs that could receive accreditation into six ar-eas: 1. Medical Rehabilitation (comprehensive inpatient, spinal cord injury, comprehensive pain management, brain injury outpatient medical rehabilitation, occupational rehabilitation), 2. Employment Services (vocational evaluation, work adjustment, community employment services, occupational skill training, job placement, work services), 3. Community Support Services (early intervention and preschool developmental programs; personal, social, and community supports and services; living supports and services; respite supports and services; family supports and services; host family supports and services), 4. Alcohol and Other Drug (detoxification services, outpatient services, residential treatment programs), 5. Mental Health (outpatient therapy, inpatient psychiatric, partial hospitalization, residential treatment, community housing, emergency/crisis intervention, case management), and 6. Psychosocial Rehabilitation. CARF's address is 4891 East Grant Road, Tucson, AZ 85712, 520-325-1044. See *physical medicine and rehabilitation.*

caries See *dental caries.*

carpal tunnel syndrome a painful compression of the median nerve in the carpal tunnel proximal to the wrist. Functionally, the individual will experience weakness, pain, tingling, burning, and aching with potential atrophy. Individuals usually also experience a sensory loss in the first three fingers, limiting their ability to function normally in activities of daily living.

case definition dividing patients into groupings based on symptoms they have in common. (CDC) In the example of chronic fatigue syndrome (CFS), a combination of symptoms, signs, and physiologic characteristics that serve to distinguish a case of chronic fatigue syndrome from other disease states.

case history a fairly detailed, retrospective reporting of a patient's medical and psychosocial history including all significant events leading up to the current admission or complaint. In strictly medical fields (e.g., medicine and nursing) a case history would emphasize unhealthy events experienced by the patient (including trauma, hospitalizations and surgery, infectious diseases, treatment and therapies received previously, and immunizations). Additional information is usually included about deaths and illnesses of the patient's significant others and about other important psychosocial and economic issues and events which may shape the patient's ability/desire to make necessary changes for health. Case histories written by therapists, while including the above information, tend to emphasize the patient's reaction and adaptation to previous health care events as demonstrated through his/her ongoing level of activities of daily living. By describing a pa-

tient's past medical case history and his/her reported level of functioning during those events, the therapist can determine more accurately the likely course of the patient's current treatment. When a case history is presented, it usually follows a specific outline:

> (Name of patient) is a (age) year old (male/female) with (list of primary diagnoses — those diagnoses which impact the patient's treatment). Patient was admitted to (service, facility, program) on (list date) and had (list scores of assessments, results of lab work, or other important measurements which were taken during the assessment process). (State a brief outline of services/treatments given to patient). Patient has responded by (give outcome of services and therapy).

While the term case history is frequently used interchangeably with *case study*, case history is more accurately the reporting of retrospective information on the patient, and a case study is the reporting of the history along with a hypothesis as to why certain events were interrelated and their significance to treatment protocols (a more global impact).

case management a way to determine the course of health care treatment and services provided to a patient. The Case Management Society of America (Wolf, 1993, p. 114) defines case management as: "A collaborative process that assesses, plans, implements, coordinates, monitors, and evaluates options and services to meet an individual's health needs through communications and available resources to promote quality, cost-effective outcomes." There is a voluntary national certification program for case managers. Case managers may work for the health care providers (e.g., the hospital), for the payer (e.g., the insurance company), or may be independent. Regardless of where they work, there are four primary responsibilities for those who manage cases (Wolfe, 1993): 1. review the patient's condition and relevant medical information to determine the medical necessity of a proposed treatment plan, 2. review and select providers and vendors and negotiate fees, 3. monitor the ongoing progress of the case, and 4. make recommendations for adding or augmenting extra contractual services (i.e., services not in the benefit plan), when they make economic and medical sense. See *medical management systems, modality-oriented clinic, rehabilitation centers.*

case mix (OBRA) When a government survey team evaluates a long-term care facility, they have a set equation that they follow to determine which resident's care plans and charts to review. This sample includes residents with a variety of care needs to determine compliance with all quality of care requirements. There are four categories in a case mix: Case Group A: interviewable residents who are relatively physically independent (light care); Case Group B: interviewable residents who are relatively physically dependent (heavy care); Case Group C: non-interviewable residents who require staff supervision or cueing to maintain independent functioning but do not require extensive or total staff assistance to perform activities of daily living (non-interviewable — light care); and Case Group D: non-interviewable residents who require extensive or total assistance to perform activities of daily living (non-interviewable — heavy care). The residents chosen as part of the sample are selected after the orientation tour. The surveyors who survey nursing homes are to include, if possible: an officer of the resident council, a resident under 55 years of age, a resident initially admitted to the facility during the month preceding the survey and a resident with mental retardation or metal illness.

case study a review of a patient's significant medical, psychosocial, and economic background to provide analysis as to why something happened. In health care, case studies are frequently used to propose/introduce a new syndrome or new treatment protocol. New syndromes or treatment protocols generally need to have their parameters discussed (and countered) then to be further defined/refined before more extensive research designs can be developed to test the validity of the new syndrome or treatment approach. See *case history.*

castration 1. removal of one or both testicles or ovaries. 2. figuratively, it means that a person's special possession or belief or a person's self-esteem has been destroyed or severely damaged. See *medical play.*

catabolic phase phase in which energy is released to the body as complex compounds are broken down into simpler ones.

cataract a common cause of reduced vision, especially in individuals over the age of 70, formed as the lens of the eye becomes harder and more opaque. In cases of cataracts where trauma or congenital pathology is not the cause, the disease usually progresses in each eye, although not at the same rate. Surgery is successful in about 98% of the individuals who undergo surgery to remove the natural lens and replace it with a plastic one. See *visual impairment.*

catastrophic responses a sudden and unexpected negative reaction to an event — an extreme overreaction. An example would be the complete emotional collapse of an individual upon hearing that s/he was going to be laid off from work.

catatonia abnormal motor movements that are not related to organic disorders or causes (such as cerebrovascular accident or cerebral palsy). Catatonia in *schizophrenia* also includes the possible symptom of extreme negativism. Catatonia usually takes the form of compulsive and motiveless resistance to all requests to change any behavior or posture (catatonic rigidity). Patient with catatonic mannerisms may demonstrate stereotyped movements, have prominent mannerisms or facial grimacing. See the table below for terms related to catatonia. See *compulsion, stereotyped behavior.*

catchment area a specifically defined geographic area which is identified as the area to be served by a health care center, usually a mental health care center. See *community mental health center.*

cath. See *catheter, catheterization.*

catharsis process of resolving unsatisfactory feelings, guilt, or otherwise relieving *stress* and *anxiety.* In many ways catharsis means an emotional cleaning that results in a feeling of peace and strength. See *Dehn's Model of Leisure Health, insight.*

catheter a tube inserted into the body to help facili-

Terms Related to Catatonia

Term	Description
Catalepsy	Referring to a position taken by the patient which s/he does not move from. Like a statue.
Catatonic Excitement	Purposeless motor activity which implies agitation but which is not related to stimuli found in the environment of the patient.
Catatonic Stupor	A retardation of motor activity to the point that the patient is motionless and unresponsive to the surrounding environment.
Catatonic Rigidity	The purposeful taking of a body stance or position by the patient who is then unwilling to change that position regardless of stimuli in the environment (including staff trying to move the patient).
Catatonic Posturing	The purposeful taking of a bizarre or inappropriate posture and holding that posture for a long period of time, regardless of the stimuli in the environment.
Cerea Flexibilitas	Literally translated to mean "waxy flexibility." The patient will allow himself/herself to be molded into a posture by another person and then maintain that position for a long period of time.

tate the addition or removal of fluids. See *indwelling catheter*.

catheterization insertion of a tube into a cavity (most commonly the bladder) to allow drainage. The therapist may need to catheterize a patient while out in the community to help reduce the symptoms of *autonomic dysreflexia*.

CAT scan See *computerized axial tomography*.

caudal end, tail, inferior to, or the bottom part; away from the head.

causalgia a neurological disorder which produces a burning sensation along specific neurological pathways, usually resulting from an injury.

cavity See *dental caries*.

CBA See *cost-benefit analysis*.

CD-ROM compact disk, read-only memory.

CDS See *controlled dangerous substance*.

CDSS See *clinical decision support system*.

CEA See *cost-effectiveness analysis*.

cellular immune response immune functions that do not involve antibodies but do involve T lymphocytes. Cellular immunity is very important for the defense against intracellular viruses, transplanted tissue, cancer cells, fungi, and protozoans.

census number of patients currently admitted to the program or facility.

centering 1. ability to consciously balance one's emotional state through self-discipline and self-knowledge. 2. ability to focus on one part or situation at a time.

Centers for Disease Control and Prevention (CDC) The Centers for Disease Control and Prevention, located in Atlanta, Georgia, USA, is an agency of the Department of Health and Human Services. The Centers for Disease Control and Prevention performs many of the administrative functions for the Agency for Toxic Substances and Disease Registry (ATSDR), a sister agency of CDC, and one of eight federal public health agencies within the Department of Health and Human Services. The Director of CDC also serves as the Administrator of ATSDR. CDC's mission is "To promote health and quality of life by preventing and controlling disease, injury, and disability." CDC's pledge to the American people: "To be a diligent steward of the funds entrusted to it. To provide an environment for intellectual and personal growth and integrity. To base all public health decisions on the highest quality scientific data, openly and objectively derived. To place the benefits to society above the benefits to the institution. To treat all persons with dignity, honesty, and respect." The CDC's core values are 1. ACCOUNTABILITY: As diligent stewards of public trust and public funds, we act decisively and compassionately in service to the people's health. We ensure that our research and our services are based on sound science and meet real public needs to achieve our public health goals; 2. RESPECT: We respect and understand our interdependence with all people both inside the agency and throughout the world treating them and their contributions with dignity and valuing individual and cultural diversity. We are committed to achieving a diverse workforce at all levels of the organization; 3. INTEGRITY: We are honest and ethical in all we do. We will do what we say. We prize scientific integrity and professional excellence. The CDC includes 11 Centers, Institutes, and Offices: 1. Office of the Director (Associate Director for Minority Health, Associate Director for Science, Freedom of Information Act Office, Information Resources Management Office, Management Analysis and Services Office, National Vaccine Program Office, Office of Communication, Division of Media Relations, Office of Global Health, Office of Health and Safety. Office of Women's Health, Technology Transfer Office and Washington D.C. Office), 2. Epidemiology Program Office, 3. National Center for Chronic Disease Prevention and Health Promotion, 4. National Center for Environmental Health, 5. Office of Genetics and Disease Prevention, 6. National Center for Health Statistics, 7. National Center for HIV, STD, and TB Prevention, 8. National Center for Infectious Diseases, 9. National Center for Injury Prevention and Control, 10. National Immunization Program, and 11. National Institute for Occupational Safety and Health, Public Health Practice Program Office.

cerebellar ataxia See *ataxic gait*.

cerebellum one of the three main parts of the brain (along with the *cerebrum* and *brainstem*). The cerebellum is located underneath and behind the cerebrum and extends to the base of the skull behind the brainstem. The cerebellum has three parts, two cerebellar lobes with the vermis to connect them. The outer layer of the cerebellum is gray and referred to as the cerebellum cortex while the core of the cerebellum is white. The cerebellum's main function is to coordinate physical/muscular movements that are voluntary in nature. See *ataxic gait, Parkinsonian gait*.

cerebral atrophy See *alcohol use*.

cerebral contusion a bruising and possible death of the tissue in the brain caused by edema and hemorrhaging usually caused by a traumatic brain injury. See *coup lesions, contrecoup lesions, traumatic brain injury*.

cerebral embolism an occlusion (blockage) of a cerebral artery; a type of *cerebrovascular accident*.

Therapy Concerns with Cerebral Palsy

Concern:	Intervention:
muscles/joint contractures	While the neurological damage causing CP is not progressive, its negative impact on the elasticity of the muscles is. The professional should help the patient develop an activity repertoire that promotes the full *range of motion* of all affected muscles and joints (either through passive and/or active movement). These activities should be varied enough to allow this range of motion a minimum of 4x a day.
positioning	Ensure that all activities and equipment are modified to reduce spasticity and encourage good posture.
constipation	A patient who uses a wheelchair, which reduces activity, has an increased chance of having chronic *constipation*. Encourage out-of-chair, gross motor activities on a daily basis.
vision, seizure, and hearing impairments	Monitor for vision, seizure, and hearing impairments. Approximately 50% of the patients with CP also have visual impairments, 45% have a seizure disorder and a smaller percentage have a hearing impairment.
developmental delays or mental retardation	Prescriptive activities to increase muscle control and coordination and a purposeful program to encourage normalizing experiences will help increase muscle control later in life and will decrease developmental delays due to physical disability. Approximately 70% of patients with CP (especially those with spastic diplegia) also are mentally retarded.

cerebral hemorrhage rupturing of a cerebral vessel with bleeding into the brain; a type of *cerebrovascular accident*.

cerebral palsy (CP) a chronic neurological disorder developed prenatally, at birth, or shortly thereafter. A patient with CP has anatomically normal muscles and nerves. The disability is caused by the brain's inability to control the muscles and nerves. The two primary functions impacted by CP are motor and communication. The range of functional impairment varies from patient to patient and, depending upon the location of the damaged brain cells, the patient may have one or more of the following: 1. spasticity, 2. dyskinesia, 3. ataxia, and 4. mixed. *Spasticity:* When there is damage to the motor cortex (surface of the brain) or damage to the nerves originating on the surface of the brain and passing through either the corticospinal or pyramidal tracks to the spinal cord, the patient will experience muscle stiffness. This stiffness is called hypertonia and produces a slowed response. *Dyskinesia:* When there is damage to the basal ganglia (which controls motor function) the patient will experience uncontrolled, jerky movements of his/her body. These jerky movements increase when the patient actively tries to execute a controlled movement or when the patient is experiencing emotional *stress*. Certain body postures will also increase the patient's tone and decrease function. There are three primary types of dyskinesia: 1. athetosis, 2. choreoathetosis, and 3. *dystonia*. Athetosis refers to a slow, writhing movement. Athetosis has a marked impact on activities as it affects the hand's and wrist's ability to perform desired movements. The "jerky" abrupt movements

seen with this disorder are called choreoathetosis. Uncontrolled, rhythmic movements are called dystonia. *Ataxia:* When there is damage to the cerebellum, the patient will exhibit an abnormal gait. Activities that require a narrow-stanced gait (gymnastics), smooth movements (some forms of dance), and good balance (ice skating, skiing) are usually very difficult for patients with ataxia. *Mixed:* About a third of the patients with CP have damage to more than one area of the brain and therefore exhibit multiple movement disorders. See the chart above for therapy concerns about cerebral palsy. See *hypertonic, developmental coordination disorder, efficiency*.

cerebral thrombosis formation of a blood clot within a cerebral artery, leading to an occlusion of the vessel, a type of *cerebrovascular accident*.

cerebrovascular accident (CVA) stroke; restricted blood supply to some part of the brain. When the brain cells do not receive the oxygen contained in the blood, they start to die. The restricted blood flow may be due to an *occlusion* (blockage) by an *embolus*, by *thrombus* (clogging of the artery), or from a cerebrovascular hemorrhage. The effects depend on two factors: 1. the location in the brain that is affected and 2. the intensity of the interruption (how much blood was cut off from the cells). The severity of the symptoms may decrease the first few days after a CVA because reduced swelling of the brain allows normal blood flow to resume in the undamaged parts of the brain. The National Stoke Association lists four primary warning signs of stroke:

1. numbness, weakness, or paralysis of face, arm, or leg — especially on one side of the body;

Treatment Implications for Patients with a Cerebrovascular Accident

Health Issue	Health Implications	Psychosocial Implications	Programming Ideas
CVA (stroke) Left-sided brain injury	Right hemiparesis/hemiplegia Language, reading/writing problems Aphasia, word finding problems Attention deficits Decreased verbal learning Difficulty distinguishing left and right Visuospatial neglect Memory deficits Lability, mood swings Low frustration tolerance Sleep disturbances Frustration with group experiences Impaired verbal math skills Lack of inhibition Behavior is slow, cautious, anxious Good attention span Underestimates ability	Isolation depending on location of CVA and degree of impairment Depression — both physiological and related to loss(es) or expectations beyond potential Impatience, frustration with new functional status and lack of speedy recovery Self-conscious about appearance and language difficulties	Involve in appropriate exercises as soon as possible after stroke Activities which stimulate cognitive functioning Body image activities Retraining cognitive and perceptual abilities Repetitive tasks and movements to achieve mastery and therefore transfer skills to other activities Sensory integration activities Sequencing activities Communication group experiences Working with significant others to identify interests and opportunities Exercise activities Opportunities for community reintegration as part of rehabilitation Life skills training Focus on strengths vs. limitations
CVA (stroke) — Right-sided brain injury	Left hemiparesis/hemiplegia Perceptual problems Poor spatial orientation and concepts of direction Gets lost easily Decrease or increase in sensation Change in vision Seizures Decreased eye-hand coordination Impaired concrete thinking Sleep disturbances Left side neglect Behavior is fast, impulsive, with lack of inhibition and verbal outbursts Short attention span Constant talking Overestimates ability		

2. loss of balance or coordination when combined with another warning sign

3. sudden blurred or decreased vision in one or both eyes; and

4. difficulty speaking or understanding language.

A list of treatment implications for a CVA may be found on the previous page. See *computerized axial tomography, diabetes, frame of reference, impulsivity, magnetic resonance imaging, neglect (visual), reflex sympathetic dystrophy, transient ischemic attack, vascular dementia, visual function.*

cerebrum one of three main parts of the brain (along with the *brainstem* and *cerebellum*) occupying the upper portion of the cranial cavity. Made up of nerve tissue and divided into two hemispheres, the cerebellum is responsible for much of an individual's *executive function, intelligence, memory,* vision, and speech. The two hemisphere are known as the right and left hemisphere. Each hemisphere is further divided into four lobes, each with its own function. The four lobes are the frontal lobe, the parietal lobe, the occipital lobe, and the temporal lobe.

certificate of need (CON) a document that provides demographics, budgetary, and geographical analysis to support the need to increase an expensive health care service. Many states require a facility to develop a CON to justify an increased number of beds, the purchase of expensive equipment (e.g., an MRI scanner), or to make a significant change in the type of care provided. The state then reviews the CON document provided by the facility and denies or approves the proposed change.

certification 1. formal recognition by a certifying body that an individual or an organization has met minimum standards of competency or outcome production. A type of professional credentialing. 2. (Medicaid certification) determination by a state agency that a facility is in compliance with HCFA Medicaid health and safety requirements. 3. (Medicare certification) recommendation by a state agency to the Regional Office of HCFA regarding provider/supplier compliance or noncompliance with HCFA Medicare health and safety requirements. See *credentialing, federal jurisdictional survey.*

certified nursing assistant (CNA) an individual who has passed the requirements for certified nursing assistants in the state in which s/he works. These requirements usually involve taking both a written and a skill test in the basics of patient care, documentation, infection control, and patient rights. The types of decisions that CNA may make independent of a nurse are very limited — they are to be supervised by a nurse, following orders for patient care.

certified therapeutic recreation specialist an individual formally trained in the field of therapeutic recreation (recreational therapy) and credentialed by the *National Council for Therapeutic Recreation Certification.*

cervical 1. referring to the neck and the cervical vertebrae. See *spinal cord injury.* 2. referring to the cervix of the uterus.

cervical lymph nodes lymphoid organs located in the neck.

CFR Code of Federal Regulations. The official document of federal laws (United States) published by the Office of the Federal Register, National Archives, and Records Administration. The CFR describes the general and permanent rules published by the federal government and is divided into fifty "titles." Each title represents a broad area of the federal law and is further divided into chapters. Chapters usually bear the name of the agency that issues the set of regulations. To cite regulations (or to find them) a standardized system has been developed. Public Health regulations are all found under title 42 of the CFR and are cited as "42 CFR." Title 42 has four volumes (or parts). The Health Care Financing Administration (HCFA) has all of its regulations in the third and fourth volume, or part, which are numbered from 400 to 429 (Part III) or 430 to End (Part IV). To cite specific parts of the CFR, the symbol "§" is placed in front of the Part number. An example would be 42 CFR §483.15(f)(1) as shown at the top of the next page. The number §483 corresponds to the federal law for conditions of participation and requirements for long-term care facilities (OBRA). The part number is followed by a period (".") followed by the number representing a specific section of regulations found within that part. In this case, ".15" refers to regulations related to Quality of Life within the *OBRA* regulations. All numbers and letters following this last number relate to the official guidelines for enforcement. Section (f) relates to "activities" and the number one (1) following the "(f)" relates to the official interpretation of what qualifies as "activities" and how the surveyor should probe to determine compliance. Interpretive guidelines are issued for each area of health care regulations. Each set of interpretive guidelines organizes the rules of compliance in segments called *"Tags."* While tags do not follow the CFR numbering system, all tags are cross-referenced to the corresponding CFR number. To obtain all of the health care laws affecting any type of agency under HCFA the reader would need to purchase 42 CFR Part III and IV from the regional federal bookstore. The CFR for all of health care is issued October 1 of each year.

Anatomy of a CFR Number

42	CFR	§483	.15	(f)	(1)
Title Number Assigned to the Specific Code of Federal Regulations This "title" number belongs to Public Health.	Code of Federal Regulations (Official publication of the laws of the United States).	Number assigned to an area of enforcement — in this case all regulations related to nursing homes.	Number assigned to a major area of compliance (frequently a condition of participation in the program) — in this case "Quality of Life Issues."	The first letter in parentheses usually corresponds to a subsection of the major area of compliance — in this case "activities."	All additional numbers and letters correspond to further regulations related to the subsection and also interpretive guidelines for determining compliance.

Updates to each edition prior to the annual publication can be found in the "List of CFR Sections Affected (LSA)," which is issued monthly or in the "Cumulative List of Parts Affected" which is found in the Readers' Aids section of the daily Federal Register. See *mandate.*

chaining a theory that states that certain actions have obvious responses and are naturally linked to other actions, e.g., you get bitten by a mosquito, you try to slap the mosquito. While many types of "training" (e.g., with individuals with lower IQs or individuals with severe brain trauma) speak about chaining tasks together, just using chaining does not work for complex tasks because there are too many possible responses.

chairbound (OBRA) in the United States, depending on a chair for mobility. This includes patients who can stand with assistance to pivot from bed to wheelchair or to otherwise transfer. The patient cannot take steps without extensive or consistent weight-bearing support from others. While this term is included in federal legislation, it is considered to be dated. A more correct way of stating this would be "person who uses a wheelchair."

change agent an object, action, or event that causes an individual to change his/her behavior. The knowledge (change agent) that failing to turn in her/her term paper on time would cause a student to fail the class may motivate a student to complete the paper (change).

charting by exception When a facility uses charting by exception, professional staff are only expected to write in the medical chart when something out of the ordinary happens. This type of charting assumes that all required services and treatment are done as ordered and when ordered. This type of charting usually does not fill the need to prove that services and treatment were provided for surveys from outside organizations such as the Health Care Financing Administration or for internal management *utilization reviews* or *quality assurance* reviews.

chart review 1. process of reading the information in the patient's medical chart to obtain information about the patient. The therapist may want to find answers to the questions below prior to writing up his/her assessment. It is not practical to write out the answers to all these questions. Note general concerns and impression after reading the chart. Medical: Restrictions and precautions should be noted. What is the person's medical history? Previous hospitalizations, surgeries? Are there coexisting illnesses? What kind of medical treatment did the person receive? Were recommendations followed? What was the response to treatment? Was there compatibility between intervention and belief system? Were traditional interventions tried? Complementary interventions? Psychiatric: Note restrictions and precautions, anniversary dates of significant events, anticipate difficult situations and prepare for them as much as possible. Is there a history of psychiatric problems, hospitalization? Was there treatment for emotional problems? Were problems present, but no treatment sought? What types of problems: personal, family, marital? Previous diagnoses? Review **DSM-IV** for specific abilities and anticipated disabilities based on the diagnoses. Social and family: What is the social background? What is the family history? Marriage, children, divorce, stepchildren? Where was the person born and raised? Educational and/or Vocational: What is the occupational history? Was retirement planned or forced? Were life-style changes anticipated? What is the educational history? How much schooling was there? Favorite subjects. Does this individual have a sense of how s/he learns best? School related problems? (Issues with authority? Peer pressure? Completion? Cooperation?) Living Situation: What is the present living situation? Where? With whom?

Upkeep of home? What is financial status, source of income, adequacy of income? Medications: What medications is the patient taking? Prescribed by, for what, how long? Over-the-counter aids? Can the patient use a medication journal or plastic pill organizer? (Nathan and Mirvis, 1997). 2. process of examining a patient's chart for the purposes of *utilization review*, *quality assurance*, or compliance with regulations (e.g., state survey).

chemokine substances that cause *chemotaxis* of specific immune cells.

chemotaxis the tendency of cells, including bacteria and other unicellular organisms, to migrate toward a chemical stimulus. Cells naturally move (chemotax) toward higher concentrations of a positive stimulus.

chemotherapy treatment of a disease using chemicals designed to kill cancer cells For example, large doses are used to help destroy a patient's diseased marrow in preparation for a marrow transplant. The chart on the right shows codes that are applied by the treatment team to describe how successful the chemotherapy session has been.

CHESS See *comprehensive health enhancement support system*.

childhood a developmental stage which comes after infancy and lasts until adolescence.

childhood injuries injuries sustained in childhood. See the Childhood Injury Fact Sheet on the next page for additional information. See *playground injuries*.

childhood psychiatric disorders The **DSM-IV** divides psychiatric disorders usually first diagnosed before the individual turns twenty-one years of age into ten categories. The chart below shows the ten categories and the specific diagnostic groups within each category.

Child Life Council (CLC) organization which represents professional child life specialists in hospitals, clinics, and universities. Once part of the *Association for the Care of Child's Health*, the Child Life Council is now a separate organization. The CLC is located at 11820 Parklawn Drive, Suite 202, Gaithersburg, MD 20852-2529, www.childlife.org. The phone number is 301-881-7090. See *child life specialist*.

Chemotherapy Code for Evaluating Progress

Rating	Description
-2	definitely worse
-1	probably worse
0	no change since last scan
+1	probably better
+2	definitely better

Psychiatric Disorders Usually First Diagnosed in Infancy, Childhood or Adolescence

Category	Diagnoses Found Within the Category
Mental Retardation	mild retardation, moderate retardation, severe retardation, profound mental retardation, and mental retardation: severity unspecified.
Learning Disorders	reading disorder, mathematics disorder, disorder of written expression, and learning disorder not otherwise specified
Motor Skills Disorder	*developmental coordination disorder*
Communication Disorders	expressive language disorder, mixed receptive-expressive language disorder, phonological disorder, stuttering, and communication disorder not otherwise specified
Pervasive Developmental Disorders	autistic disorder, Rett's disorder, childhood disintegrative disorder, Asperger's disorder, and pervasive developmental disorders not otherwise specified. See *autism*.
Attention-Deficit and Disruptive Behavior Disorders	*attention-deficit hyperactivity disorder* (predominantly inattentive type, predominantly hyperactive-impulsive type and combined type), *conduct disorder*, oppositional defiant disorder, attention-deficit hyperactivity disorder not otherwise specified, and disruptive behavior disorder not otherwise specified
Feeding and Eating Disorders of Infancy or Early Childhood	pica, rumination disorder, and feeding disorder of infancy or early childhood (*anorexia nervosa* and *bulimia nervosa* are categorized under the adult onset heading of "eating disorders.")
Tic Disorders	Tourette's disorder, chronic motor or vocal tic disorder, transient tic disorder, and tic disorder not otherwise specified
Elimination Disorders	*encopresis* and *enuresis*
Other Disorders of Infancy, Childhood, or Adolescence	separation anxiety disorder, selective mutism, reactive attachment disorder of infancy or early childhood, stereotypic movement disorder, and disorder of infancy, childhood, or adolescence not otherwise specified

Childhood Injury Fact Sheet (CDC)

Topic	Discussion
How frequently are children injured?	Each year between 20 - 25% of all children sustain an injury sufficiently severe to require medical attention, missed school, and/or bed rest. For every childhood death caused by injury, there are approximately 34 hospitalizations, 1000 emergency department visits, many more visits to private physicians and school nurses, and an even larger number of injuries treated at home. Unintentional injuries are the leading cause of death in children from 1-21 years of age. However, deaths are still a rare event. Even so, they are relatively easy to count accurately, given the sophisticated vital statistics surveillance system in the United States. These records are maintained by the National Center for Health Statistics, CDC. Nonfatal injuries are much less rare, but are more difficult to count accurately, since injured children are treated at so many types of sites by so many types of health care professionals. Very few national surveillance systems exist for such data. The Department of Transportation (National Highway Traffic Safety Administration) maintains the Fatal Accident Reporting System for fatal traffic-related events, and its companion General Estimates System to estimate the number of nonfatal traffic-related events. The US Consumer Product Safety Commission maintains the National Electronic Injury Surveillance System to monitor hospital emergency department visits for product-related injuries.
Who is at risk?	Each type of injury has a particular demographic pattern, which is determined by: 1. Developmental level of the child: physical, mental, emotional, 2. Prevalence of the threat in that community (e.g., all-terrain vehicles, backyard swimming pools, firearms, kerosene heaters, etc.), 3. Access to and use of environmental countermeasures (e.g., bike helmets, smoke detectors), and 4. Importance of supervision in avoiding the threat, relative to the degree provided (e.g., toddler living in a low-income apartment complex with an in-ground swimming pool that lacks protective fencing, with a 5-year-old supervising the toddler). Several demographic features are common to most types of injuries. The injury rates are greatest in those with: 1. Low socioeconomic status, especially urban African-American children and American Indians/Alaska Natives and 2. Males. The principal exception to this is young motor vehicle occupants before adolescence, where the male to female ratio is nearly equal.
What are the leading causes of fatal injuries?	Overall, motor vehicles, fires/burns, drowning, falls, poisoning.
What determines what body site(s) are injured?	Injury-specific. For example: 1. Motor vehicle: blunt thoracoabdominal trauma, head injuries; 2. Sports: extremity fractures, sprains, and strains; 3. House fires: body burns, inhalation injuries; 4. Near drowning: coma, brain damage; 5. Falls: head injuries, fractures, blunt trauma; 6. Poisoning: coma, kidney failure, etc. If the child was a projectile, a head injury is quite likely. Bicycle-motor vehicle collision, falling forward over the handlebars, unrestrained occupant in a motor vehicle collision, thrown forward through the windshield or ejected from the vehicle unto a roadway are all examples of accidents that cause a child to become a projectile.
Where do injuries occur most commonly?	Locations and conditions associated with possible danger are: In the home: 1. Water: kitchen, bathroom, backyard swimming pool; 2. Intense heat or flames: kitchen, backyard barbecue pit; 3. Toxic agents: under the kitchen sink, bathroom medicine chest, mother's purse, garage, and 4. High potential energy: stairwells, loaded firearms. At school: 1. Related to sports activities (especially in the absence of proper gear); 2. Carrying of weapons; and 3. Industrial arts classes. After school: 1. On the job: hostile relationships in work environment, use of machinery; 2. During transport: motor vehicle crashes (especially if unrestrained or if driver has been drinking alcohol); 3. Bicycle crashes; and 4. Pedestrian injuries.
What criteria determine the priority level for each type of childhood injury?	High mortality rate or hospitalization rate; high long-term disability rate, especially mechanisms likely to result in head and spinal cord injuries and the existence of effective countermeasure. In other words, the highest priorities are assigned to those types of injuries that are common, severe, and readily preventable.

child life specialist an individual who has trained (at the bachelor's level) and completed an internship within the specialty of child life. Child life, as a profession, addresses the negative impacts of illness and hospitalization on children, using play and other appropriate modalities to reduce or alleviate negative consequences. See *Child Life Council.*

Chlamydial infection most common type of *sexually transmitted disease* in the United States. Chlamydia is neither a bacteria nor a virus; it is an intracellular parasite of the genus Chlamydia. While Chlamydia is not a bacteria, it does share common attributes to Gram-negative bacteria and is frequently classified as a specialized bacteria. Pelvic inflammatory disease (PID) is caused by the organism Chlamydia trachomatis. PID can lead to sterility if not treated. Another Chlamydia organism, Chlamydia psittaci, is frequently carried by birds, which can transmit the disease to humans, causing a type of *pneumonia.* Birds kept as part of a pet therapy program should be removed immediately if they develop a sinus infection or seem listless. The third type of Chlamydia is Chlamydia pneumoniae, which is one of the most common infectious agents for community-acquired pneumonia. See *animal facilitated therapy, zoomatology.*

CHMIS See *community health management information system.*

cholangitis inflammation of the bile duct.

cholecystitis an inflammation of the gall bladder (either chronic or acute), often caused by a gallstone too large to pass through the cystic duct. The patient feels pain in the upper right quadrant of the abdomen and usually experiences vomiting and nausea.

cholera (CDC) an acute, diarrheal illness caused by infection of the intestine with the bacterium Vibrio cholerae. The infection is often mild or without symptoms, but sometimes it can be severe. Approximately one in 20 infected persons has severe disease characterized by profuse watery diarrhea, vomiting, and leg cramps. In these persons, rapid loss of body fluids leads to dehydration and shock. Without treatment, death can occur within hours. Although cholera can be life threatening, it is easily prevented and treated. In the United States, because of advanced water and sanitation systems, cholera is not a major threat; however, everyone, especially travelers, should be aware of how the disease is transmitted and what can be done to prevent it. A person may get cholera by drinking water or eating food contaminated with the cholera bacterium. In an epidemic, the source of the contamination is usually the feces of an infected person. The disease can spread rapidly in areas with inadequate treatment of sewage

and drinking water. The cholera bacterium may also live in the environment in brackish rivers and coastal waters. Shellfish eaten raw have been a source of cholera, and a few persons in the United States have contracted cholera after eating raw or undercooked shellfish from the Gulf of Mexico. The disease is not likely to spread directly from one person to another; therefore, casual contact with an infected person is not a risk for becoming ill. In the United States, cholera was prevalent in the 1800's but has been virtually eliminated by modern sewage and water treatment systems. However, as a result of improved transportation, more persons from the United States travel to parts of Latin America, Africa, or Asia where epidemic cholera is occurring. US travelers to areas with epidemic cholera may be exposed to the cholera bacterium. In addition, travelers may bring contaminated seafood back to the United States; food-borne outbreaks have been caused by contaminated seafood brought into this country by travelers. Cholera can be simply and successfully treated by immediate replacement of the fluid and salts lost through diarrhea. Patients can be treated with oral rehydration solution, a prepackaged mixture of sugar and salts to be mixed with water and drunk in large amounts. This solution is used throughout the world to treat diarrhea. Severe cases also require intravenous fluid replacement. With prompt rehydration, fewer than 1% of cholera patients die. Antibiotics shorten the course and diminish the severity of the illness, but they are not as important as rehydration. Persons who develop severe diarrhea and vomiting in countries where cholera occurs should seek medical attention promptly.

cholesterol (HHS) 1. (dietary) not a fat, but rather a fat-like substance classified as a lipid. Cholesterol is vital to life and is found in all cell membranes. It is necessary for the production of bile acids and steroid hormones. Dietary cholesterol is found only in animal foods. Abundant in organ meats and egg yolks, cholesterol is also contained in meats and poultry. Vegetable oils and shortenings are cholesterol-free. 2. (serum or blood) High blood cholesterol is a risk factor in the development of coronary heart disease. Most of the cholesterol that is found in the blood is manufactured by the body, in the liver, at a rate of about 800 to 1,500 milligrams a day. By comparison, the average American consumes 300 to 450 milligrams daily in foods. 3. (different types) Blood cholesterol is divided into three separate classes of lipoproteins: very-low density lipoprotein (VLDL); low-density lipoprotein (LDL), which contains most of the cholesterol found in the blood; and high-density lipoprotein (HDL). LDL seems to be the culprit in coronary heart disease and is popularly known as the "bad cholesterol." By contrast, HDL is increasingly considered desirable and is known as the "good cholesterol."

Chopart amputation an amputation at the Chopart joint. The Chopart joint is the joint between the navicular/cuboid and the talus/calcaneus bones of the foot. A Chopart amputation retains the ankle and its movement, but looses two of the three primary functions of the *ankle* and *foot*. Impaired is the ability to: 1. provide a means of mobility including being able to provide a rigid structure to push the body forward and a flexible structure to absorb the shock of foot contact with hard surfaces and 2. to provide a means of stability on even and uneven surfaces. To increase functional ability a two unit prosthetic device is used: 1. a distal weight-bearing socket and 2. a partial foot replacement.

chorea movements involuntary jerky and irregular movements of a muscle or group of muscles. These movements tend to be irregular, making the adaptation of equipment and activity a challenge for both the patient and the therapist. See *cerebral palsy, movement.*

choreoathetosis See *cerebral palsy.*

chromosomal aberrations disorders caused by chromosomal aberrations or by mutant genes. Aberrations are deviations from what would normally be expected from the combining of chromosomes. These deviations may be from the number of chromosomes or the structures of the chromosomes. Some common chromosomal aberrations are shown in the chart below.

chromosomal disorders See *chromosomal aberrations.*

chromosome (HHS) thread-like components in the cell that contain DNA and make proteins. Genes are carried on the chromosomes. These threadlike structures within the cell nucleus contain the genetic information. Chromosomes occur in pairs, originally one from each parent.

chronic referring to long term — not expected to be resolved soon; denoting a disease of slow progress and long duration. See *disorder.*

chronic disease (CDC) illnesses that are prolonged, do not resolve spontaneously, and are rarely cured completely. Chronic diseases targeted by CDC's National Center for Chronic Disease Prevention and

Common Chromosomal Aberrations

Syndrome	Characteristics
Cri du chat (cat-cry syndrome)	This syndrome is characterized by severe (developing to profound) *mental retardation*, a failure to thrive, small head, and a distinctive cry which sounds like a high-pitched mewing of a cat.
Klinefelter	This syndrome affects only males and is evidenced by long legs, hypogenitalism, a lack of masculine development, and the demonstration of poor social skill development. *Mental retardation* is also possible.
Triple X	Also known as "super female," this syndrome affects only females. Disability from this chromosomal aberration may not be evident without diagnostic work to evaluate the chromosomes. An impaired intelligence to actual mental retardation may be one of the observable symptoms. Occurs in approximately one out of 1,000 female births.
Trisomy 13	Also known as "Patau," this syndrome affects both males and females and manifests with a number of birth defects including cleft lip and palate, malformation of the ears, and mental retardation.
Trisomy 18	Also known as "Edwards'," a syndrome characterized by severe *mental retardation* and multiple physical deformities. Abnormal shaping of the skull, face (including cleft lip and palate), clenched fists, and club feet. Heart and renal defects are also common in trisomy 18. The occurrence rate is about one in every 3,000 live births; affecting females three times as often as males.
Trisomy 21	Also known as "Down," a syndrome characterized by *mental retardation* and multiple physical defects. The physical defects include the "mongoloid" faces, heart defects, short stature, and a large, protruding tongue. Individuals with trisomy 21 tend to have a greater susceptibility to respiratory infections. This is the most common chromosomal aberration occurring once in every 650 live births.
Turner	A syndrome which includes physical malformations including genital hypoplasia, cardiovascular problems, dwarfism as well as spatial disorientation, and learning disorders. Occurs in about once in every 3,000 live births of female babies. See *mental retardation.*
XYY	A syndrome in which the individual tends to grow tall but which also has a negative effect on both cognitive capabilities and social skill development. Poor coordination is also frequently evident.

Health Promotion are those illnesses that fit the broad definition of chronic disease, that are preventable, and that pose a significant burden in mortality, morbidity, and cost. The United States cannot effectively address escalating health care costs without addressing the problem of chronic diseases. More than 90 million Americans live with chronic illnesses. Chronic diseases account for 70% of all deaths in the United States. The medical care costs of people with chronic diseases account for more than 60% of the nation's medical care costs. Chronic diseases account for one third of the years of potential life lost before age 65. Chronic disease disproportionately affects women and racial minority populations. Women comprise more than half of the people who die each year of cardiovascular disease. Deaths due to breast cancer are decreasing among white women but not among African-American women. The death rate from cervical cancer is more than twice as high for African-American women as it is for white women. The five-year survival rate for men with colon cancer is 51% for African-Americans and 63% for whites. The prevalence of diabetes is about 1.7 times more among non-Hispanic African-Americans, 1.9 times more among Hispanics, and 2.8 times more among American Indian and Alaska Natives than among non-Hispanic white Americans of similar age. The death rate from prostate cancer is more than twice as high for African-American men as it is for white men. African-Americans are more likely than whites to get oral or pharyngeal cancer, half as likely to have these diseases diagnosed early, and twice as likely to die of these diseases. Practical interventions exist for controlling and preventing many chronic diseases. Implementing proven clinical smoking cessation interventions would cost an estimated $2,587 for each year of life saved, the most cost-effective of all clinical preventive services. Each $1 spent on diabetes outpatient education saves $2 to $3 in hospitalization costs. Mammography screening, when performed every two years for women aged 50–69 years, costs between $8,280 and $9,890 per year of life saved. The cost of this screening compares favorably with other widely used clinical preventive services. Cervical cancer screening among low-income elderly women is estimated to save 3.7 years of life and $5,907 for every 100 Pap tests performed. The cost of preventing one cavity through water fluoridation is about $4, far below the average $64 cost of a simple dental restoration. For every $1 spent on preconception care programs for women with preexisting diabetes, $1.86 can be saved by preventing birth defects among their offspring. Par-

ticipants in the arthritis self-help course experienced an 18% reduction in pain at a per-person savings of $267 in health care system costs over four years.

chronic fatigue and immune dysfunction syndrome (CFIDS) (CDC) a synonym for *chronic fatigue syndrome* used by some patients and physicians. It should be stressed, however, that no immune dysfunction or aberration has been persuasively linked to chronic fatigue syndrome. See *fibromyalgia*.

chronic fatigue syndrome a combination of symptoms including sore throat, chills or low-grade fever, muscle weakness, diffuse muscle pain, tender lymph nodes, joint pain without measurable swelling, headache, memory deficits, and sleep disorders which have caused the patient to reduce his/her activity level by at least 50% for over six consecutive months. The cause of the syndrome is not known and the US Centers for Disease Control and Prevention do not consider it to be contagious or fatal. See *fibromyalgia*.

chronic inflammation When a patient has long-term inflammation due to a disease like *arthritis*, the therapist must guard against promoting activities that cause the inflamed area excessive stress or cause irritation. When the affected scar tissues are in the healing and remodeling process, such stress will significantly increase the occurrence of *fibroblasts*, which in turn increase the production of *collagen*. The outcome may be an actual weakening of the affected area and a decrease in *range of motion*. The therapist will be able to tell if too much movement, stress, or irritation has occurred by noting increased *pain* and inflammation that lasts more than 2 hours after the activity. The patient may restrict movement (muscle guarding) due to pain. After a rest period the patient will experience increased stiffness and after 24 hours the patient will experience a slight loss of range of motion.

chronicity syndrome a category of patients where the patient has been out of work for at least six consecutive months as a result of an industrial injury. Data show that patients receiving workman's compensation for six consecutive months have only about a 20% chance of returning to work.

chronic lymphocytic leukemia (CLL) (HHS/-NMDP) a malignant disorder involving the overproduction of mature lymphocytes that results in the abnormal accumulation of these cells in the bone marrow, the bloodstream, and the lymph system. CLL usually involves the lymph nodes. It usually affects older persons, with an average age of 60. It is more common in men. See *leukemia*.

chronic myelogenous leukemia (CML) (HHS/-

NMDP) a malignant disorder involving the predominance of granulocytes (a particular type of white cell) of all stages of development that results in the abnormal accumulation of these cells in both the bone marrow and the bloodstream. CML may occur at any age in either sex. It is uncommon before 10 years of age, and occurs most often at an average age of 45. See *leukemia.*

chronic obstructive breathing disorder   See *chronic obstructive pulmonary disease.*

chronic obstructive lung disorder See *chronic obstructive pulmonary disease.*

chronic obstructive pulmonary disease (COPD) a group of disorders which all share a common inability of the lungs to perform the function of ventilating the body. It is the most common lung disease in the United States and is frequently grouped into five different stages (Grosvenor, 1997). The first stage, called the asymptomatic stage, will show few outwardly observable changes. While changes are taking place in the lungs, no symptoms may be present and are difficult to find during an x-ray or during pulmonary function tests. In the second stage, called the ventilatory stage, the patient coughs and produces sputum (especially when physically active) and may show signs of chronic fatigue. By the third stage, called the hypoxemic stage, the patient has increased coughing and fatigue along with a loss of appetite, possible bluing around the lips and fingernail beds (*cyanosis*) and strained breathing (trying to get more air into lungs than will fit into lungs). The fourth stage, called the hypercarbic stage, is when the lungs have failed to the point that the body can no longer get rid of all of the carbon dioxide gas. This causes organic personality and cognitive changes including *irritability,* unnatural drowsiness, decreased *attention span,* and a loss of mental "sharpness." The fifth stage, called the final stage, is when the heart is no longer able to function adequately and the patient gains weight due to *edema* (especially with excessive swelling of the legs). Also known as chronic obstructive breathing disorder and chronic obstructive lung disorder. The chart on the next page is from N. F. Gordon (1993). See *asthma, bronchitis, emphysema.*

chronic stage third and last stage of healing, maturation and remodeling after an injury or illness. For injuries to the musculoskeletal system there are two subclassifications within the chronic stage. The first involves an injury after the 21st day, when inflammation is no longer present but when the patient's functional ability has not returned to normal. The second involves a continuous state of pain or recurring episodes of pain with a suboptimal return to the patient's normal functional ability. The collagen fibers that are thickening as a result of the injury will not mature for up to 14 weeks. Up to that time the fibers and scar tissue are able to be remodeled through therapeutic activity to lessen the severity of the disability. After around 14 weeks the scar tissue resists remodeling and stretching may only be achieved through surgery or the adaptive (over) lengthening of the tissues surrounding the scar. The over lengthening of tissue around the scar should be done only under the direction of a physician or a physical therapist. See *acute stage, subacute stage.*

chronological age number of years, months, and days that have passed since the individual was born. This is different than an individual's developmental age, which refers to the age that most individuals attain the skill level demonstrated.

cineplastic amputation To help improve the use of mechanical prosthesis, the surgeon sews a skin flap into a set of muscles (usually the biceps). The contraction of the muscle then allows a prosthetic device to be operated when it is secured next to the skin. Also called kineplastic amputation.

CIP See *Community Integration Program.*

circle of Willis union of the anterior and posterior cerebral arteries, forming a loop near the base of the brain.

CircOlectric bed See *circular bed.*

circular amputation an amputation that is done to form a rounded stump.

circular bed commercially known as a *CircOlectric,* these beds are welded to a circular frame which allows a patient to be turned 360° while lying flat on his/her back. These beds actually have two mattresses with the patient placed between the two. The two mattresses are jointed at the foot of the bed and open like a clamshell, allowing more space around the patient's head. These beds are usually used for patients with extensive trauma, especially with trauma to the upper torso and head. Implications for treatment include a potential increased risk of isolation due to the massiveness of the bed, increased risk for loss of *range of motion* as it is difficult to conduct range of motion exercises around the framework of the bed and loss of eye contact (at times it may be difficult to establish and maintain eye contact with the patient when s/he is positioned with his/her face down and when the head is lower than the feet). See *bed.*

circulation path (ADA) an exterior or interior way of passage from one place to another for pedestrians, including, but not limited to, walks, hallways, courtyards, stairways, and stair landings. See *detectable warning.*

Chronic Obstructive Pulmonary Disease

Episodic (or intermittent) asthma	
Symptoms	Sudden, usually short-lived, attacks of wheezing on exhalation; breathlessness; sometimes coughing. No symptoms between attacks.
Triggers	Environmental pollutants; allergies to airborne substances or food; exposure to cold, dry air; extreme climatic changes; emotional stress; aspirin and other medications; respiratory infections such as colds; exercise.
Lung dysfunction	*Bronchospasm* (a narrowing of the bronchial tubes due to a sudden involuntary contraction of their walls); some inflammation of the lining of the bronchial tubes during attacks.
Response to therapy	Complete reversibility possible. For those with asthma caused by triggers, avoid the triggers. For those with asthma not caused by specific triggers, use medication.
Chronic asthmatic bronchitis	
Symptoms	Frequent, recurrent *asthma* attacks characterized by wheezing, varying degrees of *breathlessness*, and coughing.
Triggers	Same as for episodic asthma.
Lung dysfunction	*Bronchospasm*; thickening and inflammation of the walls of the bronchial tubes; some airflow obstruction between attacks.
Response to therapy	Partial reversibility of airflow obstruction and symptoms possible with medical therapy.
Chronic bronchitis	
Symptoms	Chronic daily cough that brings up sputum for at least three months per year for two consecutive years; accompanied by *breathlessness* and wheezing.
Triggers	Cigarette smoking.
Lung dysfunction	Inflammation of the bronchial tubes; excess mucous secretions; bronchospasm.
Response to therapy	Partial reversibility of airflow obstruction and symptoms possible with medical therapy.
Emphysema	
Symptoms	*Breathlessness*; coughing; wheezing.
Triggers	Cigarette smoking (major cause), which inhibits the action of protective enzymes in lungs; inherited deficiency of protective enzymes (for nonsmokers).
Lung dysfunction	Air sac walls lose elasticity and ability to expel air from the lungs, which results in lungs remaining over-inflated; air sac damage impedes gas exchange between lungs and bloodstream.
Response to therapy	Irreversible, but medical treatment can help relieve symptoms.

circumlocution using many words to say what could be said in a few words.

cirrhosis a chronic, degenerative disease of the liver usually caused by long-term use of alcohol but may also be caused by nutritional deprivation or *hepatitis*. Symptoms include nausea, fatigue, weight loss, and spider angiomas (small, red spots on the skin or nose with small blood vessels radiating out from the red spot like many spider legs). Symptoms do not become evident until after irreversible damage to the liver has taken place.

civil monetary penalty (CMP) a type of sanction that may used against nursing facilities that fail to meet minimum standards as authorized by Congress. This fine, levied against nursing facilities who are noncompliant, is just one of the options surveyors have to encourage facilities to meet national and state standards. CMPs apply to situations where it

has been demonstrated that there have been serious or chronic violations that harm residents.

civil rights United States civil rights laws enacted to guarantee every individual an equal opportunity to be a part of the social and economic life within the country. There are numerous civil rights laws and many court ruling that further define the laws. The chart on the next page lists only a few of the civil rights laws within the United States. See *Americans with Disabilities Act, consumer rights, interpreter, job interview, Office for Civil Rights Clearance.*

clarifying skills See *listening skills.*

claustrophobia fear of being closed in or in a small room/space, based on non-rational thoughts.

CLC See *Child Life Council.*

clear (ADA) unobstructed.

clear floor space (ADA) minimum unobstructed floor or ground space required to accommodate a

Civil Rights Laws

The Act	Description
Equal Pay Act of 1963	Originally part of the Fair Labor Standards Act of 1938, but lacked enforcement, the Equal Pay Act prohibits wage discrimination between men and women. Women who hold a similar job to men at the same company and who have the same experience and education may not receive lower pay based on their sex.
Civil Rights Act of 1964	Originally passed in 1964 and updated in 1991 (Civil Rights Act of 1991), this law prohibits discrimination based on race, color, religion, sex, and national origin.
Age Discrimination in Employment Act of 1967	Originally part of the Older Workers Benefit Protection Act, the Age Discrimination in Employment Act of 1967 prohibits employment discrimination against individuals who are over the age of forty. This Act has been partially updated through the Civil Rights Act of 1991.
Rehabilitation Act of 1973	This Act prohibits employment discrimination against individuals with disabilities. This law has been updated many times since 1973 including parts in the Americans with Disabilities Act of 1990, Civil Rights Act of 1991, and Rehabilitation Amendments of 1992.
Americans with Disabilities Act	This Act prohibits discrimination against individuals with disabilities in the area of employment and accessibility.
Civil Rights Act of 1991	Enacted in 1991, this revision of the original Civil Rights Act of 1964 corrected what some saw as inadequacies in the original law plus provided for damages in the case of intentional employment discrimination.

single, stationary wheelchair and occupant.

clear liquid diet a *diet* limited to liquids that are clear including water, clear broth, clear fruit juices, plain gelatin, tea, and coffee. Check to see if caffeine or carbonation is allowed.

cleft lip and palate a facial deformity that occurs in the second month of pregnancy. The most common presentation is on the upper lip ranging from a small notch in the lip tissue to a malformation of the soft palate, bones of the maxilla, and the premaxilla. This severe malformation causes a line of disconnected tissue and bone, so that it looks as if the child's lip (and underlying bone structure) were cut with a knife, leaving a tear from the upper lip to the nose.

client an individual who receives services. It tends to be confusing as the same individual, receiving the same services in three different settings, may be referred to by three different terms. While there may be some regional difference, the terms used for "client" in different settings are outlined in the chart.

Terms Used to Identify the Receiver of Services

Term	Setting
Client	intermediate care facilities for the mentally retarded (ICF-MRs), some psychiatric settings, drug and alcohol settings
Patient	hospitals, some psychiatric settings, outpatient settings, acute care settings, subacute and transitional care settings
Resident	OBRA regulated settings (e.g., nursing homes)

clinic a facility established primarily for the provision of outpatient physician services. Such facilities may be approved for participation in Medicare as an outpatient provider of physical, recreational, and occupational therapy services, and/or speech pathology services.

clinical care provision of health care services by credentialed providers who use some formal means to measure the quality of services being provided and who use some form of *utilization review*.

clinical decision making decisions about patient care and the types of services provided based on assessed patient needs, standards of practice, research findings, and institutional policies. Two kinds of clinical decision making are diagnoses and treatment *protocols* based on established scientific evidence. When the therapist, using his or her knowledge base and experience, but without supporting evidence from research, makes a decision, it is called a *clinical opinion*. See *clinical decision support system*.

clinical decision support (HCO) use of information to help a clinician diagnose and/or treat a patient's health problem, including information about the patient and information about the kind of health problem afflicting the patient and alternative tests and treatments for it. See *inference engine*.

clinical decision support system (CDSS) (HCO) broadly defined, the use of information to help a clinician diagnose and/or treat a patient's health problem. Two kinds of information are involved: 1. information about the patient and 2. information about the kind of health problem afflicting the patient and alternative tests and treatments for it. Clinical decision support is by no means a new phenomenon — such information traditionally has been available from several sources. However, those sources have limitations that often diminish their reliability or their accessibility at the point of care.

clinical indicators specific observations or measurements used by a treatment team (or specific discipline) to identify problems related to the delivery of services. High-risk population groups or treatments, which have an above average incidence of problems, are usually selected for review. The team identifies the threshold to be crossed. Any case that crosses the threshold (the level of acceptable performance) is examined and the causes and underlying circumstances are reviewed. An example would be the incidence of patient to staff assault. Clinical indicators would be set up to identify patient behaviors observed immediately prior to an assault and compared with the environment, treatment modality, and staffing prior to the assault to determine how to decrease the incidence of assault. Clinical indicators are used to increase the quality and effectiveness of the treatment provided to the consumer. See *quality assurance.*

clinical information system (HCO) hospital-based information system designed to collect and organize data related to the care given to a patient, rather than administrative data. Compare with *administrative data.* See *medical information bus, Regenstrief Medical Records System.*

clinical opinion belief or ideas that a professional holds regarding a patient. The opinion may be based on the use of tests and *measurements* and on the professional's experience and training but cannot be directly supported by evidence relating to the tests and measurements. Clinical opinions should be based on the therapist's *evaluation* of all available information; clinical decisions based on a therapist's synthesis of information are based on clinical opinions (Rothstein, et al. 1991, p. 925). See *prognosis.*

clinical practice guideline (HCO) an outline of broad parameters for the diagnosis, treatment, prevention, or rehabilitation of a particular health problem. See *disease management.*

clinical privileging a formal, facility-wide program used to determine when a staff person has demonstrated the minimum level of competency to practice with only minimal oversight from his/her supervisor. This privileging is usually approved by both the department/service head and the medical director. Clinical privileging has a time limitation necessitating the periodic review of the privileging status.

Typical benefits assigned to a clinically privileged staff include the ability to complete *assessments* without a cosigner, ability to complete a *treatment* plan without a cosigner, and the prestige assigned to clinically privileged staff.

clinical protocol (HCO) a rigorous, detailed model of the process of care for a particular health problem. See *protocol.*

clinical trial (HHS) experimental study of human subjects. Trials may attempt to determine whether the findings of basic research are applicable to humans, or to confirm the results of epidemiological research. Studies may be small, with a limited number of participants, or they may be large intervention trials that seek to discover the outcome of treatments on entire populations. The "gold standard" clinical trials are *double-blind*, placebo-controlled studies that employ random assignment of subjects to experimental and control groups unknown to the subject or the researcher. See *Cochrane collaboration.*

clinicians credentialed professionals who provide health care and social services.

clonic seizures rhythmic, involuntary contraction and relaxation of all muscles, loss of consciousness, and marked autonomic manifestations. See *epilepsy.*

closed amputation an amputation for which the surgical site has been sutured up and closed. Performed only when there is no infection present.

closed circuit telephone (ADA) a telephone with dedicated line(s) such as a house phone, courtesy phone, or phone used to gain entrance to a facility.

closed head injury See *traumatic brain injury.*

clubfoot a deformity of the foot caused before birth. The vast majority (95%) of children born with clubfoot have their foot turned in and down. Most of the children can regain function of the foot through splinting, although the more severe cases require a series of surgeries to correct the deformity. See *arthrogryposis.*

cluster investigation (HHS) an epidemiologic investigation mounted to determine if there has been an unexpected increase in the number or prevalence of cases of illness. The increase can be with respect to a particular time span, a location, or both.

CMHC See *community mental health center.*

coarctation of the aorta a constriction of the aorta which causes increased *blood pressure* in the blood vessels before the narrowing (leading to the upper torso and the brain) and decreased blood pressure in the blood vessels below the narrowing (leading to the lower torso).

coarse tremor See *tremor.*

cochlea snail shell shaped tube that forms part of the inner ear.

Burn's Ten Types of Cognitive Distortions (from Caudill, 1995, pp. 103-104)

Distortion	Description
All-or-Nothing Thinking	This refers to the tendency to evaluate personal qualities or situations in extreme, black-or-white categories. For example, before you developed chronic pain you used to play baseball on the weekends. Now you find yourself thinking, "If I can't play baseball, I can't enjoy the sport anymore." There is an apparent advantage to thinking in black-and-white, all-or-nothing terms. It is more predictable and creates the feeling that there is order in the world around you. This, in turn, should give you an edge to controlling your world. Unfortunately, it doesn't work that way. Uncertainty is all that we have. Living comfortably with uncertainty is possible, but it takes time to master.
Over-generalization	This refers to the tendency to see a single negative event as a never-ending pattern of defeat. Given the preceding example, you might respond, "I'll never be able to enjoy anything any more." Misery does love company, but generalizing misfortune in this way creates an exaggerated sense of rejection and loneliness.
Mind Filtering	This refers to the tendency to dwell exclusively on a single negative event, and thus to perceive the whole situation as negative. For example, you are preparing brunch for some friends and discover that you do not have an essential ingredient to make a dish you were planning to include. All you can think about is how the whole brunch will be ruined. It gives you indigestion.
Disqualifying the Positive	This refers to the tendency to take neutral or even positive experiences and turn them into negative ones. For example, a friend comes over to visit and tells you that you look great. Your immediate thought is this: "I don't feel great. She doesn't understand." Maybe not, but try a simple "thank you" first before you check it out. Maybe you don't look as bad as you feel!
Jumping to Conclusions	This refers specifically to jumping to a negative conclusion that is not justified by the facts of the situation. Two types of jumping to conclusions are mind reading and fortune telling. "Mind reading" is when you assume you know why someone else does what s/he does, and you don't bother to check it out. For example, you pass a coworker in the hallway and say, "Hi!" He doesn't respond. You think, "He must be upset with me. What did I do wrong?" When you check it out, you find that the coworker was preoccupied about a sick child he had just left at home. "Fortune telling" is when you "know" that things will turn out badly. Given your bad luck, you predict it as an already established fact. For example, you wake up with a headache. You say, "Now my whole day is ruined. I had so much to do and I'll never get it all done."
Magnification and Minification	In magnification, you exaggerate the importance of a negative event or mistake. If, for example, you experience a flare-up in your pain, you find yourself saying, "I can't stand this! I can't take this any more!" As a matter of fact, however, you can. You may not want to, and that's okay, but you can take it. In minification, conversely, you take positive personal qualities or events and deny them their importance. For example, a family member comments on how nice it is to see you at a family outing, and you reply, "A lot of good it does if I can't participate in the activities."
Emotional Reasoning	This refers to taking your emotions as evidence for the truth. If you feel that something is right, then it must be true. For example, you find yourself thinking, "I feel useless. [Therefore] I am useless.
Labeling	This refers specifically to identifying a mistake or negative quality and then describing an entire situation or individual in terms of that quality. For example, instead of seeing yourself as an individual who has a pain problem, you find yourself saying, "I'm defective, imperfect, and without any redeemable qualities."
Personalization	This refers to taking responsibility for a negative event even when the circumstances are beyond your control. For example, you and your spouse go out to eat at a fancy restaurant, but the service and food are poor. You find yourself feeling responsible for making a bad choice and "ruining" your evening together.
"Should" Statements	These are attempts to motive (or browbeat) yourself by saying things like "I should know better," "I should go there," or "I must do that." Such statements set you up for feeling resentful and pressured. They also imply that you are complying with an external authority.

Cochrane Collaboration (HCO) an international network of researchers that distributes results of systematic reviews of randomized controlled trials — or the most reliable evidence from other sources — on selected health problems. See *clinical trials.*

cocontraction involuntary contraction of both the agonist and antagonist muscles to allow the individual stability in positioning.

codec (HCO) 1. in telemedicine, an abbreviation for coder/decoder, an electronic device that converts an analog electrical signal into a digital form for transmission purposes and decodes it on the receiving end. 2. in computer-based video technology, an abbreviation for compressor/decompressor, the software that reduces the size of digitized video frames.

Code of Federal Regulations See *CFR.*

coding standard a system for assigning alphanumeric codes to specific words, concepts, or actions for the purpose of standardizing messages between computers or organizations.

coenzyme (CDC) a substance that enhances or is necessary for the action of enzymes. Coenzymes are generally much smaller than enzymes themselves.

cognition the brain's ability to process information. Obviously it takes quite a few different skills and processes to use information including: arousal, attention span, categorizing, concept formation, generalization of information across discrete tasks, memory, new learning, orientation, problem solving, recognition. and sequencing. While there are many different philosophies about what cognition is, the professional will find it useful to group cognition into three functional aspects: 1. information *processes* (which include the patient's ability to attend to the information being received, understand the information received, remember the information, and organize the information to allow for *reasoning* and *problem solving*), 2. information *systems* (which include a patient's ability to use his/her long-term and short-term *memory* in a functional manner with *executive function* skills based on learned information and reasoning), and 3. information *integration* (which includes the patient's ability to use his/her information processes and information systems to interact with the environment around him/her in a meaningful and functional manner). See *physical medicine and rehabilitation.*

cognitive deficits an inability to perform normal cognitive functions (e.g., *judgment, problem solving, communication,* interpretation of environmental stimuli, insight, ability to follow commands, *memory,* abstract thought, *attention span,* etc.) See *cognition, generalization.*

cognitive dissonance a situation where an individual becomes aware that two beliefs and/or behaviors are in conflict with each other — that both cannot be correct and/or right. A change in attitude or behavior is usually the outcome of the individual's reassessment and reinterpretation of the situation.

cognitive distortion the process of thinking about a situation in a distorted manner using half-truths, non-truths, or an unbalanced emphasis on the situation causing the individual to not see the situation as it really is. The concept of cognitive distortion is an important aspect of *cognitive therapy* and is frequently classified as negative *self-talk.* David Burns, in the chart on the previous page, has identified ten categories of cognitive distortions that lead to negative emotional states.

cognitive retraining systematic use of teaching methods to help an individual relearn information after an illness or accident. When a patient loses information that s/he once knew, it is not just a simple task of relearning the information. Frequently the part of the brain that held the information is permanently damaged or changed and cannot relearn the information in the way it did before. The staff will need to help develop a compensatory strategy for each patient that helps him/her overcome the loss of previously known information. A patient needs to regain many cognitive skills, including the basic skill of recognizing that s/he has a deficit. Other areas of cognitive retraining include *generalization* training, sequential thought training, processing, and filtering training, *problem-solving* skills, etc.

cognitive stimulation exercising an individual's thinking skills.

cognitive therapy a treatment method that emphasizes the rearrangement of a person's maladaptive processes of thinking, perceptions, and attitudes. Cognitive therapy uses discussion and directed *problem-solving* techniques to modify the patient's thinking process and behaviors. For an example of cognitive therapy, see *conflict.* Also see *extinction, physical abuse, post-traumatic stress disorder.*

cohort a group of people who share a common characteristic, life event, or interest. Men who grew up in the United States during the depression, who fought together in World War II, then engaged in similar activities after the war (e.g., fraternal organizations) would be a cohort group.

collagen a white substance found in the skin, tendon, bone, cartilage, and all other connective tissues which functions as an adhesive or glue; one of the major components of connective tissue with eleven different forms in the body. Collagen can be found in the dermis, bones, muscles, cartilage, and blood vessels. Activities that promote mild to moderate stretching of muscles over a period of 15 minutes (with frequent short periods of rest) allow breaking down of collagen crystals that may be limiting movement. A gentle, sustained stretch maintained for 15-20 minutes over 5 days will also bring about measurable change in the muscles. With daily or every other day stretching during activities, the collagen crystals will actually rebind to other collagen crystals, allowing more plasticity. Not allowing frequent rest periods or over-stressing the muscles can cause tissue failure (rupture). A lighter stretch should be used when working with older patients. As a person gets older the collagen becomes less elastic. Combined with decreased capillary blood supply due to age, the muscles are at greater risk for failure and require an increased length of time to recover. See *burn, chronic inflammation, subacute stage.*

colonization bacteria growing on a person who does not have symptoms of infection. Individuals with colonization of an infection may be carriers and can spread the infection to others. See *infection, isolation.*

colostomy a surgically placed opening in the lower abdomen which pulls the intestines to an opening (artificial anus) on the abdominal wall. This is done to correct a temporary or permanent blockage of the intestine. See *diverticulitis, ostomy.*

coma a somewhat dated term for an abnormal state of consciousness where all or most of the patient's cognitive processes, voluntary behavior, and even reflexes are diminished. The most common way to refer to a patient's depth of coma is by referring to the patient's Glasgow Coma Scale score. The use of the term "coma" is giving way to the use of "unresponsive" and "*persistive vegetative state.*" See *Glasgow Coma Scale.*

comalingering slower than expected patient recovery as a direct or indirect result of conflicting expectations from the patient's significant others, the health care providers, and the insurance agency. Symptoms of disability and an inability to return to his/her previous community and pursuits are common results.

commercial facilities (ADA) facilities whose operations will affect commerce, that are intended for non-resident use by a private entity, and that are not facilities that are covered or expressly exempted from coverage under the Fair Housing Act of 1968, as amended.

Commission on Accreditation of Rehabilitation Facilities (CARF) the organization's old name. See *CARF: the Rehabilitation Accreditation Commission.*

common use (ADA) refers to the interior and exterior rooms, spaces, or elements that are made available for the use of a restricted group of people (for example, occupants of a homeless shelter, the occupants of an office building or the guests of such occupants).

common wheelchairs and mobility aids (ADA) equipment belonging to a class of three or four wheeled devices, usable indoors, designed for and used by individuals with mobility impairments which do not exceed 30 inches in width and 48 inches in length, measured two inches above the ground, and do not weigh more than 600 pounds when occupied. The ADA accessibility guidelines for these may be found in the **Buses, Vans, and Systems Technical Assistance Manual** (US Architectural and Transportation Barriers Compliance Board).

communication (RAPs) an exchange of information. Good communication enables patients to express *emotion*, listen to others, and share information. It also eases adjustment to a strange environment and lessens social isolation and *depression*. Expressive communication problems include changes/difficulties in: speech and voice production, finding appropriate words, transmitting coherent statements, describing objects and events, using nonverbal symbols (e.g., gestures), and writing. Receptive communication problems include changes/difficulties in: hearing, speech discrimination in quiet and noisy situations, vocabulary comprehension, vision, reading, and interpreting facial expression. When communication is limited, the patient's *assessment* should focus on reviewing several factors: underlying causes of the deficit, the success of attempted remedial actions, the patient's ability to compensate with nonverbal strategies (e.g., ability to visually observe nonverbal signs and signals), and the willingness and ability of staff to engage with patients to ensure effective communication. As language use recedes with *dementia* or is lost through injury or disease, both staff and the patient must expand their nonverbal communication skills — one of the most basic and automatic of human abilities. Touch, facial expression, eye contact, tone of voice, and posture all are powerful means of communicating with the patient with dementia and recognizing and using all practical means is the key to effective communication. See *communication disorder, communication techniques, graphic input, graphic output.*

communication board a board, book, or other flat item on which pictures and words/phrases are presented/attached. Individuals who are not able to talk may use a communication board to communicate with caretakers and friends. These boards are very primitive and limited in their nature — allowing the user a very limited means to communicate. All patients with communication boards need extra time scheduled with staff to allow communication that includes more than the words on the board. If this time is not scheduled on a regular basis, the patient is at an increased risk of *depression* and sensory *deprivation*.

communication disorders a specific diagnostic grouping in the **DSM-IV**. Communication disorders include significant functional problems related to expressive *communication*, receptive-expressive communication, phonological disorders, and stuttering.

communication techniques methods of interacting with a patient. Depending on the situation, the therapist may find that s/he needs to use different techniques to communicate with the patient, his/her family, and the treatment team. Some common communication techniques are listed in the table below.

community health information network (HCO) electronic systems that facilitate community-wide exchange of clinical and administrative information among providers, payers, banks, pharmacies, public

health agencies, employers, and other participants in the health care system.

community health management information system (HCO) an electronic system similar to a community health information network that has an explicit emphasis on building a *data repository* for use in assessing the performance of health care providers and insurance plans.

Community Integration Program (CIP) a treatment program by Armstrong and Lauzen, 1994 used throughout the United States and Canada by recreational therapists and other members of the transdisciplinary team. The **CIP** has over 20 treatment modules which include a pre-test, a field trial check list, and a post-test all related to advanced daily living skills and independent function in the community.

community mental health center (CMHC) a mental health service delivery system first authorized by the federal Mental Retardation Facilities and Community Mental Health Center Construction Act of 1963, to provide a comprehensive program of mental health care to a catchment area. The CMHC is typically a community facility or a network of affiliated agencies that serves as a locus for the delivery of the various services included in the concept of community psychiatry. Current regulations governing federal support for the centers require that they

Communication Techniques

Type	Description	Example
Clarifying	Obtaining more detail and double-checking that the therapist understands what the patient said.	"You said that you like to exercise — does that mean that you go to an exercise class?"
Confronting	Calling into questioning an inconsistency between what the patient says and what the patient does.	"You tell me that you are a very busy person because you do so many leisure activities in the community and yet you can't name one location for recreation in the community. I'm confused."
Direct Questioning	Obtaining specific information.	"How many times a week did you eat out prior to your injury?"
Informing	Providing information.	"Our cooking group tomorrow night is making pizza at 5:30 p.m. You are welcome to join us."
Open-ended Questioning	Asking questions in a way that encourages the patient to answer the question using full sentences, not just "yes" or "no."	"Now, what are the types of activities you enjoyed the most these last three months?"
Reflecting	Showing the patient that you listened to him/her and encouraging him/her to explain in greater detail.	Patient: "I hate to ride the bus!" Therapist: "Why is that?"
Silence	Encouraging the patient to initiate or to continue conversation by not saying anything.	Patient: "I think that the program I signed up for isn't working for me." Therapist: (silence)
Summarizing	Giving an abbreviated summary of what the patient said.	"You said that the program you signed up for wasn't working because you find that you hate to get messy."

78

offer at least ten services: inpatient, outpatient, partial hospitalization, emergency services, consultation and education, specialized services for children and the elderly, transitional halfway house services, alcohol and drug abuse services, assistance to courts and other public agencies, and follow-up care. See *catchment, consumer rights*.

community safety skills a group of skills that are necessary to ensure a reasonable degree of personal safety within the community. Some of the skills include 1. knowledge of who "helpers" are (police, firefighters, etc.), 2. knowledge of how to contact helpers, 3. knowledge related to using a telephone, 4. ability to identify safe situations versus unsafe (using lighted pathways at night, traveling in groups, etc.), and 5. ability to problem solve emergency situations, including alternative courses of action when required. The **Community Integration Program** contains a set of modules that address community safety. See *adaptive functioning*.

Community Services Network (HCO) a project in Washington, DC, that uses communication and computer technologies to support and coordinate health and human services at the community level.

community support programs a federal effort to improve community-based services for the mentally disabled.

commuter rail car (ADA) a commuter rail car means a rail passenger car obtained by a commuter authority for use in commuter rail transport.

comorbid two or more disease conditions that occur simultaneously within the same person.

comorbidity presence of a psychiatric disorder in addition to a diagnosis of alcohol or substance-related disorders. It is believed that 76% of men and 65% of women with a diagnosis of either substance abuse or dependence also have an additional psychiatric diagnosis. The most prevalent dual diagnosis is the use of two different substances. *Mood* disorders are thought to occur after the development of substance abuse whereas *anxiety* disorders, *attention deficit hyperactivity disorders*, and *antisocial* behaviors are usually pre-existing conditions (prior to substance/alcohol abuse). Comorbidity is high among individuals with *substance abuse*, especially with individuals who are dependent on opiates and opioids. It is estimated that 90% of the individuals dependent on *opiates* or *opioids* have a comorbidity, usually with *depression*, antisocial personality disorders, anxiety disorders, or alcohol-related disorders. Other rates of comorbidity with substance abuse include 30-40% of individuals with alcohol-related disorders also have clinically significant depression, 25-50% of individuals with *alcohol-related disor-*

ders also have clinically significant anxiety disorders, 30% of individuals who seek treatment for cocaine abuse also have clinically significant depression and 20% of individuals who seek treatment for cocaine abuse also have clinically significant anxiety disorders. Also called *dual diagnosis*. See *polysubstance dependence*.

comparative survey a federal survey conducted by the Health Care Financing Administration within 60 days of the state agency survey to assess the state agency's performance in the interpretation, application, and enforcement of federal requirements. Whenever possible, comparative surveys are conducted within 30 days of the state survey. When a federal survey team walks in the door for a comparative survey, it usually means that the survey was scheduled just to evaluate the quality of work done by the state surveyors. It does not mean that the facility is in so much trouble that the federal surveyors also need to come in. In fact, it is not uncommon for the federal surveyors to conduct an extremely fair survey, coming up with more positive results than those reported by the state.

COMPASS (HCO) a local dial-up computer data network in Oregon that provides a variety of information services.

compendium 1. a summary of the main topics in an extensive collection of material. 2. a compiling of information on medications which outlines the standard for medications, including their strength, purity, and quality. In the United States there are two compendiums for medications: the **United States Pharmacopoeia** and the **Homeopathic Pharmacopoeia of the United States**.

compensation 1. process of adapting one's behaviors or movements so that a real or perceived deficit is not evident. See *coping mechanisms*. 2. payment for services, losses, etc.

compensatory skill ability to successfully complete a task using methods that overcome a disability. An example would be an individual using sign language (a compensatory skill) to communicate.

competence ability to demonstrate a desired trait, skill, or knowledge. See *clinical privileging, conservator*.

competence (professional) the holding of specific skills and knowledge which are essential for the delivery of quality services, which will produce measurable outcomes. Competence is demonstrated through performance (a combination of knowledge and skill) and the ability to complete one's responsibilities. Beyond knowledge and skill, professional competence requires the ability to observe, analyze, and then act accordingly, solving/addressing problems as they emerge. The maintenance of competence is primarily an internally driven quest. Ensuring competent staff includes: 1. pre-employment qualifications, 2. job preparation and orientation, 3. performance appraisal, and 4. maintaining and improving competence.

competency to stand criminal trial The test for competency to stand criminal trial applies to the defendant's state of mind at the time of the trial. A person is competent to stand trial when 1. s/he understands the nature of the charge s/he faces and the consequences that may result from his/her conviction and 2. s/he is able to rationally assist his/her attorney in his/her defense. Compare to *actus reus, insanity defense, forensic psychiatry.*

complaint related to *quality assurance* measurement: a complaint refers to a *verbal* expression of dissatisfaction whereas a *written* expression of dissatisfaction is usually referred to as a grievance. See *customer service, grievance.*

complaint survey on site inspection conducted by the federal regional office of HCFA or the state agency surveyors to investigate an allegation against Medicare or Medicaid providers and suppliers.

complicating condition the relationship between two separate diseases or impairments. A complicating condition is a problem that is independent of the primary problem but which negatively impacts the primary problem (e.g., second- and third-degree burns on a leg with a broken femur). Compare to *complication.*

complication a secondary problem which develops as a direct result of a medical condition or a treatment for the condition (e.g., tardive dyskinesia as a result of long-term use of antipsychotic medications or pain as a result of a femur fracture). Compare to *complicating condition.*

comprehension ability to understand thoughts, ideas, and actions.

Comprehensive Evaluation in Recreational Therapy — Physical Disabilities (CERT—Phys/Dis) This 50-item assessment measures the patient's functional ability on eight subscales: 1. gross motor function, 2. fine movement, 3. locomotion, 4. motor skill, 5. sensory, 6. cognition, 7. communication, and 8. behavior. Based on initial construct validity and years of refining by credentialed staff, this assessment is able to provide the therapist with a good measurement of the patient's functional abilities related to leisure activities. One of its strengths is that each subscale may be used independent of the others. While the entire assessment takes a full hour or more to administer (with the rehab patient frequently tiring before the assessment is completed),

the various subscales usually take less than 10 minutes. This assessment is seldom used anymore.

Comprehensive Evaluation in Recreational Therapy — Psych/R (CERT—Psych/R) This 25-item assessment is one of the most widely used assessments in the field of recreational therapy. Developed in 1975 by Parker, this quick behavioral checklist is used extensively throughout the United States to measure behavioral changes and social skill needs. The test went through minor updates in 1991 and 1996. Using a Likert scale, the therapist evaluates the patient's demonstrated functional level in the following areas: attendance, appearance, attitude toward recreational therapy, coordination, posture, response to therapist's structure (one-to-one), decision making ability, judgment ability, ability to form individual relationships, expression of hostility, performance in organized activities, performance in free activities, attention span, frustration tolerance level, strength/endurance, memory for group activities, response to group structure, leadership ability in groups, group conversation, display of sexual role in group, style of group interaction, handling of conflict in group when indirectly involved, handling of conflict in group when directly involved, competition in group, and attitude toward group decisions.

Comprehensive Health Enhancement Support System (HCO) an interactive computer system developed at the University of Wisconsin that provides information, social support, and problem-solving tools for people living with AIDS and *HIV* infection.

Comprehensive Leisure Rating Scale (CLEIRS) (Card, Compton, & Ellis, 1986) Consisting of 77 items, this assessment measures the independence level of older adults with a primary diagnosis of mental illness. The four subscales are 1. *perceived freedom*, 2. *helplessness*, 3. breadth of activity skills, and 4. depth of activity skills.

comprehensive outpatient rehabilitation facility (CORF) a non-residential facility established and operated exclusively for the purpose of providing diagnostic, therapeutic, and restorative services to outpatients by or under the supervision of a physician.

compulsion an irresistible feeling that one must perform an action that is against one's best *judgment* or desires. Different from *obsession* and *impulsivity* as shown in the chart on the next page. See *addiction.*

compulsive feeling that one must act and then taking action even if one understands the negative consequences of one's action. See *refuting irrational ideas, self-injurious behavior, thought stopping.*

compulsive drug taking behavior actions of individuals who have a problem with *substance dependence* which correlate with compulsive drug taking.

Terms Describing Underlying Causes of Actions/Thoughts

Term	Description of Term
compulsion	Action taken when circumstances cause an individual to repeatedly go against his/her best judgment or desires. May be the result of an obsession.
impulse	Action taken without much thought for what may be contrary to the individual's normal behavior. When taken, this action satisfies. Not usually a repetitive behavior.
obsession	Unlike impulsivity and compulsivity (which involve action), obsession is usually an internally driven thought which is repetitive. While obsessions may influence the individual's behavior, they do not necessarily dictate behavior.

There are five behaviors that are in part or in full, evidence of compulsive drug taking behavior: 1. using drugs in excess of expectation, 2. desire to limit use of drugs, 3. excessive amounts of time spent in seeking or using drugs, 4. other aspects of life and living are reduced or given up, and 5. the individual continues to use drugs even though s/he knows that they are harming his/her health and social life. Users who are dependent on drugs tend to take more drugs than they originally planned to each time they use (e.g., having "one for the road" after having the two s/he said was the limit). Users also tend to have tried (and failed) more than once to limit their intake or to stop using. Their whole life becomes consumed with obtaining drugs and their use. Social relationships fail, they get fired from work, and they lose an understanding of how to use free time. The user knows on some level that his/her habit has destroyed relationships, interfered with work and harmed his/her health but is unable to quit on his/her own.

computer-based patient record a compilation in digital form of all the clinical and administrative information related to the care of a single individual.

computerized axial tomography (CAT scan) The CAT scan uses x-rays and computers to visually examine the brain and other parts of the body in three dimensions. For stroke diagnosis, a CAT scan gives a clear view of the physical structure of the brain and its related arteries. Compare with *magnetic resonance imaging*.

computerized report information generated by extracting the desired elements from databases and other files to obtain information useful to the user. There are three primary types of computerized report formats available to the health care provider: "1. standardized, pre-formatted reports, in which the user can make no changes, 2. templates, in which the report is pre-defined but can be tweaked by the user to add or change certain elements, or 3. totally designed by the user, in which format and all elements are chosen (Accu-Med Services, 1998)." Computerized reports are increasingly used by health care payers to determine payment based on acuity and services provided.

concentration 1. the ability to ignore stimulating noises, sounds, and thoughts while being able to attend to the task (or thought) at hand. Concentration problems are the result of an inability to focus (visually and cognitively) and to maintain that attention. Functional skills in concentration and attention are required for mental tracking skills such as information processing, pathfinding, and other executive functions. See *psychasthenia*. 2. measurement of how much of something is contained within a defined area.

concept See *construct*.

conceptual formation or development of a set of thoughts or ideas about a specific event or object; hypothesizing why something happened.

conceptual model formal development of a reason something happened or will happen and then basing future actions on that reason/model.

concrete thinking ability to understand simple, straightforward ideas or actions. Contrast with *reasoning*. Concrete thinking accepts things just as they are seen — with little logical thought process of how they got there or why they exist. The concept of "leisure" or "free-time" is an abstract concept. Asking patients with cognitive impairments what they do for leisure or free time may too complex if they tend to think concretely. Asking those patients if they like to play cards, walk through a mall, or plant flowers is a concrete approach to determining a patient's leisure preferences. See *conservation*.

concurrent review a review of the patient's continued need for inpatient care (*utilization review*), which is different than the assessment of the patient's medical needs. This concurrent review evaluates the *appropriateness* of the placement based on cost factors or resource management principles.

concurrent validity the degree of agreement between a new test and an older, more established test for which validity has already been established. Concurrent validity measures the degree of agreement between similar characteristics shared by the two tests.

conditioning 1. a type of learning that takes place as the result of a stimulus and a related reward, such as Pavlov and his dog. There are three primary types of conditioning including classical conditioning, instrumental conditioning, and operant conditioning. 2. a physical exercise regimen designed to help the individual achieve a specified physical level of ability, strength, and/or endurance. 3. (HHS/NMDP) the process of preparing the patient to receive donated bone marrow, often through the use of chemotherapy and radiation therapy. See *desensitization, multidisciplinary pain center, operant conditioning.*

conditions of participation conditions outlined by the government that must be met (and maintained) to qualify for funds through the state or federal government (e.g., Medicare and Medicaid programs). See *effective date of participation, extended survey, home health agency.*

conduct disorder inability of a child or youth to get along with his/her peers because s/he consistently goes against normal expectations for behavior. The behaviors are evidenced in all settings (home, school, community) and must have been at least 6 months in duration. Children and youth with conduct disorders usually have low self-esteem that may be improved through formal programming (as with the **Stick Up for Yourself** curriculum, Kaufman and Raphael, 1999). For the physician to diagnose an individual as having a conduct disorder, at least three specific anti-social behaviors must have been demonstrated in the categories of aggression to people and animals, destruction of property, deceitfulness or theft, and/or serious violations of rules.

confabulation telling false information without intending to deceive; unintentional lying. See *dementia syndrome of depression, memory deficit.*

confidentiality to keep secret; to not share information with those who do not have the right to know. In health care there are strict laws concerning a patient's right to confidentiality. The professional must keep four areas of patient information confidential: 1. the patient's identity, 2. the patient's physical or psychological condition, 3. the patient's emotional status, and 4. the patient's financial situation. Confidentiality not only includes whom you can talk to about which patient, but also where you may talk. You may not discuss a patient's confidential information where another person who should not hear, can hear. That means that discussing aspects of a patient's care in the elevator, lunchroom, restaurant, or other locations may not be acceptable. There are only a few situations that allow the professional to share information without prior approval. The health care professional may break confidentiality only if s/he is reporting on a medical emergency, reporting on suspected or known *abuse*, reporting required information on a communicable disease to the health department or when required to for litigation or administrative activities. See *ethics, Kardex, privacy act, risk management.*

confirmatory typing (CT) (HHS/NMDP) a repeat tissue typing test done to confirm the compatibility of the donor and patient. This is one of the final tests done before transplant.

confirmed negativity condition (CNC) a concept first developed by Hilde Bruch in the late 1970's and early 1980's and further developed by Peggy Claude-Pierre to describe a somewhat controversial theory on the underlying condition responsible for eating disorders. The theory behind CNC is that individuals with this disorder are at war with themselves; that an internal voice destroys the individual's sense of self so that s/he becomes "tyrannical, hypercritical, destructive, and despair-confirming." Claude-Pierre further describes CNC as "the culmination of negative subjectivity turned against oneself. This...will cause the victim to interpret every comment made to her as a negative reflection on her, or it will make the victim assume blame for every event, no matter how objectively unrelated to her." (Knight-Ridders Newspapers as reported in The News Tribune (Tacoma, WA), January 7, 1998). Claude-Pierre feels that disorders such as *anorexia nervosa* are a symptom of a disorder, just as a rash is one of the symptoms of measles.

conflict presence of two opposing desires or emotional forces causing discomfort to the individual. The two main sources of conflict are anger and mistrust. Graham Scott (1990) lists five different styles of conflict: competitive, avoidant, accommodative, collaborative, and compromising. (For methods of resolving conflict, see the chart on the next two pages.) See *anger management, defense mechanism, imagery.*

confounding factor See *confounding variable.*

confounding variable an event or condition previously unknown, unidentified, or unaccounted for, which may cause the results of a research project to be wrong; (HCO) a factor other than the health service in question that may influence the *outcome* of that service; (HHS) a "hidden" variable that may cause an association that the researcher attributes to other variables.

confusion disturbed *orientation* in respect to time, place, or person.

Resolving Conflict

Questions to Ask	Strategies to Use
I. *Are emotions causing the conflict or standing in the way of a resolution? If yes:*	*Understanding and resolving emotional issues.*
a) What are these emotions?	a) Techniques to calm the feelings on both sides, so you can work out solutions/agreements.
1) Anger? If so, whose?	
a) The other person's	a) Techniques to cool down or deflect the anger, such as empathic listening, letting the other person vent his/her anger and statements to soothe hurt feelings or correct misunderstandings generating anger.
b) Your own?	b) Techniques to channel or control your anger, such as short-term venting, deflection, and *visualization* to release anger.
2) Mistrust? If so, whose? a) The other person's? b) Your own?	2) Techniques to overcome mistrust and techniques to assess the accuracy of this mistrust or deal with it openly and productively.
3) Fear? If so, whose? a) The other person's b) Your own?	a) Techniques to reduce fear. b) Techniques to assess the accuracy of this fear or deal with it openly and productively.
4) Other emotions? (i.e., jealousy, guilt, etc.) a) The other person's b) Your own?	a) Techniques to calm the other person. b) Techniques to calm yourself. See *relaxation technique.*
II. *What are the underlying reasons for the conflict?*	*Looking for real needs and wants.*
a) What does the other person really need and want?	1) Direct communication to ask the person to outline reasons, needs, and wants if possible. See *communication technique.* 2) Intuitive and sensing techniques to pick up the underlying reasons if the person isn't willing to speak or if the person isn't self-aware enough to recognize these underlying needs and wants.
b) What do you really need and want?	1) Self-examination to determine your real desires and needs if you aren't already clear about them. 2) Intuitive and sensing techniques to consider underlying goals.
III. *Is the conflict due to a misunderstanding? Whose?* a) The other person's? b) Your own? c) Both or uncertain?	*Techniques for overcoming the misunderstanding through better communication.* a) Techniques to explain and clarify. b) Techniques to be open and receptive to the other person's explanations. c) A combination of techniques to explain and clarify and to be open and receptive to the other's explanations.
IV. *Is the conflict due to someone failing to take responsibility for some actions? A past action? A future action? An agreement to do something?*	*Techniques to determine who is responsible and to gain acceptance for this responsibility.*
a) The other person's responsibility?	a) Techniques to get the other person to acknowledge responsibility and agree to do something.
b) Your own responsibility?	b) Techniques to recognize and acknowledge this.

Resolving Conflict (continued)

V. What kind of conflict styles would be most suitable to use in this situation?	*Assessing the available conflict styles and choosing between them, based on:* 1) the conflict styles you prefer; 2) the conflict styles you feel the others feel most comfortable with; 3) the conflict styles that would be most effective under the circumstances.
a) Is it possible to reach a win-win situation?	a) Using negotiation and discussion to achieve a resolution through compromise or collaboration.
b) Is the conflict worth resolving now at all?	b) Choose to avoid the issue for now.
c) Are there power considerations that can affect the resolution of the conflict?	c) Using accommodation or offers to compromise.
d) Who is more powerful? 1) The other person. 2) You.	d) Using competition or offers to compromise.
VI. Are there special personality factors to be considered in resolving the conflict?	*Understanding personality factors.*
a) Is the other person a difficult person to deal with?	a) Using techniques for dealing with particularly difficult people.
b) Do you have special personality needs you need to meet (e.g., needs for recognition)?	b) Techniques to express your needs effectively.
VII. What kind of alternatives and solutions are possible?	*Coming up with ideas yourself or getting other parties to make suggestions.*
a) What alternatives and solutions are available?	a) Brainstorming and creative visualization to come up with ideas.
b) How can this problem be turned into an opportunity?	b) Brainstorming and creative visualization.
c) What are the best outcomes?	c) Prioritizing the possibilities.

congenital existing before or at birth, though not necessarily detected at that time; may be hereditary or developed as a result of events during pregnancy. See *disorder*.

congenital disorder any disorder present at birth.

congenital heart disease (CHD) a disease in which the individual's heart was not formed correctly. This malformation was present at the time of birth. There are many types of birth defects of the heart. Listed on the following page are some of the major types of CHD that the therapist may encounter.

conical cone shaped. May refer to the shape of the end of a stump after amputation.

conjoint therapy multiple therapies or intervention types which, combined, produce a desired change. An example would be a physician prescribing a medication to reduce a patient's lack of anger impulse control while the therapist works with the patient on specific behavior/anger management skills and techniques. Both professionals are working on the same problem, share a common vision for desired outcome and work together using different approaches to help the patient reach the goal.

conjugate deviation a disorder of the nerves and/or muscles controlling eye movement that causes the eyes to persistently turn to one side when they are at rest.

conjunctivitis an infection or inflammation of the lining of the eye. Also known as "pink eye." Conjunctivitis can be caused by a virus, a bacteria, an allergic reaction, or an ingrown eyelash. Treatment includes antibiotics and/or corticosteroids. Conjunctivitis caused by infectious agents can be very contagious, as people with an inflamed eye tend to rub the eye a lot then touch other items in the environment (door knobs, telephones, etc.), passing the infectious agent to the next person's hand. When that next person rub his/her eye, s/he may be introducing the infectious agent into his/her eye. See *contact isolation*.

Major Types of Congenital Heart Disease

Type	Description
Aortic Stenosis	A narrowing of the aortic valve. The aortic valve helps control the movement of oxygen-enriched blood from the left ventricle to the aorta.
Atrial Septal Defect	A hole between the atrial chambers allows a portion of the oxygen-enriched blood to leak back into the oxygen-depleted blood in the right atrium. This leakage causes an abnormal enlargement in both the right atrium and right ventricle. The pulmonary artery is also enlarged. This enlargement (in addition to the hole) decreases the efficiency of the heart.
Atrioventricular Canal (also known as endocardial cushion defect)	Relatively common in individuals with *Down Syndrome*, atrioventricular canal refers to multiple defects of the heart, including: 1. a hole in the wall between the two ventricles, 2. a hole in the wall between the two atria, and 3. inefficient valves going between the atria and their corresponding ventricles.
Coarctation of the Aorta	A constriction of the aorta which causes increased blood pressure in the blood vessels before the narrowing (leading to the upper torso and the brain) and decreased blood pressure in the blood vessels below the narrowing (leading to the lower torso).
Hypoplastic Left Heart Syndrome (HLHS)	Usually a fatal birth defect, correctable only with a heart transplant. The left side of the heart, especially the left ventricle, is significantly underdeveloped and unable to function efficiently.
Patent Ductus Arteriosus (PDA)	Prior to birth, the fetus' heart has an opening between the aorta (oxygen-enriched) and the pulmonary artery (oxygen-depleted). This opening is used by the fetus to bypass the lungs and closes prior to birth. This defect is the failure of the fetus' heart to mature prior to birth and seal this opening. The child's heart must work harder to successfully circulate oxygen-enriched blood.
Pulmonary Stenosis (PS)	A narrowing in the proximity of the pulmonary valve causing a decreased amount of blood to reach the lungs to be oxygenated.
Tetralogy of Fallot (TOF)	A group of four birth defects of the heart which cause a mixture of oxygenated and non-oxygenated blood to be pumped throughout the body. After a series of surgeries to correct TOF, the individual should require no restrictions for physical activity.

connective tissue (CDC) the supporting tissues of the body, such as tendons, ligaments, bone, and cartilage.

connective tissue disorder a variety of inflammatory diseases of connective tissue, the most common of which is rheumatoid arthritis. Conventionally this disease is attributed to autoimmune processes, although some suggest the involvement of mycobacteria.

conscious in a psychoanalytical sense, the part of the mind that is aware of thoughts and purposefully causes actions.

consensual validation a term used by Harry Stack Sullivan to describe the mutual comparisons of thoughts, feelings, and the perceptions of others in such a manner as to test one's perception of reality.

consensus standard (HCO) a non-proprietary technological standard developed through an open, participative process under the aegis of a standards development organization.

consent voluntary agreement by a patient or representative of an incapacitated patient to accept a treatment or procedure. *Informed consent* is the voluntary agreement by a patient or a representative of a patient who is incapacitated to accept a treatment or procedure after receiving all information that is material to their decision concerning whether to accept or refuse any proposed treatment or procedure. See *conservator, consumer rights, durable power of attorney, right to appeal, right to refuse treatment.*

conservation a cognitive stage of development described by Piaget. Conservation occurs along with *concrete thinking* and refers to the process of a child learning that a cup of water is still the same amount of water if it is in a coffee cup or if it is spilled on the floor. Even though it looks like a different amount of water when it is spilled, the child can comprehend that the volume is still the same.

conservator a person who has assumed control over financial and/or personal affairs for an individual who is found to be incompetent or disabled to the point of not being able to assume reasonable control. The area of competency is complicated and there is no one standard definition of it as a general legal term. Each state sets its own standard. Ultimately, however, the courts rule on "competency" and assign the conservator. See *competence, conservatorship, consumer rights, guardian.*

conservatorship in most jurisdictions, a status where the conservatee (patient) is under the control of another person or person (*conservator*) with respect to fiscal or contractual affairs but not with respect to the physical person or body (as with consent to medical or surgical treatment). See *durable power of attorney.*

constancy ability to or act of staying the same, of maintaining traits, regardless of the angle which one uses to look at the object. Also refers to the maintenance of behavior over a period of time — a skill very important for the therapist to have when working with individuals with a cognitive loss.

constipation hard bowel movements, pain upon defecation, and abdominal cramping. Cause: There are three main causes of constipation: 1. neurogenic bowels (lack of voluntary bowel control), 2. inactivity, and 3. medication side effects. Impact on functional ability: Constipation is associated with the development of hemorrhoids (causing pain), increased abdominal discomfort, irritability, and decreased appetite. An individual experiencing the discomfort associated with constipation will be less inclined to engage in activity. Irritability induced by the discomfort of constipation may increase the incidence of behavioral outbursts. The ironic consequence is that frequently individuals who are on medications to control behavior are then placed on higher doses of medication to control the inappropriate behavior caused by constipation. Most of these medications have a side effect of constipation. See the table below for therapy concerns about constipation. See *autogenics, bed rest, cerebral palsy, diverticulitis.*

constraints on leisure perceptions and environmental structures that cause the individual to limit his/her participation and enjoyment of *leisure.* (Also referred to as "barriers.") Jackson (1993) identified six general areas of constraint, which are summarized in the table on this page. An individual's age tends to play an important part in the impact of all of

Constraints on Leisure Participation

Area of Constraint	Indicators
Social Isolation	• lacks knowledge of resources • lacks knowledge of how to take part • lacks ability to find others to participate with
Accessibility	• lacks cost of transportation • lacks transportation • lacks opportunity within reasonable distance
Personal Reasons	• lacks physical ability • lacks confidence in social situations • involvement medically contraindicated
Costs	• lacks cost of equipment • lacks cost of admission fees and other charges
Time Commitments	• lacks time due to work • lacks time due to family
Facilities	• facilities/areas overcrowded • facilities/areas poorly kept • facilities/areas not available

the factors except for facilities. (A lack of adequate facilities is a factor for all age groups.) Not surprisingly the constraints of cost and accessibility generally decline with age. The constraint of time commitments has the greatest impact on individuals who are middle aged. Social isolation tends to be a greater constraint in those who are young and those who are elderly while constraints based on personal reasons tend to increase with age. See *Dehn's Model of Leisure Health.*

construct a description of how different elements fit together to make one concept. Being able to take a concept, such as the concept of "mental health," and apply it to a patient, requires the therapist to answer the question, "What things are necessary for mental

Constipation, Concerns for Therapy

Concern	Intervention
decreased activity	Motion through activity is one of the best treatment modalities for constipation.
irritability	Prior to providing intervention through medications or other means of behavior modification, the professional may want to recommend a trial period of two to three weeks of daily physical activities which are enjoyable to the patient.
constipation inducing diets	Provide educational sessions to help the patient identify satisfying snacks that promote bowel health, which can be found at many different community recreation centers, the grocery store, gas stations, or food marts.

Constructs Related to Leisure Categories

Testing Tool	Construct of the Categories of Activities which Make Up "Leisure"
Leisurescope Plus	Games, Sports, Nature, Collection, Crafts, Art & Music, Entertainment, Helping Others/Volunteering, Social Affiliation, and Adventure
Leisure Diagnostic Battery	Outdoor/Nature, Music/Dance/Drama, Sports, Arts/Crafts/Hobbies, and Mental Linguistic
Leisure Interest Measure (1991)	Physical, Outdoor, Mechanical, Artistic, Service, Social, Cultural, and Reading
Leisure Step Up	Community Spectator, Expressive Leisure, Physical Leisure, and Cultural Leisure
STILAP	Physical Skills/Solitary; Physical Skills/with Others, Regardless of Skill Level; Physical Skills/Requiring More than One Participant; Outdoor Environment; Physical Skills not considered to be Seasonal; Physical Skills with Carryover Opportunity for Later Years; Physical Skills with Carryover Opportunity and Vigorous Enough for Cardiovascular Fitness; Mental Skills/Solitary; Mental Skills/Two or More; Observation or Passive Response; Creative Construction or Self-expression through Manipulation, Sound or Visual Media; Enables Enjoyment/Improvement of Home Environment; Social Situations; and Community Service

health?" A construct for mental health would describe the attributes an individual needs to have to be mentally healthy. Once the therapist has the different elements of mental health defined, it is easier for him/her to evaluate the patient's mental health status and to address areas of need in mental health. See the table on this page for Constructs Related to Leisure Categories used by some recreational therapy assessment tools.

construct validity a measure of how well an assessment tool matches the underlying concepts that it intends to assess. All testing tools must begin with a solid construct or else all other types of validity and reliability are meaningless. Solid constructs begin with a good definition of the topic followed by the division of that topic into commonly recognized groupings. Construct validity determines if what the test is designed to measure actually agree with the already established definitions and divisions, a much broader perspective than content or criterion validity. Construct validity looks at how well the idea that the tool is measuring was developed; how much integrity the idea itself has. There are three questions that are generally asked for construct validity: 1. How well have the relationships between the concepts been defined and simplified so information can be easily collected as data? 2. How well does the test collect, analyze, or evaluate the data? and 3. Does the manner in which the data is summarized or interpreted help clarify the concepts being measured? One example of a construct would be the classification of fruit types. If the people writing a test divide the fruit samples by color (Group 1/Yellow = bananas, pears, apples; Group 2/Red = strawberries, apples, plums; Group 3/Green =

grapes, apples, and kiwi), the results of the test would be relatively meaningless as most people divide fruit by type (apples, pears, grapes, etc). A testing tool construct that divides fruit by color would be of little worth, regardless of how well the questions were written (content validity) or how likely it is that different people would come up with the same answer (inter-rater reliability). And results obtained by using this test would be hard to compare with the results of tests that divide fruit by type and not color. One area of measurement, which has problems with construct validity, is the area of the acceptable categories of leisure involvement. The professionals who study "leisure" have not reached a definitive agreement on the actual categories. As a result, the major testing tools measured similar, but different divisions. (See the table above.) Construct validity is one of the most important attributes for a testing tool because without it the professional cannot be sure what s/he is measuring. Construct validity looks at the theoretical framework on which the testing tool is based. It is better to rely on clinical impression then to use a testing tool with poor or questionable content validity. See *face validity*, *Delphi technique*.

consulting physician physicians who are not the patient's attending (main) physician, but who have been asked to give their advice on certain aspects of the patient's care or problems.

consumer rights for individuals with disabilities Prior to the 1960's in the United States individuals who had a disability were frequently ostracized and denied the basic rights afforded to the other "normal" individuals living in our society. Since the 1960's a series of laws have been enacted and test-case litigation filed which have greatly expanded the rights of individuals who are disabled. Through the work of groups such as the *ARC*, the Mental Health Association, and Veteran's Groups, as well as the support of numerous patients, change has taken place. The charts below describe the laws that granted the rights. See *conservator, normalization, Protection and Advocacy for the Mentally Ill Individual Act, psychiatric admissions.*

consumer skills skills needed to consume resources within the community. Some consumer skills include: 1. ability to manage money, including knowledge of coins/bills, adding/subtracting, using checks, credit cards, and cash, 2. ability to use store directories, yellow pages, and other types of directional and instructional materials, 3. ability to find prices of objects, and 4. ability to make/maintain lists. See *advanced activities of daily living.*

Consumer Rights for Individuals with Disabilities

Basic Right	Description
Consumer Bill of Rights	While lacking any enforcement rights, a proclamation called "Consumer Bill of Rights" was read by President John F. Kennedy which stated that all Americans had the right to be informed, the right to safety, the right to choose, and the right to be heard.
Community-Based Care	1963 *Community Mental Health Centers* Act (Public Law 88-164) authorized funding for community-based facilities for the treatment and rehabilitation of individuals with mental illness.
Entitlement for Health Care	Social Security Act, which included Social Security disability insurance, Supplemental Security Income (SSI), and Medicaid.
Freedom from Architectural Barriers	The "Federal Architectural Barriers Act of 1968," as revised, required that architectural barriers be eliminated in all new buildings, but lacked enforcement, so therefore was not very effective.
Education Rights for Minority Groups (including disabled)	*Brown v. Board of Education* (347 US 483 1954) Even as late as 1971, only sixteen states had requirements that outlined the public education rights of children who were disabled. Within five years another thirty-two states enacted legislation ensuring access to education for children with disabilities. Chief Justice Earl Warren went on record as saying, "Education is perhaps the most important function of state and local governments. It is the very foundation of good citizenship … the principle instrument in … helping the child to adjust normally to his environment. In these days, it is doubtful that any child may reasonably be expected to succeed in life if he is denied the opportunity of an education."
Right to Refuse Treatment	*Winters v. Miller*, 446 F.2d 65 (2d Cir. 1971) was a case in which the judge decided that an individual institutionalized against his/her will had the right to refuse treatment based on religious beliefs.
Right to Due Process to Fight for Access to Appropriate Education	Two lawsuits at a state level set the precedent that children with a disability had the right to sue a school district to obtain an education. The first case was the *Pennsylvania Association for Retarded Children (PARC) v. Pennsylvania* (334 F. Supp. 1257 [ED Pa 1971]). This case set two standards: 1. that children with mental retardation (regardless of severity) had the right to an appropriate public education and 2. if it was felt that the public education being provided was inappropriate or inadequate, there was a legitimate right to appeal. The second case was *Miller v. Board of Education* (348 F. Supp. 866 [DDC 1972]). It extended the *PARC v. Pennsylvania* ruling from just those with mental retardation to children with any type of significant disability that negatively impacted their ability to benefit from public education.
Freedom from Architectural Barriers	This was a lawsuit that sought to establish the requirement that the stations and trains for Washington, DC's new subway must be accessible. This case was a precursor to the Americans with Disabilities Act — *Urban League v. WMATA, Civil No. 776-72* (DDC plaintiffs' motion for summary judgment granted October 9 order issued October 24, 1973).

Consumer Rights for Individuals with Disabilities (continued)

Basic Right	Description
Human Subjects Protection	The Congress of the United States set up a commission in 1974 with the job of setting standards for the use of human subjects in research. This commission was called the National Commission for the Protection of Human Subjects of Biomedical and Behavioral Research.
Right to Treatment	Bryce Hospital, a 5,000-bed facility for patients with psychiatric disorders was an unhealthy place to be. The buildings originally built in the 1850's housed the patients with psychiatric disorders as well as 1,000 patients who were diagnosed as being mentally retarded and over 1,500 patients who were considered to be geriatric patients. This facility had only three physicians (non-board certified in psychiatry) and one PhD level psychologist. The food was worse than poor and the buildings were filled with insects, mice, and rats. The patients were just being "housed," not receiving treatment. In 1971 a class-action suit was initiated, *Wyatt v. Stickney*, 325 F. Supp. 781(MD Ala. 1971), 334 F. Supp. 1341 (MD Ala. 1971), 344 F. Supp. 373, 387 (MD Ala., 1972). The judge ruled that patients confined against their will had the basic constitutional right to receive appropriate, individualized treatment (*individualized treatment plan*).
Right to Fair Compensation	A class action suit, *Souder v. Brennan*, 367 F. Supp. 808 (DDC 1973) ruled that individuals who were institutionalized were covered under the 1966 Amendments to the Fair Labor Standards Act and, therefore, must receive the minimum hourly wage and other standard rights granted to workers under this law. A further court case in 1976 threw out the requirement that patients receive the federal minimum wage, while upholding the requirement that patients still qualified for the state minimum wage if they lived in state-run facilities (*National League of Cities v. Usery*, 44 USLW 4974 June 24, 1976).
Right to Protection from Harm	Based on the Constitution's Eighth Amendment prohibition against cruel and unusual punishment, a class action suit was brought on behalf of the 5,209 patients of the Willowbrook Developmental Center in New York State, *New York State Association for Retarded Children v. Carey* (393 F. Supp. 715 (EDNY 1975)). The judge in this case ruled that the facility must outline, in detail, the steps, standards, and procedures required to protect patients from *abuse* (e.g., seclusion, use of *restraints*, corporal punishment, degradation, and medical experimentation). In addition to the ruling on the patient's right to freedom from harm, additional steps were taken to reduce the inhumane treatment of the patients, replacing it instead with training, treatment, and transfer to smaller, community-based group homes.
Freedom from Architectural Barriers	An act passed in 1972 specified that only metropolitan transportation systems that provided accommodations for individuals with disabilities would qualify for an 80% federal match on money for the project. This act was called the Federal Urban Mass Transportation Act of 1972. This law had little "bite" and did not require architectural accessibility for individuals who used walkers or wheelchairs.
Right to be Free from Discrimination	The *Rehabilitation Act of 1973* (*Section 503* and *Section 504*) made it illegal to discriminate against individuals due to a disability. This law called for affirmative action programs for the hiring of individuals with disabilities and for the prohibition of discrimination against individuals with disabilities (the penalty being the loss of federal funds).
Education for All Handicapped Children Act	President Ford signed a bill in 1975 that mandated each state to provide an education for all children, regardless of disability. This was called the *Education for All Handicapped Children Act* (Public Law 94-142). Public Law 94-142 provided a formula for federal and state governments to share in the cost of educating children who were disabled.

Consumer Rights for Individuals with Disabilities (continued)

Basic Right	Description
Right to Consumer Education	In 1975 President Ford added the right for consumer education to President John F. Kennedy's basic consumer rights.
Right to Emancipation	As early as 1975 the states of California, Colorado, New York, Washington, and West Virginia had laws that required the assessment of actual capability for emancipation in various areas prior to the removal of these rights. Often individuals with *mental retardation* (or others in institutions for most of their lives) are considered to be totally incompetent to make decisions concerning their care, their finances and are considered incapable to vote, drive, or exercise other freedoms associated with adulthood and emancipation. Instead of automatically assuming that these individuals are incompetent, many states have set up laws that require a formal review of the individual's actual competency level. In addition, sweeping decisions concerning incompetency are not allowed in some states, requiring separate decisions about the right to vote and the right to decide about one's own health treatment and training goals. See *conservator, psychiatric admissions, right to refuse treatment.*
Right for Attorney Fees in Valid Cases of Discrimination	Many lawyers were hesitant to take on litigation concerning the violation of the civil rights of an individual with a disability because they seldom got paid for their services. The Civil Rights Attorney Fees Act (Public Law 94-559) (1976) authorizes federal courts to order the payment of attorney fees if it is found that the claimant had, indeed, been discriminated against due to his/her disability.
Civil Rights Associated with Disability	Prior to the *Americans with Disabilities Act of 1990* (ADA), individuals with a disability had little legal recourse to end discrimination based on their disability. The ADA provided a clear and comprehensive mandate to eliminate barriers caused by discrimination and set up enforceable standards, which were lacking in earlier efforts.
Right to Self-Determination	The Patient Self-Determination Act of 1990 required health care facilities to explain to patients, staff, and families that patients had the legal right to make decisions about their own medical and nursing care, including right-to-die directives. With this Act, health care facilities and staff must actively promote the rights of each patient.

contact isolation a specific type of isolation precaution used when patients have acute respiratory infections; *conjunctivitis*; influenza; multiply-resistant bacteria, infection, or colonization of specific bacteria; pneumonia (viral); rubella; scabies; and skin, wound, or burn infection. The specific isolation procedures are 1. masks are indicated for those who come close to patient, 2. gowns are indicated if soiling is likely, 3. gloves are indicated for touching infective material, 4. hands must be washed after touching the patient or potentially contaminated articles and before taking care of another patient, and 5. articles contaminated with infective material should be discarded or bagged and labeled before being sent for decontamination and reprocessing. The sign for contact isolation is always orange.

content validity the degree to which items on an instrument or scale reflect the content that an instrument is designed to measure. Content validity frequently looks at two aspects of the content. First, the question is asked if the individual items, when compared to each other and as a whole, represent a balanced approach to measuring the desired skill, object, or idea. An example may be a test which says that, if a student is able to demonstrate all the skills listed on the test, then s/he will be able to independently shop at the grocery store. If the test measures how well the student can find items in the grocery store and how well the student can push the grocery cart without running into things, but asks nothing about the student's math skills or knowledge of money, the test would have poor content validity. (It does not have an reasonable balance of questions related to all the skills required to independently shop for groceries.) The second part of content validity asks the question whether the test is measuring what is says it is measuring (e.g., grocery shopping) or if it is really measuring how much the student understands the words being used in the test. An example would be asking a student in which aisle s/he would find grains. The student may fail this item because s/he doesn't know what a "grain" is but could easily find the cereals. In this case the test would actually be measuring the student's vocabulary and not his/her skills associated with finding cereal. Content validity looks at the scope, balance, and wording of the testing tool.

contextual orientation ability to cognitively process events in one's environment and/or the ability to identify objects. See *disorientation, orientation.*

Continuing Survey of Food Intake of Individuals (CSFII) (HHS) a part of the National Nutrition Monitoring System, which was the first nationwide dietary intake survey, designed to be conducted annually. The survey is conducted by the USDA.

continuity of care providing an uninterrupted flow of intervention regardless of where the therapy is being provided (e.g., inpatient, outpatient, day treatment center, home health care). Many health care systems are providing services by their own staff all the way from acute care (hospital) to nursing home, to outpatient, to home health care. Both NCQA and CARF standards call for an umbrella of care provided without any noticeable breaks in the care regardless of how many different corporate entities are providing the services. Compare to *aftercare.* See *continuum, risk management.*

continuous quality improvement (HCO) a method of analyzing and improving processes for manufacturing products or delivering services to meet customer needs and expectations. See *quality assurance, disease management, exposure control plan,*

continuous tube feedings a type of feeding schedule for patients who use a *feeding tube* that has a small volume of liquid nourishment provided continuously to the patient, usually 1.5 ml per minute. An electric feed pump is usually used, requiring the patient who is ambulatory to "drag" along an IV pole and pump. The reduced volume delivered continually may be allowed to bypass digestion in the stomach (delivery right into the small intestine) thus reducing risk of vomiting and aspiration.

continuum flow from one end to the other, from one extreme to the other. The concept of a continuum is used to describe many aspects in health care such as the continuum from total health to death, from birth to old age, from being totally independent to totally dependent. An individual's status is frequently described by where s/he fits into a continuum. Frequently the type of intervention proposed is based on the individual's location on the continuum. See *continuity of care, Joint Commission, Recreation Service Model, Therapeutic Recreation Service Model.*

contract an agreement between two or more people that clearly states what behaviors are expected and what other attributes can be expected to be brought forth over a period of time. It is common for the treatment team to have contracts with patients over behavioral issues. The patient agrees to specific behavior and can expect a benefit as a result.

contracture reduction of normal mobility and/or flexibility of a body part caused by a shortening or tightening of the skin, fascia, muscle, or joint capsule. Contractures may be caused by immobility, injury, or scarring and, depending on the cause and degree of involvement, may require surgery to correct. The professional's best approach to contractures (especially in long-term care settings) is prevention. Assisting the patient in identifying enjoyable activities that allow the daily range of motion of all body parts reduces the chance of contracture development. Contrast with *ankylosis.* See *burn, Dupuytren's contracture, Jobst, physical restraint, tightness.*

contraindication indicates that a treatment or action should not be taken because the situation does not call for it. In fact, the treatment or action may actually make the patient's condition worse. In other words, an identified reason not to provide a procedure that would otherwise be recognized as beneficial. In the past the phrase "counter indications" has been used. Compare to *indication.*

contralateral on or from the opposite side. In injuries to the brain, the origin of the disability is on the opposite side of the body from where the trauma is located. For example, damage to the right side of the brain from a stroke will usually affect the left side of the body.

contralateral associated movement movement of a paralyzed body part that is caused by a voluntary active movement on the non-paralyzed side. See *movement.*

contrecoup lesions lesions caused by the brain's hitting the skull wall after its initial impact (counter bounce) due to a significant acceleration or deceleration of the head. Because the brain is encased but free-moving inside the skull, it will impact the skull initially when the head impacts an object and then rebound in the opposite direction to impact the opposite side of the skull. The lesions are caused by the impact of hitting the skull. These lesions may translate to reduced neurological functioning for months to years after the injury. See *brain-skull differential, coup.*

control group (HHS) the group of subjects in a study to whom a comparison is made in order to determine whether an observation or a treatment has

Developmental Levels of Cooperation

Level	Description
1. Self As Agent	When the therapist asks the patient to convince two peers who are in wheelchairs to go through a door, the patient will take himself/herself through the door. The intent is to follow directions and the patient is able to regulate his/her own behavior but not the behavior of others.
2. Passive Recipient	When the therapist asks the patient to convince two peers who are in wheelchairs to go through a door, the patient will push one or both peers through without using any communication and without monitoring the approval or disapproval of the peers. The intent is to follow directions and the patient is able to regulate his/her own behavior and able to influence the movement of their peers, but is not monitoring the peer's responses.
3. Single Active Agent	When the therapist asks the patient to convince two peers who are in wheelchairs to go through a door, the patient will attempt to influence one of the peers either with gestures and/or physical movements and/or by giving verbal orders for one peer to go through the door. The intent is to influence the behavior of the peer through the use of "one way" orders (patient to peer) without the obvious monitoring of the peer's reaction.
4. Dual Active Agents	When the therapist asks the patient to convince two peers who are in wheelchairs to go through a door, the patient will make awkward attempts at monitoring and influencing each peer's behavior. The intent is to influence the behavior of each peer individually (dyad interaction) and some monitoring of the peer's response is noted.
5. Dual Active Agents with Communication	When the therapist asks the patient to convince two peers who are in wheelchairs to go through a door, the patient will interact with both peers (small group interaction) with obvious, observable monitoring and influencing flowing between the patient and peers.

an effect. In an experimental study it is the group that does not receive a treatment. Subjects are as similar as possible to those in the test or treatment group.

controlled dangerous substance (CDS)   chemicals (medications) which the Food and Drug Administration (USA) have identified as having a high potential for misuse and/or harm and therefore are highly regulated. See *Drug Enforcement Agency.*

controlled experiment   (HHS) In this type of research, study subjects (whether animal or human) are selected according to relevant characteristics, and then randomly assigned to either an experimental group or a control group. Random assignment ensures that factors known as variables, which may affect the outcome of the study, are distributed equally among the groups and therefore could not lead to differences in the effect of the treatment under study. The experimental group is then given a treatment (sometimes called an intervention), and the results are compared to the control group, which does not receive treatment. A placebo, or false treatment, may be administered to the control group. With all other variables controlled, differences between the experimental and control groups may be attributed to the treatment under study.

convalescent diet   See *diet, light diet.*

Cooley's anemia   (HHS/NMDP) another name for thalassemia major. See also *thalassemia.*

cooperation   a complex skill that has three primary components: 1. the ability to define, monitor, and regulate one's own behavior, 2. the ability to define, monitor, and influence another person's behavior, and 3. the awareness of external standards of behavior (Bullock & Luthenhaus, 1988 and Eckerman & Stein, 1982). The fundamental framework to demonstrate cooperation is obtained by the age of 30 months (Brownell & Carriger, 1990). From the age of 2.5 (30 months) an individual will have formed the basic skills for cooperation and will spend the rest of his/her life fine-tuning those skills. For the therapist who is concerned about a patient's apparent lack of cooperation, s/he must first try to discern whether the patient has reached the developmental age of 30 months in the area of cooperation. Some individuals, especially those with learning disabilities, may never have mastered the skills to cooperate. The emergence of cooperation has been documented by Brownell and Carriger (1990) to consist of five developmental levels as shown in the chart above.

coordination   ability to perform tasks using more than one body part or function in a harmonious manner. To coordinate multiple functions to achieve a desired *outcome.* See *developmental coordination disorder.*

coordination of benefits   (HCO) determination of primary payer, that is, the payer whose coverage is applied first. A secondary payer reimburses, subject to the terms of its contract, that portion of a claim unpaid by the primary payer. See *reimbursement.*

coordination of clinical care coordination of information on each patient (e.g., current condition and treatment received) to ensure that each professional has knowledge of and takes into account all relevant information so that the entire treatment team and the patient can work together. Compare with *concurrent review.*

COPD See *chronic obstructive pulmonary disease.*

coping the means by which an individual cognitively evaluates the relative threat or stressors (internal and in the environment) and process the negative emotions that are created by this evaluation. The better the individual's ability to assimilate the stress in a positive, healthy manner, the better his/her coping skills.

coping mechanisms behaviors and thought patterns that help an individual with survival and getting through stressful events. There are five main behavior/thought patterns or styles when coping as shown in the chart below.

coping skills training a type of *relaxation* and self-management technique. Also known as "stress inoculation." Coping skills training was formulated by M. Godfried (1973) and Suinn and Richardson (1971). The basic premise is that when stressed, individuals react with a series of learned behavior patterns, which may include *anxiety*, anger, *fear*, etc. In coping skills training the individual inventories times of successful coping and identifies how s/he did it. Then additional strategies are also learned and practiced. Coping skills training seems to work well for helping individuals manage general anxiety, phobias, and anger/stress. Mastery usually involves the mastery of *progressive relaxation* first, then about a week or two of daily practice with coping skills training. This is an important sequence for therapists to remember when working with patients in need to developing *anger management* skills. See *coping skills, self-control.*

coping techniques techniques used to cope with a stressful event that will depend on what the event is and what causes the event. There are six important actions to take to control or eliminate the impact of the stressful event: 1. get information about the best methods to control or eliminate the *stress* itself, 2. help your body out by practicing deep *relaxation*, 3. keep physically fit by following a regular program of exercise, 4. learn to identify and express your feelings, especially feelings related to anger and sadness, 5. eliminate stimulants (especially with psychosocial stresses) such as caffeine, sugar, and nicotine, and 6. use positive *self-talk* to strengthen your inner self. See *conflict resolution, desensitiza-*

Coping Mechanisms

Style	Description
Compensation	Making the decision to accept a similar and obtainable goal in place of the unobtainable but desired goal. An example would be a patient with a type of seizure activity that can only be controlled with a moderately high doses of medication (with side effects) accepting that reality and letting go the desire to be medication and side effect free (but with serious seizure activity as a result). This is a relatively positive type of coping mechanism. See *compensation.*
Denial	Refusing to accept or believe the information or situation. An example would be a patient with a newly acquired C5 complete lesion saying that s/he would be walking by the end of six months.
Displacement	Directing one's thoughts and emotions about a given, stressful situation away from the situation and directing those thoughts and emotions to a third object or situation. An example would be a spouse's anger at the physical abuse by her partner, displacement would have her lash out at the police officers arresting her partner instead of directing that anger toward her partner/abuser.
Rationalization	Using cognitive messages to one's self to justify why the current stressful situation may actually be acceptable. An example would be a patient with a traumatic brain injury waiting to be accepted into a specific group home but getting turned down. Rationalization behavior would include the patient deciding that a placement at another group home may actually be better because it would place him closer to his favorite recreation center. This is a relatively healthy type of coping mechanism.
Repression	To cognitively ignore (or try to ignore) the situation. This is different than denying the situation; the individual has on some level accepted that the situation has some truth. An example would be a woman who was recently gang raped consciously or unconsciously being unable/unwilling to recall events that took place during the traumatic event.

tion.

corporate alliances (FB) a term used in the *Health Security Act* that referred to entities created by employers with 5,000 or more employees to provide health insurance. Corporate alliances would have had to enroll all eligible persons and provide comprehensive benefit packages. They would have had to offer a choice of at least three health plans, one of which would be a *fee-for-service* plan.

correlation the degree to which a prediction can be made about how a change in one object, idea, or action will be reflected in another. Correlations range from −1.0 (movement in opposite directions) through 0.0 (no relationship) to +1.0 (movement in the same direction). The greater the degree of confidence in being able to predict (e.g., the further from "0.0") the better the correlation. An example would be the relationship between room temperature and how fast a block of ice melts. You should find a high, positive correlation between room temperature and how much ice melts in a ten-minute period (i.e., a hotter room will cause more ice to melt). While in this example it is the high temperature that is causing the ice to melt, correlation does not necessarily imply any direct cause and effect relationship.

cortex layer of gray matter that covers the surfaces of the *cerebrum* and of the *cerebellum.*

cortisol a diurnal steroid hormone that is produced by the adrenal cortex in response to stress. Cortisol is highest at around 8 a.m. with its low point around midnight. The known essential features of cortisol include the maintenance of glucose production from protein as well as facilitation of fat metabolism. Individual levels of cortisol found in plasma, urinary, and saliva samples can be used to determine endocrine responses to stressful stimuli.

cost-benefit analysis (HCO) a comparison of the net costs of an intervention with the net savings. See *human capital approach, willingness to pay approach.*

cost-effectiveness analysis (HCO) a structured, comparative evaluation of two or more health care *interventions.*

cost sharing (FB) provisions of a health benefit plan that require the enrollee to pay a portion of the cost of services covered by the plan, typically exclusive of premium cost-sharing (sharing the cost of a health care plan premium between the sponsor and the enrollee). Usual forms of cost sharing include deductibles, coinsurance, and co-payments. These payments are made at the time a service is received or shortly thereafter, and are only made by insured people who seek treatment.

cost shifting (FB) condition that occurs when health care providers are not reimbursed or not fully reim-bursed for providing health care. This results in increased charges for those who do pay.

counselor an individual who helps another individual: 1. identify and define a problem, 2. develop a vision of what it would look like to solve the problem, and 3. determine the decisions to be made, skills to be developed, and actions to be taken to resolve the problem. A counselor provides information meant to alleviate the emotional strain surrounding an event or series of events. Counseling may consist of a one-time visit or may involve ongoing contact, providing the opportunity for a patient to express feelings of loss, sadness, depression, etc., and to help cope or problem solve. There are many different theories and methods used by therapists to help an individual achieve the desired changes and results. See *problem solving.*

counter indication a dated term that has been replaced by *contraindication.*

countertransference therapist's response to the patient and the patient's needs where the response is a result of the conscious or unconscious needs of the therapist. Countertransference is exhibited in the emotional involvement of the therapist in what the patient is saying or doing. Depending on the psychoanalytical theory one adheres to, the countertransference can either be harmful to the patient or benign to the therapy process. See *transference.*

coup any injury caused by a blow but usually referring to lesions of the brain resulting from initial impact. In open-head injuries the damage is from the striking object. In closed-head injuries the brain is damaged when it hits the skull as a result of a sudden change in the individual's velocity (e.g., sudden stop as a result of one's car hitting a bridge support). The skull tends to stop faster than the brain in such cases causing the brain tissue to impact the inside of the skull at the site of the blow. Additional injuries, often on the opposite side of the brain are called *contrecoup lesions.* See *brain-skull differential.*

covered entity When used in a federal law, covered entity refers to "an employer, employment agency, labor organization, or joint labor management committee" (ADA 1630.2(b)).

CPT See *Current Procedural Terminology.*

crash cart a cart that contains all of the emergency supplies required to quickly respond to a medical emergency. Each crash cart is stocked with equipment such as antiseptics, suction devices, analgesics, sutures, defibrillators, surgical needles, sponges, swabs, retractors, hemostats, and trachea tubes. The idea is that each crash cart is quickly and readily available to medical staff in the case of an emergency such as a heart attack. Because of the types of medical supplies stored on a crash cart, crash carts often have the supplies "borrowed" by staff who intend to replace the equipment later. Sometimes items are simply stolen. To prevent loss, crash carts are often, and incorrectly, locked up. Staff may also store equipment in front of the closet door where the crash cart is stored. Health care surveyors often consider a locked up or blocked crash cart an immediate threat to patient safety.

craving related to *substance dependence*, having a strong desire, need, or longing for a drug of abuse.

creatinine (HHS) a component of urine, and the final breakdown product of creatine, which is an important molecule for building energy reserves, for example, in muscle cells.

creativity ability to create objects, emotions, or traits in others through the use of one's knowledge, imagination, and understanding of others.

credentialing process by which an individual or an agency is formally recognized as having met minimum standards. The ability to meet predefined levels of education, licensure, professional experience, and compliance with professional and ethical standards are all part of the initial credentialing process. Health care credentialing must also contain mechanisms to review the individual's or group's continued ability to meet minimum standards on a regular basis, usually every three to seven years. Types of credentialing are shown below. See *Pew Health Professions Commission, professional, professional misconduct.*

Credé's maneuver a maneuver to help empty the bladder for patients with either retention or overflow *incontinence*. With the patient sitting on a toilet leaning slightly forward, have the patient place his/her palms on the skin below the navel and slowly apply downward pressure as the hands are moved downward to the pubic hair.

credible allegation of compliance a credible allegation is a statement made by a provider/supplier of Medicare or Medicaid that deficiencies have been corrected. The allegation of compliance must be realistic in terms of the provider's/supplier's ability to correct the deficiencies between the survey date and the date of the allegation. See *deficiency.*

cri du chat See *chromosomal aberrations.*

criminal responsibility a defendant's state of mind at the time of the alleged crime. A person cannot be convicted of a crime if it can be proved that s/he lacked the ability to formulate a criminal intent at the time of the alleged crime because of criminal insanity. Also known as the *insanity defense.* See *actus reus, competency to stand trial, mens rea.*

crisis intervention a brief therapeutic interaction for the purpose of helping control or reduce the immediate crisis. It is not intended to address the underlying causes or to necessarily prevent the crisis from happening again.

criteria a set of written statements containing measurable standards that are used to determine the appropriateness of 1. the health care decision making process, 2. the services delivered, and/or 3. the outcomes achieved. See *measurement.*

criterion related validity the degree to which a test-

Types of Professional Credentialing

Type	Description
Certification	Certification is a credentialing process that may include minimum educational qualifications, specifically defined professional experience and an examination. Certification may be run by either a governmental body or a designated agency. While certification restricts others from using the professional title, it does not restrict others from practicing within the scope of practice of the certified profession.
Licensure	Licensure is the most stringent type of credentialing available for health care professionals. Based on educational background, experience, and other measurements of competency, licensure is granted by a governmental agency. Licensure is developed for professional groups whose scope of practice has a high likelihood of causing harm to the public health if not provided by a well-qualified individual. Not only does licensure recognize individuals who have demonstrated competency but it also restricts the practice of that profession. In the United States (1987) there are 490 occupations (not just health care) that require the professional to become licensed. (Connolly, 1997).
Registration	Registration is probably one of the least stringent and simplest of all professional credentials. In many cases, individuals are required to do little more than file their name with a designated agency. In some cases, the designated agency may have a minimum educational requirement to become registered. In 1987, there were 643 occupations that required registration in the United States (Connolly, 1997).

ing tool measures an object, idea, process, or other item (e.g., ability to control one's temper). This is done by judging how closely the scores on the test are able to correctly describe an object, an idea, or process. An example would be using a checklist test to determine if the dinosaur fossils you found scattered across a field belonged to a Tyrannosaurus Rex. Let's say that you have a checklist that says that if you are able to check off all of the items as "true," then the fossils you found belong to a Tyrannosaurus Rex. If you checked off as "true" all of the criteria listed and yet, after putting the fossils together, it is obvious that your fossils belonged to a Triceratops, the criterion-related validity of your checklist would be poor. The list did not describe the object well enough to correctly do what it said it was going to do. Examples of criterion related validity:

- If a testing tool's intent is to identify patients who are likely to have significant problems in managing their anger outbursts, do patients who score poorly on that test, in fact, have significant social handicaps due to their anger outbursts?
- If a testing tool's intent is to identify patients who will be independent in toileting, does passing the test in the hospital correctly predict that the patient is independent in toileting after discharge?
- If the testing tool's intent is to measure the patient's barriers to leisure, do the results match the patient's actual experiences with barriers while in the community?

Criterion related validity looks at the testing tool's ability to predict or describe. A testing tool with poor criterion-related validity is a waste of both the therapist's and patient's time. Even worse, it may lead to treatment interventions that are unnecessary or even harmful to the patient. See *construct validity*.

critical pathway a clinical guide to care using a systematic sequence of treatments and *interventions* delivered within an established length of stay. Critical pathways are developed as a result of using *quality assurance* measurements and actual patient/functional *outcomes*. By having a pre-established method of approaching a specific patient problem and using previously identified successful intervention strategies, the treatment team can better predict the patterns of treatment and allocate resources appropriately. Originally developed in the 1970's, critical pathways will become an increasingly important part of the *managed care* system. Critical pathways are taking the place of *care plans* in some facilities. See *medically complex*.

Cronbach's Alpha Reliability Coefficient Using a complex mathematical equation, all of the elements (questions) of the testing tool are compared to each other to establish the strength of its internal consistency. The benefits of Cronbach's Alpha are 1. you need to administer the test only one time, 2. your reliability is not impacted by either a practice effect or a memory effect, and 3. your reliability testing is not dependent upon a single split (as in split-half reliability) so your procedure produces a more stable measure of reliability. Cronbach's Alpha (also referred to as just Alpha) is considered to be the "standard" or "best practice" choice for determining a testing tool's reliability. Cronbach's Alpha works when the answers to the questions on the testing tool use a scale with at least three levels (e.g., a Likert scale with "almost never, sometimes, almost always"). When the testing tool has only two choices (e.g., yes/no, pass/fail), you would want to use Kuder-Richardson 20 or Kuder-Richardson 21 computation instead. A .6 or higher is considered to be a reasonable Cronbach's Alpha.

cross-sectional study (CDC) in epidemiology, a study in which participants are examined a single time to see if they exhibit or have the characteristic being studied. Cross-sectional studies try to measure the prevalence of a characteristic within a population.

cross slope (ADA) slope that is perpendicular to the direction of travel. See *running slope*.

crutch a prosthetic device used for support. May also refer to a means of supporting an individual emotionally or psychologically. Patients who use either an axillary or Canadian crutch will generally use the "crutch stance." In the crutch stance, the patient's body is in the standing position with the shoulders down but not hunched, the pelvic area is in line with the head and the base of the crutch is positioned a couple of inches in front and a couple of inches to the side of either foot. While the weight of the patient's body is supported on the palms of the hands, the crutch top is about two inches below the armpit and the elbows are bent to between 25 and 30 degrees. For patients who have weakened abdominal, back, or hip muscles and use a *swing-to gait*, a *swing-through gait*, or a drag-to gait the "tripod position" is generally recommended. The tripod position places the patient's weight forward onto the crutches. The tips of the crutches are about 8 to 10 inches in front of and to the side of the feet. The patient's weight is borne under the arms while standing, allowing some use of the hands for activities. The therapist will need to observe the patient for *fatigue* when using the tripod position, as this position is more stressful on the body than the crutch stance.

Types of Crutches

Type	Description
Axillary	Also known as the underarm crutch, this is the most common type of crutch used. The crutch has a foam or rubber pad placed on top of the body of the crutch which forms a modified upside down triangle. In the middle of this triangle is a cross bar which the patient grasps with his/her hand. The crutch then tapers down to a single shaft, which is capped with a rubber cap to decrease slippage. These crutches are adjusted at the cross bar (for appropriate distance from the armpit to the foam pad at the top of the crutch) and at the point where the modified triangle is connected to the single shaft. Properly fitted axillary crutches should allow a two-inch space between the armpit and the rubber pad as the patient stands in the "crutch stance."
Canadian (also known as Lofstrand)	This crutch has a vertical metal cuff for the patient's lower arms (about 1 - 2 inches below the elbow) with a handle for the hand to allow weight bearing.
Platform	Crutches that have a horizontal support or trough for the patient's arm, which bears the weight of the patient's body (instead of having the palm bear the weight as in both the Canadian and the auxiliary crutch).

When working with patients who use crutches, the therapist will want to establish the patient's functional performance in a variety of activities, including:

- general *static balance* and *dynamic balance*
- balance with only one crutch
- balance when using one crutch as a striking implement
- balance during upper trunk movement
- general motor movement function with crutch use
- positioning flexibility of upper and lower extremity segments
- degree of independence for transferring to different surfaces and planes
- integrity of skin and degree of risk for *pressure sores*
- ability to maintain own crutches

Common types of crutches are listed above. See *four-point gait*.

CSN See *community services network*.

CT scan See *computerized axial tomography*.

cueing prompting, usually with words or gestures, for the purpose of stimulating an activity or directing behavior. See *behavior modification, diversional program, FIM, following directions, grooming, pathfinding, visual cues*.

culture a group of people who share common origins, customs, and living styles. This group usually also shares a common language and has a general sense of common identity. This shared lifestyle and identity helps develop a sense of group values, expectations, beliefs, and perceptions. Rituals tend to be shared by the group for all major life events from

Comparison of Common Cultural Values

Anglo-American	Other Ethnocultural Groups
Mastery over nature	Harmony with nature
Personal control over the environment	Fate
Doing — activity	Being
Time dominates	Personal interaction dominates
Human equality	Hierarchy/rank/status
Individualism/privacy	Group welfare
Youth	Elders
Self-help	Birthright inheritance
Competition	Cooperation
Future orientation	Past or present orientation
Informality	Formality
Directness/openness/honesty	Indirect/ritual/"face"
Practicality/efficiency	Idealism
Materialism	Spiritualism/detachment

birth to death. Modifying Schilling and Brannon's work, Randall-David (1989) developed the chart on the previous page. See *acculturation, disenfranchised*

Culture-Free Self-Esteem Inventories (CFSEI) (Second Edition) (James Battle, 1992) a series of self-report scales used to determine the level of self-esteem in children and adults. In addition to providing total scores, the CFSEI measures children's self-esteem in five areas: general, peers, school, parents, and lie (defensiveness) scales. Four areas are measured for adults: general, social, personal, and lie scales. CFSEI-2 results clearly show the relationship of self-esteem to proper behavioral-social, emotional, and academic functioning. The test is designed to screen for possible intervention, to measure therapeutic progress, and to suggest when treatment may be discontinued. This testing tool has gone through extensive reliability and validity testing (N=5,000). Reliability and validity have been thoroughly established: test-retest coefficients are generally over .80 and correlations with other recognized measures of self-esteem also revealed coefficients of .80. Results from 60 research studies are presented in over 100 tables in the examiner's manual. The CFSEI-2 is untimed but can generally be administered and scored for individuals and groups in 15 to 20 minutes. There are three forms for administration: Form A for children contains 60 items; Form B for children contains 30 items (extracted from Form A); Form AD for adults contains 40 items. Responses (simple yes-or-no answers) may be either written or spoken. Conversion tables give t scores and percentiles for total and all subscale scores. The CFSEI-2 may be used with individuals from age 5 through adult. This testing tool is available in English, French, and Spanish.

cunnilingus oral intercourse consisting of stimulation of the labia or clitoris with the tongue or lips. When working with youth or adults who have been sexually abused some of the "slang" terms for cunnilingus include: "eat-me," "fur-burger," and "eat-pussy."

curb ramp (ADA) a short ramp cutting through a curb or built up to it.

curiosity desire to find new or novel objects, experiences, and thoughts. This desire to experience part or all of one's environment is a critical component to new learning. To be able to demonstrate curiosity, the individual must have: 1. an awareness that his/her *environment* exists, 2. knowledge that s/he can influence and interact with the environment, 3. the ability to recognize something as novel, 4. the desire to experience the novel, and 5. the ability to

derive pleasure from the experience.

current population survey (CPS) (FB) sponsored by the Department of Labor's Bureau of Labor Statistics and the Department of Commerce's Bureau of the Census, a continuing monthly cross-section survey of about 60,000 US households. Data collected includes labor force status for ages 15 and older. The March CPS includes supplementary questions on income, employment status, and health insurance coverage during the previous calendar year.

Current Procedural Terminology (CPT) name of a health care billing code system developed and maintained by the American Medical Association (AMA). The AMA publishes the book every year with updates. Most therapists will find the CPT codes for therapy listed under the Physical Medicine section. These codes are not occupation specific (e.g., OT or RT) but treatment specific (e.g., mobility). In each case, when a CPT code is used, the therapist must be present during the treatment. CPT codes are considered "Level One" (primary) codes by the United States Government. HCPCS (*Health Care Financing Administration's Common Procedure Coding System*) are considered "Level Two" (secondary) codes by the United States Government.

custodial care care given to individuals who are not capable of meeting their own basic needs.

customer service broadly defined as whatever it takes to make a customer satisfied. Davidow and Uttal (1989) state that "satisfaction, or lack of it, is the difference between how a customer expects to be treated and how he or she perceives being treated (p. 19)." Many health care facilities have been able to provide good customer service in the past, but little formal structure has been offered to provide a systematic approach to providing good quality service. Just as the development of formalized quality control systems received definition from such leaders as Deming, Juran, and Crosby, formalized systems of customer service are being developed today. Davidow and Uttal (1989) divided customer service into six components. By using these six components, professionals are able to develop statistical and organizational methods to quantify customer service. See the table titled "Six Components of Customer Service" (burlingame, 1998a) on the next page, which provides an overview. Programs and processes that are implemented to increase the quality of services for individuals who are consuming the services include:

1. information on how to obtain and use the services available

2. information on how to express concerns, *com-*

Six Components of Customer Service

Principle Area	Description
Design	Products and services should be designed from the beginning to make access to and use of the services and products easy, with little "down time" due to being out of service or otherwise not functioning.
Infrastructures	Support, both in human resources and physical structures, should be well thought out to provide efficient and timely support for the services and products. Infrastructures include staff education, building space, and stock on hand for the customer and support staff.
Leadership	The best customer service tends to be possible when the staff having face-to-face contact with the customer have the greatest discretion to modify the service or product to meet that specific customer's needs. The type of leadership that promotes this must be willing to let go of the need to follow rules and regulations and trust each staff person's judgment.
Measurements	Three types of measurements are taken regularly to quantify customer service: 1. *process measures* (comparing staff performance to standards of quality and quantity), 2. *product measures* (also known as outcomes of treatment), and 3. *satisfaction measures* (customer perceptions compared to customer expectations).
Personnel	The staff who meet with the customer face-to-face are a critical component of good customer service. All other components of customer service must be geared toward supporting front-line personnel in their quest to provide quality customer service. Motivated, well-trained, and respected staff provide management with satisfied customers, a low staff turnover rate, and good outcomes.
Strategy	The first step toward organizing a facility's customer service program is to develop a strategy. Strategies that focus resources into similar services tend to produce better customer satisfaction than taking a "shotgun approach." Grouping rehabilitation services in one place and general medicine services in another tend to increase customer satisfaction over mixing differing needs together.

plaints, and compliments about the services available/received

3. information on how to receive extra information about accessing and understanding the services available

4. systems that facilitate this communication including special 800 phone numbers, short (if any) time "on hold," staff receiving and responding to messages

5. staff behavior that demonstrates a desire to meet the consumer's perceived and real needs.

See *medical management systems*.

cutaneous pertaining to the skin.

cutaneous sensation awareness of contact with the dermis (skin). See *sensation*.

CVA See *cerebrovascular accident*.

cyanosis a bluish tint to the skin caused either by an excess of deoxygenated hemoglobin in the blood or by a structural defect in the hemoglobin molecule. See *chronic obstructive pulmonary disease*.

cyst a sac or pouch which contains fluid or solid material. Cysts are abnormal but are not treated unless the body of the cyst is causing undue pressure and discomfort or is blocking a passage within the body.

cystic fibrosis (CF) a disorder of the exocrine system that causes a thickening of saliva, mucus, and sweat. This inherited disorder has two primary im-

Cystic Fibrosis, Concerns for Therapy

Concern	Intervention
Interrupted lifestyle	The individual should be assisted in the development of a variety of activities that can be enjoyed in a variety of settings, including the hospital.
Abnormal cardiovascular ability	Swimming is one of the healthiest activities for the individual with CF to participate in. Not only does swimming multiple times a week increase the individual's cardiovascular health, but the moisture from the water also helps thin the mucus accumulating in the lungs.
Self-esteem	Youth, especially adolescents, are concerned if their body looks "different" than their peers. Activities that help increase self-esteem are indicated.

pacts on the patient's functional ability: 1. recurrent infections of the lungs due to thickened mucus that lines the lungs, trapping bacteria and 2. small stature due, in part, to abnormal mucus secretions that interfere with the flow of digestive enzymes (incomplete digestion). Cause: CF is a recessive genetic trait and requires that both parents be carriers of the CF recessive gene. Impact on functional ability: The chronic lung infections and the abnormal digestive action cause the youth with CF to have less energy than most of his/her peers and to miss a fair amount of school and other activities due to time spent in the hospital. The older the youth gets, the more frequent the hospitalizations become. Few individuals with CF live past their 20's. See the previous page for some concerns for therapy.

cytokine (CDC) proteins manufactured by cells of various lineages that, when secreted, drive specific responses (e.g., proliferation, growth, or maturation) in other susceptible cells.

cytomegalovirus (CMV) (CDC) one of the eight known types of human herpes viruses, also known as human herpes virus 5 (HHV-5). It belongs to the beta subfamily of herpes viruses. CMV can cause severe disease in patients with immune deficiency and in newborns when the virus is transmitted in utero. It is also a cause of pneumonia in post bone marrow transplant patients.

D

dance therapy also known as movement therapy. Dance therapy uses movement as a modality to increase or maintain *flexibility* and *strength* as well as a means to express and explore emotions in a therapeutic setting. A dance therapist helps the patient maintain or increase *range of motion*, build strength, increase or maintain balance, and gain an awareness of body position in the environment. Psychosocially, dance therapy can help the patient explore his/her emotionally volatile issues in a nonverbal, often less threatening manner, increase *self-esteem* and provide opportunities for *socialization*. For further information contact the American Dance Therapy Association, Inc., 2000 Century Plaza, Suite 108, 10632 Little Patuxent Parkway, Columbia, MD 21044, 410-997-4040, www.adta.org.

data an accumulated set of information used to help facilitate the evaluation of an event over a predetermined period of time. In experimental settings, the information collected is based on a predetermined set of criteria which describes what is to be measured. This information may be either numerical or non-numerical in nature but is compiled in an organized manner. See *Recreation Participation Data Sheet, research, run-length encoding, secondary data, structured data entry, transmission control protocol.*

database the structured collection of information about a defined group. Usually the term "database" is used in the context of computer-stored information. Databases in health care have three components: input data, process data, and outcome data (Niemeyer, 1998). When using a database to obtain treatment outcomes, Niemeyer defines input data which includes some type of identifying code for each entry (e.g., patient identification), the programs or facilities involved in care, demographics, referral and payment source, information on diagnostic groupings including scope and severity, background/medical history including prior functions and roles experienced by the patient, and the psychosocial environment. Process data contains information about actions taken while the patient was admitted to the program including the frequency and duration of treatment, the types of services provided, treatment types and intensities, and the use of critical pathways (if any). The information included in the input and process data lead to a result, which is described in the outcome data. This includes changes in the patient's functional status between admission and discharge; the patient's status related to independent living, community integration skills, and ability to return to work; the patient's satisfaction with the service; the patient's quality of life; and the cost of the services. See *online analytic processing, primary database, rehabilitation centers regional database.*

data distillation (HCO) an informal label for the process of deriving meaning from raw data.

data repository (HCO) component of an information system that accepts, files, and stores data from a variety of sources. See *community health management information system.*

day treatment program outpatient programs that provide the patient with intensive, interdisciplinary *treatment* on a time-limited basis. These programs are designed to maximize function and independent living through a structured program of treatment *protocols.* A day treatment program is not intended to provide long-term adult daycare or to provide a sheltered workshop for supportive employment. See *adult daycare centers, partial hospitalization.*

DEA See *Drug Enforcement Agency.*

debilitation loss of previous *skills* or wellness.

debridement removing foreign material or contaminated cells through cleansing, usually once every shift. Debridement is frequently extremely painful, especially when associated with "tubbing" for patients with *burns.* The four primary goals of debridement are

1. to keep the injured area clean
2. to remove dead tissue
3. to remove bacteria
4. to remove caked antimicrobials

There are three means of debriding a burn: 1. mechanical (as in scrubbing), 2. surgical (as in the surgical cutting away of dead tissue), and 3. enzymatic (using enzymes to dissolve the dead tissue).

decerebrate rigidity an extension and internal rotation of the upper extremities along with a forceful extension of the joints of the lower extremity due to a contusion of the *brainstem.*

decision making process of selecting one option over another. This requires recognizing the purpose and use of each option, picturing the consequences of using each one, and weighing the pros and cons of the possible *outcomes* from each option. (RAPs) The patient's ability to make everyday decisions about the tasks or *activities of daily living*. Examples of daily decisions include choosing items of clothing; determining mealtimes; using environmental cues to organize and plan (e.g., clocks, calendars, posted listing of upcoming events); using awareness of one's own strength in regulating the day's events (e.g., ask for help when necessary). See *dependent personality disorder.*

decision support See *clinical decision support.*

decompensation literally meaning to not compensate or correct for changes or challenges. In mental health, decompensation refers to the failure of an individual's defense mechanisms. This failure usually leads to an exacerbation of the individual's underlying condition (e.g., schizophrenia, substance addiction, anxiety).

deconditioning a decrease in the combined functional ability of the circulatory system, cognition, neuromuscular movement, and metabolic system as a direct result of prolonged immobility and/or *bed rest* (usually two weeks or longer). This decrease is a direct result of inactivity and not a result of an injury or illness. Typical loss of abilities include:

1. decreased brain wave activity caused by bed rest or chair rest (which produces the same EEG patterns as individuals placed in environments which promote sensory *deprivation*)
2. noted decrease in cognitive ability including verbal fluency, color discrimination, reversible figures, and distorted awareness of time
3. potential decrease in thermo-regulation
4. noted increase in *anxiety*, irritability, *depression*, and possible hallucinatory experiences
5. decrease in *balance* (after 2 to 3 weeks on bed rest)
6. increase in resting heart rate (by the end of 3 weeks morning heart rate can increase by 21%, evening by 33%, or an average of 1 heartbeat per 2 days of bed rest)
7. decrease in oxygen uptake (anticipated 15% to 30% decrease in uptake after just 3 weeks bed rest). (burlingame and Blaschko, 1997, p. 3)

See *hallucination, intermittent claudication, tilt table.*

decubitus ulcer See *pressure sore.*

deductive approach to test construction a technique used to isolate the major theoretical trends, issues, and research findings associated with the elements to be measured by a testing tool.

deductive reasoning a mature thought process where the individual starts with known principles to reach a conclusion using thought and logic. Deductive reasoning usually starts to emerge around the age of seven. In deduction, if the original principles are correct, the conclusions will be correct. See *inductive reasoning.*

deemed status 1. a facility that has met minimum expectations and can receive government funding for its services. 2. a health care facility that participates in the Medicare/Medicaid program by virtue of its accreditation by a national accrediting organization, whose standards have been determined to be at least equivalent to those of Medicare/Medicaid.

defense mechanism conscious and unconscious reactions to reduce *anxiety* and *conflict*; the process of using *magical thinking*, defensive positions, and other actions to reduce the discomfort a situation is causing. See *coping mechanisms.*

deficiency 1. lack of ability to meet some part of a law. In health care a provider or supplier violation of an applicable program as outlined in HCFA regulations. See *credible allegation of compliance, effective date of participation, exit conference, nonrenewal, reasonable assurance.* 2. lack of an important chemical, enzyme, or other element that, in turn, leads to compromised health.

degenerative disease a disease which is anticipated to become worse, to reduce the individual's function and overall health over a period of time.

degenerative joint disease a breakdown of cartilage and formation of bony outgrowths without evidence of inflammation over a period of time. This is the most common type of *arthritis*, also called osteoarthritis. The most common areas involved are the hips and knees, generally not becoming clinically evident until after the individual has reached the age of 40. Osteoarthritis causes a deep, aching joint pain usually evident after exercise or weight bearing. Relief usually comes with rest. Moderation is the key to helping the individual maintain normal life activities. Planned periods of rest throughout the day, adequate sleep, and regular *range of motion* exercises prescribed by a physical therapist will help prolong normal activity.

Dehn's Model of Leisure Health Dave Dehn (1995) theorizes that leisure is more than just what individuals do in their "free time." Through leisure, individuals learn basic social, motor, and cognitive skills, as well as provide themselves with the physical exercise they need. When individuals do not have these basic skills and experiences either through lack of knowledge or because of other barriers, they risk developing or complicating illnesses or disabilities. Like the need for balanced nutrition,

Dehn feels that individuals need a balanced leisure lifestyle to promote and maintain basic health. He developed a model based on the earlier work of Nash (1953) that outlines a hierarchy of choices which lead from lost freedom (hospitalization, incarceration, or death) to *catharsis*. The chart below shows the nine levels of Dehn's model. See *constraints on leisure.*

dehydration loss of fluid (and usually electrolytes) from body tissues that can cause other serious physical problems. Restoring fluid volume and electrolytes should be done as quickly as possible. See *dia-*

betes.

delayed sensation awareness that happens some time after the initial contact. See *sensation.*

delegation in health care, the formal process of contracting with a subcontractor to deliver specific services. A home health care agency may contract with a recreational therapist in private practice to provide home-based recreational therapy services in its south county area. The therapist would bill the home health care agency instead of the patient (or patient's insurance). When an agency delegates service delivery to a subcontractor, the agency still has the

Dehn's Model of Leisure Health

Leisure Level Model The activities that I choose to participate in during my free time.	Cathartic Level	**My Choice/My Behavior.** My participation reaches a point of catharsis. My participation makes a measurable change in my life. **Examples:** vacation, climbing a mountain, prayer, ropes course, watching an event, achieving the goal, etc.
⇑	Level 4	**My Choices/My Behavior.** I am creative, inventive, imaginative, taking nothing, and making something. Not following a plan or instruction. **Examples:** Poetry, drawing, painting, crafts, cooking, sculpting, music, prayer, etc.
⇑	Level 3	**My Choices/My Behavior.** I am active physically, socially, and/or cognitively. Activity follows instruction, a plan, rules, with participation on an emotional level. **Examples:** Crafts, cooking, bike riding, sports participation, intense laughter (internal jogging), dancing, games, skateboarding, reading, physical workout, relaxation therapy, etc.
⇑	Level 2	**My Choices/My Behavior.** I am a spectator emotionally involved. There is a personal investment, true entertainment. **Examples:** TV, radio, watching others participate in Level 3 and 4 activities.
Healthy Positive Choices	Level 1	**My Choices/My Behavior.** I am a spectator with no emotional involvement. Participation lacks personal investment, *positive* activities with nothing else to do. **Examples:** Watching TV, listening to the radio, watching others participate in Level 3 and 4 activities.
⇑	Level 0	**My Choices/My Behavior.** I am preoccupied in thought or feeling and just going through the motions of the activity. Participation could be forced, obligated, duty, with no internalization of participation. **Examples:** Preoccupation during participation in Level 1, 2, 3, or 4 activities.
⇓	Level -1	**My Choices/My Behavior.** I am harmed physically, mentally, or emotionally. **Examples:** Substance abuse, dangerous high risk activities, self-abuse, negative thinking, poor dietary choices, too much or not enough sleeping, eating, exercising, relaxing, etc.
Unhealthy Negative Choices	Level -2	**My Choices/My Behavior.** I affect others in a harmful or hurting manner. This includes physical, emotional, or mental harm to my family, friends, or community. **Examples:** Substance abuse, inappropriate competition, gossip, threatening, name calling, fighting, hurting animals, breaking the law (minor), no family time, etc.
⇓	Lost Freedom	**My Choices/My Behavior.** I harm myself or others. My behavior causes a loss in freedom to choose my own leisure. Often the victim's and/or family's leisure are also affected. **Examples:** Crime, gang involvement, vandalism, fighting, suicide gestures, breaking the law (major: rape, self-abuse, sexual abuse, substance abuse, etc.).

© 1995 Dave Dehn and Idyll Arbor, Inc.

responsibility for the quality of services provided by the contractor. An example would be a situation where the recreational therapist provided substandard care. The Health Care Financing Administration in that situation would hold the agency, not just the therapist, responsible for the citation and fine. A therapist in private practice or a therapy group which contracts with agencies to deliver services is professionally responsible for ensuring that it meets all of the regulatory and other *standards* which apply to the agency. In most cases, this means that the subcontractor's patient charts, policies and procedures, personnel files, and accounting records must be available upon request (and all are to be up-to-date and comply with standards of practice and regulations).

delirium a state of cognitive dysfunction where the patient appears confused, has a decreased ability to attend to stimuli in the environment, and may experience a disconnection with reality (from a mild inability to correctly interpret events to full *hallucinations*). Delirium may mimic other types of organically caused brain disorders, however, delirium and *dementia* are not the same thing. (RAPs) Delirium (acute confusional state) is a common indicator or nonspecific symptom of a variety of acute, treatable illnesses. It is a serious problem with high rates of *morbidity* and *mortality*, unless it is recognized and treated appropriately. Delirium is never a part of normal aging. Some of the classic signs of delirium may be difficult to recognize and may be mistaken for the natural progression of dementia, particularly in the late stages of dementia when delirium has high mortality. Thus, careful observation of the patient and review of potential causes are essential. Delirium is characterized by fluctuating states of consciousness, disorientation, decreased environmental awareness, and behavioral changes. The onset of delirium may vary, depending on the severity of the cause(s) and the patient's health status; however, it usually develops rapidly, over a few days or even hours. Even with successful treatment of cause(s) and associated symptoms, it may take several weeks before cognitive abilities return to pre-delirium status. See *alcohol-induced disorders, attention span, dementia, deprivation, orientation, physical restraint, psychotropic drugs.*

delirium tremens an acute, and sometimes fatal, reaction to the sudden lack of alcohol intake when the patient has been used to excessive amounts on a regular basis over a long period of time. The acute phase of withdrawal usually lasts from three to six days followed by days of deep sleep and depressed mood. The acute phase initially starts with a lack of appetite and restlessness. This is followed by severe *agitation*, coarse tremors of the extremities and tongue, mental confusion, vivid *hallucinations*, and cognitive disorientation. In addition, the person experiences a high *fever*, stomach upset, sweating, and an increased heart rate. Once the delirium tremens subsides, the patient sleeps for days, often experiencing deep *depression* and regretfulness. Delirium tremens is a medical emergency that requires medical attention and, frequently, *suicide* precautions. The *length of stay* is so short on many psychiatric, *dual diagnosis* units that therapists have little opportunity to see patients prior to their discharge. The first three to five days of delirium tremens usually require the patient to be in a low stimulation environment, ruling out most types of therapeutic *intervention*. See *orientation.*

Delphi technique a method of gathering expert opinion on an issue and then fine tuning the opinion by summarizing the results and asking the experts again for a response and possible consensus. Through this multiple-cycle process of polling the experts, the Delphi process helps achieve some group consensus among the experts. The Delphi technique consists of four distinct steps in each cycle: 1. developing the questionnaire, 2. distributing the questionnaire to a group of experts, 3. tallying the returned questionnaires, determining areas of agreement and disagreement, 4. statistically summarizing (obtaining a *mean*) for each item presented to the experts for their opinion and then providing feedback to the experts. Once this first cycle is completed, the panel of experts is asked to respond again to the same items. Each expert is allowed to review the statistical summary that accompanies each successive round of the questionnaire. Experts tend to revise their responses on the basis of this feedback to help achieve a consensus within the field. Delphi technique is a type of *face validly* and one means of establishing initial *construct validity.*

delusion a false belief firmly held despite incontrovertible and obvious proof or evidence to the contrary. Further, the belief is not one ordinarily accepted by other members of the person's culture or subculture. See *bipolar disorder, Global Assessment of Functioning Scale, schizophrenia.*

delusional disorder (HHS) a psychiatric disorder characterized by states of heightened self-awareness and a tendency toward paranoia. The **DSM-IV** requires that non-bizarre delusions be exhibited for at least one month, that the delusions are not related to hallucinations, that the behavior does not qualify as schizophrenia, that delusions are not acted out in a bizarre manner, and that the behaviors are not the physiological effect of a substance or other general medical condition. There are eight subcategories of delusional disorder shown in the accompanying chart.

Subcategories of Delusional Disorders

Type	Description
Erotomanic Type	The unfounded belief that another individual is in love with oneself. The object of this delusion often is of a higher status (economically, socially, or otherwise).
Grandiose Type	The overexaggeration of one's abilities or status (economically, socially, or otherwise).
Jealous Type	Holding an overwhelming belief, not based on fact, that one's significant other cares for someone else and has been unfaithful.
Persecutory Type	Holding the unsupported belief that an individual, group, or organization has treated oneself unfairly or with the intent to harm.
Somatic Type	Unsupported believing that physical or mental illness or conditions exist.
Mixed Type	Holding unsupported beliefs that contain elements of two or more of the above listed types of delusions and that don't obviously fall into just one category.
Unspecified Type	Holding delusional beliefs that don't fit into the other six categories.

demand management (HCO) a method of controlling health care costs by controlling access to health care services.

demand response systems (ADA) a system which transports individuals, including the provision of designated public transportation service by public entities and the provision of transportation service by private entities, including but not limited to specific public transportation service, which is not a *fixed route system*. The ADA accessibility guidelines for demand response systems may be found in the **Buses, Vans, and Systems Technical Assistance Manual** (US Architectural and Transportation Barriers Compliance Board).

dementia an illness or condition which is marked by a progressive loss of intellectual functions. The individual will demonstrate an up and down course of cognitive ability on a day-to-day and even hour-to-hour basis with an overall decrease in ability month by month. The ability to use information stored in

memory will decrease, as will the patient's ability to exercise good *judgment, executive function*, and *abstract reasoning*. Family members are usually the first to identify dementia because they notice a change in the patient's personality and an increased tendency to be "forgetful." Dementia in the past was usually referred to as senile onset (after the age of 65) or presenile onset (before the age of 65). Since the term "senile" is no longer politically correct, the terms "early onset" (before age 65) and "late onset" (after age 65) are now used. Dementia does not include a loss of cognitive ability due to *delirium* or *depression* — although both may mimic aspects of dementia. (RAPs) Approximately 60% of patients in nursing facilities exhibit signs and symptoms of decline in intellectual functioning. Recovery will be possible for less than 10% of these patients — those with a reversible condition such as an acute confusional state (delirium). For most patients the syndrome of cognitive loss or dementia is chronic and progressive and appropriate care focuses on enhancing *quality of life*, sustaining functional capabilities, minimizing decline, and preserving *dignity*. Confusion and/or behavioral disturbances present the primary complicating care factors. Identifying and treating acute confusion and behavior problems can facilitate assessment of how chronic cognitive deficits affect the life of the patient. For patients with chronic cognitive deficits, a therapeutic *environment* is supportive rather than curative and is an environment in which licensed and non-licensed care staff are encouraged (and trained) to comprehend a patient's experience of cognitive loss. With this insight, staff can develop *care plans* focused on three main goals: 1. to provide positive experiences for the patient (e.g., enjoyable activities) that do not involve overly demanding tasks and stress, 2. to define appropriate support roles for each staff member involved in a patient's care, and 3. to lay a foundation for reasonable staff and family expectations concerning a patient's capacities and needs. See *communication, dementia syndrome of depression, diminished, disoriented, focus, intelligence, Pick's disease, sunsetting, vascular dementia, visual function.*

dementia syndrome of depression a cognitive impairment found in geriatric patients as a secondary result of a distressed emotional state such as depression or a depressed physical state due to a side effect of medication or a temporary illness. It is not true dementia. Dementia syndrome of depression is commonly known as *pseudodementia*. The difference between true dementia and pseudodementia may be hard to distinguish. About 15% of elderly patients who are depressed show signs of dementia syndrome of depression and over 25% of elderly patients with true dementia also have clinically significant depression. The main distinction is that patients with pseudodementia are less likely to have a language deficit or to confabulate than patients with true dementia. Patients with pseudodementia are more likely to answer with "I don't know" to questions on reality *orientation* tests than patients with true dementia. See *confabulation, self-hypnosis.*

DEMPAQ See *Developing and Evaluating Methods to Promote Ambulatory Care Quality.*

dendrite a branched, protoplasmic extension of a nerve cell. A dendrite conducts impulses from adjacent cells towards the cell body. A nerve can have many dendrites.

denial 1. non-approval of a prospective provider's or supplier's initial request to participate in the Medicare or Medicaid program. See *reconsideration.* 2. subconscious defense mechanism used by an individual to delay needing to address a discomforting situation; a denial of part of reality. See *coping mechanisms.*

dental caries (HHS) popularly known as cavities. Dental caries occur when bacteria in the mouth feed on fermentable carbohydrates and produce acids that dissolve tooth enamel. Various conditions affect this process, such as heredity and the composition and flow of saliva. Any fermentable carbohydrate (starches and sugars) can serve as food for cavity-causing bacteria. The amount of carbohydrate is not as important as how often these foods are eaten and how long they stay in the mouth. Widespread use of *fluoride* in water supplies and oral health products is credited with the dramatic decline in dental caries among children and adults alike over the past 20 years.

Denver Developmental Screening Test (DDST) a screening tool used to measure a child's developmental level between six weeks and six years. The categories of *functional ability* measured are *gross-motor, fine-motor,* language, and personal social skills. The test classifies the child's score into one of three levels: "normal," "questionable," or "*abnormal.*" The DDST is the most commonly used preschool screening test in the United States even though it has been highly criticized. The process of interviewing the child's caregiver instead of having the therapist measure the child's functional ability leaves the results of the test open to question. This is the same problem that both the *General Recreation Screening Tool* (GRST) and the *Recreation Early Development Screening Tool* (REDS) have when the information is obtained from the patient's *caregiver.*

There is less of a problem if the testing is used only as a general placement indicator, also using other tests that have better *reliability.* See *General Recreation Screening Tool, Recreation Early Developmental Screening Tool.*

Departmental Appeals Board Department of Health and Human Services appeal entity to which states may appeal a disallowance of Medicaid *Federal Financial Participation* (FFP).

Department of Health and Human Services (DHHS) department within the United States government that oversees policies, procedures, and programs related to the nation's health. The *Health Care Financing Administration* (HCFA) is one part of DHHS. The organizational chart of the Department of Health and Human Services is shown below (D'Antonio-Nocera, DeBolt, and Touhey, 1996). See *Office of Civil Rights Clearance, regulatory agency.*

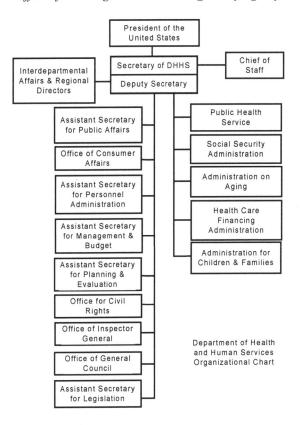

Department of Health and Human Services Organizational Chart

dependency act of being dependent or of relying on someone or something for support, satisfaction, or survival. Compare with *autonomy.*

dependent state of having to rely on another person or an object for emotional support (love, security, definition of self, etc.), physical support (ambulation, feeding, dressing, etc.), or cognitive support (reminders, language, problem solving, etc.) There is a psychiatric diagnosis termed *dependent* *personality disorder.* See *FIM.*

dependent personality disorder DSM-IV diagnosis referring to an individual who passively allows others to make most of the decisions for him/her. Individuals who have dependent personality disorder tend to lack an awareness of the skills they possess to take care of themselves and also lack *self-esteem* and self-confidence in the abilities that they do acknowledge they have. Health care workers can help decrease a patient's likelihood of developing dependent personality disorder not only by allowing patients to take care of themselves as much as possible but also by supportively encouraging them to do so. See *decision making.*

dependent position relaxed position of a limb, which is hanging downward, held in place by gravity.

depersonalization feeling that one is just part of a larger group, that the individual does not have an independent identity.

depression a feeling of sadness or grief. In patients with *cerebrovascular accidents* (CVA), this depression can be psychological and/or physiological. Depression is a mood state with many different possible diagnoses; some describing the severity and some describing a cause. To meet the criteria (**DSM-IV**) for a "major depressive episode" the patient needs to have demonstrated a change in his/her emotions such as a "down" mood or a loss of interest in life for at least two weeks. Additionally, at least five of the following nine symptoms must be present: 1. reports (or others report) a down mood lasting almost continuously, 2. significant decrease in interest in events around him/her evident almost continuously, 3. a change in eating habits that leads to a 5% loss or gain in weight, 4. a change in sleep patterns which lead to a significantly greater need for sleep or a significantly decreased need for (or ability to) sleep, 5. observable difference in motor activity (either greater as in fidgeting or lesser as in being a "couch potato"), 6. loss of energy on a regular basis, 7. overstated (not based on fact) feelings that s/he is not worth anything or excessive feelings of guilt on an almost daily basis, 8. noticeable decrease in the ability to concentrate or to make decisions during this period of time, and 9. recurrent thoughts about dying (suicidal ideation). The observed and felt symptoms must not be explained by a *bipolar disorder*, physiological effects of alcohol or other substances, and not explained by a general medical condition such as *hypothyroidism.* (Bereavement for a lost loved one is generally considered "normal" and only in certain situations is it considered to be a major depressive episode.) These symptoms must also be significant enough to negatively impact the patient's ability to function at work, school, socially, or in other important areas of the patient's life. A *dysthymia disorder* is similar to a major depressive disorder with the primary exception that the symptoms have lasted almost continuously for two or more years. General medical conditions may also be responsible for depression. Studies have found that over 50% of patients with CVAs have clinical depression. The closer the CVA is to the left frontal pole of the brain, the greater the risk for severe depression. Without intervention, this depression directly caused by the CVA will normally last 9 to 12 months. See *anhedonia, anorexia nervosa, autonomy, breathing, bulimia, communication, comorbidity, deconditioning, dementia, dementia syndrome of depression, dual diagnosis, electroconvulsive treatment, initiation, meditation, Minnesota Multiphasic Personality Inventory, mood state, post traumatic stress disorder, progressive relaxation, refuting irrational ideas, suicide.*

deprivation removal or reduction of a desirable or positive object or stimulus. The human body is meant to be bombarded with sensory input from all the senses during waking hours. A short period of sensory deprivation can be very therapeutic for individuals who frequently experience high levels of stimulation. *Relaxation techniques* are a healthy, self-initiated type of sensory deprivation. For individuals who are restricted to environments that provide an unhealthy sensory environment (e.g., hospitals, nursing homes, other residential institutions), one of the most important treatment *interventions* for the professional is to offset the harm done by the lack of healthy stimulation in the environment. A patient will be at an increased risk to develop *delirium* and other cognitive disorders after as little as two days in an unhealthy sensory environment. Fred Rogers (Mr. Rogers on TV) goes as far as to suggest that every person would be healthier if they were exposed to the natural stimulation found out of doors one to two hours a day, every day of the year. An individual who has an impaired ability to *focus* may also experience deprivation due to an inability to take in appropriate stimulation. See *bed, bronchopulmonary dysplasia, communication board, deconditioning.*

depth perception ability to perceive that objects have three dimensions and to be able to distinguish between objects which are close at hand and those that are distant.

dermal graft graft that uses only a thin layer of the dermis. The epidermis and subcutaneous fat have been removed prior to positioning the graft.

Types of Dermatitis

Type	Description
chronic dermatitis	variety of causes; variety of lesion types, may follow long remission periods
contact dermatitis	due to contact of skin with irritants; may be an allergic response
exfoliative dermatitis	usually a progression of an existing skin dermatitis; symptoms include large loss of the top layer of skin and inflammation; may require hospitalization with protective isolation
localized neurodermatitis	a chronic scratching or rubbing of a lesion or insect bite, intense itching, lesions may disappear two weeks after scratching stops
nummular dermatitis	due to stress, dryness of skin/air, contact irritants, or prolonged scratching; coin shaped lesions on easily accessible body parts (e.g., legs, arms)
seborrheic dermatitis	dermatitis of unknown causes, stress thought to be a factor, lesions usually erupt on scalp, face, and trunk area; dandruff may be a mild case of seborrheic dermatitis
stasis dermatitis	a secondary effect of peripheral vascular disease; usually limited to lower legs; starts as dusky red spots, develops into edema, redness, and scaling of skin

dermatitis an inflammation of the skin. There are many different kinds of dermatitis. At the top of the page are some of the major categories of dermatitis. Compare to *eczema*.

dermis a layer of the skin that lies just beneath the *epidermis*. See *skin*.

desensitization an effective treatment technique of immediate or gradual exposure to a stimulus that evokes fear. Desensitization is applied in a repetitive manner and can be classified using the following criteria: 1. in vivo (in life) or contact desensitization, 2. systematic desensitization or reciprocal inhibition deconditioning, 3. cognitive/behavioral strategies such as cognitive restructuring and assertiveness training, 4. implosive therapy or flooding. See *coping techniques*.

designated public transportation (ADA) a transportation system that is run by a public entity (other than public school transportation) by bus, rail, or other conveyance (other than transportation by aircraft or intercity or commuter rail transportation) that provides the general public with general or specific service, including charter service, on a regular and continuing basis. The ADA accessibility guidelines for designated public transportation may be found in the **Buses, Vans, and Systems Technical Assistance Manual** (US Architectural and Transportation Barriers Compliance Board).

detectable warning (ADA) a standardized surface feature built in or applied to walking surfaces or other elements to warn people who are visually impaired of hazards on a circulation path. See *circulation path*.

Detroit Tests of Learning Aptitude (DTLA) (multiple versions available) The Detroit Tests of Learning Aptitude are usually administered by a psychologist or special education instructor. The results obtained by this assessment help the team know the person's verbal/non-verbal, attentional, and motor ability compared to his/her peers. The DTLA-P:2 is for children ages 3-9 and the DTLA-3 is for children ages 6 - 17. Once the therapist knows the person's scores from the Detroit Tests of Learning Aptitude and the person's activity preferences, s/he should be able to develop an activity-based treatment intervention which will help the person increase skills through fun or meaningful activities.

Developing and Evaluating Methods to Promote Ambulatory Care Quality (DEMPAQ) (HCO) a set of performance indicators for ambulatory care providers that is being developed by HCFA for its Medicare program.

development ongoing changes (cognitive, emotional, social, and physical) as a result of physiological and environmental influences. These changes can be measured both quantitatively and qualitatively and generally follow expected patterns of growth or development. Developmental norms are used to determine if a person is developing as expected. See *magical thinking, medical play*.

developmental age age at which the skills an individual has are normally obtained.

developmental coordination disorder a formal diagnosis in the **DSM-IV** under the general category of disorders usually first diagnosed in infancy, childhood, or adolescence. An individual is considered to have a developmental coordination disorder if s/he is significantly less coordinated, displays substantially slower progress in physical skill/motor tasks than his/her peers of a similar age and intelligence ability. These impairments must be great enough to make a difference in the child's performance at school and in basic ADLs. If the lack of physical *coordination* is due to any known medical diagnosis such as *cerebral palsy, muscular dystrophy*, or *paralysis* the correct diagnosis would be the medical

Diabetes, Concerns for Therapy

Concern	Implications
decreased ability to assimilate sugars	Exercise is an important component of treatment for individuals with diabetes. To help assist in balancing the insulin hormone in the body, the individual should develop a balanced pattern of activities using physical movements. This balance allows for easier control of diet and insulin requirements and helps avoid ketoacidosis (serious imbalance of insulin in the body causing *dehydration*, electrolyte imbalance, acidosis, *coma*, and then death).
insulin use during activity	Insulin is absorbed faster in muscles that are used extensively (therefore putting individuals who depend on insulin therapy at greater risk of depleting the insulin too quickly). The professional may want to evaluate the muscle groups used in any newly learned leisure or vocational activity to insure that any significant increase in the activity of muscles near the typical injection site is not going to increase activity enough to cause risk. A simple solution is to arrange for the insulin site to be changed.
decreased sensation	The professional should assess the degree to which decreased *sensation* in the lower extremities caused by microvascular disease will increase the individual's risk during activities. Ill-fitted shoes, water, or air temperatures in either extreme or breaks in skin integrity could be hazardous. Add to these problems a diagnosis of *mental retardation* or *traumatic brain injury* and the individual is at increased risk.

diagnosis and not developmental coordination disorder. See *activities of daily living, intelligence.*

developmental disability a disability caused by an individual's abnormal developmental growth and/or experiencing the world differently than others. An individual with an acquired C3 quadriplegia at age two years will experience a developmental delay related to spatial awareness because s/he is not able to purposefully move himself/herself around his/her environment and is not able to explore the environment in the same manner as his/her peers. See *bronchopulmonary dysplasia, cerebral palsy, Public Law 94-103, visual impairments.*

developmental sequence incremental steps of learning experienced by the majority of the population. For the most part, individuals learn tasks and knowledge in similar qualitative and quantitative patterns of growth and *development.*

DHHS See *Department of Health and Human Services.*

diabetes also known as diabetes mellitus. A disorder in the body's production and use of insulin and in the body's use of blood sugar resulting in a high blood glucose level. Diabetes has both short-term and long-term consequences. Individuals with diabetes have a disorder that causes the abnormal metabolism of carbohydrates, fats, and proteins. Diabetes is divided into three groups: 1. non-insulin dependent also known as "Type II" (the vast majority of individuals), 2. insulin dependent also known as "Type I," and 3. maturity-onset diabetes of youth, also known as "MODY." All three types of diabetes are treated through use of an appropriately balanced diet, exercise, and in the case of individuals who are insulin dependent, insulin. There are a few diseases that are a direct result of diabetes, which the professional may want to be familiar with:

1. Macrovascular disease is the development of enlarged blood vessels. This enlargement affects the metabolism of carbohydrates leading to a significantly increased likelihood of a *cerebrovascular accident* and an increased likelihood of a heart attack.
2. Microvascular disease is a disorder of the smaller blood vessels in the body. Individuals with diabetes may develop problems with nephropathy (disease of the kidneys), retinopathy (ongoing damage to the small vessels which provide blood to the eyes), and neuropathy (degenerative/pathological changes in the peripheral nervous system which decreases function).

The chart above shows some of the concerns for therapy. See *aerobics, arteriosclerotic disease, diet — prescribed, neuropathy, visual impairment.*

diabetic acidosis (HHS) a condition in diabetic patients in which the levels of alkali are reduced relative to the level of acids.

diabetic ketoacidosis (HHS) a form of acidosis in diabetic patients caused by the enhanced production of ketone bodies.

diabetic nephrosclerosis (HHS) a condition in diabetic patients marked by hardening of the kidney from overgrowth and contraction of the connective tissue of the organ.

diagnosis art and science of distinguishing one *disease* or *disorder* from another. Most diagnoses have

Recommended Diet for Chronic Pain Patients (Rook, 1995)

Foods that are Allowed	Food to be Avoided
Fresh fruit	Soft drinks with sugar
Fresh vegetables	Ice cream
Fish (backed or broiled)	Syrups
Fowl (skinned and not fried)	Canned fruits packed in syrup
Diet drinks (no caffeine or sugar)	Cakes and cookies
Freshly squeezed juices	Donuts
Veal	Candies
Lean roast beef	Bologna
Lobster and shrimp (no butter)	Salami
Skim milk	Hot dogs
Tuna (water packed)	Bacon
Oatmeal (plain)	Fried foods
Cereals (low sugar)	Potato chips
Low-fat cheeses	Butter, margarine, and mayonnaise
Low-fat yogurt (and fresh fruit)	
Olive oil for cooking	

commonly known, standardized definitions for what symptoms are present (and not present). Once a diagnosis has been assigned, the treatment team will be able to work with a common understanding of the patient's needs, limitations, and strengths. For mental disorders the professional will find it extremely helpful to read the **DSM-IV** (**Diagnostic and Statistical Manual of Mental Disorders, Fourth Edition**) published by the American Psychiatric Association (1994). This book lists the functional skills lacking in individuals with each disorder. After confirming with the **DSM-IV,** the professional may find it easier to formulate *assessment* plans and treatment *objectives* for patients with psychiatric diagnoses. The other publication that lists the standardized diagnoses is the **ICD 9 CM** (*International Classification of Diseases 9th Revision Clinical Modification*) published by the US Department of Health and Human Services. The **ICD 9 CM** contains the recognized medical diagnoses. See *admission/discharge record, dual diagnosis, process, sign, therapy.*

Diagnostic and Statistical Manual of Mental Disorders, Fourth Edition See **DSM-IV.**

Diagnostic and Statistical Manual of Mental Disorders, Third Edition, Revised See **DSM-III-R.**

diagnostic related groups a type of reimbursement payment strategy also known as the *prospective payment system* (PPS). Diagnostic related groups (DRGs) puts patients with similar *diagnoses* and needs into a single group. Groupings take into consideration primary and secondary diagnoses, primary and secondary procedures, patient age, and typical length of inpatient stay. Payment for patients within that group is determined by a national and regional history of previously approved services. (HCO) a class of health problems derived from sets of diagnoses and procedure codes and used by HCFA to determine reimbursement for treatments.

DIAPPERS an acronym used to list the most common causes of transient urinary incontinence: delirium, infection, atrophic urethritis/vaginitis, pharmaceuticals, psychological (especially severe depression), excess urine output, restricted mobility, and stool impaction.

DICOM See *digital imaging and communications in medicine.*

diet — for pain a diet that seems to reduce the amount of pain a patient experiences. Based on the idea that certain types of food are responsible for increased pain. See the Recommended Diet for Chronic Pain Patients above.

diet — prescribed types of food a patient is allowed to eat. There are six primary types of diet prescribed for patients. It is important that the therapist is aware of the type of diet prescribed for each patient, as well as specific dietary and fluid restrictions. Common types of prescribed diets are shown on the next page.

differentiation ability to 1. identify the unique aspects or elements of an object or event, 2. compare those aspects and elements to another object or event, and 3. identify the differences between the objects or events.

digital imaging and communications in medicine (DICOM) (HCO) a standard for communications among medical imaging devices.

Common Types of Prescribed Diets

Type	Description
Clear Liquid	A diet limited to liquids that are clear, including water, clear broth, clear fruit juices, plain gelatin, tea, and coffee. Check to see if caffeine or carbonation is allowed.
Full Liquid	Thick fluids including different kinds of juices (e.g., pureed vegetable and fruit juices), milk, ice cream, gelatin, custards, and other non-alcoholic drinks that generally accompany a meal.
Light or Convalescent	This diet may include most foods, the difference is in how the food is prepared. Raw and fried foods are usually not allowed. Foods that are high in fat, which produce fat, or which are hard to digest are not allowed.
Mechanical Soft	Similar to the light or convalescent diet, this food differs only in that it needs to be prepared for individuals who are not able to chew the food (e.g., those with no teeth). Whole meats are avoided because they require chewing.
Regular or General	A diet that allows most kinds of foods, provides a balanced nutritional intake, allows the patient to make some choices of foods and which totals about 1400 calories in every 24-hour period.
Special Therapeutic	A diet which is selected to meet the patient's specific needs due to *allergies*, caloric intake (high or low), *diabetes*, or for patients needing particular amounts of specific types of food (e.g., reduced salt, fat, fiber, high or low protein).

digital palpitation the use of one's fingers to feel and assess a body part.

digital signal processor (HCO) a special-purpose computer processor customized to make rapid calculations associated with audio or video data streams.

dignity (OBRA) Federal law in the United States requires that all staff treat patients with dignity. This means that in their interactions with patients, staff carry out activities that assist the patient to maintain and enhance his/her self-worth. For example:

- *Grooming* patients as they wish to be groomed (e.g., hair combed, beards shaved/trimmed, nails clean and clipped);
- Assisting patients to dress in their own clothes appropriate to the time of day and individual preferences (See *dressing.*);
- Promoting patient independence and dignity in dining in long-term care facilities including such things as avoidance of day-to-day use of plastic cutlery and paper/plastic dishware, dining room conducive to pleasant dining, aides not yelling;
- Respecting patient's private space and property (e.g., not changing radio or television station without patient's permission);
- Respecting patient's social status, speaking respectfully, listening carefully, treating patients with respect (e.g., addressing the patient with a name of the patient's choice); and
- Focusing on patients as individuals when they talk to them. (Guidance to Surveyors, Tag 241)

See *dementia, physical restraint*

dimension I-IV See *mental retardation.*

diminished loss of a previously gained skill or skills. Individuals with dementia have diminished cognitive skills. See *cognition, disintegration, dysfunction, regression.*

diminished sensation a subnormal awareness of contact. See *sensation.*

diplegia paralysis of the same part on both sides of the individual's body (e.g., paralysis of both arms).

diplopia double vision; seeing two of the same object.

directionality skill to be able to determine direction — where you just came from, the way back, the way to specific locations; an element of both short and long-term *memory*. See *pathfinding.*

director of nursing services (DNS) nurse who is the manager over the nursing services in a facility.

disability (ADA) legally defined, a physical or mental impairment that substantially limits one or more of the *major life activities* of an individual; where there is a record of such an impairment; or being regarded as having such an impairment. The term disability does not include 1. transvestitism, transsexualism, *pedophilia*, exhibitionism, voyeurism, gender identity disorders not resulting from physical impairments, or other sexual behavior disorders; 2. compulsive gambling, *kleptomania*, or *pyromania*; or 3. psychoactive substance use disorders resulting from current illegal use of drugs. See the table on the next page, Worker's Compensation Disability Levels, for levels of disability recognized in the United States. See *substance abuse, idiopathic.*

disability rating a standardized system to rate the degree of functional loss caused by a disability. See *functional ability.*

Worker's Compensation Disability Levels (United States)

Level	Description
Temporary Total Disability	This category addresses the period immediately after the injury, when the patient is convalescing and receiving aggressive medical care. If the employer is unable to provide work that allows for the employee's disability, then temporary total disability is continued. Payment is rendered for the employee's loss of wages.
Temporary Partial Disability	This category indicates that the employee is able to return to work part-time after the work-related injury and that the inability to work full-time is the result of that injury. A percentage of temporary total disability benefits is paid.
Permanent Partial Disability	This category applies when the determined healing period has ended (e.g., when the condition is stable and it is thought that further treatment will have no substantial effect). Permanent partial disability can reflect permanent impairment due to a *scheduled injury* or *nonscheduled injury*.
Permanent Total Disability	A person is designated as permanently totally disabled when s/he is judged to be permanently impaired and unable to return to work at any time in the future. Benefits in this situation are paid weekly and are determined on a state-by-state basis.

disarticulation removal of a part of the body by cutting through a joint. See *amputation.*

discharge 1. act of terminating a patient's active status of receiving services. See *right to appeal.* 2. drainage of fluids from an opening in the body.

discharge abstract See *admission/discharge record.*

discharge plan a written plan that contains the criteria for discharge, resources, equipment, and contacts required before and after discharge. The plan is written in the first few days after admission and modified as the patient's status changes. See *alternative disposition plan, elopement, intake assessment.*

discharge summary a report that the professional writes when s/he will no longer be treating the patient. This report may be seen by another health care professional the same day that the report is written or it may be reviewed by a health care professional years later. To help make the discharge summary useful and easy to understand, it is recommend that:

- Whenever possible, refer to the specific instead of the general; be concrete instead of abstract.
- Take care with what you say and how you say it. Avoid fancy or obscure words, abbreviations, or words that overstate. Avoid qualifiers such as "rather, very, little, pretty."
- When you write, be clear, document sequentially; be brief but do not take short cuts that might leave out key information.
- Whenever possible, write your statements in the positive, e.g., "patient was able to ambulate 45 feet between stores before needing to rest" versus "patient was not able to ambulate between stores before needing to rest." The second sentence also leaves the reader wondering if the patient had functional ambulation skills or if the patient could go 50 feet before needing a rest – two very different cases. While being positive,

do not be reluctant to provide realistic or negative findings.

- If the treatment was as a result of a *referral,* make sure that all issues addressed in the referral are answered in the discharge summary.
- It will not be helpful to future readers of the discharge summary if you include just raw data from your *assessments.* Include a concise interpretation of all data presented.
- Whenever you make a recommendation, make sure that the justification for that recommendation can be found in your discharge summary.
- Without being long-winded, include an alternative recommendation or an alternative course of action, if it is appropriate for the situation. (See *alternate disposition plan.*)
- Make your recommendations realistic for the patient, his/her cultural, social, and economic background and for his/her discharge destination.
- Remember that the discharge summary is just that, a summary. All of the information presented should be brought together in a way that presents the entire picture of all the pertinent information. (Armstrong & Lauzen, 1994 and Zuckerman, 1994)

discretionary time time during which the individual is free of obligations and can make decisions about the use of that time. Contrast with *leisure.*

discrimination See *consumer rights.*

disease a pathological progression with commonly recognized characteristics which have identifiable *signs* and symptoms. Not the same as *disorder.* See *diagnosis, etiology, exacerbate, idiopathic.*

disease management (HCO) a method of managing the care of a specific health problem (usually a chronic and costly disease) that employs the principles of *continuous quality improvement*, including the use of *clinical practice guidelines*, *outcome* measurement, and *feedback* to providers and insurance plans.

disease model (also known as *medical model*) theory that states the origin of most psychiatric disorders can be found in *disease* states. This is generally the opposite of the *behavioral model*, which looks at psychological disorders more as a behavioral or thought pattern dysfunction and not a disease state.

disease state having a disease.

disenfranchised feeling of being separate from one's *culture*. See *acculturation*.

disengagement theory a theory on aging that was popular in the 1960's, which stated that as a person, aged, s/he tended to withdraw from the community and social systems in preparation for death.

disequilibrium a loss of part or all of one's *equilibrium*.

disintegration generally meant to be a substantial loss or disorganization of one's behavioral, psychological, moral, personality, cognitive, or other systems of functioning in the world. More severe than *diminished*. See *dysfunction*.

dislocation displacement of a bone from its correct alignment in the joint.

disorder a disability caused by a specific event or stimuli. Disorders generally fall into one of three types: *congenital*, chronic, or acute. Disorders may arise from congenital malformation, movement dysfunctions, postural syndromes, or traumatic injuries.

See *diagnosis, disease, etiology, exacerbate, mixed*.

disorientation temporary (due to drugs, alcohol, etc.) or permanent (due to *dementia*, *CVAs*, etc.) inability to understand and use informational stimuli in one's environment. Disorientation may be divided into three areas: 1. temporal — the inability to tell and use time (time of day, time of year, time of life, etc.), 2. spatial — the inability to distinguish between and use both visual and non-visual information (e.g., proprioception, a mental map of where one is in relationship to room, etc.), and 3. contextual — the inability to cognitively process events in the environment and/or identify objects (including oneself). See *memory deficit*.

displacement a defense mechanism, operating unconsciously, in which emotions, ideas, or wishes are transferred from their original object to a more acceptable substitute; often used to allay *anxiety*. See *coping mechanisms*.

disproportionate share hospitals (FB) hospitals that serve a relatively large volume of low-income patients and therefore receive a payment adjustment under the prospective payment system from Medicare and Medicaid.

dissociation process of separating one's emotions from what one is doing or experiencing. Severe dissociation may cause painful memories to be "forgotten" by the individual. Severe dissociation, called "dissociative reaction" is different from forms of *schizophrenia*, as the individual still stays generally based in reality.

Dissociative Disorders

Type	Description
Dissociative Amnesia	Usually as a result of a traumatic or stressful event (or events), an individual is not able to recall personal information. The degree of forgetfulness is beyond what would normally be expected.
Dissociative Fatigue	An inability to recall who one is, often associated with a sudden and unexpected break from normal patterns and travel away from home, work, and other normal activities. The individual may take on an new identity without remembering his/her past identity.
Dissociative Identity Disorder	The presence of two or more different personalities assumed by the individual, each "sharing" the individual, and each taking over the individual's behavior when it is "present." The individual is unable to recall events and information acquired while in one role when s/he is in another role. This inability to use the memory obtained while in one personality when assuming another personality cannot be explained by normal forgetfulness. This disorder used to be called multiple personality disorder.
Depersonalization Disorder	The feeling of being detached from one's body or mind while still retaining the ability to be cognitively present and without assuming another personality. This feeling is persistent and recurring.
Dissociative Disorder Not Otherwise Specified	This type of dissociative disorder is for individuals with symptoms that meet the general definition of a dissociative disorder but whose behavioral and cognitive presentation does not fit comfortably into any of the other four types.

dissociative disorders a group of five psychiatric disorders that all share the feature of a break in normally integrated aspects of personality. With dissociative disorders an individual may demonstrate intermittent inability to act with one identity. In the past this set of disorders was referred to as multiple personality disorders. See the chart on the previous page.

distal opposite of close; away from the center or midline of the body. The fingers are more distal to the chest than the shoulder. Compare with *proximal.*

distinct part a component within a facility that furnishes a different level or type of service covered under Medicare or Medicaid. A distinct part component must be recognizable or distinguishable as separate. An example would be a wing of a hospital that is being used as a nursing home.

distractibility ease with which an individual's attention is drawn away from a task. Distractibility is a result of a conscious or unconscious lack of filtering out stimuli in the environment. See *attention span, bipolar disorder.*

diuretics medications or natural substances that cause the body to produce extra urine, often by causing the fluid between cells to drain toward the kidneys. Typically patients with congestive heart failure, hypertension, or edema will be placed on diuretic medication. One of the common side effects of most diuretic medications is electrolyte imbalance and hypovolemia, causing patients to feel lightheaded and more prone to falls. If a patient with one of those three disorders demonstrates balance problems during activity, the therapist should contact the patient's physician to help rule out diuretic medications as the cause of the balance problems.

diversional program a program of activities that diverts the patient's attention from discomfort or stressful thoughts. May or may not be medically indicated, therefore in only a few cases is it therapeutic and billable. A card game because a patient is bored is a non-therapeutic filling of time. A card game to allow the patient practice waiting (objective: decrease *impulsivity*) and practice overcoming left neglect with a therapist present to provide *cueing* is a therapeutic *treatment.* See *electroconvulsive treatment, neglect — visual.*

diverticulitis a disease of the small sacs that form the wall of the large intestine. Weak intestinal walls allow sections of the intestinal wall to push through surrounding muscles causing pockets. This process causes an irritation to the wall of the colon, reducing flow, and causing stagnation of food or feces in the pockets. While it is estimated that up to 40% of elderly Americans have some form of this disease, only the most severe forms show any symptoms. In the acute stage, the patient may experience inflammation of the peritoneum and formation of an abscess. The typical symptoms are pain in the lower left side between the waist and the hipbone with alternating problems of *constipation* and diarrhea along with flatulence. A low-grade *fever* may develop. Severe cases may require surgical correction including bowel resection or *colostomy.* More and more elderly are being admitted to the hospital to be treated for this condition. Diverticular disease is thought to be due, in part, to a lack of roughage in the patient's diet. The therapist may want to educate and encourage good selection of food (especially fresh fruit and vegetables) that contain roughage. Fluid intake is also important. Watch for electrolyte imbalance during treatment; strictly adhere to fluid intake and output measurement requirements. If patient is currently experiencing internal bleeding as a result of the disease, avoid having the patient flex his/her legs at the groin unless told to do so by the physician.

DNA (HHS) deoxyribonucleic acid; the molecule that carries the genetic information for most living systems. The DNA molecule consists of four bases (adenine, cytosine, guanine, and thymine) and a sugar-phosphate backbone, arranged in two connected strands to form its characteristic double helix.

DNR orders See *Do Not Resuscitate orders.*

DNS See *director of nursing services.*

documentation written information about events that others may read, which provides a record of treatment and services; the process of making a permanent record. Initial health care documentation includes prior medical history, a baseline for initial patient function, a description of function anticipated at discharge, the specific diagnosis (disease, illness, or disability) addressed, and the treatment that is used to address the diagnosis to achieve the desired outcome. Documentation also includes the patient's insight into treatment needs. To be considered complete, documentation related to treatment must also include information relating to, or implying, the medical necessity of the service, the skill provided, and the outcomes (patient function) seen as a result of the service. On-going documentation includes information related to the areas addressed during specific treatment sessions, the patient's response to the treatment, and changes in the patient's status. Common rules for writing in a medical chart are shown in the chart on the next page. See *discharge summary, narrative style, PIE, problem-oriented record, problem list, progress notes, quarterly notes, risk management, SOAP, uniform data system.*

doff to take off. Usually referring to a patient's abil-

Common Rules for Documentation in a Medical Chart

Topic	Discussion
Abbreviations	The only abbreviations that may be used in the medical chart are the pre-approved abbreviations found in the facility's policy and procedure manuals. Therapists who work as consultants should obtain a copy of the approved abbreviations from each facility in which they consult to ensure that only the abbreviations pre-approved for that facility are used in the medical chart. If the consultant wants to have abbreviations added to the approved list, s/he should approach the medical records department of that facility to have specific abbreviations added to the "official" list.
Accurate	Entries should be made that are objective (what the therapist has observed through seeing, hearing, smelling, or touching) and factual (events and actions that the therapist can attest to because s/he directly observed them). Subjective comments (statements by others) may be recorded only as direct quotes with the source of the quote attributed in the documentation.
Adverbs and Adjectives	The therapist should use adverbs and adjectives to better describe the patient's function and response to treatment (e.g., <u>inconsistent</u> short-term memory during session, <u>abrupt</u> gait used when ambulating in the community, <u>apprehensive</u> affect during bingo).
Content	The content of the documentation should be concise, including enough detail to clearly describe.
Continuity of Documentation	The author of a progress note should always read his/her last two entries (or the last two entries of his/her service, i.e., the entry of the therapist in the same department who saw the patient last) to make sure that all notations for follow-through have been addressed. This check-back helps increase the continuity of care.
Corrections of Errors	If an error is made in documentation, the author of the error should draw one horizontal line through the error (allowing the error to still be readable) and then place the date the line was drawn through (month/day/year) and his/her initials above the crossed out material. Never erase or use white out in medical charts.
Date	Each entry in the medical chart should be dated, and in some facilities, a time noted using *military time*.
Format	The format used to document in the medical chart should follow the facility's policies and procedures for documentation. The *narrative style of documenting* tends to be the most popular, however, *SOAP Notes* are still used in many facilities.
Frequency	The frequency of documentation is set by each facility but generally follows a specific schedule (e.g., once a week or each contact) or event (with measurable change, as each treatment goal is obtained, after each team meeting).
Penmanship	All entries in the medical chart should be easily read by everyone who needs to read the chart.
Signing Note	The therapist should sign each entry in the medical chart with his/her full name followed by his/her title or professional credential.
Writing Instrument	It is standard to write using only a black ink ballpoint pen. Never use pencils. Magic markers tend to "bleed" to the back side of the progress note, making other entries hard to read.

ity to undress himself/herself or to take off a piece of adapted equipment by himself/herself. See *dressing, dressing skills*.

don to put on. Usually referring to a patient's ability to dress himself/herself or to put on a piece of adapted equipment by himself/herself. See *dressing, dressing skills*.

do not resuscitate orders (DNR orders) a medical order, backed up by a legal document signed by the patient or legal guardian allowing staff to refrain from applying life saving measures to restore breathing or heartbeat. See *durable power of attor-*

ney, no code.

dopamine a neurotransmitter. Dopamine works as an inhibitor for various functions, is a factor in motor control systems in the body and impacts *behaviors* and *emotional*/motivational reactions. A neurosynaptic transmitter found in the central nervous system, specifically associated with some forms of psychosis and abnormal movement disorders. See *tardive dyskinesia*.

Doppler-Ultrasound a test used to check for turbulent blood flow caused by narrowing in the arteries, which may be the cause of transient blockage of blood flow to the brain.

dorsiflexion moving a body part closer to the center plane of the body by flexing or bending. To dorsiflex the foot, the patient would flex the toes toward the body. To dorsiflex the hand, the patient would cock his/her hand back over the wrist, exposing the palm.

double-blind, placebo-controlled study (HHS) In a double-blind, placebo controlled study, neither the researchers nor the participants in the study are aware of which subjects receive the treatment under study and which subjects receive the placebo until after the study is completed. The study design is intended to remove bias on the part of both researcher and study subject. See *blind experiment*.

Down syndrome a chromosome disorder (trisomy 21) which usually includes *mental retardation*, distinctive facial features, and congenital heart defects. A good testing tool to measure the incremental developmental progress of youth with Down syndrome is the *Denver Developmental Screening Tool*. See *atrioventricular canal, chromosomal aberrations, inclusive recreation*.

drainage/secretion precautions isolation an isolation procedure for patients with infectious diseases that are producing an infective purulent material, drainage, or secretions. The isolation procedure includes: 1. masks are not indicated, 2. gowns are indicated if soiling is likely, 3. gloves are indicated for touching infective material, 4. hands must be washed after touching the patient or potentially contaminated articles and before taking care of another patient, and 5. articles contaminated with infective material should be discarded or bagged and labeled before being sent for decontamination and reprocessing. The sign for drainage/secretion precautions is always green.

dressing coverings applied to wounds or diseased tissue to protect it from further injury, to absorb secretions, and to reduce the risk of infection. See *wet-to-dry dressing*.

dressing putting on clothing. For a patient to be considered independent in dressing s/he would need to be able to complete the following tasks without cueing or other assistance:

1. ability to determine appropriate clothing for the situation, activity, and weather,
2. ability to identify where the clothing is kept and then obtain the clothing,
3. ability to *don* (put on) and *doff* (take off) clothing, shoes, and appliances in a sequential fashion,
4. ability to manipulate buttons, zippers, ties, etc. as needed for clothing and appliances.

While the patient's initial training in these skills will most likely come from an occupational therapist, the recreational therapist will need to supervise, assist, and evaluate the patient in his/her skills related to dressing while on community integration outings. (OBRA) This refers to the patient's ability to put on, fasten, and take off all items of street clothing, including donning or removing *prostheses* (e.g., braces and artificial limbs). In the United States, many facilities routinely set out clothes for all patients. If this is the case and this is the only assistance the patient receives, the patient is still considered to be independent in dressing. However, if a patient receives assistance with donning a brace, elastic stocking (e.g., *Jobst*), a prosthesis, and so on, securing fasteners, or putting a garment on, this patient is counted as needing assistance in dressing.

dressing skills one aspect of *advanced activities of daily living*, advanced dressing skills are skills which allow the patient to use good *judgment* in the selection of appropriate clothing (e.g., swimsuit for pool, winter coat for snow skiing), allow the patient to use *executive function* and knowledge of social expectations to dress socially appropriately (fashion awareness), and allow the patient to manipulate buckles, ties, and other aspects of *fine motor* and *gross motor* movement to *doff* or *don* clothing and equipment.

DRG See *diagnostic related group*.

drug abuse improper and/or illegal use of drugs usually implying that this use is in excess of the normal dosage, that it is harmful and socially or legally unacceptable. See *substance abuse*.

Drug Enforcement Agency (DEA) federal agency that, among other things, issues the licenses to prescribe and to dispense controlled substances. See *controlled dangerous substance*.

drug-resistant Streptococcus pneumoniae disease (DRSP) one of the possible infectious agents responsible for pneumonia, bacteremia, otitis media (OM), meningitis, peritonitis, and sinusitis. (CDC) Five sero-types (6B, 9V, 14, 19A, and 23F) account for most DRSP. Since 1987, the incidence of DRSP has increased in the United States. Each year, S. pneumoniae infections cause 2,600 meningitis cases, 63,000 bacteremia cases, 100,000-135,000 hospitalizations for pneumonia, and 7 million OM cases. Of these infections, 10%-40% are caused by DRSP. Prevalence of DRSP shows wide geographic variation. Death occurs in 14% of hospitalized adults with invasive disease. *Neurologic sequelae* occur in meningitis patients. Learning disabilities and/or hearing impairment can result from recurrent OM. DRSP is associated with increased costs due to use of antimicrobial agents, recurrent disease, surveillance, education, and new antimicrobial drug development. Person-to-person transmission with a symptomatic carriage in the nose and throat is common. Persons who attend or work at child-care centers and persons who recently used antimicrobial agents are at increased risk for infection with DRSP. Prevalence of strains resistant to multiple classes of drugs is increasing. Outbreaks of DRSP have been reported in nursing homes, institutions for HIV-infected persons, and child-care centers. Widespread overuse of antimicrobial agents has contributed to emerging resistance. Some clinical laboratories have not adopted standard methods (NCCLS guidelines) for identifying and defining DRSP. Campaigns for more judicious use of antibiotics may slow or reverse emerging drug resistance. Prevention of infections could improve through expanded use of 23-valent polysaccharide vaccine. The newly developed pneumococcal conjugate vaccine, licensed in February 2000, is effective in infants and young children. Among children < 5 years of age, it elicits protection against ~80% of invasive pneumococcal isolates that are not susceptible to penicillin.

DS-0, DS-1, DS-3 (HCO) digital telecommunications channels capable of transmitting 64 kilobits, 1.544 megabits, and 45 megabits per second, respectively. The higher capacity connections are suitable for high-volume voice, data, or compressed video traffic.

DSM-III-R Diagnostic and Statistical Manual of Mental Disorders, Third Edition, Revised published by the American Psychiatric Association in 1987. This is not the most current edition and many of the disorders listed in this version are no longer considered accepted diagnoses (e.g., *organic brain syndrome*, multiple personality disorder).

DSM-IV Diagnostic and Statistical Manual of Mental Disorders, Fourth Edition published by the American Psychiatric Association in 1994. This edition of the **DSM-IV** contains the most current diagnostic classifications for psychiatric disorders.

DTs See *delirium tremens.*

dual certification simultaneous participation of a facility as a *provider* or supplier of two types of Medicare or Medicaid services. An example is a facility that is a nursing home (*OBRA*) for adults with *mental retardation* or *learning disabilities* (*intermediate care facility for the mentally retarded*). See *dual participation.*

dual diagnosis a patient description which indicates that the patient has more than one major diagnosis; each of the major diagnoses must be addressed together as there is a *comorbidity* (causal or medical connection) between them. The most common type of dual diagnosis includes a combination of mental illness and *substance abuse*. Studies have frequently reported the connection between *antisocial personality disorder* and alcohol or substance abuse-related disorders. Whether one is a precursor to the other has not been established to the point of general acceptance. A full 30% to 40% of individuals with *alcohol-related disorders* also meet the **DSM-IV** criteria for mood disorders, most commonly *depression*. Studies report that between 25% and 50% of individuals with diagnosable *anxiety* disorders also have alcohol-related disorders. Some feel that this may be the case because individuals often use alcohol to calm themselves. The dual diagnosis with alcohol and anxiety are most common with individuals who have *phobias* or *panic disorders*. Many researchers feel that the suicide rate of 10% - 15% of individuals with alcohol-related disorders is a very under-reported statistic. Even higher is the incidence of *suicide* among individuals with substance abuse disorders. An individual who has a substance abuse dependence is twenty times more likely to die from suicide than the "normal" population. See *antisocial personality disorder, delirium tremens, mental retardation.*

dual option when an employee has more than one option to chose from for his/her health care benefits. These options may include an indemnity insurance plan, a managed care plan, or a health care organization plan. Typically the employees are offered an opportunity to switch plans once a year, if they so choose, without penalty. See *office enrollment.*

dual participation simultaneous participation of a facility in the Medicare and Medicaid programs.

due process process of appealing a decision. The rights of appeal afforded *providers* and suppliers of Medicare or Medicaid who are the subjects of *adverse action* taken by the state or HCFA. See *exit survey.*

Dupuytren's contracture a thickening of the fascia and the resulting contracture around the palmar fascia of the hand. This type of contracture produces flexion deformities of the fingers. Early surgical intervention to remove the excess tissue can restore full use of the hand.

durable power of attorney a legal, written agreement that states that an individual gives permission for another person to make health care decisions for him/her. The person granting permission may indicate limitations on the scope of decisions the other person is allowed to make. See *conservatorship, do not resuscitate orders, guardian.*

duration length of time that an event lasts.

dwelling unit (ADA) a single unit that provides a kitchen or food preparation area, in addition to rooms and spaces for living, bathing, sleeping, and the like. Dwelling units include a single family home or a townhouse used as a transient group home; an apartment building used as a shelter; guest rooms in a hotel that provides sleeping accommodations and food preparation areas; and other similar facilities used on a transient basis. For purposes of these guidelines, use of the term "dwelling unit" does not imply the unit is used as a residence.

dyad, dyadic referring to a one-on-one relationship.

dying (stages of dying — Kübler-Ross) Elisabeth Kübler-Ross (1969) developed a theory of the stages that an individual goes through when they know that they are dying. The five stages are 1. denial and isolation, 2. anger, 3. bargaining, 4. depression, and 5. acceptance. These five stages are well laid out in her book **On Death and Dying**.

dynamic balance ability to remain balanced while moving. See *static balance, crutch.*

dynamic splint a splint that allows some movement of the splinted body part through the use of springs, rubber bands, electricity, or carbon dioxide. Compare to *orthosis.*

dysarthria loss of function in the muscles used for speech and voice production. The speech produced is difficult to understand. The individual may have all other language and comprehension centers intact, but be unable to physically produce speech.

dysesthesia alteration of any sense, but particularly the sense of touch. This is usually experienced as pain and/or pinpricks. Often caused by *spinal cord injuries.* Compare with *hyperesthesia.* See *hypoesthesia, sensation.*

dysfunction a malfunctioning of a body part; a subfunctional performance of a social, psychological, cognitive, or physical skill required for healthy integration into one's community. See *diminished, disintegration.*

dyskinesia an impairment in voluntary *movement.* See *cerebral palsy, tardive dyskinesia.*

dyspepsia a feeling of epigastric discomfort that takes place after a person has eaten. Symptoms include an uncomfortable feeling of fullness, potentially heartburn and nausea. These symptoms tend to increase with *stress.* Dyspepsia is a common sign of underlying disorders which may include *ulcers* or others intestinal disorders.

dysphagia difficulty swallowing, due to loss of neurological function.

dyspnea an abnormal shortness of breath. See *breathlessness.*

dyspraxia a loss of functional ability to perform voluntary movement not directly caused by a loss of motor or sensory input and function.

dysrhythmia a change in the normal rhythm. An abnormal change in the patient's speech rate due to illness or disability or a change in a patient's heartbeat due to illness or excessive activity are types of dysrhythmias. See *aerobic, panic.*

dyssocial behavior below normal, antisocial, and/or criminal social behavior that is not considered to be part of a clinical diagnosis of mental illness (e.g., *antisocial personality disorder*). A person with dyssocial behavior is an individual whose behavior (e.g., gang behavior) is contrary to behavior that benefits the community and yet is not caused by true mental illness.

dysthymia a type of mood disorder which has persisted for at least two years which decreases the individual's interest in activities because of a persistent feeling of sadness, of being "down in the dumps" or being "blue." The severity of the mood is not sufficient enough to warrant a diagnosis of *depression* but severe enough to impact activities. Individuals with dysthymic disorder tend to have low *self-esteem*, a feeling of hopelessness, and a tendency to self-criticize. This is a formal psychiatric disorder found in the **DSM-IV**. See *anhedonia.*

dystonia muscle tone impairment. See *cerebral palsy.*

dystonic movement a slow, gross motor movement with athetoid characteristics. See *movement.*

dystrophic gait movement is achieved by rolling the hips from side to side producing a pronounced waddling or penguin gait. Because of the nature of this gait, the patient's ability to run or to climb stairs or hike up inclines is impaired. The most common reason for this gait is *muscular dystrophy* but it is also seen in a variety of *myopathies.*

E

eating See *feeding.*

eccentric lengthening exercises prescriptive exercise program which:
1. uses equipment to provide a pulling force on actively contracting muscles
2. lengthens and strengthens the muscles.

echolalia involuntary repeating of words, phrases, or sentences; seen in patients with *autism, schizophrenia,* and brain injuries. See *stereotyped behavior, cardiovascular accident, traumatic brain injury.*

eclectic approach use of more than one type of treatment or the use of *protocols* that come from different theoretical bases to provide the best intervention.

E. coli O157:H7 (CDC) a bacterial pathogen that has a reservoir in cattle and other similar animals. Human illness typically follows consumption of food or water that has been contaminated with microscopic amounts of cow feces. The illness it causes is often a severe and bloody diarrhea and painful abdominal cramps, without much fever. In 3% to 5% of cases, a complication called hemolytic uremic syndrome (HUS) can occur several weeks after the initial symptoms. This severe complication includes temporary anemia, profuse bleeding, and kidney failure.

ECT See *electroconvulsive treatment.*

eczema a skin disease which is not contagious, tends to be chronic, and causes the skin to blister and develop dry scales. Eczema is different from *dermatitis,* which is a short-term inflammation of the skin.

edema excessive accumulation of fluid in the body's soft tissue causing swelling and discomfort. This swelling is controlled by:
1. positioning (using gravity to drain fluids)
2. pressure wraps (like ace bandages)
3. medications

The professional should be aware of the strategies used to reduce edema in the patient and ensure that the leisure and vocational activities that the patient engages in are not *contraindicated.* The use of ace bandages on extremities or pressure clothing (like *Jobst*) may be required during activities, even passive ones. See *burn, cerebral contusion, chronic obstructive pulmonary disease.*

EDI See *electronic data interchange.*

ED-NET (HCO) a statewide network created by the State of Oregon in 1989 that offers a full range of services for those who have a need to communicate.

education, appropriate See *consumer rights.*

Education for All Handicapped Children Act a federal law, passed in 1975, which required each state to provide a minimum level of free and appropriate education in the *least restrictive* environment for children with disabilities. Children with special educational needs between the ages of 5 years and 21 years were included in this legislation also known as *Public Law 94-142.* See *consumer rights, Individuals with Disabilities Education Act.*

Education of the Handicapped Amendments of 1986 an amendment to the *Education for All Handicapped Children Act of 1975* which extended downward the age of eligibility to three years and added emphasis on the development of services for at-risk and handicapped infants and toddlers. (Public Law 99-457.)

EEG See *electroencephalogram.*

effective date of participation When all federal and, as applicable, state requirements are met on the date of the survey, the effective date of participation can be no earlier than the last day of the on site survey or the date the current agreement expires. If all *conditions of participation* are met, but there are *deficiencies* below the condition level, the effective date of the provider agreement would be the earlier of the following: the date the facility submits an *acceptable plan of correction* or approvable waiver request or both; or the date all deficiencies have been corrected.

effective listening See *listening skills.*

efferent outward movement of fluid or of a nerve impulse. Compare *afferent.*

efficiency 1. degree to which an individual is able to complete a task measured against the amount of energy and work required from the body to complete the task. Usually a modification of movement to decrease unneeded movement combined with increased endurance will result in increased efficiency. Individuals with neuromuscular disorders like *cerebral palsy* may require significant modifications of an activity or equipment to reduce *tone* or to eliminate undesired movement to be able to increase efficiency. 2. degree to which a facility or group can provide services or produce *outcomes* measured against the human resources, time, and material resources required.

ego *Freud* described three elements of a person's psyche, which constantly battle to influence the individual's behavior. Ego is the term given to the *reasoning* and *problem solving* aspect of a person's consciousness. The other two are *id* and *superego*.

ego states three competing psychological aspects of each person's personality as described by *Freud*. See *ego, id, superego*.

eigenvalues the results of a *factor analysis*. Eigenvalues are the results of mathematical procedures that help determine how well the individual questions match the categories in the test or how important a specific item is to the integrity of the category or the test as a whole. Eigenvalues are frequently used to determine which questions to drop from the initial version of the testing tool.

EKG See *electrocardiogram*.

elasticity ability of soft tissue to return to its normal state after a period of gentle, passive *stretching*. Muscles are made up of bundles of fibers called *myofibril*. Each myofibril is made up of shorter, overlapping fibers called sarcomere made up of actin and myosin filaments. During contraction the actin and myosin filaments slide closer together (overlap more) causing the muscle fibers to contract. When the muscle is relaxed, the actin and myosin filaments pull apart a little, allowing the muscle to lengthen. When a patient remains immobile (or experiences a decrease in normal movement) over a period of time, the amount of connective tissue produced by the muscles will increase. At the same time the body increases its absorption of sarcomere fibers. This undesirable physiological event may be stopped and/or reduced through the prescriptive use of activities. The therapist should ensure that the activities prescribed are enjoyable to the patient while, at the same time, they adequately exercise all of the appropriate muscles. This exercise regimen may require combining numerous activities. See *escharotomy*.

elasticity of demand (FB) percentage change to be expected in the demand for an economic good in response to a specified percentage change in one or more of its determinants, such as price or income.

elbow disarticulation an amputation through the elbow joint. Functional ability is improved through the use of a five unit prosthesis:

1. Specially made socket trimmed to allow maximal shoulder *range of motion*
2. Figure 8 harness
3. External elbow hinges with a locking device
4. Wrist unit
5. Terminal device

Cosmetically the patient may be concerned with the extensive appearance of the device. An elbow disarticulation is abbreviated "ED."

electrical interference Humans and biofeedback sensors pick up electrical signals or noise from a variety of environmental sources including power lines, motors, lights, electrical equipment, and radio stations. Most of this electrical interference falls rhythmically at around 60 hertz (cycles per second).

electrocardiogram (EKG) a non-invasive test which measures the electrical activity of the patient's heart. The results are printed out on a graph.

electroconvulsive treatment (ECT) use of electric current to induce convulsive *seizures*. Most often used in the treatment of *depression*. First introduced by Cerletti and Bini in 1938. Modifications are electronarcosis, which produces sleep like states and electrostimulation, which avoids convulsions. Used with anesthetics and muscle relaxants. While the use of ECT has fluctuated over the years due to the controversy over the treatment, it remains one of the few effective treatments for individuals with severe, persistent depression. Patients usually receive ECT as an inpatient, as short-term *memory* is severely impaired during the 24 hours after ECT. Many patients will not benefit from therapy groups during this time but should still be offered *diversional* activities. Arts and crafts activities are especially indicated during the 24 hours after ECT. Taking short walks outside with constant staff supervision may also be indicated as long as the patient is not experiencing balance problems.

electroencephalogram (EEG) a test that records the brain's spontaneous bioelectrical activity. The bioelectrical activity being recorded by the numerous electrodes produces patterns on a print out. Certain patterns are associated with *seizure* activity, tumors, infections, or other metabolism dysfunctions. See *epilepsy, metabolic disorders*.

electroencephalographic biofeedback a rapidly growing separate field of biofeedback calling for specialized certification. Electroencephalographs measure the frequency, amplitude, and duration of electrical activity of the brain: theta (4-10 hertz), alpha (8-13 Hertz), and beta (13 Hertz or greater). Excessive theta activity and lack of beta activity are the prime neurological characteristics of ADHD. EEG biofeedback has numerous other indications including the treatment of addictions and ADHD as well as many emotional and cognitive disorders.

electromyography (EMG) an electrical correlate of muscle contraction. It measures electrical output of contracting muscles. EMG is measured in microvolts (one millionth of a volt) and provides quantitative information. Indications for EMG biofeedback include muscle re-education (e.g. incontinence training, pain management, and relaxation).

electronic data interchange (HCO) application-to-application interchange of business data between organizations using a standard data format.

electronic mailing lists (HCO) free, subscription-based, electronic mail communications on the Internet or commercial online services focused on defined topics.

element (ADA) an architectural or mechanical component of a building, facility, space, or site, e.g., telephone, curb ramp, door, drinking fountain, seating, or water closet.

elopement purposeful running away from a treatment group or hospital unit against medical advice (*AMA*) and without arranging a *discharge*. Elopement is of special concern to therapists who take voluntary inpatient clients on walks. A voluntary patient has the right to elope. If the therapist feels that a patient is considering elopement, s/he should recommend that the patient not go on the walk. The patient should talk to the appropriate case manager or staff person instead. See *psychiatric admission.*

embolism sudden blocking of an artery by a blood clot or foreign material that has been brought to that site by the blood (an embolus). See *occlusion.*

emergency admission admission of a patient to a facility against his/her wishes. Due to perceived danger to self or others, a person may be institutionalized for 48-72 hours (the length of time depends on state law). See *involuntary admission, psychiatric admissions.*

emergency preparedness See *environment of care.*

emesis vomit.

emotion feelings an individual has which are expressed in the environment of the mind, felt by the body (as with *stress*), and usually tied to behavioral actions. *Mood* and *affect* are part of an individual's emotions. See *communication, dissociation, dopamine, empathy, equilibrium.*

emotional baggage usually negative components of personality based on the sum of one's personal and interpersonal experiences that accompany an individual throughout his/her life. People tend to react or act based on their past experiences. See *frame of reference.*

empathy cognitive or vicarious awareness of another person's feelings or emotions. Empathy is an important attribute for the therapist to demonstrate but also one that is fraught with potential problems related to conduct. It is appropriate for the therapist to demonstrate awareness of the patient's feelings or emotions but how the therapist acts on them has to be carefully thought out. The therapist should exam-

ine his/her motives and understand the consequences of any action that s/he takes, both for the patient and for himself/herself. When in doubt, consult with a supervisor. Empathy is not the same as sympathy or feeling sorry for someone. See *intake assessment, listening skills.*

emphysema a chronic disease which affects the ability of the patient's lungs to exchange gases. Generally, the elasticity of the lung walls has been destroyed resulting in a chronic shortness of breath, *dyspnea*, and coughing along with potential restlessness and confusion secondary to a lack of oxygen. See *breathlessness, chronic obstructive pulmonary disease.*

empirical knowledge which has been obtained through experience and observable events but which has not been obtained through other forms of scientific studies.

employee malfeasance actions taken by an employee that harm the employer. Employee malfeasance can be divided into two different categories: 1. clear cut crimes (bribery, theft, fraud, vandalism) and 2. counterproductive behaviors (on-the-job alcohol or drug abuse, misuses of absences or tardiness, and misuses of sick leave). Employers have three primary methods of identifying and screening employees (or potential employees) who may exhibit employee malfeasance: 1. polygraph examinations (almost totally outlawed in 1988 with the Employee Polygraph Protection Act), 2. background checks (required by law in almost all states for human service and teaching positions), and 3. paper and pencil integrity tests (including the Employee Attitude Inventory, the Reid Survey III, and the Wilkerson Employee Input Survey). Prior to the 1990's *integrity tests* were referred to as *honesty* tests. Rogers (1997) reports that employee malfeasance is a big problem for American businesses (p. 264): "Yearly losses in the United States due to employee theft may be as high as $25 billion dollars. Significant percentages of employees admit to stealing from their employers: 36% in manufacturing and 40% in retail. The incidence of employee theft is only getting worse, with the rate of employee theft increasing 15% a year. It is estimated that approximately 30% of mall-business failures are due to employee pilferage."

employer The *Americans with Disabilities Act* defines an employer as: 1. In general, the term "employer" means a person engaged in an industry affecting commerce who has fifteen or more employees for each working day in each of twenty or more calendar weeks in the current or preceding calendar year and any agent of such person, except that, from July 26, 1992 through July 25, 1994, an employer means a person engaged in an industry affecting commerce who has 25 or more employees for each working day in each of 20 or more calendar weeks in the current or preceding year and any agent of such person. 2. Exceptions, the term employer does not include — (i) the United States, a corporation wholly owned by the government of the United States or an Indian tribe; or (ii) a bona fide private membership club (other than a labor organization) that is exempt from taxation under Section 501(c) of the Internal Revenue Code of 1986. ADA 1630.2 (e).

empowerment feeling that one can influence one's own life and the events surrounding it. Many therapists are assigned the job of helping the patient to feel empowered. By the nature of empowerment, this cannot be done through talking or self-help programs. Empowerment only comes from the actual experience of being able to control a significant aspect of one's environment. See *self-esteem.*

empty-nest syndrome a feeling of emotional loss and sorrow when one's children grow up and leave home. Pop psychology coined this phrase to describe a specific situation in which an adult has a major change in lifestyle without being prepared to replace a lost responsibility (the daily nurturing of a child) with a new freedom (more time for oneself). A 1999 study funded by the MacArthur foundation found that this was a misperception, that very few individuals felt extreme sorrow when their children left home. Part of this misperception was influenced by the acceptance of the thought that a *midlife crisis* happens at the same age span in which one's children usually leave home.

encephalitis an inflammation of the brain usually caused by mosquito-borne arbovirus. May also be caused by lead poisoning.

encoder (HCO) decision support systems used to facilitate accurate assignment of codes for clinical procedures.

encopresis an incontinence of the feces. See *childhood psychiatric disorder.*

encounter group a form of sensitivity training promoted by J. L. Moreno that promoted self-awareness through supportive interactions with others within the group.

endemic disease a disease that is continually present in the environment or community even with aggressive efforts to fight the disease. See *infection.*

endocrine system a network of structures and ductless glands that secrete hormones into the bloodstream. The *hormones* affect specific processes in the body including metabolism and growth. Organs that are part of the endocrine system include the thy-

roid, the parathyroid, the anterior and posterior pituitary, the gonads, the suprarenal glands, and the pancreas. See *adrenal gland.*

endogenous 1. created in a tissue, cell, or organism. **2.** a feeling or thought originating from the person himself/herself. Opposite of *exogenous.*

endogenous cause variation See *variation.*

endogenous infection an infection whose origin comes from within the individual (e.g., e. coli bacteria from the intestines being introduced into the mouth due to poor handwashing). See *infection.*

endorphin chemical produced in the body that has effects similar to morphine. Endorphins act on the central and peripheral nervous systems to reduce *pain.* "Runner's high," the enjoyable sensation caused by exercise, is partially from the production of endorphins. See *opioids.*

endotracheal airway When the patient requires assisted ventilation (usually for no more than 7 days), a tube is slipped down the trachea (windpipe) into the lungs. This tube may be placed into the trachea through the nose (nasotracheal), through the mouth (orotracheal), or through an existing hole (stoma) in the trachea. See *tracheostomy.*

endotracheal tube See *artificial airway, endotracheal airway.*

end stage renal disease (ESRD) stage of renal impairment that appears irreversible and permanent and requires a regular course of dialysis or kidney transplantation to maintain life. See *hospital insurance, Medicare.*

endurance ability of:
1. the muscle to resist *fatigue* even with repeated contractions over a period of time,
2. the cardiovascular system to resist fatigue through efficient delivery of oxygen over a period of time,
3. the neuropsychological system to resist fatigue allowing the performance of cognitive functions over a period of time, and/or
4. the general ability to sustain low intensity activity over a period of time.

See *efficiency, physical therapy.*

enhance to help make better. To enhance a patient's skill or environment or positive feelings is an important aspect of all who work in health care settings. In the United States, *OBRA* expects all staff to work on the enhancement of a patient's life. This is considered to be a standard service.

enkephalin (from the Greek "in the head") a five-amino-acid peptide that binds to an opiate receptor, causing analgesia and exercise-induced euphoria sometimes referred to as a "runners high." The brain's morphine.

ENT medical specialty for ear, nose, and throat disorders.

enteric precautions an isolation procedure for patients with amebic dysentery, cholera, diarrhea, *gastroenteritis*, *hepatitis* (viral, type A), and other specifically listed diseases. The isolation procedures include: 1. masks are not indicated, 2. gowns are indicated if soiling is likely, 3. gloves are indicated for touching infective material, 4. hands must be washed after touching the patient or potentially contaminated articles and before taking care of another patient, 5. articles contaminated with infective material should be discarded or bagged and labeled before being sent for decontamination and reprocessing. The sign for enteric precautions is always brown.

enterovirus (CDC) a genus of RNA viruses with over 70 types identified in humans. They reproduce in the intestinal tract, and various members can cause a variety of human diseases including poliomyelitis, aseptic *meningitis*, *hepatitis*, inflammatory heart disease, and rhinitis.

entitlement programs (FB) programs that provide benefits paid out automatically to all who qualify unless there is a change in underlying law. These programs may or may not require an annual appropriation by Congress. Social Security and Medicare, for example, are autonomous trust funds that possess the authority to pay benefits without annual appropriation by Congress. Many other individual benefit programs such as Medicaid, Supplemental Security Income, and Aid to Families with Dependent Children programs, are all considered entitlements by Congress. See *Agreement (1864).*

entrance (ADA) any access point to a building or portion of a building or facility used for the purpose of entering. An entrance includes the approach walk, the vertical access leading to the entrance platform, the entrance platform itself, vestibules if provided, the entry door(s), or gate(s), and the hardware of the entry door(s) or gate(s).

entrance conference initial meeting between the *provider*/supplier (usually the administrator) and survey team upon the survey team's arrival at the facility. This conference sets the tone for the entire survey. The survey team and the provider/supplier should be well prepared, make requests not demands, and treat everyone with courtesy. The survey team leader will explain the purpose, time schedule, and procedures the survey team will follow during the survey. The staff at the facility can make the surveyor's experience a more positive one during the survey process if they have a surveyor's orientation pack ready. (Most state and federal surveys are

unannounced — in fact, there may be a $5,000 fine levied on anyone who releases the survey schedule — so update the pack regularly!) This packet should contain the names, phone numbers, and normal work schedule of each department director; important information about the facility (and don't forget the locations of staff bathrooms, pop machines, and cafeteria); newspaper clippings of awards the facility or staff have received in the last year; and a list of favorite, modestly priced restaurants near the facility. See *survey process.*

enuresis urinary *incontinence* while sleeping; bedwetting. See *childhood psychiatric disorders.*

environment a term borrowed from the French that means to encircle. A general term that refers to all stimuli and objects in the proximity of the individual. See *curiosity, dementia, developmental disability, environment of care.*

environmental assessment generally, the measurement of how well an individual (or a group) fit into his/her (their) environment; specifically in health care, an evaluation of the ability of the environment to be able to accept the patient and his/her disabilities/illnesses and equipment. Kane and Kane (1981) report that most measurements of person-environment fit contain five themes commonly found in these testing tools: "1. the degree of perceived control, freedom, choice, autonomy, or individuality permitted to the individual by the environment; 2. structure, rules, and expected behavior imposed by the environment on the individual; 3. relationships between the individual and caregivers in the environment; 4. perceptions of activity and stimulation levels; and 5. expressed satisfaction with various aspects of the environment. (p. 192)" See the chart on the next page for an example of an environmental assessment.

Environmental Protection Agency (EPA) (HHS) The EPA's mission is to protect human health and safeguard the natural environment, air, water, and land upon which life depends. Through regulation, EPA tries to ensure the human population and the environment are protected from environmental risks and exposures.

environment of care one of the *Joint Commission's* concepts of quality patient care, the "environment of care" describes the management of facilities, equipment, and support services. The expectation is that each individual working within the facility will know his/her role. The therapist will need to understand his/her role in the facility's fire plan, understand how to determine which of the supplies s/he uses may be hazardous and what to do in the event of a spill or exposure, how to work with equipment

Assessments and Recommendations for Environmental Assessment

Area	Assessment	Recommendations
Outside	Path: condition; lighting; obstacles; surface type	Ensure good repair, adequate lighting (consider photosensitivity), keep shrubs, etc., trimmed and back from walk, level, non-slippery surface, arrange for assistance with snow/ice removal if needed
	Stairs and doorway: handrails; condition of steps; contrast of nosing; doormat; door opening allows adequate room	Repair loose or damaged stairs, ensure adequate lighting, contrast strip along nosing, handrail extends beyond first step, remove loose doormats, consider removing outer door if inadequate room to swing open.
Transition Areas	Lighting; room for donning/doffing clothing; surface	Light switch readily available, non-slip surface, no loose mats, adequate time and space for adjustment to changes in lighting, remove objects to allow as much room as possible, use chair or bench to allowing sitting when donning/doffing clothing and footwear
Living Area	Thick pile or worn carpet; area rugs; height, depth, angle, supportiveness, arms present on frequently used chairs/couch; location of frequently used objects, e.g., phone; loose or fragile furniture; electric cords; lighting	Low pile carpet advised; remove area rugs; recommend most appropriate chair be used; ensure frequently used objects within easy reach of chair; remove or alert to unsafe furniture; remove clutter; secure electric cords; light switches easily accessible; curtains available for windows which might result in glare.
Bedroom	As for living area plus: bed height; firm mattress; bedclothes out of way when turned back; closets; footwear	As for living area plus: adjust bed height; recommend light, non-trailing bedclothes; arrange closets to avoid reaching; recommend shoes rather than slippers.
Bathrooms	Floor surface; toilet seat height; tub transfers; use of sink or towel bars for support; clutter; storage; ability to clean	Avoid highly polished surfaces; recommend adaptive devices if needed; advise avoiding use of sink, towel bars as grab bars; arrange storage to avoid bending and reaching; minimize clutter; consider help for cleaning if needed; and suggest long-handled sponges, etc. to avoid reaching.
Kitchen	Area rugs; storage; oven/stove: height, location of controls, weight of door, ability to clean; refrigerator: storage, ability to clean; countertops used for support, clutter	Remove area rugs; rearrange storage to avoid reaching, bending including refrigerator; recommend assistive devices if needed; minimize clutter.
Stairs	Lighting; condition; contrast of nosing; handrail; surface	Ensure adequate lighting with 2-way switch; handrail should extend beyond first stair, non-slip surface; good contrast.
Laundry and Garbage	Accessibility; lighting; transporting materials	Advise about the best location; ensure adequate lighting; recommend small loads, use of wheeled garbage cans; recommend assistance if needed.

From Merla & Spaulding, ©1997, The Haworth Press. Used with permission.

and utility systems within the facility (including problem solving supply or equipment problems), and understanding how to respond to disasters (internal or external) using the facility's disaster plan. Managing the environment of care includes seven functions. These are listed on the next page. The areas covered under JCAHO's Management of the Environment of Care are similar to the Health Care Financing Administration's immediate jeopardy guidelines. Comparison of the two documents is suggested. See *accident prevention plan, hazardous materials, life safety code, immediate and serious threat.*

enzyme a protein or large peptide that functions to catalyze chemicals hundreds to thousands of times faster than would be possible otherwise. (HHS) Spe-

JCAHO's Management of the Environment of Care

Function	Description
Emergency Preparedness	Management and implementation of the process to ensure that the facility is fully prepared to respond to a disaster situation, whether the disaster is internal or external.
Hazardous Materials and Waste Management	Management and implementation of the process by which materials are safely handled including the proper techniques used to clean spills. This also includes the function that ensures that waste is disposed of properly.
Life Safety Management	Management and implementation of the process by which the building systems and the structural features of the building are kept safe in the event of a fire.
Medical Equipment Management	Management and implementation of the process that ensures that all patient care technologies and other medical equipment are monitored, repaired and maintained to ensure safe and proper operation.
Safety Management	Management and implementation of the process for creating, monitoring, and otherwise ensuring that the environment within and around the facility is safe for patients.
Security Management	Management and implementation of the process for monitoring and insuring that the facility's environment is secure for the provision of patient care.
Utility Systems Management	Management and implementation of the process by which utility systems are monitored and maintained. Utility systems include the heating and electrical systems including patient call lights.

cialized proteins that act as catalysts for virtually all of the necessary chemical reactions that take place within the body. Like all catalysts, enzymes are unchanged by the reactions they promote, and initiate many reactions until they are degraded (usually by another enzyme). Enzymes can restructure the body's fabric by both creating larger molecules and breaking them down.

eosinophil (HHS) a white cell of the category known as granulocytes. These cells contain numerous dense granules in their cytoplasm that comprise a battery of highly active digestive chemicals and toxins. Their chief role is thought to be in combating large parasites, although occasionally their activity may be triggered by other agents, potentially leading to damage of normal tissues. See *eosinophilia myalgia syndrome*.

eosinophilia myalgia syndrome (EMS) (HHS) a disease caused by marked promotion of *eosinophil* activity, resulting in a symptom complex of severe pain, inflammation of the tendons, fluid build-up in the muscles, and skin rash. The disorder has been linked to a contaminant of some commercial preparations of the amino acid L-tryptophan.

epicondyle referring to a bony prominence on the top of a condyle of a bone. An example would be the bump felt on the top of the femur on the outside of the hip. Skin tissue covering epicondyles are prone to *pressure sore*s caused by pressure, sheer, inactivity, and poor circulation. The eight epicondyle locations on the body are

1. external epicondyle of femur
2. external epicondyle of humerus
3. internal epicondyle of femur
4. internal epicondyle of humerus
5. lateral epicondyle of femur
6. lateral epicondyle of humerus
7. medial epicondyle of femur
8. medial epicondyle of humerus

epicritic function highly developed sensitivity to touch, taste, pain, and temperature; usually referring to the nerve fibers supplying the skin and oral mucus membranes which allow for the greatly expanded sensitivity of those areas.

epidemic disease a disease that is affecting a greater number of the population than would be statistically expected. See *infection*.

epidemiology multi-level study of the origin of a disease, how that disease is transmitted, what in the environment (the person's body and where s/he lives) strengthened or weakened the disease, and other factors that may influence the development and spread of the disease. See *infection*.

epidermis the top layer of the skin which is exposed to the environment. The epidermis is made of three layers or strata: the stratum basale, stratum spinosum, and stratum granulosum. The microscopic connections that hold the stratum basale and the stratum spinosum together are called desmonsomes.

epigastric sensation referring to "that sinking feeling" produced by worry or *fear*; felt in the stomach. See *sensation*.

epilepsy disorders of the central nervous system (CNS) that are manifested by *seizure* activity that must meet all three of the following criteria: 1. the seizure activity is of rapid onset, 2. the actual dura-

Classification of Epileptic Seizures

Seizure Type	Characteristics
Simple partial seizures	Various manifestations, without impairment of consciousness, including convulsions confined to a single limb or muscle group (Jacksonian motor epilepsy), specific and localized sensory disturbances (Jacksonian sensory epilepsy), and other limited signs and symptoms depending on the particular cortical area producing the abnormal discharge.
Complex partial seizures or Partial seizures secondarily generalized	Periods of confused behavior, with impairment of consciousness, with a wide variety of clinical manifestations, associated with bizarre generalized EEG activity during the seizure but without evidence of anterior temporal lobe focal abnormalities even in the inter-seizure period in many cases. See *electroencephalogram.*
Absence seizures	Brief and abrupt loss of consciousness associated with high-voltage, bilaterally synchronous, 3-per-second spike-and-wave pattern in the EEG usually with some symmetrical clonic motor activity varying from eyelid blinking to jerking of the entire body, sometimes with no motor activity.
Atypical absence seizures	Seizure activity with slower onset and cessation than is usual for absence seizures, associated with a more heterogeneous EEG.
Myoclonic seizures	Isolated clonic jerks associated with brief bursts of multiple spikes in EEG.
Clonic seizures	Rhythmic clonic contractions of all muscles, loss of consciousness, and marked autonomic manifestations. See *clonic seizures.*
Tonic seizures	Opisthotonus (arching of the back), loss of consciousness, and marked autonomic manifestations.
Tonic-clonic seizures (grand mal)	Major convulsions, usually a sequence of maximal tonic spasm of all body musculature followed by synchronous clonic jerking and a prolonged depression of all central functions.
Atonic seizures	Loss of postural tone, with sagging of the head or falling.

tion of the seizure activity is short in *duration* and 3. the reoccurrence of the seizure activity is chronic. This grouping of brain disorders affects about 2% of the population of the United States (Goldenson et al, 1978) and seems to be evenly distributed between males and females and all ethnic groups. Cause: The brain uses nerve cells to transmit information through coordinated electrical charges. Individuals with epilepsy have periods when this coordination of the nerve cells breaks down, allowing an overproduction of electrical energy. Impact on functional ability: The amount of impairment depends on the extent of the over-production and the location of the brain where this overproduction occurs. It ranges from little to no impact to a severe impact on functional ability. The Epilepsy Foundation of America estimates that with good medical care and prescription medications, up to 80% of the individuals with epilepsy will experience little or no impact on their functional ability. The table above (Julien, 1992) lists different seizure types associated with epilepsy. See *biofeedback.*

epinephrine a *hormone* whose effects mimic that of a stimulation of the sympathetic division of the autonomic nervous system including arousal and cardiac stimulation. The vernacular term for epinephrine is adrenalin. See *adrenal gland.*

Epstein-Barr virus (EBV) (CDC) one of the eight known types of human herpes viruses, also known as human herpes virus 4 (HHV-4). It belongs to the gamma subfamily of herpes viruses. It commonly causes acute mononucleosis, and less commonly chronic mononucleosis. In some populations EBV is causally associated with life-threatening malignancies (Burkitt's lymphoma, nasopharyngeal carcinoma).

equilibration generally referring to the balancing of two opposing forces whether they be the balance between assimilating a new idea (*assimilation*) and accommodating the new idea (*accommodation*) (Piagetian theory) or the general process of growth and development.

equilibrium achieving a balance of physical position, of biochemical relations within one's body or of the *emotions.* See *disequilibrium, kinesthetic.*

eremophobia irrational fear of being alone. Not an official psychiatric diagnosis.

ergonomics science of designing work and living environments to enhance human performance and to reduce the incidence and severity of injury. See the table on the next page for Basic Ergonomic Risk Factors to consider when designing a workplace.

Basic Ergonomic Risk Factors

Risk	Discussion
Posture	Postures that are awkward require the individual to experience stress placed on joints and surrounding tissue. This leads to extra muscle and tendon fatigue and joint soreness. This added stress is thought to contribute to an increased likelihood of musculoskeletal disorders.
Repetition	A repetitive motion is an action that is repeated many times with a cycle time of less than 30 seconds or when the basic cycle accounts for 50% or more of the total work cycle (OSHA, 1995). This repetitive action can lead to accelerated muscle fatigue and increased risk of muscle-tendon damage. Tasks that are very repetitive do not allow for adequate tissue recovery.
Force	The greater the force needed to complete the task, the greater the physiological stress to the body (muscles, tendons, and joints).
Mechanical Compression or Contact Stress	Mechanical compression refers to pressure points created when an object places uneven pressure on the body such as a garden shovel would place extra stress on the tissue in the palm of the hand at the points that the handle of the shovel contacts the hand. Mechanical compression can impede blood flow and interfere with nerve function.
Duration	Duration refers to the length of time that the body is exposed to a stress in the environment. Increased length of exposure can lead to increased impact on the immediate area of exposure as well as increasing a general fatigue response. Generally, the greater the duration of exposure to a stressful risk factor the greater the length of time it takes the body to revert to its baseline of function.
Vibration	Vibration types can be impact, oscillation, or combined impact and oscillation. Vibration can also be categorized as localized (e.g., vibration of the hand) or whole body (riding in a semi-truck). National vibration threshold standards have been set for some aspects of the workplace to limit the neurological and fatigue factors associated with vibration.
Temperature	The lower a temperature goes, the greater the loss of dexterity, sensitivity, and grip force. Also, a lower temperature can make the impact of vibration worse. OSHA (1995) recommends that metal surfaces be above 59° F as temperatures below this point decrease dexterity. Metal surfaces below 44.6° F may lead to numbness. The ACGIH (1995) recommends the following exposure limits: for sedentary work, 60° F; for light work, 40° F; and for moderate work (fine motor dexterity not required), 20° F.

See *physical activity, side effect, work hardening*.

Erikson, Erik (1902-1994) a German-born psychoanalyst who immigrated to the United States in 1933. His main contributions were his extensive research into psychological development of humans. In his classic book *Childhood and Society* (1950) he presented a model of development which was based on an individual's ongoing relationship between one's body (biological impact) and one's society. This model of development contained eight stages, each listing what Erikson considered to be the main task or challenge of that stage. His eight stages are: *Stage One:* Basic Trust, *Stage Two:* Autonomy vs. Shame and Doubt, *Stage 3:* Initiative vs. Guilt, *Stage 4:* Industry vs. Inferiority, *Stage 5:* Identity vs. Role Diffusion, *Stage 6:* Intimacy vs. Isolation, *Stage 7:* Generatively vs. Stagnation, and *Stage 8:* Integrity vs. Despair. See the section at the end of the book (p. 350) for additional information on models of growth and development.

eschar thick crust formed by coagulation and dead cells that develops after a thermal or chemical *burn* to the skin.

escharotomy surgical incision in scar tissue to allow *elasticity* in the skin. Especially in patients with *burns* encircling an entire body part (e.g., arm, abdomen), the non-elastic scar tissue is incised (cut) the length of the scar tissue, through the complete depth of the scar. This allows greater movement. Escharotomy is especially important for patients who have burns encircling the torso to allow the expansion of the thoracic cavity for *breathing*. The procedure leaves especially disfiguring scars, usually causing the patient concerns about cosmetic issues. The use of activities to help increase feeling of self-worth and control over one's environment are extremely important. Extremities with circumferential burns will experience a tightening of the scar tissue throughout the hospitalization. The patient is at risk for a restricted blood flow below the circumferential scar. Peripheral pulses may be cut off, requiring immediate medical attention. The therapist should be skilled in taking extremity *pulses* in patients with burns or know what to look for to avoid further complications.

ESP See *extrasensory perception*.

ESRD See *end stage renal disease*.

essential tremor See *tremor*.

ethics a system of values held by a group of people that outline acceptable and non-acceptable behavior. Technical knowledge may allow a professional to provide a therapeutic intervention (e.g., teach anger management skills) but ethics guides the professional in how to manage the therapy environment to implement his/her technical knowledge. The ethical implementation of a technical skill includes the use of modalities which are known to be beneficial and not harmful to the patient, the appropriate training and skill level of the practitioner to use the modalities, the maintenance of an honest and respectful communication with the patient throughout the treatment, and the on-going maintenance of *confidentiality* after the treatment has occurred. The origin of the word "ethics" is from the Greek word "ethos" which means "customary." See the chart below for more information about some of the terms used in discussions of ethics. See *Joint Commission, modality*.

etiology study of where a *disease* or *disorder* originates, how it progresses, and what other factors and effects result from the disease or disorder.

etregenous a cognitive processing deficit characterized by an inability to respond appropriately in a conversation. The patient's response to a topic is somehow twisted by the internal mental state of the patient so that the response is not appropriate to the topic at hand. A conversation may be mutually etregenous when the two parties cannot find any common cultural references. See *interpersonal skills*.

euphoria an exaggerated sense of well-being; a (usually unrealistic) sense of being free from *stress, pain,* or psychological discomfort. See *mood*.

euthanasia act of assisting a terminally ill person in his/her death. The assistance may be *active* (taking some actions to cause immediate death) or *passive* (not taking an action which would prolong life).

evaluation a *clinical opinion* as a result of the professional's review of data and assessment results. Evaluation is not the same as an *assessment*. See *measurement, modality-oriented clinic, physical activities, test, therapy process*.

eversion turning outward of a body part.

exacerbate to make a disease or disability worse. A lifestyle that does not involve active movement throughout each day may exacerbate (make worse) a *pressure sore* in an elderly patient.

excitatory bringing about an increase of the thought processes or the physical functions of the body due to stimulation.

exclusion (Prospective Payment System) There is a limited group of hospitals and hospital units excluded from the *prospective payment system*. There are two types of exclusions. A hospital is either excluded in its entirety or a specific unit of an otherwise non-excluded hospital is excluded. Hospital and hospital units which may be excluded from prospective payment include: psychiatric, rehabilitation, children's, and long-term care hospitals and psychiatric and rehabilitation units of hospitals.

executive function cognitive functions that are considered the "higher" functions (*problem solving, abstract reasoning, judgment*, interpretation of social cues, adapting to the environment, planning skills, *initiation* skills, sequencing, monitoring skills, *inhibition* of inappropriate behavior, etc.). A person's ability to walk and complete other motor activities has been compared to the engine of a car and the ability to decide where to go and what to do (executive function) has been compared to the steering system of a car. The car can still run without the steering system but it does not get where the driver

Differentiation of Terms Used in Discussions of Professional Ethics (White and Wooten, 1986)

Ethics	Concepts and standards held by individuals or groups concerning the values surrounding the rightness and wrongness of models of conduct in human behavior and the result of human behavioral actions.
Laws	A system of social rules, norms or standards of behavior, concerning the right and wrong of human conduct that is put in codes enforced by sanctions imposed through recognized authority.
Norms	Ideas, conceptualizations, beliefs, or statements enforced by the sanctions of members of a group concerning their behavioral rules, patterns, and conduct, which is referenced in the form of what should be done, what ought to be done, what is expected, and the level of action or expectation under specific circumstances.
Science	A body of knowledge that is characterized by the use of the scientific method, which seeks out goal-oriented information through systematic, unified, and self-correcting processes.
Values	Beliefs or ideals held by individuals or groups concerning what is good, right, desirable, or important in an idea, object, or action.

wants to go, safely, without the steering system. The same can be said of a patient who lacks executive function skills (due to a *traumatic brain injury*, *dementia*, etc.). The patient may be able to walk about but not to do so in a goal-directed manner. See *alcohol-induced disorders, cognition, knowledge.*

exercise exertion for the sake of training or improvement. Regularly engaging in exercise gives the body a higher level of energy and reduced susceptibility to illness. Frequency should be 3 to 5 times a week for at least 20 minutes of uninterrupted exercise. Some patients may need to have this modified depending on their condition. There are three different types of exercise that patients can engage in: *aerobic, stretching,* and toning exercises. Patients' ability to stick to an "exercise" program tends to increase when the exercise is achieved through a leisure activity such as yoga, basketball, or dance. See *gout, intermittent claudication, kinesthetic.*

existentialism a school of psychology using commonly understood metaphors to describe behavior. The focus of existentialism is personal choice based on the immediate reality of the individual's world; not necessarily structured to follow strict social rules. This is an important philosophical movement that is between social idealism and objective materialism.

exit conference a discussion of survey findings by the state or federal survey team given to the *provider*/supplier at the conclusion of a survey. This is also the beginning of the *due process* in that providers/suppliers have the first opportunity to present additional information in response to cited deficiencies. Exit conferences may be videotaped or audio taped as long as the survey team is provided with copies of the tapes upon leaving the facility. In addition, providers are allowed to have an attorney present. The attorney may function only as an observer. Any questions the attorney asks must be for clarification purposes, rather than for the purpose of challenging the findings and attempting to turn the proceedings into a hearing. See *deficiency, survey process.*

exogenous a thought, action, feeling, or substance which originates from outside a person. Opposite of *endogenous.*

exogenous cause variation See *variation.*

exogenous infection an *infection* whose origin comes from environmental pathogens (e.g., typhoid).

experimental group (HHS) the group of subjects in an experimental study that receives a treatment.

exposure control plan a management tool, required by federal law, which outlines the facility's plan to reduce an employee's exposure to *blood-borne pathogens* and *OPIMs* (other potentially infectious materials). All workplaces must have an exposure control plan and exposure determination if any employees might be exposed to blood or other potentially infectious materials in the course of their work. This, for all intents and purposes, includes every workplace in the United States. The exposure determination contains the following information:

1. A list of all job classifications in which all employees have *occupational exposure.*
2. A list of job classifications in which some employees have occupational exposure.
3. A list of all tasks and procedures or groups of closely related tasks and procedures in which occupational exposure occurs and that are performed by employees in the job classifications listed above.

The exposure determination is made without regard to use of *personal protective equipment.* Employees are considered exposed even if they ordinarily wear protective equipment. All therapists with direct patient contact should be considered to be in the "exposed" groups. Considering the general recreational field, any person working in a facility for people who are developmentally disabled who is responsible for first aid and CPR would have a job listed in the first category. The secretary in a park office would have limited exposure and therefore his or her job would be listed in the second category. The employer must list all jobs and determine which fit into each category. The exposure control plan, in addition to the exposure determination, must contain the policies and procedures for carrying out the control of exposure as well as a system of *continuous quality assurance.* These policies must define the engineering controls that are in place to isolate or remove blood-borne pathogen hazards from the workplace. They also list personal protective equipment available and state how it is to be used. Housekeeping practices are outlined. The procedure for obtaining *hepatitis B* vaccine and for post-exposure evaluation must be detailed as well as signs that must be used to warn employees of exposure to potentially infectious materials. Finally, documentation of employee training and record keeping must appear in the exposure control plan. In case of exposure, the exposure control plan outlines the steps taken to investigate the actual exposure incident and a mechanism for making necessary changes to reduce further risk. The exposure control plan must be kept current (reviewed and updated at least annually) and must be accessible to employees and available for inspection by regulatory agencies.

Extensors of the Hand and Foot

extensor	Description
extensor digitorum longus and brevis	the two muscles which pull the lesser toes into extension and stabilize the lesser metatarsophalangeal joints
extensor hallucis longus and brevis	the two muscles that pull the great toe into extension and stabilize the first metatarsophalangeal joint
extensor retinaculum	along with the flexor retinaculum, the thickened deep fascia of the muscles of the forearm which become tendons as they move into the hand, forming a superficial fascia over the wrist
extensor wad of three	the set of three muscles that extend the wrist and flex the elbow: brachioradialis muscle, extensor carpi radialis longus, and extensor carpi radialis brevis

exposure determination rating of exposure risk to infectious pathogens for specific occupational groupings. See *exposure control plan*.

expressive communication See *communication*.

extended admission an admission to a facility that is against the patient's wishes. After the emergency and/or temporary admission the patient and psychiatrist reconvene with the court. Depending on the state, the psychiatrist may ask for an extension of the involuntary admission for 60-120 days. Federal law requires that individuals be confined in the *least restrictive* treatment setting possible. See *psychiatric admission*.

extended care facility a dated term used to describe a facility where a patient is admitted for months to years.

extended survey (OBRA) further evaluation of a facility after a standard survey. In the process of conducting a patient-centered survey (standard survey), the surveyors determine that the facility may have provided substandard care in any of the *conditions of participation* including the areas of admission, transfer, and discharge rights; patient assessment; dietary services; specialized rehabilitative services; dental services; pharmacy services; *infection control*; and/or physical environment. It is not an indication of a good survey to have to go into a partially extended survey. See *standard survey*.

extensibility See *flexibility*.

extension straightening or unbending a flexed limb. Moving two ends of a jointed part away from each other. Opposite of *flexion*. See *full arc extension, range of motion*.

extensor muscles that assist in the extension of a body part. See the chart above.

external locus of control See *locus of control*.

external powered flexor-hinge splint use of external power to provide prehension of the splinted body part.

extinction (of behaviors) ending of undesirable traits or *behaviors*. Extinction of behaviors usually follows a modification of the environment and changes in consequences that, in turn, motivate the individual to change his/her behavior. Depending on the type of behavior, a simple *cognitive therapy* approach may work (e.g., explaining to a child that s/he is to say "hello" instead of "what" when first answering the phone). For other, more deeply ingrained habits like smoking, a variety of approaches may be necessary.

extrapyramidal pertaining to the structures that coordinate involuntary motor movement directed by the central nervous system, especially postural, static, and locomotor mechanisms.

extrasensory perception (ESP) ability to know or sense something without using the six *senses*: vision, taste, touch, smell, hearing, or proprioception. ESP is generally not accepted by the established scientific community and includes such paranormal phenomena as telepathy and clairvoyance.

extrasystemic cause variation See *variation*.

extrinsic actions taken as a result of the influence of others. A patient who joins an activity because the therapist wants him/her to is joining for extrinsic reasons. The patient who joins an activity because s/he wants to gain the benefits of the activity is joining for *intrinsic* reasons. See *behavior modification program, locus of control*.

extrinsic muscles referring to muscles that are located outside of the part that they move.

F

face validity an initial means to establish the degree of truthfulness or correctness of a defined concept (construct) that is to be measured. One of the first steps in determining the quality of a testing tool is to have a group of experts review the contents. The experts are asked to judge how appropriate the contents of the new testing tool seem compared to what they know about the subject. Face validity is typically used during the initial phases of test development because of its inherent subjectivity. Once the testing tool's face validity has been established, the more rigorous *content validity* testing is conducted. See *Delphi technique*.

facilitator an individual who is making a group's job easier by suggesting structure and choices as the group process goes forward. The facilitator contributes to an activity by promoting an atmosphere that is conducive to productivity (i.e., a safe and intimate environment that encourages the sharing of ideas and feelings). In this type of group dynamics, the group is as responsible for the *outcome* of the group process as the leader/facilitator. This *leadership* role is different from the role of a leader whose job is to make the decisions and be responsible for the outcome of the group.

facility building(s) in which services are being provided. In health care the term "facility" usually means the buildings used to provide specific type(s) of services. The group of buildings is usually accredited or licensed as one entity (e.g., "psych" facility, "long-term care" facility, "rehab" facility). It is not uncommon for people to use the term "facility" to mean both the buildings and the services provided. (ADA) all or any portion of buildings, structures, site improvements, complexes, equipment, roads, walks, passageways, parking lots, or other real or personal property located on a site.

faciotomy an incision through a fascia into a muscle compartment to reduce the risk of swelling that would reduce blood flow.

factor analysis a general term in the field of test development and statistics that refers to many different types of procedures used to determine how well items on a test fit together. By allowing items to be grouped together, some variables or different items can be combined with others that are statistically similar, thus reducing the amount of data that needs to be analyzed. The information obtained by group-

ing items through factor analysis often makes the information obtained easier to apply. An example would be a testing tool designed to help high school students decide on career choices. A very large testing tool could be developed which explores the students' degree of interest in 200 different occupations. This would be a very long test to take and the reliability of the student's reported interests might be influenced as much by his/her fatigue in answering so many questions as by his/her actual preferences. By grouping similar occupations together, the test taker would be able to take a much shorter test. The results would allow a broader generalization to occupations with similar profiles.

factor loadings a factor analysis that helps measure the strength of a relationship between a test item and a specific test scale. The higher the factor loading value, the more the factor stands out as being prominent.

FACTR See *Functional Assessment of Characteristics in Therapeutic Recreation*.

failure to thrive (FTT) usually, lack of normal growth and development during infancy. Causes include disease, malnutrition, and psychosocial deprivation (especially maternal). FTT also applies to children and adults in conditions where they are not able to take in enough fluids and nutrition to sustain life. (RAPs) Cognitively impaired patients can reach the point where their accumulated health/neurological problems place them at risk of clinical complications (e.g., *pressure sores*) and death. As this level of disability approaches, staff can review the following:

- Do emotional, social, and/or environmental factors play a key role?
- If a patient is not eating, is this due to a reversible *mood* problem, a basic personality problem, a negative reaction to the physical and interactive environment in which eating activity occurs, or a neurological deficit such as a deficiency in swallowing or loss of hand coordination?
- Could an identified problem be remedied through improved staff education, trying an antidepressant medication, referral to OT for training, or an innovative counseling program?
- If causes cannot be identified, what reversible clinical complications can be expected as death

approaches (e.g., fecal impaction, urinary tract infection, diarrhea, *fever*, *pain*, pressure sores)?

- What interventions are or could be in place to decrease complications?

falls For older adults who are still in their homes, daytime is the most common time for falls. The most common rooms for falls include the living room, bedroom, and stairs. The greatest risk of falling and severe injury occurs with older adults who are just beginning to experience cognitive or physical decline. They are less likely to realize and acknowledge their new limitations. The most common

time of day for falls for institutionalized adults is during the evening. Of great concern to health care facilities (and *risk management* programs) is the incidence of patient falls. All patients should be assessed for their fall risk and appropriate documentation concerning the need to supervise, assist, or restrain each patient should be noted. Inpatient programs to reduce falls (in addition to appropriate identification of patients at risk) include policies concerning floors, windows, and beds. Floors should be kept clean and dry without excess wax. Caution signs (e.g., "slippery when wet") should be used

Falls and Hip Fractures Among Older Adults (CDC)

Topic	Discussion
How serious is the problem?	In the United States, one of every three adults 65 years old or older falls each year. Falls are the leading cause of injury deaths among people 65 years and older. In 1997, about 9,000 people over the age of 65 died from fall-related injuries. Of all fall deaths, more than 60% involve people who are 75 years or older. Fall-related death rates are higher among men than women and differ by race. White men have the highest death rate, followed by white women, black men, and black women.
What other health outcomes are linked with falls?	Among older adults, falls are the most common cause of injuries and hospital admissions for trauma. Falls account for 87% of all fractures for people 65 years and older. They are also the second leading cause of spinal cord and brain injury among older adults. Each year in the United States, one person in 20 receives emergency department treatment because of a fall. Advanced age greatly increases the chance of a hospital admission following a fall. Among older adults, fractures are the most serious health outcomes associated with falls. About 3% of all falls cause fractures. The most common are fractures of the pelvis, hip, femur, vertebrae, humerus, hand, forearm, leg, and ankle.
Where are people most likely to fall?	For adults 65 years old or older, 60% of fatal falls happen at home, 30% occur in public places, and 10% occur in health care institutions.
What is the impact of hip fractures?	Of all fractures from falls, hip fractures cause the greatest number of deaths and lead to the most severe health problems. In 1996, there were approximately 340,000 hospital admissions for hip fractures in the United States. Women sustain 75% – 80% of all hip fractures. People who are 85 years or older are 10-15 times more likely to experience hip fractures than are people between the ages of 60 and 65. Most patients with hip fractures are hospitalized for about two weeks. Half of all older adults hospitalized for hip fractures cannot return home or live independently after their injuries. In 1991, Medicare costs for hip fractures were estimated to be $2.9 billion. Because the US population is aging, the problem of hip fractures will likely increase substantially over the next four decades. By the year 2040, the number of hip fractures is expected to exceed 500,000.
What factors increase older adults' risk of falling?	Factors that contribute to falls include problems with gait and balance, neurological and musculoskeletal disabilities, psychoactive medication use, dementia, and visual impairment. Environmental hazards such as slippery surfaces, uneven floors, poor lighting, loose rugs, unstable furniture, and objects on floors may also play a role.
What can older adults do to reduce their risk of falling?	Maintain a regular exercise program. Exercise improves strength, balance, and coordination. Take steps to make living areas safer. Remove tripping hazards and use non-slip mats in the bathtub and on shower floors. Have grab bars put in next to the toilet and in the tub or shower, and have handrails put in on both sides of all stairs. Ask their doctor to review all of their medicines in order to reduce side effects and interactions. Have an eye doctor check their vision each year. Poor vision can increase the risk of falling.

when needed. Broken or cracked surfaces should be repaired and all foreign materials that are tripping hazards should be removed immediately. Windows should contain (where appropriate) safety glass and should be designed to reduce the chance that a patient may fall from an open window. Falls from beds are one of the main causes of falls in health care. *Beds* and bed rails should be maintained in good working condition, as should all call lights. (RAPs) Falls are a common source of serious injury and death among the elderly. Each year 40% of nursing home patients fall. Up to 5% of falls result in fractures, an additional 15% result in soft tissue injuries. Moreover, most elders are afraid of falling and this fear can limit their activities. In about one-third of falls, a single potential cause can be identified; in two-thirds, more than one risk factor is involved. Risk factors that are internal to the patient include the patient's physical health and functional status. External risk factors include medication side effects, use of appliances and *restraints*, and environmental conditions. See the tables: Falls and Hip Fractures Among Older Adults and The Costs of Fall Injuries Among Older Adults for the CDC's information about falls. See *activities of daily living, ambulatory, cognitive deficits, foam mattress bed, gait, institutional settings, physical restraint.*

False Claims Act a federal law that allows a private citizen to take an individual or a corporation to court if they feel that they can prove the person or corporation is fraudulently billing the federal government. This law is better known as the "Whistle Blower" law. If the individual making claim of fraud proves his/her case in court, s/he is able to keep part of the money regained. This amount is usually substantial. The Whistle Blower law has recently been applied to nursing homes that provide substandard care and then bill the federal government for the provision of this care through Medicare or Medicaid.

The Costs of Fall Injuries Among Older Adults (CDC)

Topic	Discussion
The problem	Falls are a serious public health problem among older adults. In the United States, one of every three people 65 years and older falls each year. Older adults are hospitalized for fall-related injuries five times more often than they are for injuries from other causes. Of those who fall, 20-30% suffer moderate to severe injuries that reduce mobility and independence, and increase the risk of premature death.
Calculating cost estimates	The cost of fall-related injuries is usually expressed in terms of direct costs. Direct costs include out-of-pocket expenses and charges paid by insurance companies for the treatment of fall-related injuries. These include costs and fees associated with hospital and nursing home care, physician and other professional services, rehabilitation, community-based services, the use of medical equipment, prescription drugs, local rehabilitation, home modifications, and insurance administration. Direct costs do not account for the long-term consequences of these injuries, such as disability, decreased productivity, or quality of life.
The costs of fall-related injuries	In 1994, the average direct cost for a fall injury was $1,400 for a person over the age of 65. The total direct cost of all fall injuries for people age 65 and older in 1994 was $20.2 billion. By 2020, the cost of fall injuries is expected to reach $32.4 billion.
Fall-related fractures	The most common fall-related injuries are osteoporotic fractures. These are fractures of the hip, spine, or forearm. In the United States in 1986, the direct medical costs for osteoporotic fractures were $5.15 billion. By 1989, these costs exceeded $6 billion. Over the next 10 years, total direct medical costs for osteoporotic fractures among postmenopausal women will be more than $45.2 billion.
Hip fractures	Of all fall-related fractures, hip fractures are the most serious and lead to the greatest number of health problems and deaths. In the United States, hospitalization accounts for 44% of direct health care costs for hip fracture patients. In 1991, Medicare costs for this injury were estimated to be $2.9 billion. Hospital admissions for hip fractures among people over age 65 have steadily increased, from 230,000 admissions in 1988 to 340,000 admissions in 1996. The number of hip fractures is expected to exceed 500,000 by the year 2040. A recent study found that the cost of a hip fracture, including direct medical care, formal non-medical care, and informal care provided by family and friends, was between $16,300 and $18,700 during the first year following the injury. Assuming 5% inflation and the growing number of hip fractures, the total annual cost of these injuries may reach $240 billion by the year 2040.

Family APGAR Scale a screening tool to help the professional determine if the patient needs extra staff or volunteer time. The Family APGAR with its five categories is given below. Read each statement and then determine a score by using "0" (zero) for "almost always," "1" for "some of the time," and "2" for "hardly ever." Total the scores for the five questions. Total scores over 3 (out of a possible 10) are considered a problem. Patients with a score of five or more may be good candidates for extra volunteer and/or staff time. See *Apgar*. The questions below are adapted from Smilkstein (1978).

    Adaptation: In my family we help each other out. If we can't find the help we need within the family, we have places and people in the community to help.

    Partnership: In my family we make decisions by talking things out and then reaching an agreement.

    Growth: In my family we help each other achieve our desires and support each other so that we can grow and change.

    Affection: In my family we are able to share all kinds of feelings with each other including love, anger, and sorrow.

    Resolve: In my family we share what we have including our time, our space, and our money.

    Note: If some of the patients do not have family close by but have a good support network of friends, use the Family APGAR using the statement "My friends and I" instead of "In my family we."

family council an organization within a long-term care facility that is run by and for families and friends of the patients. It is independent of the hospital administration, is self-determining and organized to meet the individuals' needs and interests of the group. Unlike the *resident council*, the family council is not required by federal law.

family of origin referring to the family that one was born to.

family therapy treatment of more than one member of a family simultaneously in the same session. The treatment may be supportive, directive, or interpretive. The assumption is that a dysfunction in one member of a family may be a manifestation of disorder in other members and may affect interrelationships and functioning.

Fanconi's anemia (HHS/NMDP) a rare form of aplastic anemia. Bone marrow transplantation for Fanconi's anemia would require a less intense conditioning regime than other diagnoses.

fatigability referring to the patient's increased sus-

ceptibility to *fatigue*, requiring additional rest times throughout the activity and throughout the day. The patient's *functional ability* usually drops as s/he becomes more fatigued.

fatigue decreased ability of an individual to complete a task because of a lack of oxygen delivery, protective influences of the central nervous system, or a depletion of potassium in the elderly. The use of a muscle past the point of fatigue may lead to *strain* or to overuse syndrome. The idea of "No Pain, No Gain" is a phrase that the professional probably wants to avoid. Too frequently it leads to over fatigue of a muscle. The intensity of exercise should cause a gentle "pulling" sensation in the tight tissue and not pain (Kisner and Colby, 1990, p. 679). With patients who have experienced a recent prolonged reduction in normal activity, the professional may need to help the patient develop a schedule of modified activity until the appropriate level of *endurance* and *strength* can be achieved. See *aerobic, baclofen, crutch, fatigability, Parkinson's disease, postural dysfunction, progressive relaxation.*

fats (dietary) (HHS) Fats are referred to in the plural because there is no one type of fat. Fats are composed of the same three elements as carbohydrates: carbon, hydrogen, and oxygen. However, fats have relatively more carbon and hydrogen and less oxygen, thus supplying a higher fuel value of nine calories per gram (versus four calories per gram from carbohydrates and protein). One molecule of fat can be broken down into three molecules of fatty acids and one molecule of glycerol. Thus, fats are known chemically as triglycerides. Fats are a vital nutrient in a healthy diet. Fats supply essential fatty acids, such as linoleic acid, which is especially important to childhood growth. Fat helps maintain healthy skin, regulate cholesterol metabolism, and is a precursor of prostaglandins, hormone-like substances that regulate some body processes. Dietary fat is needed to carry fat-soluble vitamins A, D, E, and K and to aid in their absorption from the intestine.

fatty acid (HHS) Fatty acids are generally classified as saturated, monounsaturated, or polyunsaturated. These terms refer to the number of hydrogen atoms attached to the carbon atoms of the fat molecule. In general, fats that contain a majority of saturated fatty acids are solid at room temperature, although some solid vegetable shortenings are up to 75% unsaturated. *Fats* containing mostly unsaturated fatty acids are usually liquid at room temperature and are called oils. See *fats, hydrogenation.*

FDA See *Food and Drug Administration.*

fear a combined physiological and psychological

response to a real or imagined threat. See *coping skills training, epigastric sensation, hypochondriasis, medical play.*

febrile pertaining to a *fever.*

Federal Financial Participation (FFP) the federal government's share of money paid to the state for services furnished to state Medicaid recipients as well as for administrative costs related to the operation of the Medicaid program in the state. The FFP share is determined by a formula based on the state's per capita income. See *departmental appeals board, Section 1905 (d).*

federal jurisdictional survey a federal survey to assess provider performance and to determine whether a provider/supplier meets all applicable program requirements. These surveys are the basis for certification of providers in situations where no state agency has jurisdiction. Certification surveys conducted by federal personnel include: Indian Health Service hospitals, Commonwealth of the Virgin Islands, and end-state renal disease facilities in Veteran Administration Hospitals.

federal monitoring survey surveys of Medicare and/or Medicaid participating facilities performed by a federal team to assess state agency performance in certifying providers and suppliers. A monitoring survey is generally conducted within 60 days of a state survey and may be a full or partial survey. A survey is selected on a sample or focused basis. See *survey process*

feedback information given back to an individual (or other entity) on how his/her behavior/actions/words affected another person or the environment. An evaluation of performance by someone other then oneself. See *disease management, listening skills.*

feeding the act of obtaining nutrition. For a patient to be considered independent in feeding s/he would need to be able to complete the following tasks without cueing or other assistance:

1. order and/or obtain and set up food and drink,
2. successfully and appropriately use regular or adapted tableware, utensils, and cups,
3. bring food and drink from the table or eating surface to mouth,
4. adequately chew food and swallow food/liquids so that threat of choking is not evident.

While the patient's initial training in these skills will most likely come from either the occupational therapist or the speech therapist, the recreational therapist will often supervise, assist, and evaluate the patient in his/her skills related to feeding and eating while on community integration outings.

feeding and eating disorders of infancy or early

childhood a specific category of developmental disorders in the **DSM-IV** characterized by on-going *feeding/eating* difficulties. Included in this grouping are *pica* and rumination disorder. See *childhood psychiatric disorders.*

feeding tube certain patients are not able to take nutrition through their mouths, so they need to be fed through tubes. On the next page are charts that review the more common feeding tubes and methods of tube feeding.

fee-for-service a medical payment plan where the patient is billed for each therapy session or procedure as opposed to having the cost of those services included as part of the fees for a *health maintenance organization* or rolled into the *roomrate.* See *average adjusted per capita cost, corporate alliances.*

festination gait a gait in which the individual takes small steps while leaning forward. Due to the foreword position of the patient's center of gravity, the gait becomes steadily faster as the patient tries not to fall foreword. This gait is frequently seen in individuals with *Parkinson's disease.* See *falls.*

fetal alcohol syndrome (FAS) a group of disabilities that are seen in children born to women who drank heavily during pregnancy. Between 3% and 6% of all births have this syndrome. The three predominate features are 1. below normal growth patterns, 2. delayed *fine motor* and *gross motor* development, and 3. identifiable facial features. See *mental retardation.*

fever elevated body temperature. A person with a fever is said to be febrile. See *vital signs.*

Normal Body Temperature

Tempera-ture Scale	Oral Site	Rectal Site	Axillary Site
C	37.0°	37.5°	36.4°
F	98.6°	99.5°	97.6°

FFP See *Federal Financial Participation, Section 1905(d).*

fiber (HHS) parts of fruits, vegetables, grains, nuts, and legumes that can't be digested by humans. Meats and dairy products do not contain fiber. Studies indicate that high-fiber diets can reduce the risks of heart disease and certain types of cancer. There are two basic types of fiber, insoluble and soluble. Soluble fiber in cereals, oatmeal, beans, and other foods has been found to lower blood cholesterol. Insoluble fiber in cauliflower, cabbage, and other vegetables and fruits helps move foods through the stomach and intestine, thereby decreasing the risk of cancers of the colon and rectum.

fibrillation limited involuntary contraction of small

Types of Feeding Tubes

Type	Description	Notes
Gastric gavage	A tube that is inserted into the nasal passage and then pushed down into the stomach (nasogastric) or into the intestines (nasointestinal).	• Best for patients who do not have a disruption in the ability to digest food but are not able to take enough nutrition through their mouths to meet their needs. • May be left in for up to 4 weeks.
Jejunostomy Tube	A tube inserted directly into the mid-portion of the small intestine. A gastrostomy device is required.	• Least risk of aspiration. • Small intestines do not usually tolerate the high caloric content of most formulas so the formula must be watered down. • Delivered using a pump to provide consistent and slow delivery of formula.
Hyperalimentation Tube	Parenteral hyperalimentation tubes go directly into the bloodstream from a catheter placed through the subclavian vein into the superior vena cava.	• For patients who cannot eat, digest, or absorb nutrition adequately. • Since catheter goes directly to the heart, activity must be limited to activities that do not risk disturbing or displacing the catheter.

Methods of Tube Feeding

Type	Description	Notes
Bolus Tube Feedings	A large amount (250 to 400 ml) of liquid nourishment is placed into the patient's stomach over the period of a few minutes.	• Repeated four to six times a day. • Allows freer movement of patient, as patient can clamp end of tube and move about. • Patients who are unconscious or who take a long time to digest the food are at greater risk of vomiting and aspiration.
Intermittent Tube Feedings	Usually gravity driven, a large amount (250 to 400 ml) of liquid nourishment is fed into the patient's stomach over a period of 30 to 60 minutes.	• Reduced bloated feeling by stretching out delivery time of liquid. • "Normalizes" feeding time, as feeding times usually mimic the frequency and duration of normal meal times.
Continuous Tube Feedings	A small volume of liquid nourishment is provided for the patient (approximately 1.5 ml per minute).	• Electric feed pump is usually used, requiring the patient who is ambulatory to "drag" along the IV pole and pump. • Reduced volume delivered continually may be allowed to bypass digestion in stomach (delivery right into small intestine) thus reducing risk of vomiting and aspiration.

groups of muscles due to an irritation at the root of the nerve. Fibrillation of the heart can disrupt the normal pumping action.

fibroblasts cells that produce the material necessary for the development of new connective tissues. See *chronic inflammation.*

fibromyalgia The American College of Rheumatology in 1990 developed two criteria to diagnosis fibromyalgia: 1. a history of widespread pain for at least three months and 2. pain in 11 of 18 tender point sites on *digital palpation.* Fibromyalgia may share some of the same symptoms as other diseases, including *thyroid disease, lupus,* and rheumatoid *arthritis* and is usually not chosen as a diagnosis until other, similar diseases are ruled out. Fibromyalgia is not just a disease of the musculoskeletal system because frequent secondary complaints include headaches, short-term memory problems, intermittent blurred vision, irritable bowel and/or bladder, and painful menstrual periods. Two secondary aspects of this disorder are depression and disturbances in normal sleeping patterns. Also known as fibrositis, myofascial pain, post-viral fatigue syndrome, chronic fatigue syndrome, tension myalgia, and generalized tendomyopathy.

fibrosis 1. development of fibrous tissues in response to damage to the body. 2. abnormal replacement of smooth muscle tissue or organ tissue with fibrous connective tissue.

fibrositis See *fibromyalgia.*

fibrotic adhesion contractures When a patient experiences chronic inflammation, as with arthritis, the soft tissues involved tend to become more fibrotic. These changes cause tissues to adhere to each other, significantly reducing range of motion. Fibrotic adhesions are extremely difficult, if not impossible, to reduce through general activity.

field 1. a defined area or space. 2. the part of a computerized form which is to be filled in by the individual entering data into the system. An example would be a computerized form that asks for the patient's name. After the word "name" would be a space (usually marked by shading) in which the patient's name would be typed.

field cut decrease or loss of a portion of a person's field of vision following a stroke or some other types of brain injury. See *neglect, visuospatial neglect.*

filtering See *listening skills.*

FIM-FRGs See *function related groups.*

FIM Scale one of the most common coding systems used in assessment and charting is the Functional Independence Measure or the "FIM." The FIM is a seven-point scale that is divided into two basic levels of ability: *independent* and *dependent.* Shown

below. See *spinal cord injury, uniform data system.*

fine motor movement which require delicate, well-controlled movement, usually of the hands. See *Denver Developmental Screening Tool, dressing skills, General Recreation Screening Tool, manual dexterity.*

fine tremor See *tremor.*

firewall (HCO) computer hardware and software that block unauthorized communications between an institution's computer network and external networks.

firms trial (HCO) a form of randomized controlled trial in which patients are randomly assigned to similar ("parallel") providers who use different health services, rather than to different groups that receive different services from the same provider.

fiscal intermediary an organization (usually an insurance company) that has an agreement under Medicare Part A to process *provider* claims and perform other functions.

fish mouth amputation skin flaps are left to extend below the amputated bone.

five a day (HHS) refers to the dietary recommendation to consume five servings of fruits and vegetables every day. The tagline, 5 A Day, became a promotional message in campaigns to increase fruit and vegetable consumption.

fixed route systems (ADA) systems that provide transportation for individuals on vehicles (other than aircraft) that are operated along a prescribed route according to a fixed schedule. The ADA accessibil-

---

Functional Independence Measure (FIM)

© Copyright 1987 Research Foundation — State University of New York

Independent — Another person is not required for the activity (No Helper).

7 Complete Independence All of the tasks described as making up the activity are typically performed safely without modification, assistive devices, or aids and within reasonable time.

6 Modified Independence Activity requires any one or more than one of the following: an assistive device, more than reasonable time, or there are safety (risk) considerations.

Dependent — Another person is required for either supervision or physical assistance in order for the activity to be performed or it is not performed (Requires Helper).

Modified Dependence The subject expends half (50%) or more of the effort. The levels of assistance required are

5 Supervision or Setup Subject requires no more help than standby, *cueing,* or coaxing, without physical contact. Or, helper sets up needed items or applies *orthoses.*

4 Minimal Contact Assistance With physical contact the subject requires no more help than touching and subject expends 75% or more of the effort.

3 Moderate Assistance Subject requires more help than touching or expends half (50%) or more (up to 75%) of the effort.

Complete Dependence — The subject expends less than half (less than 50%) of the effort. Maximal or total assistance is required or the activity is not performed. The levels of assistance required are

2 Maximal Assistance Subject expends less than 50% of the effort, but at least 25%.

1 Total Assistance Subject expends less than 25% of the effort.

ity guidelines for fixed route systems may be found in the **Buses, Vans, and Systems Technical Assistance Manual** (US Architectural and Transportation Barriers Compliance Board).

flaccid a muscle or limb that is weak, lacks *tone* and lacks voluntary control. See *lower motor neuron lesion.*

flaccid bladder a bladder that has a weakened capability to retain fluid without artificial help. See *incontinence.*

flaccid gait See *hemiplegic gait.*

Flesch grade level To help determine the degree of difficulty (or ease) in reading text, an index was developed called the Flesch Grade Level Index. Through research, it was found that by determining the average number of words in a sentence and the average number of syllables per 100 words, a person could predict who could understand the material. After conducting normative studies, a grade level reading equivalent was determined. The number before the decimal indicates the grade level of the text. The number after the decimal indicates the number of months the average reader in that grade would have been in that grade before being able to read the written text. (The **Community Integration Program's** Module 3B Grocery Store has a Flesch grade level of 6.4, which means a reader in the fourth month of sixth grade could understand the material.) See *graphic input.*

flesh-eating bacteria See *group A streptococcus, necrotizing fasciitis.*

flexibility body's or mind's ability to yield (bend, move, change stance) when required. Muscles and other soft tissues respond when challenged with stretching force, the mind responds when challenged to format thoughts in a different manner. The maintenance of flexibility usually requires an individual's involvement in multiple activities on a regular basis. Flexibility is important. Being flexible allows the patient to maintain better *balance* and posture, decreases the chance of injury, and relieves *stress* (Karam, 1989, p. 1). See *dance therapy.*

flexible spending account (FB) a reimbursement account under which participating employees are reimbursed for medical expenses or other nontaxable employer-sponsored benefits. A flexible spending account can either be part of a *cafeteria plan* or a stand-alone benefit plan.

flexion moving two ends of a joint closer together. Opposite of *extension*. See *Dupuytren's contracture, full arc extension, hyperflexia, hypoflexia, range of motion.*

flooding See *implosive therapy.*

fluent aphasia speech that is fluent with paraphasic

errors (words may be unrelated to the current topic or unintelligible). Auditory comprehension, reading comprehension, and writing comprehension are impaired. See *aphasia, cerebrovascular accident.*

fluid intelligence a group of cognitive skills related to higher functioning cognition including associative *memory*, figural relationship, and *inductive reasoning.*

fluid reality a psychiatric condition, frequently associated with non-productive coping, in which an individual redefines his/her feelings and interpretations about events or relationship depending on his/her current situation instead of on the event/relationship itself. Individuals who exhibit fluid reality tend to have poorly defined self-images and frequently flip-flop the meaning of things in their lives.

fluoride (HHS) a compound of fluorine (an element with atomic number 9); a natural component of minerals in rocks and soils. Widespread use of fluoride in water supplies and oral health products is credited with the dramatic decline in *dental caries* among children and adults alike. All water contains fluoride, but it is sometimes necessary to add it to some public supplies to attain the optimal amount for dental health. Fluoride makes tooth enamel stronger and more resistant to decay. It also prevents the growth of harmful bacteria and interferes with converting fermentable carbohydrates to acids in the mouth.

foam mattress bed commercially known as "Egg Crate," "Geo-Matt," "Spencegel Pad," these mattresses are used for patients who have intact skin or lower grade (stage one or a small area stage two) *pressure sores*. They provide a slightly more therapeutic surface for skin at risk than regular mattresses. These are frequently placed over an existing mattress. Implications for treatment include a potentially increased risk of *fall* (patient not used to mattress height) or decreased bed *mobility* (patient may need a firm surface to move in bed). See *bed.*

focus primary interest of one's actions or attention. The ability to focus on one thought or task requires complex skills and is frequently limited or lost with brain damage or *dementia*. The loss of the ability to focus greatly increases the risk of sensory deprivation. See *deprivation.*

focused reviews a term used in *quality assurance* programs. A focused review is a review of all or a majority of cases within one very specific aspect of practice. Focused reviews are usually selected because of the high-risk nature of the treatment, the high volume of the patient diagnostic group, or the high incidence rate of problems within the aspect of practice. An example is a review of all patients who refuse to attend required treatment groups.

Foley catheter a tube inserted into the urethra to allow continuous emptying of the bladder. The amount of fluid (and how it looks) is an important indicator of patient health. The therapist is expected to empty the Foley catheter bag and accurately record the amount and appearance of the urine. Often a patient who has progressed to the point of being able to leave the hospital for short periods of time will still rely on a urine collection device. There are many different options for urine collection (especially for outings of three hours or less). Because Foley catheter bags hang on the side of a wheelchair, the patient's urine is visible for all to see. The therapist should work with the rest of the treatment team and the patient to come up with a more normalizing alternative. Patients with burns usually have both an intravenous line (IV) and a catheter due to the amount of intravenous fluid loss.

folic acid (HHS) folic acid, folate, folacin, all form a group of compounds functionally involved in amino acid metabolism and nucleic acid synthesis. Good dietary sources of folate include leafy, dark green vegetables, legumes, citrus fruits and juices, peanuts, whole grains, and fortified breakfast cereals. Recent studies show that if all women of childbearing age consumed sufficient folic acid (either through diet or supplements), 50 to 70% of birth defects of the brain and spinal cord could be prevented, according to the US Centers for Disease Control and Prevention. Folic acid is critical from conception through the first four to six weeks of pregnancy when the neural tube is formed. This means adequate diet or supplement use should begin before pregnancy occurs. Recent research findings also show low blood folate levels can be associated with elevated plasma homocystine and increased risk of coronary heart disease.

following directions The ability to follow directions is frequently referred to as the ability to follow one-step, two-step, or three-step commands. The ability to follow the number of steps given in directions is an indicator of cognitive function. Patients who are able to follow only one-step commands are considered very impaired and usually require frequent cueing to function in the facility or in the community. A one-step command (direction) might be "Pick up the phone." Patients who are able to follow only two-step commands are considered to be moderately impaired and usually require some support (from another person or from a memory book) to function in the facility or community. A two-step command might be "Pick up the phone and call your doctor's office." Patients with little or no impairment should be able to follow three-step commands with little or

no cueing support. A three-step command might be "Pick up the phone and call your doctor's office for an appointment sometime near the end of next week." It is not customary to talk about four (or more) step commands. Generally it is assumed that patients who are able to follow three-step commands (directions) are able to function independently. For patients who have exceptional ability, the therapist might report the ability to follow complex directions independently. See *cognition*.

Food and Drug Administration (FDA) (HHS) part of the Public Health Service of the US Department of Health and Human Services. It is the regulatory agency responsible for ensuring the safety and wholesomeness of all foods sold in interstate commerce except meat, poultry, and eggs (which are under the jurisdiction of the US Department of Agriculture). The FDA develops standards for the composition, quality, nutrition, safety, and labeling of foods including food and color additives. It conducts research to improve detection and prevention of contamination. It collects and interprets data on nutrition, food additives, and pesticide residues. The agency also inspects food plants, imported food products, and feed mills that make feeds containing medications or nutritional supplements that are destined for human consumption. And it regulates radiation-emitting products such as microwave ovens. The FDA also enforces pesticide tolerances established by the Environmental Protection Agency for all domestically produced and imported foods, except for foods under USDA jurisdiction.

food-borne disease (CDC) a disease caused by consuming contaminated foods or beverages. Many different disease-causing microbes, or pathogens, can contaminate foods, so there are many different food-borne infections. In addition, poisonous chemicals, or other harmful substances can cause food-borne diseases if they are present in food. More than 250 different food-borne diseases have been described. Most of these diseases are infections, caused by a variety of bacteria, viruses, and parasites that can be food-borne. Other diseases are poisonings, caused by harmful toxins or chemicals that have contaminated the food, for example, poisonous mushrooms. These different diseases have many different symptoms, so there is no one *syndrome* that is food-borne illness. However, the microbe or toxin enters the body through the gastrointestinal tract, and often causes the first symptoms there, so nausea, vomiting, abdominal cramps, and diarrhea are common symptoms in many food-borne diseases. Many microbes can spread in more than one way, so we cannot always know that a disease is food-borne. The distinction matters, because public health authorities need to know how a particular disease is spreading to take the appropriate steps to stop it. For example, Escherichia coli O157:H7 infections can spread through contaminated food, contaminated drinking water, contaminated swimming water, and from toddler to toddler at a day care center. Depending on which means of spread caused a case, the measures to stop other cases from occurring could range from removing contaminated food from stores, chlorinating a swimming pool, or closing a child day care center. The most commonly recognized food-borne infections are those caused by the bacteria *Campylobacter, Salmonella,* and *E. coli O157:H7,* and by a group of viruses called calicivirus, also known as the Norwalk and Norwalk-like viruses. Some common diseases are occasionally food-borne, even though they are usually transmitted by other routes. These include infections caused by Shigella, *hepatitis* A, and the parasites Giardia lamblia and Cryptosporidia. Even strep throats have been transmitted occasionally through food. In addition to disease caused by direct infection, some food-borne diseases are caused by the presence of a toxin in the food that was produced by a microbe in the food. For example, the bacterium Staphylococcus aureus can grow in some foods and produce a toxin that causes intense vomiting. The rare but deadly disease *botulism* occurs when the bacterium Clostridium botulinum grows and produces a powerful paralytic toxin in foods. These toxins can produce illness even if the microbes that produced them are no longer there. Other toxins and poisonous chemicals can cause food-borne illness. People can become ill if a pesticide is inadvertently added to a food, or if naturally poisonous substances are used to prepare a meal. Every year, people become ill after mistaking poisonous mushrooms for safe species, or after eating poisonous reef fishes. See *food poisoning.*

Food Guide Pyramid (HHS) a graphic design used to communicate the recommended daily food choices contained in the Dietary Guidelines for Americans. The information provided was devel-

oped and promoted by the US Department of Agriculture and the US Department of Health and Human Services. See a copy of the pyramid on the next page.

food irradiation (HHS) the exposure of food to sufficient radiant energy (gamma rays, x-rays, and electron beams) to destroy microorganisms and insects. Irradiation is used in food production and processing to promote food safety.

food poisoning a noxious and/or destructive microbe or other element that is introduced into a person's body through food or drink. The most common microbes that cause food poisoning in the United States are campylobacter, salmonella, E. coli O157:H7, vibrio species, and listeria. See the chart below. See *food-borne disease.*

foot See *ankle and foot.*

footdrop gait a *gait* where the patient slaps the foot to the ground after lifting the knee high on the affected side only. This gait causes increased jarring to the body and limits, to some degree, the patient's ability to achieve a high skill level in physical activities that require highly coordinated foot and leg movements. Frequently due to weak or paralyzed dorsiflexor muscles.

forensic psychiatry a specialty within psychiatry which addresses the legal issues of mental illness, including a determination whether the patient is mentally competent to stand trial and treatment for those who are not mentally responsible for their actions. See *actus reus, competency to stand trial, mens rea.*

formal operations last stage of Piagetian theory that describes the ability to think logically and to demonstrate a grasp of abstract concepts. This stage is usually reached by 12 to 15 years of age.

four-point gait use of two *crutches* in addition to the use of two weight-bearing legs in ambulation. By alternating the movement of the crutches and the legs the patient is able to move while always having at least three points of support. This gait provides maximal support with stability but causes significant limitations to activities. This type of gait is usually

Common Types of Food Poisoning	
Type	**Foods Most Often Effected**
Campylobacter	Poultry, raw milk, untreated water. Occurrence is 4,000 illness per 100,000 per year.
E. coli O157:H7	Ground beef, raw milk, unpasteurized cider and apple juice, lettuce. Occurrence is 25 illnesses per 100,000.
Listeria	Processed, ready-to-eat foods such as deli foods and soft cheese. Occurrence is 1.5 illnesses per 100,000.
Salmonella	Eggs, poultry, meat, and fresh produce. Occurrence is 2,000 illnesses per 100,000 per year.
Vibrio species	Seafood, especially raw shellfish. Occurrence is 10 illnesses per 100,000.

Food Guide Pyramid

A Guide to Daily Food Choices

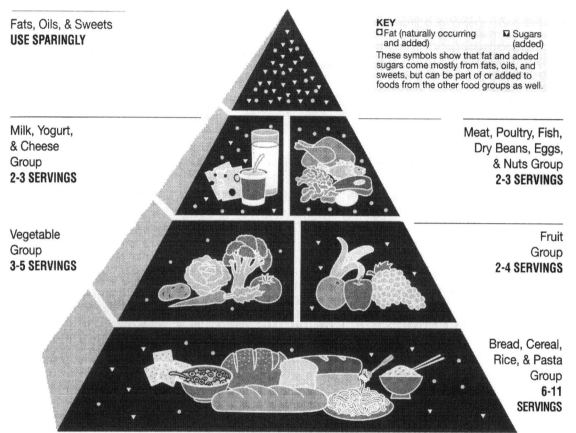

Fats, Oils, & Sweets
USE SPARINGLY

KEY
☐ Fat (naturally occurring   ▨ Sugars
and added)   (added)
These symbols show that fat and added
sugars come mostly from fats, oils, and
sweets, but can be part of or added to
foods from the other food groups as well.

Milk, Yogurt,
& Cheese
Group
2-3 SERVINGS

Meat, Poultry, Fish,
Dry Beans, Eggs,
& Nuts Group
2-3 SERVINGS

Vegetable
Group
3-5 SERVINGS

Fruit
Group
2-4 SERVINGS

Bread, Cereal,
Rice, & Pasta
Group
**6-11
SERVINGS**

SOURCE: U.S. Department of Agriculture/U.S. Department of Health and Human Services

Use the Food Guide Pyramid to help you eat better every day. . .the Dietary Guidelines way. Start with plenty of Breads, Cereals, Rice, and Pasta; Vegetables; and Fruits. Add two to three servings from the Milk group and two to three servings from the Meat group.

Each of these food groups provides some, but not all, of the nutrients you need. No one food group is more important than another — for good health you need them all. Go easy on fats, oils, and sweets, the foods in the small tip of the Pyramid.

slower than other types of gaits and requires the use of the hands, providing limited or no use of the hands during activities while ambulating. Backpacks are frequently used by patients who ambulate using the four-point gait. The therapist may need to educate the patient on appropriate and safe ways of *donning* and *doffing* the pack, as well as how to determine a good pack weight and balance. See *ambulatory.*

frame of reference set of beliefs and knowledge on which an individual bases his/her actions. Frame of

reference can be very important for the therapist to consider when addressing treatment issues for a patient. The author once had a patient from a tropical island whose culture felt that any illness was due to being possessed by "the devil." With this frame of reference and the patient's cognitive disorder from a *cerebrovascular accident*, the patient tended to lash out physically at other patients, trying to literally kill all those "possessed by the devil." While this is an unusually extreme case of a frame of reference impacting the patient's ability to respond to *treatment*, it does point out that the therapist will be more successful in providing treatment if s/he understands the patient's frame of reference.

frame relay (HCO) a fast networking protocol in which data are packaged in variable-length frames for shuttling between computer networks.

frank an indication that a sign of clinical significance is obviously evident. "Frank" blood in the stool indicates that freshly lost blood is in the fecal matter.

Frankel Neurological Assessment for Spinal Cord Injury one type of *scale* to help indicate ability or to measure changes in functional ability. (Shown below.) This scale has been replaced by the American Spinal Injury Association's modification shown in *spinal cord injury*.

Frankel Neurological Assessment for Spinal Cord Injury

Complete (A)	No motor power below site of lesion.
Sensory (B)	No motor power but some sensory awareness below site of lesion.
Motor Useless (C)	Some motor power below the site of lesion but not enough to provide functional ability to patient.
Motor Useful (D)	Adequate motor power below site of lesion to allow functional ability to patient.
Recovery (E)	Full motor power, adequate to normal sensory awareness, no sphincter impairment; may have subnormal reflexes.

fraud (Medicare) (HCFA/Questions) an intentional deception or misrepresentation that someone makes, knowing it is false, that could result in an unauthorized payment. Keep in mind the attempt itself is fraud, regardless of whether it is successful. See *abuse (Medicare)* for a discussion of process and penalties.

Freedom of Information Act a federal law in the United States that establishes the right of the public to have access to numerous types of government-held information. There is an established procedure for using the Freedom of Information Act and most state agencies have a person specifically identified to handle all Freedom of Information Act requests. The information obtained through the Freedom of Information Act is not free; a charge is determined by the amount of copying required, as well as the amount of staff time required to find the information.

Free Time Boredom Measurement a 20-item measurement of boredom developed by Ragheb and Merydith (1995). The purpose of the Free Time Boredom Measurement is to identify the degree to which the patient is bored in each of the four components of *boredom*: 1. meaningfulness (focus or purpose during free time), 2. mental involvement (adequate number of things to think about and thoughts that are emotionally satisfying), 3. speed of time (enough purposeful and satisfying activity to fill time), and 4. physical involvement (adequate amount of physical movement to satisfy). See *scales*.

Frenkel's movement movement exercises prescribed for patients with *ataxia* to help restore functional ability. See *movement*.

frequency 1. repetitions within a fixed period of time, such as number of breaths per minute. 2. (in biometry) how often a characteristic is observed in a population expressed as the fraction of the population that has the particular characteristic. 3. (in electronics) the number of cycles (Hertz) or completed alterations per unit time of a wave oscillation.

Freud, Sigmund a neurologist who lived between 1856 and 1939 and developed many theories associated with human behavior. One of his primary theories was about the unconscious mind and how the unconscious mind influenced behavior. He is also known for his theory that events experienced in early life significantly influence behaviors later in life and that *aggression* and sexuality are the main causes of *motivation* for all types of human behavior. See *genital phase, ego, id, superego, latency phase, libido*.

frontal cortex forebrain; the outer layer of gray matter that covers the cerebral cortex located just behind the forehead. The frontal cortex is the most evolved of all brain structures, is present only in primates, and is involved with higher functioning such as understanding and communication.

fructose (HHS) a monosaccharide (single sugar) found naturally in fruits, as an added sugar in a crystalline form and as a component of high-fructose corn syrup (HFCS).

fruit (HHS) the edible reproductive body of a seed plant, especially one having a sweet pulp associated with the seed.

frustration an emotional response to being unable to achieve one's goal or to be satisfied in such a manner as to threaten one's self-esteem or perception of security or to cause a feeling of unwanted isolation.

FTT See *failure to thrive*.

Principles for Selecting and Performing Functional Assessments

Principle	Description
Objectivity	Testing protocols that reduce the therapist's subjectivity produce a stronger legal document if the test must be defended in court. Two therapists should be able to test the same patient and get the same results.
Standardization	The same patients, tested on the same equipment, should produce the same results.
Methodology	How the test is conducted must be consistent from test to test, from instructing the patient to analyzing the results. Protocols should be written and followed with consistency.
Information Processing	The processing and reporting of data must be standardized.

full arc extension movement of a joint from *flexion* to *extension*. Some activities that may promote full arc extension are creative dance and swimming. See *dance therapy.*

full liquid diet a prescribed *diet* which consists of thick fluids including different kinds of juices (both pureed vegetable and fruit juices), milk, ice cream, gelatin, custards, and other non-alcoholic drinks that generally accompany a meal.

full service continuum ability to provide the services a patient needs through his/her health care continuum, which would include everything from emergency room services and intensive care to *home health* and wellness care.

full-thickness graft a graft that contains the epidermis and the dermis of the skin, but does not contain the subcutaneous fat.

functional ability ability to perform a task well enough to have some measured success; to be able to complete enough of a task to achieve the desired outcome. See *Denver Developmental Screening Tool, disability rating, fatigability, generalization, habilitation, helplessness, maneuver, mastery, physical activities, scales.*

functional aquatic activities also known as basic water safety skills. These are specific activities related to the water environment including but not limited to supine to stand, prone to stand, lateral rotation, vertical rotation, sit to stand, treading water, blowing bubbles, and rhythmic breathing. The actual technique of performing these skills may vary depending on an individual's abilities, but the basic steps are the same. Basic water safety skills do not include safety awareness.

functional assessment a measurement of the patient's ability to perform a set of pre-determined tasks (specific functional skills). Each facility may develop their own "in-house" functional capacity assessment or use a standardized, commercial assessment. (The **Community Integration Program's** (Armstrong and Lauzen, 1994) modules all contain functional assessments.) In either case, the assess-

ment should have the four specific attributes shown above (Wieder-Singer, 1994). Functional assessments are different from attitudinal assessments, which ask for the patient's impression or opinion. See *intake assessment.*

Functional Assessment of Characteristics of Therapeutic Recreation - Revised (FACTR-R) (Peterson, Dunn, Carruthers, 1983/1996) 33-item screening tool which is used to help prioritize the patient's *treatment* objectives. Once the therapist has reviewed the patient's chart and observed the patient in a few activities, s/he should be able to fill out the FACTR-R score sheet. The scoring technique used helps pinpoint the functional domain (physical, cognitive, social/emotional) with the greatest need and ability to be improved. It helps the therapist identify the areas most likely to improve through the services of recreational therapy. Originally developed for use in the Veteran's Administration system, this assessment was intended to be used by both non-credentialed and credentialed staff. The FACTR-R is used as a screening tool, to supplement the assessments that the therapist is using to determine treatment priorities. When combined with the clinical judgment of the therapist and the results of other assessment tools, it can be a helpful tool. The original 1983 version contained some problems with content validity, which were corrected in the 1996 version. Interrater reliability is known to be greatly improved with the use of credentialed staff.

functional foods (HHS) foods that may provide health benefits beyond basic nutrition. Examples include tomatoes with lycopene, thought to help prevent the incidence of prostate and cervical cancers; *fiber* in wheat bran and sulfur compounds in garlic also believed to prevent cancer.

functional imaging (HCO) medical image modalities that portray the function (such as oxygen uptake) as well as the morphology of anatomical features.

Functional Independence Measure The Functional Independence Measure or the "FIM" is a standardized, seven-point scale used to document a patient's degree of independence in performing any observable skill. See *FIM scale.*

functional treatment   *treatment* that directly addresses the patient's specific functional deficits.

Function Related Groups (FIM-FRGs)   a billing system developed to help accurately reflect the intensity of treatment in billing/reimbursement rates.

In general medicine, billing and actual cost of services are relatively easy to predict. In rehabilitation the impact of acquired disability and loss of function can vary (especially in traumatic brain injury). The FIM-FRGs system is meant to try to correct the problem of billing inequalities. FIM-FRGs stands for Functional Independence Measurement — Function Related Groups. See *FIM scale.*

G

gait referring to the body mechanics and movement patterns used by a patient when ambulating. See *arthogenic gait, ataxic gait, dystrophic gait, festination gait, flaccid gait, footdrop gait, four-point gait, gastrocnemius-soleus gait, hemiplegic gait, homolateral gait, listing gait, Parkinsonian gait, swing-through gait, swing-to gait, three-point gait.*

gall stone a stone made up of cholesterol and/or bile pigments and/or calcium salts which forms in the biliary tract of the gallbladder. Also known as biliary calculi.

galvanic skin response (GSR) a measurement of the amount of electricity allowed to pass through the skin when it is applied in small amounts to areas saturated with sweat glands (e.g., volar surface of the fingers or the palmar surface of the hand). Since stress increases perspiration and water is an excellent conductor of electricity, increased electrical current can show when a person becomes stressed by some factor. This is one of the processes used for "lie detectors."

gamma (g) glutamyl transferase (HHS) one of a family of enzymes involved in transporting amino acids from the exterior to the cytoplasm of a cell. High serum levels of this enzyme serve as an indicator for liver disease.

gastric gavage feeding tube a tube that is inserted into the nasal passage and then pushed down into the stomach (nasogastric) or into the intestines (nasointestinal). These tubes are best for patients who do not have a disruption in the ability to digest food but are not able to take enough nutrition through their mouths to meet their needs. They may be left in for up to four weeks. See *feeling tube, gavage feeding, jejunostomy.*

gastrocnemius-soleus gait an abnormal *gait* where the affected side is dragged along due to the lack of heel lift on push off. Activities that involve going up inclines are most affected. Since this gait is usually due to weakened gastrocnemius and/or soleus muscles, a strengthening program involving activities which mildly stress those muscles may lead to an increase in function.

gastroenteritis an inflammation of the stomach and intestinal lining. Symptoms may include an upset stomach, diarrhea, cramping, and vomiting. See *enteric isolation.*

gastronomy (HHS) the study and appreciation of good food and good eating; a culture's culinary customs, style, and lore; any interest or study of culinary pursuits as relates essentially to the kitchen and cookery, and to the higher levels of education, training, and achievement of the chef apprentice or professional chef.

gatching positioning the patient's hospital *bed* in such a manner to allow the patient's knees to be bent when s/he lies down.

gatekeeper an individual who works for the facility or provider who determines the appropriate services for the patient based on need and standards of practice. See *appropriateness, managed care.*

gavage feeding nutrition supplied to the patient through a tube inserted into the stomach. See *feeding tube, gastric gavage feeding tube.*

gel cushion bed See *bed.*

gene (HHS/NMDP) basic unit of inheritance that controls for specific characteristics such as eye color or tissue type. Genes are located on the chromosome and consist of segments of DNA.

General Adaptation Syndrome (GAS) a term first used by Selye (1982) to describe the nonspecific result of psychological or somatic demands placed on the body.

general diet See *regular diet.*

generalizability (HHS) the extent to which the results of a study are able to be applied to the general population of people that is comparable to the population studied.

generalization ability to understand that one behavior or skill can be modified to work in a different situation or setting. This is a skill that is frequently impaired in patients who have experienced a *traumatic brain injury* or have other significant *cognitive deficits*. For community integration to be successful, the patient needs to be taught how to generalize the skills learned while in an institution or hospital to the *functional abilities* required in the community. The therapist will want to ensure that 1. the patient has the perception that the *problem solving* strategies taught during therapy were helpful, 2. the patient has learned specific techniques to enhance generalization of the problem solving strategies, and 3. (the therapist had determined that) the problem solving strategy will work for that patient.

generalized tendomyopathy See *fibromyalgia.*

generally recognized as safe (HHS) the regulatory status of food ingredients not evaluated by FDA prescribed testing procedures. It also includes common food ingredients that were already in use when the 1959 Food Additives Amendment to the Food, Drug, and Cosmetic Act was enacted.

General Recreation Screening Tool (GRST) a screening tool that helps the therapist estimate the patient's functional ability in eighteen areas related to leisure. The eighteen areas are 1. *gross motor*, 2. *fine motor*, 3. eye-hand coordination, 4. play behavior, 5. play structure, 6. language use, 7. language comprehension, 8. understanding of numbers, 9. object use, 10. following directions, 11. *problem solving*, 12. *attending behavior*, 13. possessions, 14. emotional control, 15. imitation play, 16. people skills, 17. music, and 18. stories/drama. The tool looks at developmental milestones between birth and ten years of age. The tool is usually used by a recreational therapist who then selects a second tool to obtain more specific functional ability. The test is abbreviated GRST and pronounced "grist," rhyming with fist. See *Denver Developmental Screening Test, Recreation Early Development Screening Tool*.

genital phase final psychosexual developmental phase outlined by *Freud* which states that pleasure is based on genital-to-genital contact. The phase is usually reached during puberty.

genome (HHS) the total hereditary material of a cell, containing the entire chromosomal set found in each nucleus of a given species.

genotype (HHS/NMDP) the actual genetic makeup of an individual. For example, a person with brown eyes may have inherited a brown eye color gene (Br) from one parent and a blue eye color gene (Bl) from the other. This person's genotype would be Br/Bl. Contrast with *phenotype*.

geriatrics having to do with the physiology and psychology of aging.

gerontology study of all aspects of aging.

gestures non-verbal actions which are meant to communicate a person's intent or thoughts.

Glasgow Coma Scale (GCS) a measurement used to describe the severity of a *coma* and subsequent injury by grading eye, motor, and verbal responses. The numerical values of the *scale* run from 3 (low) to 15 (normal). The total score of a patient's GCS means: 3-8 = severe coma, 9-12 = moderate coma, and 13-15 = mild coma. A newer Glasgow-type scale has been developed for children, which allows more accurate measurement of the early recovery in young children (under the age of three years). This assessment is called the Children's Coma Scale (CCS). The standard documentation style to record the Glasgow Coma Scale score is EMV (<u>e</u>yes, <u>mo</u>tor, <u>v</u>oice) with the score following the letter, dropped half a line: $E_3M_4V_3$.

glaucoma a disease of the eye that produces increased intraocular pressure. Prolonged periods of increased pressure without treatment may lead to *visual impairment* and eventually blindness. See *visual function*.

Global Assessment of Functioning Scale (GAF Scale) quick rating scale conceptualized by Luborsky (1962) and now part of the Multiaxial Assessment System outlined in the **Diagnostic and Statistical Manual of Mental Disorders, Fourth Edition (DSM-IV)**. The GAF Scale (shown on the following page) is a continuum that estimates the individual's psychological, social, and occupational health on a zero (worst) to 100 (best) point scale. (Used with permission from the American Psychiatric Association. Found on page 32 in the **DSM-IV**.) See *multiaxial system, scales*.

globulin (HHS) a family of proteins found in abundance in plasma. They include the gamma globulins, which in turn include the various antibody molecules produced by the immune system.

glomerulonephritis (HHS) kidney disease characterized by bilateral inflammatory changes in the glomeruli (tufts of capillary loops associated with the nephrons, the functional units of the kidney). The disorder is not caused by infection. It is considered an autoimmune disease.

glucose (HHS) a simple sugar that is actively transferred into the blood following the digestive breakdown of starch and other carbohydrates in the gut. This sugar is most commonly in the form of dextroglucose. It occurs naturally, has about half the sweetening power of regular sugar, and does not crystallize easily. Glucose comes from grape juice, honey, and certain vegetables, among other things.

glutamate (HHS) an amino acid. It is necessary for metabolism and brain function, and is manufactured by the body. Glutamate is found in virtually every protein food we eat. In food, there is "bound" glutamate and "free" glutamate. Glutamate serves to enhance flavors in foods when it is in its free form and not bound to other amino acids in protein. Some foods have greater quantities of glutamate than others. Foods that are rich in glutamate include tomatoes, mushrooms, Parmesan cheese, milk, and mackerel.

glycerol (HHS) a colorless, odorless, syrupy liquid; chemically, an alcohol that is obtained from fats and oils and used to retain moisture and add sweetness to foods.

goal an outcome that an individual will strive for,

Global Assessment of Functioning (GAF) Scale

Consider psychological, social, and occupational functioning on a hypothetical continuum of mental health-illness. Do not include impairment in functioning due to physical (or environmental) limitations.

100 91	Superior functioning in a wide range of activities, life's problems never seem to get out of hand, is sought out by others because of his/her many positive qualities. No symptoms.
90 81	Absent or minimal symptoms (e.g., mild anxiety before an exam), good functioning in all areas, interested and involved in a wide range of activities, socially effective, generally satisfied with life, no more than everyday problems or concerns (e.g., an occasional argument with family members).
80 71	If symptoms are present, they are transient and expectable reactions to psychosocial stresses (e.g., difficulty concentrating after family argument), no more than slight impairment in social, occupational, or school functioning (e.g., temporarily falling behind in schoolwork).
70 61	Some mild symptoms (e.g., depressed mood, mild insomnia) OR some difficulty in social, occupational, or school functioning (e.g., occasional threatening or theft within the household), but generally functioning pretty well, has some meaningful interpersonal relationships.
60 51	Moderate symptoms (e.g., flat affect and circumstantial speech, occasional panic attacks) OR moderate difficulty in social, occupational, school functioning (e.g., few friends, conflicts with co-workers).
50 41	Serious symptoms (e.g., suicidal ideation, severe obsessional rituals, frequent shoplifting) OR any serious impairment in social, occupational, or school functioning (e.g., no friends, unable to keep a job).
40 31	Some impairment in reality testing or communication (e.g., speech is at times illogical, obscure, or irrelevant) OR major impairment in several areas such as work, school, family relations, judgment, thinking, or mood (e.g., man who is depressed, avoids friends, neglects family, and is unable to work; child who frequently beats up younger children, is defiant at home, is failing school).
30 21	Behavior is considerably influenced by delusions or hallucinations OR serious impairment in communication or judgment (e.g., sometimes incoherent, acts grossly inappropriately, suicidal preoccupation) OR inability to function in almost all areas (e.g., stays in bed all day, no job, home, friends).
20 11	Some danger of hurting self or others (e.g., suicide attempts without clear expectation of death, frequently violent, manic excitement) OR occasionally fails to maintain minimal personal hygiene (e.g., smears feces) OR gross impairment in communication (e.g., largely incoherent or mute).
10 1	Persistent danger of severely hurting self or others (e.g., recurrent violence) OR persistent inability to maintain minimal personal hygiene OR serious suicidal act with clear expectation of death.

stated in a general way, not clearly measurable. An example of a goal would be; "Patient will increase his time management skills." Objectives are statements that define how the various aspects of meeting the goal will be measured. See *modality, objective*.

goal setting and time management a relaxation and life management technique. Individuals who have difficulty managing their time well and making choices based on previously set goals tend to experience high levels of *stress*. For many patients, even if they are able to develop good relaxation states using a variety of techniques, life is still stressful because of mismanaged time. By improving goal setting skills the patient should be able to reduce his/her basic level of stress. See *relaxation techniques*.

gonorrhea a *sexually transmitted disease* caused by the organism Neisseria gonorrhoeae.

gout a painful, destructive joint disease which is caused when the body inadequately deals with the build up of uric acid. The crystals formed from the excess uric acid are deposited around joints, causing painful swelling. Chills and *fever* are also common. The disease gets progressively worse from year to year unless interventions (dietary modifications, medications, and *exercise*) are implemented.

governing body individuals who make up the group that is ultimately responsible for the overall operations of the facility or agency. The group is defined by a pre-determined method of selecting and identifying individuals who will have the power, authority, and responsibility to make decisions.

graciousness a category of social skills that include "higher level" or more advanced interaction skills. The ability to be so sensitive to others that those around the gracious person feel emotionally comfortable and safe without even realizing that the person is creating the safe environment. The judicious exercising of one's power and privilege to allow for the choices of others. The opposite of the forceful imposition of legitimate power and privilege.

graft implantation or transplantation of tissue or organ. See *allograft, cadaver graft, dermal graft, full-*

Clinical Grading System for Graft-Versus-Host Disease (Pyle, 1996, p. 196)

Grade	Description of Symptoms
Clinical Grade 1	Mild skin rash (generally maculopapular). No gastrointestinal or liver function abnormalities.
Clinical Grade 2	Moderately severe skin rash. Mild gastrointestinal symptoms. Slight increase in bilirubin and perhaps also in liver enzymes.
Clinical Grade 3	Moderately severe skin rash, gastrointestinal symptoms, and liver function abnormalities.
Clinical Grade 4	Severe peeling and flaking of the skin, severe gastrointestinal symptoms, and liver function abnormalities.

thickness graft, granulation, heterodermic graft, isologous graft, mesh graft, pedicle graft, split thickness graft.

graft-versus-host disease (GVH) a potential side effect of a graft, usually referring to a *bone marrow transplant*. Graft-versus-host disease is the body's rejection of the newly transmitted bone marrow that usually starts developing three to five weeks after the transplant. Damage usually occurs to the recipient's skin, intestines, and/or liver. The primary symptoms are a rash, fever, and diarrhea. See the table above for a clinical grading system for GVH.

grains (HHS) the seeds or fruits of various food plants including cereal grasses. The examples of wheat, corn, oats, barley, rye, and rice provide a partial list. Grain foods include bread, cereals, rice, and pasta.

grandiosity an exaggerated statement or belief of one's abilities, possessions, achievements, or importance. The **DSM-IV** lists grandiosity (grandiose type) under the diagnostic category of delusional disorder.

grand mal seizure See *seizure, epilepsy.*

granulation normal, healthy reaction of the body to tissue damage. Small blood vessels increase significantly at the site of a wound to help promote healing. Granulation tissue is eventually replaced by normal tissue but at first it appears red and raw. Granulation tissue is a desired tissue type to *graft* skin onto.

graphesthesia ability to recognize a number or letter traced on one's skin though *tactile* sensation alone.

graphic input (reading) ability to read symbols (e.g., letters, numbers). *Traumatic brain injuries* often impact a patient's ability to read. Once the patient is able to recognize words and to consistently scan from left to right, s/he is ready to progress to reading safety and other information on community integration outings. Patients tend to progress from being able to find concrete information in reading passages (as found in menus) to being able to figure out implied abstract information (such as satire or subtle meanings found in parks program bulletins). In-house therapy along with actual experience on community integration outings with the therapist helps the patient understand any visual/spatial deficits that s/he might have and how to compensate for them. It is important that reading speed and accuracy increase together.

graphic output (writing) ability to write (generate) symbols (e.g., letters, numbers). Written *communication* is one of the key skills required of adults. Whether it is writing a check, filling out an insurance form, or just writing a letter to a friend, the use of the written word is vital to independence in the community. One of the primary uses of the written word prior to discharge is a *memory book*. The purpose of the memory book is to provide the patient with a visual reminder of his/her schedule as well as to provide a place to write down thoughts and questions that should not be forgotten. Patients who require the use of a memory book usually have difficulty with spelling, punctuation, sentence formation, and paragraph organization. Unless these skills will be required soon (because of vocational or educational needs), it is best to focus on the content of the material and not the manner in which it is written.

GRAS See *generally recognized as safe.*

grievance formal process of notifying the facility or the health care provider that an individual feels that s/he has been "wronged" and is seeking a satisfactory resolution to his/her concern. See *complaint.*

grieving, stages of See *dying.*

grooming For a patient to be considered independent in grooming, s/he would need to be able to complete the following tasks without cueing or other assistance:

1. identify and obtain the supplies needed for such activities as donning and doffing makeup, shaving, nail care, hair care, applying deodorant, etc.
2. perform all required grooming tasks on a socially acceptable schedule and in a socially acceptable manner.
3. identify the appropriate care and placement (storage) for grooming supplies.

See *dignity, mental retardation.*

gross motor use of the large muscle groups for coordinated action and strength to complete a task. See *Denver Developmental Screening Tool, dressing skills, General Recreation Screening Tool.*

ground floor (ADA) any occupiable floor less than one story above or below grade with direct access to grade. A building or facility always has at least one ground floor and may have more than one ground floor as where a split level has been provided or where a building is built into a hillside.

group A streptococcus (CDC) a bacterium often found in the throat and on the skin. People may carry group A streptococci in the throat or on the skin and have no symptoms of illness. Most GAS infections are relatively mild illnesses such as "strep throat," or impetigo. On rare occasions, these bacteria can cause other severe and even life-threatening diseases. These bacteria are spread through direct contact with mucus from the nose or throat of persons who are infected or through contact with infected wounds or sores on the skin. Ill persons, such as those who have strep throat or skin infections, are most likely to spread the infection. Persons who carry the bacteria but have no symptoms are much less contagious. Treating an infected person with an antibiotic for 24 hours or longer generally eliminates his/her ability to spread the bacteria. However, it is important to complete the entire course of antibiotics as prescribed. It is not likely that household items such as plates, cups, or toys spread these bacteria. Infection with GAS can result in a range of symptoms: no illness, mild illness (strep throat or a skin infection such as impetigo), or severe illness (necrotizing fasciitis, streptococcal toxic shock syndrome). Severe, sometimes life-threatening, GAS disease may occur when bacteria get into parts of the body where bacteria usually are not found, such as the blood, muscle, or the lungs. These infections are termed "invasive GAS disease." Two of the most severe, but least common, forms of invasive GAS disease are *necrotizing fasciitis* and Streptococcal Toxic Shock Syndrome. Necrotizing fasciitis (occasionally described by the media as "the flesh-eating bacteria") destroys muscles, fat, and skin tissue. Streptococcal toxic shock syndrome (STSS), causes blood pressure to drop rapidly and organs (e.g., kidney, liver, lungs) to fail. STSS is not the same as the "toxic shock syndrome" frequently associated with tampon usage. About 20% of patients with necrotizing fasciitis and more than half with STSS die. About 10%-15% of patients with other forms of invasive group A streptococcal disease die. About 10,000 cases of invasive GAS disease occurred in the United States in 1998. Of these, about 600 were STSS and 800 were necrotizing fasciitis. In contrast,

there are several million cases of strep throat and impetigo each year. Invasive GAS infections occur when the bacteria get past the defenses of the person who is infected. This may occur when a person has sores or other breaks in the skin that allow the bacteria to get into the tissue, or when the person's ability to fight off the infection is decreased because of chronic illness or an illness that affects the immune system. Also, some virulent strains of GAS are more likely to cause severe disease than others. Few people who come in contact with GAS will develop invasive GAS disease. Most people will have a throat or skin infection, and some may have no symptoms at all. Although healthy people can get invasive GAS disease, people with chronic illnesses like cancer, diabetes, and kidney dialysis, and those who use medications such as steroids have a higher risk. GAS infections can be treated with many different antibiotics. Early treatment may reduce the risk of death from invasive group A streptococcal disease. However, even the best medical care does not prevent death in every case. For those with very severe illness, supportive care in an intensive care unit may be needed. For persons with necrotizing fasciitis, surgery often is needed to remove damaged tissue. The spread of all types of GAS infection can be reduced by good *hand washing*, especially after coughing and sneezing and before preparing foods or eating. Persons with sore throats should be seen by a doctor who can perform tests to find out whether the illness is strep throat. If the test result shows strep throat, the person should stay home from work, school, or day care until 24 hours after taking an antibiotic. All wounds should be kept clean and watched for possible signs of infection such as redness, swelling, drainage, and pain at the wound site. A person with signs of an infected wound, especially if fever occurs, should seek medical care. It is not necessary for all persons exposed to someone with an invasive group A strep infection (i.e. necrotizing fasciitis or strep toxic shock syndrome) to receive antibiotic therapy to prevent infection. However, in certain circumstances, antibiotic therapy may be appropriate.

grouper (HCO) software used to deduce DRGs from sets of *diagnostic related groups* and procedure codes, or to analyze the grouping decisions of medical coders for consistency and thoroughness. See *grouper software.*

grouper software a software database system specifically developed for use in nursing homes, which analyzes the resident information, entered into the *Minimum Data Set* (MDS). The grouper software then crunches the data by using a case mix analysis to assign the resident to one of the predetermined classifications used by the *Health Care Financing Administration* (HCFA). The predetermined classifications, called the *Resource Utilization Group System* (RUGS), are used by HCFA to determine reimbursement levels for each resident. See *grouper*.

group psychotherapy application of psychotherapeutic techniques to a group, including utilization of interactions of members of the group. Usually six to eight people constitute a group and sessions typically last 75 minutes or longer.

GRST See *General Recreation Screening Tool*.

guardian individual or corporation which has obtained the legal right to make decisions concerning the patient's care because the patient has been determined unable to make his/her own decisions. See *durable power of attorney, conservatorship*.

guided imagery the process of mentally and consciously changing body functions by the internal representations of events that involve the senses.

Guillain-Barré syndrome a quickly spreading paralysis which starts at the feet and then progresses toward the head. This *paralysis* may occur over a period as short as a few hours. At some point the spread of the paralysis stops and given rest and treatment, may reverse itself, possibly leaving little functionally measurable paralysis after a couple of months.

guillotine amputation an amputation that is cut straight through the limb, leaving a flat stump.

gustatory pertaining to the sense of taste.

H

habilitation development of maximum independence in activities of daily living and maintenance of an individual's current health status and *functional ability*.

HACCP See *Hazard Analysis and Critical Control Points*.

hairy cell leukemia (HCL) (HHS/NMDP) a rare type or variant of chronic leukemia, primarily a disease of middle-aged men. HCL infrequently requires bone marrow transplant as a treatment. See *leukemia*.

Halliwick This ten-step process developed by James McMillan, an engineer, was historically considered a method of swimming instruction. Used for clinical purposes, it is the application and analysis of developmental sequences of movement in water. Halliwick targets an individual's abilities and exploits those strengths using the complementary recreational and therapeutic aspects of a water medium.

hallucination a sensory perception in the absence of an actual external stimulus. May occur in any of the *senses*. A hallucination is a perception that an event has taken place — an event that has no basis in the physical environment. The individual has a strong sensory impression that the event has taken place and, because a hallucination tends to affect one sense more than the others, hallucinations generally have an adjective added (e.g., auditory hallucination). There are two sensory events that are similar to a hallucination but are not considered pathological. They are hypnagogic and hypnopompic events as described in the table below. See *delirium, delirium tremens, Global Assessment of Functioning Scale, illusion, schizophrenia*.

halo a splinting/traction device that has a metal ring placed around the head of a patient who has a *spinal cord injury*. The mental ring has supporting "arms" which extend down to the patient's torso to help stabilize the head. There are metal pins extending from the metal ring into the patient's skull to help further stabilize the vertebra and spinal cord. The use of a halo allows the patient to regain mobility faster than if s/he were placed in traction in bed.

handicap 1. an attitude or environmental barrier that stops an individual from performing "normally." 2. (outdated) a disease or disability which impairs an individual's ability to engage in activities (now termed a "*disability*"). 3. a level of classification found in the **International Classification of Impairments, Disabilities, and Handicaps** (World Health Organization's, 1980) that addresses impairments related to the application of skills within the community. See *Recreation Service Model*.

handwashing process of cleansing one's hands. This is the most important infection control technique. *Infection control* is extremely important to prevent nosocomial infection. Therapists should wash their hands between contacts with patients. Proper handwashing technique is described below. See *hepatitis, nosocomial infection*.

Handwashing Technique

1. Wet and lather hands to wrists.
2. Scrub lathered hands (including nail areas) for 10 seconds.
3. Rinse hands under *running* water for a minimum of 10 seconds or until all the soap residue is gone — whichever takes longer.
4. Dry hands — turn off water using paper towel so that faucet controls don't come into contact with cleaned hands.

Terms Related to Hallucination

Term	Description
hallucination	A perception that an event has taken place that has no basis in the physical environment and that frequently interferes with an individual's ability to function normally in the community.
hypnagogic	Very short hallucination — sensations that may be experienced as the individual makes the transition from wakefulness into sleep. Hypnagogic illusions are usually experienced as dreams but do not happen during REM (rapid eye movement) sleep. Unlike true hallucinations, which may indicate a mental illness, hypnagogic illusions are considered "normal."
hypnopompic	Very short hallucination — sensations that may be experienced as the individual makes the transition from sleep to wakefulness. Unlike true hallucinations, which may indicate a mental illness, hypnopompic illusions are considered "normal."

handwriting recognition (HCO) conversion of script or block letting to computer based text.

Hansen's disease (leprosy) (CDC) a chronic infectious disease usually affecting the skin and peripheral nerves but with a wide range of possible clinical manifestations. Patients are classified as having paucibacillary or multibacillary Hansen's disease. Paucibacillary Hansen's disease is milder and characterized by one or more hypopigmented skin macules. Multibacillary Hansen's disease is associated with symmetric skin lesions, nodules, plaques, thickened dermis, and frequent involvement of the nasal mucosa resulting in nasal congestion and epistaxis. Hansen's disease is caused by a bacillus, Mycobacterium leprae, that multiplies very slowly and mainly affects the skin, nerves, and mucous membranes. The organism has never been grown in bacteriologic media or cell culture, but has been grown in mouse footpads. An estimated 500,000 new Hansen's disease cases are identified each year, with about 300 of these occurring in the United States. Most cases come from 55 countries where disease continues to be endemic. In 1998, WHO listed those countries reporting the most cases as Bangladesh, Brazil, India, Indonesia, Myanmar, and Nigeria. Worldwide, 1-2 million persons are permanently disabled as a result of Hansen's disease. However, persons receiving antibiotic treatment or having completed treatment are considered free of active infection. Although the mode of transmission of Hansen's disease remains uncertain, most investigators think that M. leprae is usually spread from person to person in respiratory droplets. Infection is thought to come from close contacts with patients with untreated, active, predominantly multibacillary disease, and persons living in countries with highly endemic disease. Hansen's disease is nationally notifiable in the United States. Incidence/prevalence has remained relatively stable in the United States. There are decreasing numbers of cases worldwide with pockets of high prevalence in certain countries. The main challenges for Hansen's disease elimination efforts are to reach populations that have not yet received multi-drug therapy services, improve detection of disease, and provide patients with good quality services and free drugs.

haplotype (HHS/NMDP) one half of a *genotype*; the gene inherited from one parent.

haptic referring to the sense of touch, of *tactile* awareness.

Harrington rod a rod surgically implanted into the spine used to help fuse the spine of patients with *scoliosis* or some types of spinal fractures.

Hazard Analysis and Critical Control Points (HACCP) (HHS) The underlying approach under HACCP for preventing food-borne illness and promoting quality is to identify the danger spots and try to avoid them. Instead of putting the burden on the government to discover that a food safety problem exists, HACCP shifts responsibility onto the industry to ensure that the food it produces is safe. Food producers will have to prevent bacterial contamination from occurring in the first place. HACCP works by the following principles: Identify the likely health hazards to consumers in a given product, identify the critical points in the processing where the hazards may occur, establish safety measures to prevent the hazard from occurring, monitor to make sure the safety measures are working, establish an appropriate remedy if monitoring shows a problem, establish detailed record keeping to document monitoring and remedies taken, verify that the whole system is working. See *food-borne disease.*

Hazard Communication Standards a federal law, more commonly known as the employee's "right to know" law, which states that employees have the need and right to know about harmful chemicals in the workplace. Employers are required to inform employees about hazardous chemicals as well as the appropriate protective measures needed to remain safe. Employers are also required to provide protective equipment and ongoing training at no cost to the employee. Blood-borne pathogens protection is part of the Hazard Communication Standards regulations. See *blood-borne pathogens, hazardous materials.*

hazardous materials chemicals or elements in the work place environment that may cause illness or injury. Chemicals are considered to be liquids, solids, gases, vapors, fumes, mists, dusts, and exhaust fumes. Any company that sells materials that could be considered harmful is required to provide the purchasing facility with a Material Safety Data Sheet (MSDS). These sheets include the chemical and the common names used for the chemical, the physical and chemical characteristics and known hazards, appropriate emergency and first aid procedures, applicable precautions for safe use and handling (including required *personal protective equipment*), a contact number for more information, and the publication date of the MSDS. See *environment of care, hazardous communication standards.*

HCFA See *Health Care Financing Administration.*

HCPCS See *Health Care Financing Administration's Common Procedure Coding System.*

head injury a general term for trauma to the brain or skull. See *traumatic brain injury, coup lesion, contrecoup lesion, executive function.*

Health Care Financing Administration (HCFA)
The Health Care Financing Administration is part of the *Department of Health and Human Services* in the United States. HCFA has the responsibility to oversee Medicare and Medicaid programs. Combined, these two programs provide health care services to over 67 million individuals. Over 17,000 facilities qualify to receive funds from HCFA. While HCFA funnels health care funds to each facility to help pay for services of individuals who qualify for funding, it also is responsible for conducting surveys to determine that each facility which receives funding meets minimum standards. See *Department of Health and Human Services, Medicare, Medicaid, peer review organizations, survey process.*

Health Care Financing Administration's Common Procedure Coding System (HCPCS) a health care billing code system which contains more than 2,600 codes. Most of these codes are used for billing supplies, services, and procedures to Medicare and Medicaid programs across the United States. HCPCS codes are considered to be secondary codes, with *Current Procedural Terminology* (CPT) being the primary source of billing codes. Pronounced "hick pick," these codes were developed in the early 1980's to complement the codes used by the American Medical Association (CPTs). CPTs were designated as the Level One or primary codes. HCPCS (National Codes) were then created to serve as the second level of codes. Level Two (HCPCS) codes start with a letter of the alphabet (A - V) and are followed by four numbers (e.g., Q0082: Activity Therapy furnished with partial hospitalization). To adjust for local and regional differences, a third level of codes was allowed by the Health Care Financing Administration. This third level includes local HCPCS codes. Level Three Codes start with the letters W, X, Y, or Z. A modifier to HCPCS codes is available and is signified by using two letters after the four numbers.

health care function Health care organizations perform a variety of functions, with the overall goal to improve the quality of health and life of their patients. Health care functions can be divided into two primary categories: caring for patients and managing the organization. Patient-focused functions include patient *assessment*, patient care, and patient education along with focus on the rights, responsibilities, and *ethics* of both patients and staff. Organization-focused functions include providing leadership; improving organizational performance; managing the *environment of care*; managing human resources; managing information; and providing surveillance, prevention, and control of infection. The informa-tion a health care organization needs to manage includes the clinical records, aggregate information, expert information (standards, regulations, professional journals, etc.), and comparative data.

Healthcare Information Standards Planning Panel (HCO) a body created by American National Standards Institute to coordinate standards development efforts among the various standards bodies in health care.

Health Care Quality Improvement Act of 1986 Peer review (having a group of professionals from outside your facility) has been a popular and effective way to evaluate the quality of services being provided. An honest review points out both strengths and weaknesses of a service delivery system. Peer reviews may even find areas where the facility is providing substandard or harmful care. During the 1970's and 1980's malpractice lawyers picked up on these results and increasingly used these quality assurance measures against the facilities. In 1986, the United States Congress passed the Health Care Quality Improvement Act to provide limited immunity from damages and litigation as a result of peer reviews done to help improve the quality of services. See *peer review organization, quality assurance.*

Health Evaluation through Logical Processing (HCO) a clinical information system at LDS Hospital in Salt Lake City, Utah.

health level 7 (HCO) an application-level interface specification for transmitting health-related data transactions, generally used within a single institution.

health maintenance organization (HMO) a legal entity that provides or arranges for the provision of prepaid basic and supplemental health services to its members in the manner prescribed by and operated in accordance with Section 1301 of the Public Health Services Act. Also known as *managed care.* See *capitated, fee-for-service, rehabilitation centers.*

health plan and employer data set (HCO) a set of performance indicators for managed care plans, developed by the *National Committee for Quality Assurance.*

Health Protection/Health Promotion Model for Therapeutic Recreation Service Delivery developed by Austin, the model is "based on the humanistic assumption that human beings have an overriding drive for health and wellness." (Austin, 1997, p. 135) The model emphasizes the provision of three distinct service components, "prescriptive activities," "recreation activities," and "leisure." For individuals experiencing low levels of health (i.e., limited functional capacity as a result of illness or disability) and in need of a health-protection focus, the therapist utilizes prescriptive activities to assist in returning the individual to a healthier state. Prescriptive activity affords what Austin refers to as a "stabilizing tendency" which promotes healing and protects the health of the individual. "Recreation" is used within the model as a means to move from services that protect and stabilize health toward health-promoting services. While still in need of some level of stabilizing, the therapist transitions the individual into recreation experiences and activities that have an "actualizing tendency" and a greater focus on self-determination and health promotion. The third activity component is "leisure." Leisure is a considered to be intrinsically motivated and a state of self-actualization where an individual is self-directed and engages in health-promotion activities.

Health Security Act (HR 3600/S 1757) (FB) a proposal devised by the Clinton Administration that would have required all persons to obtain a comprehensive health benefits package from large insurance purchasing cooperatives called health alliances. Health plan premiums would have been paid through a combination of employer and individual contributions, supplemented by federal subsidies for some types of firms, early retirees, and persons with incomes below certain levels. A national health care budget would have been established for expenditures for services covered under the comprehensive package. This budget plan limited both initial premiums and the year-to-year rates of increase that could be charged by health plans participating in the alliances. Ultimately, premiums could grow no faster than the rate of growth in per capita gross domestic product, unless Congress specified a different inflation factor. This Act did not pass but has served as a basis for further national discussion on what the United States should provide for individuals' health care.

hearing See *audition.*

hearing aid a mechanical device inserted into the patient's ear to enhance hearing. Therapists should be familiar with the steps for inserting a hearing aid, as they may need to assist a patient with the process. First, examine the ear that the aid is to be inserted into. Is there an accumulation of cerumen (ear wax)? If so, the ear should be cleaned before the hearing aid is put in. Test the hearing aid before it is inserted. Does the volume adjust up and down correctly? Is the battery okay? It is normal for a functioning hearing aid to produce a whistling sound when not inserted into the ear. Next, turn down the volume and turn off the hearing aid before inserting it into the ear. Gently grasp the ear lobe and exert a

slight downward pull on the lobe as you insert the hearing aid, pressing the hearing aid gently inward. Hearing aids are shaped to fit snugly into the ear so that they won't fall out with normal activity. A hearing aid that is not inserted all the way in may produce an irritating, shrill feedback sound once it is turned on. Once it is correctly inserted into the ear, the hearing aid may be turned on and the volume adjusted. Talk normally with the patient during this process so that s/he can help judge when the volume is correctly adjusted. Remember to turn off the hearing aid and restore it to the correct container when it is taken out. See *bed rest.*

hearing deficit below normal ability to sense sound. A set of standardized criteria has been developed to measure hearing deficits. Because hearing deficits are measured by the decibel level of the sound necessary before the individual can hear the sound (e.g., passing the individual's hearing threshold), the six levels of hearing loss are measured in decibels (dB). See *hearing impairment.*

Levels of Hearing Loss

Hearing Loss Category	Range
normal	0-25 dB
mild	25-40 dB
moderate	40-55 dB
moderately/severe	55-75 dB
severe	75-90 dB
profound	90 dB and higher

hearing impairment a decreased ability to hear sounds. The sensation of hearing is made up of two components: 1. the ability to perceive a range of volumes (loud to soft) and 2. the ability to perceive a range of pitches (do-ra-me-fa-so-la-te-do). When a professional sees an individual with a hearing loss, the loss will be described by the part of the ear that is damaged: 1. conductive (damage to the outer or middle ear), 2. sensorineural (damage to the inner ear or to the auditory nerve), or 3. mixed (a combination of both conductive and sensorineural). A sensorineural hearing loss is seldom correctable by medication and/or surgery, requiring instead the use of a hearing aid and/or sign language. A loss of the ability to hear sounds in one's environment is a significant loss. The primary concerns to be addressed by the professional are 1. social isolation, 2. communication impairment, and 3. loss of normal (hearing) development, even with early intervention. See *audiometrist, auxiliary aides and services, hearing deficit.*

heart attack See *myocardial infarction.*

heart rate variability (HRV) a highly accurate measurement of stress. When heart rate is analyzed by both time and frequency analysis, several important characteristics emerge. One component, respiratory sinus arrhythmia (RSA) can be seen at the high end of the frequency scale and represents respiratory influences on the heart. Another characteristic of heart rate recorded at the very low end of the frequency scale is called pulse wave velocity (PWV). When analyzed mathematically RSA, PWV coupled with a time analysis of heart rate, represent a quantitative multidimensional measure of autonomic activity and cardiac function.

heat exhaustion The body's mechanism to cool an overheated body is to pump extra blood to the skin surface to help cool the blood. This causes a reduction in the amount of blood available to vital organs, including the brain. Symptoms include nausea, heavy perspiration, dizziness, rapid breathing, and rapid pulse. The individual's temperature is normal. Quick cooling of the body and lowering the head (to increase blood to the brain through gravity) are important first aid steps.

HEDIS See *health plan and employer data set.*

HELP See *health evaluation through logical processing.*

helper T lymphocytes cells that stimulate the production of immunoglobulins by B lymphocytes.

helplessness a term first developed by M. Seligman to describe the loss of *functional ability* in basic life skills that an individual develops after continual exposure to uncomfortable, noxious situations that s/he is not able to escape or get free from. While the noxious situation may be present in only one aspect of the individual's life (e.g., an abusive marriage), the learned helplessness generalizes over all aspects of the patient's life and skills. This generalization is caused by a chemical reaction inside the body to noxious stimulation. The professional's intervention consists of structuring a situation where the individual actually has control over a part of his/her life that is important to him/her and is able to achieve success with that aspect of his/her life. The chemicals produced inside the patient as a direct result of this honest feeling of success will eventually be able to overcome the chemical/emotional reaction of learned helplessness. This intervention is more successful if the noxious situation can be diminished or removed from the patient's life. See *Brief Leisure Rating Scale, Comprehensive Leisure Rating Scale.*

hematologic (HHS) having to do with the blood.

hematoma an accumulation of blood within tissue as a result of trauma. As the trauma heals, the hematoma becomes a "black and blue mark."

hematopoietic (HHS/NMDP) blood forming; of, or pertaining to, the formation and maturation of blood cells and their derivatives.

hemianopsia defective vision or blindness in half of the visual field. This is an anatomical problem. (Also called hemianopia.) Contrast with *visual neglect.*

hemimelia a birth defect that involves the absence of part or all of the lower half of a limb.

hemiparesis weakness of one side of the body.

hemipelvectomy an amputation at the hip joint that also includes removal of the ischial tuberosity. Functional ability is improved with a four unit prosthetic device:
1.   a specially molded socket which distributes the weight through the torso by utilizing what is left of the pelvic bone, the ribs, and remaining musculature
2.   cosmetic socket (to "normalize" body form)
3.   mechanical hip and knee joints
4.   prosthetic foot

hemiplegia paralysis of one side of the body. See *reflex sympathetic dystrophy.*

hemiplegic gait also known as a flaccid gait. This gait has two primary elements:
1.   a swinging (circumduction) or pushing of the affected leg forward
2.   forefoot strike with a missing heel strike on the affected leg.

This gait is usually noted with patients who have a measurable difference in leg length or a deformity of one leg.

hemoglobin oxygen carrying element of blood. See *lead poisoning.*

hemophilia a hereditary disorder in which the individual experiences excessive and prolonged bleeding because s/he is missing specific blood clotting factors. Prevention of cuts and bumps (bruising) through counseling and education is a key factor in helping the individual with hemophilia. Treatment includes the infusion of blood products containing clotting factors. Because of the need to use blood products to treat hemophilia, many individuals contracted *HIV* or hepatitis in the early to mid 1980's.

hemorrhage escape of a large amount of blood from a ruptured vessel.

hepatic relating to the liver.

hepatitis an inflammation of the liver due to a viral infection. There are three primary types of hepatitis, type "A," type "B," and type "C." The table on the following page is from **Facts About Hepatitis**, Washington State Department of Social and Health Services (1988). See *blood/body fluid precautions, blood-borne pathogens, cirrhosis, enteric isolation, exposure control plan, OPIMs.*

Facts About Hepatitis

	Who Gets	Symptoms Are	It Is Spread By	Treatment	Prevention
Hepatitis A	This virus usually infects children and young adults.	Sudden lack of energy — diarrhea, fever, nausea, abdominal discomfort, often followed by yellow color to the whites of the eyes or skin (jaundice) and darkening of urine. Incubation period is 15 to 45 days after exposure. The disease varies from mild illness (one to two weeks), to more severe cases (four to six weeks) to recover. Many cases in children have no symptoms.	The Hepatitis A virus is present in the feces of an infected individual. Person-to-person contact occurs when persons are careless about hand washing after going to the restroom. Hepatitis A is spread by eating uncooked food prepared by an infected person. Among toddlers, the virus is spread during play, sharing toys, and other close contact. Hepatitis A is not infectious prior to the onset of symptoms. There are no chronic carriers.	If symptoms suggest the possibility of hepatitis, contact your physician or community clinic for advice or diagnosis and treatment, if necessary.	Careful attention should be paid to personal cleanliness, particularly to the thorough washing of hands with soap and water after going to the toilet and before handling food and beverages. Immune serum globulin can help prevent Hepatitis A if administered within 14 days of exposure.
Hepatitis B	Most common among adults, especially gay and drug-using communities, but can infect all ages, including infants. Also common in Asian and Pacific Islander populations.	Begins slowly — lack of appetite, abdominal discomfort, nausea, and vomiting, often followed by yellow color to the whites of the eyes or skin (jaundice). Incubation period is 30 to 90 days. Many cases have no symptoms.	Very minute amounts of infected blood are able to spread this virus. Contaminated needles, syringes, razor blades, or other equipment used to pierce the skin may also spread the virus. It is possible to transmit the virus to a newborn at delivery. Sexual contact and needle sharing are the most common modes of spreading in adults. About 10% of cases become carriers and remain infectious indefinitely. Chronic hepatitis develops in over 25% of carriers.	If symptoms suggest the possibility of hepatitis, contact your physician or community clinic for advice or diagnosis and treatment, if necessary.	Tests are administered to all prospective blood donors to screen out those whose blood is positive for Hepatitis B. Other methods of prevention include proper sterilization of all instruments used for piercing the skin and avoiding sharing needles or other instruments that may be contaminated with blood. Responsible sexual activity, including the use of condoms, can minimize the transmission of Hepatitis B virus. A vaccine is available for people who are at high risk of Hepatitis B infections. (Three injections are required.)
Hepatitis C	Most commonly in transfusion recipients but can affect the same groups as Hepatitis A and B.	Lack of appetite, abdominal discomfort, nausea, and vomiting, chronic liver disease can occur after this infection.	Primarily spread through transfusion, but has been seen after sharing needles and in sexually active individuals. More needs to be known about this infection. Research is ongoing to discover more about transmission.	Contact your physician or community clinic for advice or diagnosis and treatment, if necessary.	For non-transfusion-related cases, prevention strategies are similar to Hepatitis B. Vaccines are not available at this time.

hepatitis A virus a slow onset virus primarily affecting children and young adults. The virus is spread through fecal contamination from an infected person. In the US this is often from poor handwashing.

hepatitis B virus (HHS) a small DNA virus capable of causing both acute and chronic liver disease, possibly by eliciting tissue damage by the immune system. The virus may also be a risk factor for hepatic carcinoma. It is often transmitted through sexual activity or through exposure to contaminated blood.

hepatitis C virus (HHS) an RNA virus related to the pestiviruses and flaviviruses. It is capable of causing both acute and chronic liver disease. As with hepatitis B, the liver damage resulting from this infection may be the result of immune reactivity against virus-infected liver cells. This condition is marked by excessive secretory activity of the thyroid gland.

hepatitis D virus (HDV) (CDC) a defective single-stranded RNA virus that requires the helper function of *hepatitis B virus* (HBV) to replicate. HDV requires HBV for synthesis of envelope protein composed of HBsAg, which is used to encapsulate the HDV genome.

hepatitis E virus (HEV) (CDC) the major etiologic agent of enterically transmitted non-A, non-B hepatitis worldwide; a spherical, non-enveloped, single-stranded RNA virus that is approximately 32 to 34 nm in diameter. Based on similar physico-chemical and biologic properties, HEV has been provisionally classified in the Caliciviridae family; however, the organization of the HEV genome is substantially different from that of other caliciviruses and HEV may eventually be classified in a separate family.

herbicides (HHS) a class of crop protection and specialty chemicals used to control weeds on farms and in forests, as well as in non-agricultural applications such as golf courses, public tracts of land, and residential lawns.

hereditary (HHS/NMDP) the genetic transmission of characteristics from parents to children.

hernia a protrusion of part of the intestinal tract or other organ through a weak spot in the surrounding muscular wall.

herpes a group of large DNA viruses that cause recurring infections with blisters and painful lesions. Cold sores, chicken pox, and shingles are all caused by herpes viruses.

hertz the International System of Units official unit of frequency, equal to one cycle per second (after Heinrich Rudolf Hertz).

heterodermic graft a temporary skin graft taken from a donor of a different species than the recipient.

heterozygous antigens (HHS/NMDP) presence of different alleles on each chromosomes, one inherited from each parent.

heuristic 1. a desire that one acts upon to learn more about a subject. 2. a teaching method which may enhance the patient's ability to discover ways to adjust to a newly acquired disability.

high-fructose corn syrup (HFCS) (HHS) formulations generally containing 42%, 55%, or 90% fructose (the remaining carbohydrate being primarily glucose) depending on the product application. HFCS are used in products such as soft drinks and cake mixes.

High Performance Computing and Communications (HCO) an advanced technology program involving several agencies of the federal government, including the National Library of Medicine and the National Institute for Standards and Technology.

high speed rail (ADA) an intercity type rail service which operates primarily on a dedicated guideway or track not used, for the most part, by freight, including, but not limited to, trains on welded rail, magnetically levitated (meglev) vehicles on special guideways, or other advanced technology vehicles, designed to travel at speeds in excess of those possible on other types of railroads. The ADA accessibility guidelines for high-speed rail may be found in the **High Speed Rail Cars, Monorails, and Systems Technical Assistance Manual** (US Architectural and Transportation Barriers Compliance Board).

hip disarticulation an amputation at the hip joint that retains the ischial tuberosity. Functional ability is improved with a four unit prosthetic device:
1. plastic socket
2. mechanical hip and knee joints
3. prosthetic foot

The socket is molded to provide maximal direct support through the ischial tuberosity and uses the gluteal musculature for additional stability. A hip disarticulation is abbreviated "HD."

Hirschsprung's disease a congenital disorder of the intestines, which lack the necessary autonomic ganglia nerves in the smooth muscle of the intestines to move fecal matter through. See *ostomy*.

HISPP See *Healthcare Information Standards Planning Panel*.

histiocytosis (HHS/NMDP) a rare and frequently fatal blood disease that affects the body's immune system, allowing a type of white blood cell called a histiocyte to multiply wildly and attack vital body organs. Its cause is unknown and its progression is unpredictable.

histocompatibility (HHS/NMDP) referring to the similarity of tissue between different individuals. The level of histocompatibility describes how well matched the patient and donor are. The major histocompatibility determinants are the *human leukocyte antigens* (HLA). HLA typing is performed between the potential marrow donor and the potential transplant recipient to determine how close an HLA match the two are. The closer the match, the less the donated marrow and the patient's body will react against each other. See *graft-versus-host disease.*

histology study of microscopic anatomy of the body's cells, tissue, and organs.

HIV/AIDS HIV, also known as the human immunodeficiency virus, is a virus that attacks and impairs the person's immune system. AIDS, also known as acquired immune deficiency syndrome, is the end stage of an HIV infection. HIV works over a long period of time to weaken an individual's defenses against infections and cancers. Because of this impairment of the immune system, people who are HIV positive develop infections and cancers that would not normally develop in people without HIV. It may take ten or more years for a person who is HIV positive to progress to the last stage, AIDS. Individuals usually live two to four years after being diagnosed with AIDS. "HIV is transmitted when infected blood, semen, vaginal fluids, or breast milk enter the body through the mucous membranes of the anus, vagina, penis (urethra), or mouth, or through cuts, sores, or abrasions in the skin." (Seattle - King County Department of Public Health, 1994) A person may remain without any symptoms of HIV for ten years yet still be able to infect others with the virus. Signs of the advanced stages of HIV/AIDS include persistent swollen lymph nodes, unintentional weight loss, persistent dry cough, night sweats, yeast infections, unexplained skin spots, unexplained diarrhea, severe pelvic infections, unusually large numbers of genital warts, or persistent fever. See *blood-borne pathogens, blood/body fluid precautions, Comprehensive Health Enhancement Support System, hemophilia.*

HL7 See *health level 7.*

HMO See *health maintenance organization.*

Hodgkin's disease (HHS/NMDP) a *lymphoma* most frequently occurring in young adults. Hodgkin's disease not responding to chemotherapy may be treated by autologous bone marrow transplant and less frequently by allogeneic bone marrow transplant.

holistic approach awareness that illness is not just a disease state and that an individual's social, emotional, economic, and physical states are all connected. When all these elements of an individual's life are taken into account as part of providing *treatment*, the treatment is considered to be using a holistic approach.

home and community-based waivers a method for funding providers for home and community-based Medicaid services for individuals who would otherwise require care in a skilled nursing facility or an intermediate care facility. Under waivers, states can provide medical services and certain non-medical services not covered in their Medicaid state plan.

home health agency (HHA) a public or private organization primarily engaged in providing skilled nursing and other therapeutic services in the patient's home. The HHA must meet certain *conditions of participation* that ensure the health and safety of the individuals to whom it furnishes services.

home health care provision of medical care in a patient's home has increased significantly over the last decade. Not only can home health care be cost-effective but it also allows the patient to be in a familiar environment with all of its social and emotional supports. Treatments such as IV therapy, rehabilitation therapy, post surgery recovery, and respiratory treatment can all take place in the home. See *full service continuum.*

homeostasis physiological process of maintaining a *balance*, achieved by the body's coordinated process of regulation of systems.

homolateral gait a gait that is identified by the turning of the head, thorax, and pelvis toward the flexing side of the body with the contralateral extremities extending.

homozygous (HHS/NMDP) presence of identical alleles on both chromosomes, one inherited from each parent.

honesty a personality trait of telling the truth and acting truthfully. While honesty is a socially desired attribute, from a clinical standpoint it is not supportable. The US Congressional Office of Technology Assessment (1990) concurs with Hartshorne & May (1928) that honesty is an unstable personality trait, which cannot be reliably measured. Additionally, since "honesty" is revered so much, prejudice against individuals labeled "dishonest" is so severe that many practitioners feel uncomfortable (or refuse) to assign that label. Currently, the term *integrity* is used instead of honesty in clinical settings. See *integrity testing.*

hookworm (CDC) an intestinal parasite of humans that usually causes mild diarrhea or cramps. Heavy infection with hookworm can create serious health problems for newborns, children, pregnant women, and persons who are malnourished. Hookworm infections occur mostly in tropical and subtropical climates and are estimated to infect about 1 billion people (about one-fifth of the world's population). One of the most common species, Ancylostoma duodenal, is found in southern Europe, northern Africa, northern Asia, and parts of South America. A second species, Necator americanus, was widespread in the southeastern United States early in this century. The Rockefeller Sanitary Commission was founded in response, and hookworm infection has been largely controlled. People can become infected by direct contact with contaminated soil, generally through walking barefoot, or accidentally swallowing contaminated soil. Hookworms have a complex life cycle that begins and ends in the small intestine. Hookworm eggs require warm, moist, shaded soil to hatch into larvae. These barely visible larvae penetrate the skin (often through bare feet), are carried to the lungs, go through the respiratory tract to the mouth, are swallowed, and eventually reach the small intestine. This journey takes about a week. In the small intestine, the larvae develop into half-inch-long worms, attach themselves to the intestinal wall, and suck blood. The adult worms produce thousands of eggs. These eggs are passed in the feces (stool). If the eggs contaminate soil and conditions are right, they will hatch, molt, and develop into infective larvae again after 5 to 10 days. People who have direct contact with soil that contains human feces in areas where hookworm is common are at high risk of infection. Children (because they play in dirt and often go barefoot) are at high risk. Since transmission of hookworm infection requires development of the larvae in soil, hookworm cannot be spread person to person. Contact among children in institutional or child care settings should not increase the risk of infection. Itching and a rash at the site of where skin touched soil or sand is usually the first sign of infection. These symptoms occur when the larvae penetrate the skin. While a light infection may cause no symptoms, heavy infection can cause anemia, abdominal pain, diarrhea, loss of appetite, and weight loss. Heavy, chronic infections can cause stunted growth and mental development. Hookworm can cause serious health problems. The most serious results of hookworm infection are the development of anemia and protein deficiency caused by blood loss. When children are continuously infected by many worms, the loss of iron and protein can retard growth and mental development, sometimes irreversibly. Hookworm infection can also cause tiredness, difficulty breathing, enlargement of the heart, and irregular heartbeat. Sometimes hookworm infection is fatal, especially among infants.

hormone a group of chemical substances produced by the body that initiates or regulates the functions of body organs or groups of cells. See *adrenal gland, endocrine system, epinephrine.*

horticultural therapy use of plant and natural materials to help remediate, rehabilitate, or to provide palliative care. Horticultural therapy is also used successfully as a type of vocational training for individuals requiring a sheltered or supported work environment. Horticulture as a modern therapeutic modality was first conceptualized by Alice W. Burlingame and Ruth Mosher in the late 1940's. An individual who is professionally trained as a horticultural therapist may be registered through the American Horticultural Therapy Association, 909 York St., Denver, CO 80206-3799, www.ahta.org.

hospice an entity that provides an alternative way of caring for terminally ill individuals, stressing palliative care (medical relief) from pain as opposed to curative or restorative care. Hospice care usually encourages home care instead of institutional care when practical.

hospital an institution that is primarily engaged in providing, by or under the supervision of physicians, to inpatients: 1. diagnostic services and therapeutic services for medical diagnosis, treatment, and care of injured, disabled, or sick persons or 2. rehabilitation services for the rehabilitation of injured, disabled or sick persons.

hospital insurance generally, an insurance policy which helps pay for all or part of a beneficiary's hospital bill. For those receiving *Medicare*, hospital insurance is known as Medicare Part A. This is an insurance program providing basic protection against the cost of hospital and related post hospital services for individuals who are age 65 and over and are eligible for retirement benefits under the social security or railroad retirement systems; or individuals under age 65 who have been entitled for not less than 24 months to disability benefits under the Social Security Act or railroad retirement systems; and for certain other individuals who are medically determined to have *end stage renal disease* (ESRD) and are covered by the Social Security Act or railroad retirement systems.

hospital insurance tax (FB) The Medicare program consists of two parts; the hospital insurance (Part A) program and the supplementary medical insurance (Part B) program. The hospital insurance program is financed primarily through the hospital insurance payroll tax contributions paid by employers, employees, and the self-employed. For wages paid in 2001, the total hospital insurance tax rate is 2.9% of wages. One half of the tax is imposed on the employee and one half on the employer.

HOST Healthcare Open System and Trials Consortium.

HPCC See *high performance computing and communications.*

Human Activity Profile (HAP) a quick screening tool that measures the general physical activity level of a patient compared to norm groups. The HAP contains 94 items, which include activities covering a broad range of energy requirements based on estimated metabolic equivalents (METS). The HAP is to be used with adults between the ages of 20 and 79 and should take less then 10 minutes for the patient to complete.

human capital approach (HCO) a valuation technique used in *cost-benefit* analysis that assigns a monetary value to a human life based on an estimate of the individual's projected future earnings.

human herpesvirus 6 (CDC) a virus of the herpesvirus beta-subfamily, discovered in 1985, that infects more than 95% of people by the age of 2 years. It has been causally associated with *roseola*, mononucleosis-like illness, and inflammation of lymph glands. There is also suggestive evidence for a role in *multiple sclerosis.*

human immunodeficiency virus See *HIV/AIDS.*

human leukocyte antigens (HLA) (HHS/NMDP) proteins found on the surface of white blood cells and other tissues that are used to match donor and patient. Patient and potential donor have their white blood cells tested for three antigens, HLA-A, B, and DR. Each individual has two sets of these antigens, one set inherited from each parent. For this reason, it is much more likely for a brother or sister to match the patient than an unrelated individual, and much more likely for persons of the same racial and ethnic backgrounds to match.

Huntington's chorea a hereditary disease characterized by the progressive deterioration of the patient's cognitive ability and also an erratic deterioration of the patient's involuntary muscle movements. There is no cure for the disease at this point although there is a test to determine if an individual is carrying the gene for the disease.

hydrocephalus a usually treatable increase of fluid inside the skull causing increased pressure, dilation of the cerebral ventricles, thinning of the brain itself, and possibly, separation of the cranial bones. Treatment usually involves the placement of a *shunt* (valve and tube) leading from the brain to the chest cavity to drain the excess fluid. Without warning the shunt may become clogged, causing some loss of cognition, and a potential change in personality. Therapists working in the schools and other social and health departments should be especially obser-

vant of patients with shunts and maintain an objective measurement of the patient's social and cognitive skills (*baselines* plus quarterly or half yearly re-evaluations). See *macrocephaly, neurofibromatosis.*

hydrogenation (HHS) the process of adding hydrogen molecules directly to an unsaturated fatty acid from sources such as vegetable oils to convert it to a semi-solid form such as margarine or shortening. Hydrogenation contributes important textural properties to food. The degree of hydrogenation influences the firmness and spreadability of margarines, flakiness of piecrusts and the creaminess of puddings. Hydrogenated oils are sometimes used in place of other *fats* with higher proportions of saturated fatty acids such as butter or lard.

hydrophysics factors that influence water or a body in water such as hydrostatic pressure, buoyancy, water temperature, viscosity, resistance, streamline flow, surface tension, and osmosis.

hydrotherapy "use of water by external applications either for its pressure effect or as a means of applying physical energy to the tissue." (Stedman's Medical Dictionary, 26th Edition, 1995, p.818). This term often refers to the use of water in wound management, such as whirlpool baths, but can be used interchangeably with the term "aquatic therapy."

hydroureter nephrosis a clinical condition which may develop as a result of a blockage of the urine causing a backup of urine in the ureter (ureter distention).

hyperactivity (general definition) abnormally high levels of physical activity; the inability to keep one's body quiet in a manner that would normally be expected for one's age group. Behaviors associated with hyperactivity include restlessness, fidgeting, squirming, off-task behaviors, unnecessary movements, and excessive physical activity (e.g., running instead of walking). The hyperactivity demonstrated by patients is usually caused by either an internally driven force or by a side effect of medications. Internally caused hyperactivity is frequently paired with a sensory deficit (e.g., lack of ability to process incoming visual, tactile, or auditory stimulation) or neurological problems. The therapist may need to evaluate how different types of sensory input affect the patient before being able to provide effective treatment. Once it has been determined how sensory input affects the patient, the therapist should be able to control input (modify environment) as well as to teach the patient specific attending skills. (specific definition) The **DSM-IV** defines hyperactivity as having at least one of the following nine symptoms for at least six months, the symptoms being developmentally inappropriate. Hyperactivity includes

Blood Pressures and Hypertension

Diastolic Blood Pressure	Category	Systolic (When DBP < 90 mm HG)	Category
≥ 115	Severe hypertension	≥ 160	Isolated systolic hypertension
105 - 114	Moderate hypertension	140 - 159	Borderline isolated
90 - 104	Mild hypertension	<140	Normal blood pressure
85 - 89	High normal		
<85	Normal blood pressure		

impulsivity and has nine possible symptoms: (hyper-activity) a. often fidgets with hands or feet or squirms in seat, b. often leaves seat in classroom or in other situations in which remaining seated is expected, c. often runs about or climbs excessively in situations in which it is inappropriate (in adolescents or adults, may be limited to subjective feelings of restlessness), d. often has difficulty playing or engaging in leisure activities quietly, e. is often "on the go" or often acts as if "driven by a motor," f. often talks excessively (impulsivity), g. often blurts out answers to questions before the questions have been completed, h. often has difficulty awaiting turn, and i. often interrupts or intrudes on others (e.g., butts into conversations or games). See *attention deficit, bipolar disorder, lead poisoning, mental retardation, metabolic disorders.*

hyperalimentation insertion of a tube into the subclavian vein to allow the infusion of nutrition, medication, and hydration. A parenteral hyperalimentation tube goes directly into the bloodstream from a catheter placed through the subclavian vein into the superior vena cava. These tubes are best for patients who cannot eat, digest, or absorb nutrition adequately. Since the catheter goes directly to the heart, activity must be limited to activities that do not risk disturbing or displacing the catheter.

hyperendemic a disease which is endemic to the area and which is occurring at a significantly higher rate of infection than would normally be expected. See *infection.*

hyperesthesia abnormal, increased sensitivity of the skin or an organ to stimuli. Compare with *dysesthesia.* See *sensation, spinal cord injury.*

hyperflexia excessive *flexion* of a joint or joints.

hyperplasia an abnormal acceleration of cell growth that significantly increases the size of the organ or body part but which does not form a tumor. Different from *hypertrophy.*

hypersensation an abnormal increased awareness of contact. See *associated features, baroreceptor sensitivity, hyperesthesia, sensation, tactile defensiveness.*

hypersensitivity allergy, or an enhanced response by the immune system to a foreign substance that leads to pathological tissue changes. Hypersensitivity can occur as an immediate response, in minutes; well know examples are asthma, hay fever, and hives.

hypertension (HHS) the persistently elevated arterial blood pressure. It is the most common public health problem in developed countries. Emphasis on lifestyle modifications has given diet a prominent role for both the primary prevention and management of hypertension. See the chart above. See *biofeedback, blood pressure, coarctation of the aorta, meditation, progressive relaxation.*

hypertonic an increased level of tension in a muscle or limb. See *cerebral palsy.*

hypertrophic scarring excessive growth of *scar* tissue. See *Jobst.*

hypertrophy enlargement of all or part of an organ beyond its normal size as long as the enlargement is not caused by a tumor or a proliferation of cells (*hyperplasia*).

hypervigilant the excessive attention to all stimuli, both internal and external, frequently seen in individuals who have been sexually abused or who are in delusional or paranoid states. The individual is usually demonstrating this behavior because s/he does not perceive that s/he is personally safe in the current situation.

hypnagogic illusion a very short hallucination — experienced as the individual makes the transition from wakefulness into sleep. Hypnagogic illusions are usually experienced as dreams but do not happen during REM (rapid eye movement) sleep. Unlike true hallucinations that may indicate a mental illness, hypnagogic illusions are considered "normal." See *hallucination.*

hypnopompic illusion a very short hallucination — sensations that may be experienced as the individual makes the transition from sleep to wakefulness. Unlike true hallucinations that may indicate a mental illness, hypnopompic illusions are considered "normal." See *hallucination.*

hypnosis a subconscious condition in which the objective manifestations of the mind are more or less inactive, accompanied by abnormal sensibility to suggestions made by the hypnotist. Hypnosis has been shown to be efficacious in treating psycho-physiological conditions such as pain, anxiety, and phobias.

hypoactivity abnormally low levels of physical activity. Compare with *anhedonia*.

hypochondriasis a psychological condition in which the patient has imagined or highly exaggerated complaints of physical illness. The patient's concern about his/her heartbeat, sweating, breathing, or bowel/bladder functions interferes with normal day-to-day activities. An official **DSM-IV** diagnosis, hypochondriasis has six criteria: 1. a belief or fear that one has a serious illness 2. even though there is not medical evidence to support the illness, 3. even though the belief or fear exists, the patient is able to verbally, but reluctantly, admit that s/he might be mistaken, 4. the belief or fear caused the patient to have impaired or interrupted function or to exhibit measurable and clinically significant signs of *stress*, 5. this belief or fear has lasted at least six months, and 6. is not better identified as another psychiatric disorder. See *Minnesota Multiphasic Personality Inventory.*

hypoesthesia a functional decrease in the ability to sense touch. See *dysesthesia, hyperesthesia, sensation.*

hypoflexia less than normal *flexion* of a joint or joints.

hypoglycemia a condition in which the patient does not have adequate blood sugar levels to sustain normal health and activity. See *metabolic disorders.*

hypomanic episode episodes of mania that are not severe enough to warrant a manic diagnosis (lasting up to four days and, while behavioral changes are noted, the changes do not cause significant functional problems). See *bipolar disorder, mania, Minnesota Multiphasic Personality Inventory.*

hypoparathyroidism (HHS) a condition caused by the reduction or absence of secretions of the parathyroid gland.

hypoplastic left heart syndrome (HLHS) usually a fatal birth defect, correctable only with a heart transplant. The left side of the heart, especially the left ventricle, is significantly underdeveloped and unable to function efficiently.

hypotension blood pressure well below what is considered normal. An individual with hypotension may experience dizziness if s/he stands up quickly. See *blood pressure, hypertension.*

hypothesis a statement that serves as a tentative explanation for why something happens. When a therapist is trying to determine if a specific *treat-*ment protocol provides good *outcomes*, s/he would start with a hypothesis followed by a testing of the hypothesis. The author worked with children with traumatic brain injuries on a rehab unit and was responsible for evaluating the patient's *tolerance* to stimuli while on community outings. It soon became apparent that it is psychologically traumatizing to the patient when s/he is taken out to the community too soon because it can cause a devastating lack of ability to handle the situation due to being overstimulated. Noticing a parallel between the level of stimulation complexity on the computer games played on the unit and the patient's tolerance to the stimulation at the local hamburger restaurant, the author developed the following hypothesis: "Patients who are able to tolerate fifteen minutes on computer games rated at 5.0 or greater on the burlingame software scale (burlingame, 1990) will be able to tolerate 20 minutes at the local hamburger restaurant." A formal comparison of the patient's tolerance of the stimulation on the computer games and their ability to tolerate the stimulation at the local restaurant was made. The author then found that the hypothesis proved to be true approximately 70% of the time — a moderate predictor. By developing hypotheses about specific treatment programs and then analyzing the data collected, each individual therapist will both increase the effectiveness of treatment and advance his/her field.

hypothyroidism a disorder in which the thyroid activity is deficient causing a reduced basal metabolic rate, *lethargy*, and sensitivity to cold. In women (it affects a higher percentage of women), hypothyroidism may also lead to menstrual disturbances. See *depression.*

hypovolemia an abnormally low volume of blood circulating through the body caused by a significant loss of blood, a circulatory problem, and/or inadequate tissue perfusion (the allowing of body fluids to evenly pass through cell tissue or organs). Patients with hypovolemia may have lowered blood pressure, light-headedness, decreased urine output, clammy skin, faster than normal breathing, and/or *tachycardia*. Severe hypovolemia (hypovolemic shock) is a life-threatening event.

I

iatrogenic caused by procedures related to diagnosis or treatment; a disorder caused by exposure to health care treatment or the health care environment. *Nosocomial* infections are a type of iatrogenic disorders.

ICD-9-CM See *International Classification of Disease, Ninth Revision, Clinical Modification*.

ICF-MR See *intermediate care facility for the mentally retarded*.

id *Freud* described three elements of a person's psyche that constantly battle to influence the individual's behavior. Id is the term given to the most basic drives of the individual — satisfying his/her own basic needs. The other two elements, *ego* and *superego*, control the id's drives.

IDEA See *Individuals with Disabilities Education Act*.

ideational apraxia an inability to connect the method or purpose for doing something with the desired *outcome*. Motor movement itself is not impaired. See *apraxia*.

identification 1. process of selectively comparing an object to other objects, noticing differences and similarities, and then determining what the object is. 2. process of empathizing or feeling similar to another. There are two terms that refer to the process of an individual copying the another's actions. Identification refers to unconscious patterning of oneself after another individual. *Imitation* refers to conscious patterning of oneself after another person.

identity a person's perception of himself/herself as compared to others in the community. Quite often a newly acquired, severe disability will leave a person without an identity (or at least with the realization that his/her past identity is not completely valid). This causes a crisis within the individual, a crisis that may be more severe than the actual disability itself. Therapists must be sensitive to a patient's need to develop a new or modified identity and help facilitate development of a realistic, positive identity.

ideomotor apraxia loss of the ability to perform movements or gestures upon demand (when they are asked to). This type of *apraxia* does not affect the individual's ability to perform automatic routine movements or gestures.

idiopathic a combination of the Greek word *idios* which means "originating from oneself" and *pathic*, which means "a disease state." Idiopathic refers to a disease or disorder that originates from within the individual. In health care the term idiopathic also implies a disease or disorder of unknown origin that originates within the person. Autism is idiopathic while hepatitis is not.

idiosyncratic particular to that individual. In health care idiosyncratic behavior tends to imply unusual mannerisms that deviate from customary behavior. Idiosyncratic behavior may extend from being curious to eccentric to outright bizarre. Children with *autism* often are described as demonstrating idiosyncratic behaviors.

IDS See *integrated delivery system*.

Idyll Arbor Leisure Battery a battery made up of four separate instruments used to measure how a patient relates to leisure: 1. *Leisure Attitude Measurement*, 2. *Leisure Motivation Scale*, 3. *Leisure Satisfaction Measure*, and 4. *Leisure Interest Measure*. The Idyll Arbor Leisure Battery was developed by Ragheb and Beard (1990, 1991a, 1991b, 1991c). See the figure on the next two pages for more information about each instrument.

IEP See *individualized education program*.

IITF Information Infrastructure Task Force.

ileostomy an ostomy placed in the ileum (small intestine). See *ostomy*.

illusion a perception that an object exists but that object cannot necessarily be proven to exist through an analysis of the existing physical environment. The therapist should not confuse illusion with *hallucination* or *delusion* as described below.

Comparisons with Illusion

Term	Description
delusion	A perception or belief that the patient holds to regardless of physical and cognitive proof that the perception or belief is incorrect.
illusion	A perception which is the result of retinal and/or cortical processing of a stimuli which is unexpected and not proven through an analysis of the existing physical environment.
hallucination	A perception that an event has taken place — an event that has no basis in the physical environment. The individual has a strong sensory impression that the event has taken place.

IDYLL ARBOR LEISURE BATTERY - EXECUTIVE SUMMARY

Description of Instrument	Interpretation of Scores

LEISURE ATTITUDE MEASUREMENT
 	
The **Cognitive** component of leisure attitude gathers information in the following areas:
  a) general knowledge and beliefs about leisure,
  b) beliefs about leisure's relation to other concepts such as health, happiness, and work, and
  c) beliefs about the qualities, virtues, characteristics, and benefits of leisure to individuals such as: developing friendship, renewing energy, helping one to relax, meeting needs, and self-improvement.
 	
The **Affective** component of leisure attitude is designed to take into account the individual's:
  a) evaluation of his/her leisure experiences and activities,
  b) liking of those experiences and activities, and
  c) immediate and direct feelings toward leisure experiences and activities. This component generally reflects the respondent's like or dislike of leisure activities.
 	
The **Behavioral** component of leisure attitude is based on the individual's:
  a) verbalized behavioral intentions toward leisure choices and activities, and on self-reports of current and past participation
	LEISURE ATTITUDE MEASUREMENT
	
	Score Intervention
	
	    Cognitive — education about the need for leisure in society and one's life.
	
	Less than "2.5" Affective — provision of positive experiences related to interests, values, needs.
	
	    Behavioral — education about the importance of leisure activities for improving quality of life.

LEISURE INTEREST MEASURE
 	
Measures how much interest the client has in each of the eight domains of leisure interest.
 	
Areas Measured:
 	
  1. Physical   5. Service
  2. Outdoor   6. Social
  3. Mechanical 7. Cultural
  4. Artistic   8. Reading
	LEISURE INTEREST MEASURE
	
	Score Intervention
	4 or more High degree of interest.
	    Ensure opportunity to participate in activities of interest.
	
	2 or less Low interest.
	    May need education, instruction.
	
	"2" Needs education and instruction in areas of interest and development of skill competence.

163

IDYLL ARBOR LEISURE BATTERY - EXECUTIVE SUMMARY

Description of Instrument

LEISURE SATISFACTION MEASURE

Measures which areas of leisure provide the most satisfaction for the individual.

1. **Psychological:** Psychological benefits such as: a sense of freedom, enjoyment, involvement, and intellectual challenge.
2. **Educational:** Intellectual stimulation and learning about self and surroundings.
3. **Social:** Rewarding relationships with other people.
4. **Relaxation:** Relief from the stress and strain of life.
5. **Physiological:** A means to develop physical fitness, stay healthy, control weight, and otherwise promote well being.
6. **Aesthetic:** Aesthetic rewards. Individuals scoring high on this part derive satisfaction from the places where they engage in their leisure activities because they find them pleasing, interesting, beautiful, and generally well-designed.

LEISURE MOTIVATION SCALE

The **Intellectual** component of leisure motivation assesses the extent to which individuals are motivated to engage in leisure activities that involve mental activities such as learning, exploring, discovering, creating, or imagining.

The **Social** component assesses the extent to which individuals engage in leisure activities for social reasons. This component measures two basic needs. The first is the need for friendship and interpersonal relationships, while the second is the need to be valued by others.

The **Competence-Mastery** component assesses the extent to which individuals engage in leisure activities in order to achieve, master, challenge, and compete. These activities are usually physical in nature.

The **Stimulus-Avoidance** component of leisure motivation assesses the need to escape and get away from overstimulating life situations. Some individuals need to avoid social contacts, to seek solitude and calm conditions while others seek to rest and unwind.

Interpretation of Scores

LEISURE SATISFACTION MEASURE

Score	Intervention
4 or more	High satisfaction. Ensure opportunities to participate in activities.
2 or less	Low satisfaction.
"2"	Education/opportunities to increase satisfaction level. Review results of LAM, LIM, LMS.
	Determine if low score is having negative impact on client's ability to make progress on treatment objectives.

LEISURE MOTIVATION SCALE

Score	Intervention
highest	Primary motivating force.
	• Ensure opportunity to participate in activities with motivating dimensions.
	• Activity analysis modify/adapt.
lowest	Least motivating force.
	• Provide choice.
	• Avoidance behavior.
	• Modify, adapt, and adopt new activities.

164

imagery picturing something in your head; the process of developing an image. The image developed is seldom static — that is, the image is cognitively manipulated into taking some kind of action. Imagery can be a powerful tool in therapy as the therapist can help the patient guide the imagery to help *problem solve* and to resolve *conflicts* without the patient actually having to physically experience that action first. These "dry runs" help the patient gain confidence (*self-esteem*) by anticipating problems, developing strategies, and picturing himself/herself as successful before having to encounter the actual *stress*-producing event. Imagery is also one of the main techniques used in relaxation and stress reduction work. See *guided imagery, relaxation techniques.*

imaging tests (CDC) any of a variety of methods for observing the internal anatomy of the body, ranging from simple x-rays to complex three-dimensional scanning techniques using nuclear magnetic resonance, positron emission, and other techniques.

imitation act of copying the movements of others; a conscious attempt to duplicate another person's actions. Compare with *identification*, the unconscious act of duplicating another person's actions.

Immediate and Serious Threat to Patient Health and Safety title of the federal regulation on patient safety which applies to almost all health care settings in the United States. This law supersedes other health care laws, as it is the law that is intended to protect the consumer from the most damaging health care situations. A surveyor may "call" an Immediate and Serious Threat even if no patient has been injured; only the likelihood that one will be injured. The chart on the following page lists the five sections of this law (referred to as "Core Statements") and the subsections of each Core Statement (referred to as Operational Definitions).

immune globulin (CDC) a crude preparation of antibody molecules collected from pooled multiple blood donations, used as a means for passively transferring antimicrobial resistance to susceptible individuals. See *antibodies.*

immune suppressants (CDC) agents that block or restrict the activity of one or more components of the immune system, usually leading to increased susceptibility to infectious disease.

impaired adjustment a patient's inability to modify his/her style/behavior in a manner that is consistent with a change in his/her health status. The patient may either choose to not recognize the change through lack of acceptance or be unaware of the change. Due to this impaired adjustment, the patient will probably demonstrate a lack of movement to-ward independence; experience an extended period of shock, disbelief, or anger toward his/her health change; or demonstrate an impaired ability to make plans for the future. See *independence, insight.*

impetigo an infection of the skin which is very contagious that causes redness of the skin progressing to pruritic vesicles and then produces a honey-colored crust over the eruptions. The infections are usually found on the face. See *group A streptococcus.*

implosive therapy a technique for overcoming avoidance behavior by, paradoxically, increasing fear, sometimes by placing a person in close proximity to the fear-producing stimulus. Also known as flooding.

important aspects of care a health care quality assurance term. Important aspects of care are services or treatments that:
1. involve a high volume of patients,
2. expose the patient to a significant risk, and/or
3. have a higher-than-normal history of causing problems for either the patient or the staff.

Because of the significance of these aspects of care, they are frequently selected for monitoring and evaluation in the agency's *quality improvement program.* See *quality assurance.*

impotence an inability to engage in sexual intercourse due to a variety of reasons. Impotence is frequently a side effect of medications or of poor health. There are three different types of functional impotence: 1. the inability to develop and sustain an erection (erective impotence), 2. the inability to eject seminal fluid (ejaculatory impotence) or 3. the inability to have a full orgasm (orgasmic impotence). Some individuals do not feel that orgasmic impotence is a true impotence because the male can achieve coitus. Secondary impotence is the term given to individuals whose impotence stems from a psychological disorder. For diagnostic purposes, males are considered to have a secondary impotence if they are not able to achieve coitus during 25% or more of their attempts.

impulse control disorders inability or failure to resist an impulse or temptation that could harm oneself or others. Patients with these disorders tend to have a growing feeling of tension or sense of arousal prior to taking the impulsive action, then experience relief, pleasure, gratification afterwards. Patients do not necessarily experience feelings of guilt, regret, or self-reproach afterwards. Impulse control disorder is an official category in the **DSM-IV** and contains six specific disorders: *intermittent explosive disorder, kleptomania, pyromania, pathological gambling, trichotillomania,* and impulse-control disorder not otherwise specified. See *impulsivity.*

Immediate and Serious Threat To Patient Health and Safety

Core Statement	Operational Definition
I. Failure to Protect Patients from Disease and Infection	1. Failure to protect from *nosocomial infections* and/or communicable diseases. 2. Failure to maintain sterile technique during invasive procedures.
II. Failure to Provide Care or Services Essential to Maintaining or Improving Patient Health	1. Failure to protect patients from bodily harm. 2. Failure to ensure that patients receive medications as prescribed. 3. Failure to ensure that patients do not suffer from undue adverse medication consequences. 4. Failure to ensure that patients receive prescribed nutrition/hydration in the amount, type, and consistency needed to support and maintain health. 5. Failure to perform reliable and accurate lab tests which lead to treatment/non-treatment that adversely affects patient care. 6. Failure to administer blood products safely. 7. Failure to employ a system that ensures that the facility will correctly identify patients. 8. Failure of provider to furnish supervision or monitoring consistent with patient needs. 9. Failure to apply appropriate mechanical/orthotic devices used to achieve proper body alignment safely. See *orthosis.* 10. Failure to provide initial medical screening of emergency patients and women in active labor. 11. Failure to monitor patient status to identify conditions or changes in conditions that potentially could lead to patient harm and/or deterioration. 12. Failure to react and/or take remedial action in response to identified conditions or changes in conditions that could lead to patient harm and/or deterioration. 13. Failure to ensure the safe transfer of patients to another facility.
III. Failure to Maintain Equipment and Supplies at an Acceptable Level to Ensure Health and Safety.	1. Failure of provider to maintain or have available emergency equipment and supplies, appropriate to type of health care entity. 2. Failure to maintain and monitor use of equipment and supplies, appropriate to type of health care entity.
IV. Failure to Prevent Situations/Conditions in Environment or Physical Plant Which Would Present a Hazard and Would Jeopardize Patient Health and Safety See *environment of care.*	1. Failure to ensure that fire/smoke will be contained to site of fire. 2. Failure to ensure that equipment, furnishings, or supplies do not present hazards to patients. 3. Failure to maintain operative smoke detection and fire alarm system. 4. Failure to maintain a means by which patients can summon help. 5. Failure to ensure staff can deal effectively with emergency situations. 6. Failure to maintain fire extinguishment systems. 7. Failure to maintain means of egress. 8. Failure to prevent exposure of patients to hazardous wastes. 9. Failure to prevent widespread infestation of insects/rodents. 10. Failure to store, prepare, maintain, and serve food to ensure against the growth/transmission of pathogens. 11. Failure to control temperature of hot water used by patients (max. 110 degrees Fahrenheit). 12. Failure to provide power in emergencies. 13. Failure to provide appropriate heating, air conditioning, and ventilation. 14. Failure to take necessary precautions to ensure patients are not harmed by patients, staff, or visitors. 15. Failure to maintain physical plant in a safe condition.
V. Failure to Uphold Patient Rights Whereby Violations Can Result in Harm or Injury	1. Inappropriate *restraints.* 2. Inappropriate *psychiatric seclusion.* 3. *Neglect.* 4. *Mental abuse.* 5. *Physical abuse.*

impulsivity   act of carrying out an action without forethought of the consequences and without prior anticipation of all of the equipment/supplies needed for the action. It is common for individuals who have sustained a *traumatic brain injury* or a right-sided *cerebrovascular accident* to exhibit impulsive behaviors. While impulsivity in social situations may be aggravating for others (e.g., patient decides on the way to a party to go to a movie instead when she was bringing the potato chips), it can also be life threatening. More than one individual has parked his/her car next to a hiking trial because the late afternoon was so pleasant — only to find himself/herself a mile from the trail head at dark without a coat or flashlight. It is not uncommon for patients with an impulse disorder to also have problems with *lability*, so once they discover their error due to impulsivity, they tend to overreact with excessive emotional responses making a difficult or dangerous situation even worse. Contrast with *inattention*. See *compulsion, diversional program, hyperactivity, inhibition, kleptomania.*

IM system   See *indicator measurement system.*

inattention   as defined by the **DSM-IV**, inattention has nine possible symptoms: 1. often fails to give close attention to details or makes careless mistakes in schoolwork, work, or other activities, 2. often has difficulty sustaining attention in tasks or play activities, 3. often does not seem to listen when spoken to directly, 4. often does not follow through on instructions and fails to finish schoolwork, chores, or duties in the workplace (not due to oppositional behavior or failure to understand instructions), 5. often has difficulties organizing tasks and activities, 6. often avoids, dislikes, or is reluctant to engage in tasks that require sustained mental effort (such as school-work or homework), 7. often loses things necessary for tasks or activities (e.g., school assignments, pencils, books, or tools), 8. is often easily distracted by extraneous stimuli, and 9. is often forgetful in daily activities. For symptoms of inattention to be part of a diagnosis of attention deficit hyperactivity disorder, other elements must also be present. Contrast with *impulsivity*. See *attention deficit hyperactivity disorder.*

incidence   the number of times the event or object being measured occurred during a specific time period; (HHS) the number of new cases of a disease during a given period of time in a defined population.

incident report   a management tool used by facilities to record potentially harmful events, including the suggested cause of the incident, the action(s) taken by staff, the immediate consequences/outcomes, and follow-up actions. Incident reports are helpful in determining areas of risk and areas that would benefit from *quality improvement*. See *risk management, psychiatric seclusion.*

inclusive education   a program in public schools (previously called "mainstreaming") that has experienced limited success. While implemented with good intentions, teachers tend to have too large a classroom size (25-35 students) without adequate support staff, adapted equipment, and limited training in addressing the educational needs of children with disabilities. This causes resentment (and helps develop prejudicial attitudes) when the group's work is continually interrupted. Some individuals have gone to referring to this kind of mainstreaming as "intrusive" education. Inclusive education and *inclusive recreation* can produce positive experiences for all involved and are generally the "desired" types of programs. The key is to engage those who are interested; who, given the ability to use adaptations, can meet minimum skill requirements; and to use staff who are skilled in being able to use appropriate accommodations. There is no reason that inclusive recreation needs to experience the drawbacks that inclusive education has. See *normalization.*

inclusive recreation   recreation programming which has a mix of individuals who are disabled and individuals who are not disabled. While inclusive recreation clearly meets the general intent of non-discrimination and the *Americans with Disabilities Act* (ADA), a closer look shows that it can be fraught with problems if not done carefully. A recreation program is truly inclusive if:

1. Participants have a desire to be in the recreation program.
2. Participants have the general ability to actively participate in the group — even if this requires extra equipment and staffing.
3. The leader(s) of the recreation program have the knowledge of how each of the disabilities represented affects the individual's performance and what adaptations and equipment help resolve the resulting deficits.
4. The leaders can clearly state why an individual is appropriate or inappropriate for a recreation program and can offer alternative suggestions for recreation programming.

Denial of the right to participate in a specific program should be based on minimum skill requirements (may use adapted equipment) and basic safety principles. Safety includes psychological as well as physical safety. Examples of inclusive recreation are shown in the chart on the next page. See *normalization.*

Examples of Inclusive Recreation

Program	Minimum Skills	Adapted Equipment	Inclusion in Group?
bridge club	• able to follow three-step commands • basic math, ability to wait for turn • moderate impulse control	• aide to provide cues • memory book listing steps involved in game • card holder	• individual with *Down syndrome* who is able to demonstrate minimum skills with or without aide - YES - include in group.
diving lessons	• ability to reach diving board • ability to swim one length of the pool	• long pants for individuals with paraplegia (to reduce skin tears as s/he scoots along to end of diving board) • appropriate devices to insure urinary and bowel continence as needed	• individual with L5 total paralysis who meets all minimum requirements - YES - include in group. • Individual who is not disabled but not able to swim length - NO - do not include in group

incontinence inability to control when one urinates (urinary incontinence) or defecates (fecal incontinence). There are many factors that influence incontinence and many degrees of incontinence. Some individuals only have a limited leakage during episodes of coughing or sneezing. Such limited incontinence is usually not a limiting factor for activities. Many of the products on the market work well at providing a barrier to leakage and smell. (RAPs) Nationally, 50% of nursing home patients are incontinent. Incontinence causes many problems, including skin rashes, *falls*, isolation, and *pressure sores* and the potentially troubling use of *indwelling catheters*. In addition, continence is often an important goal to many patients and incontinence may affect patients' psychological well-being and social interactions. Urinary incontinence is curable in many elderly patients but realistically not all will benefit from an evaluation. Catheter use increases the risk of life-threatening infections, bladder stones, and cancer. Use of catheters also contributes to patient discomfort and the needless use of toxic medications often required to treat the associated bladder spasms. For many (but not all) patients, urinary incontinence is curable and safer and more comfortable approaches are often practical for patients with indwelling catheters. See *catheter, Credé's maneuver, enuresis, flaccid bladder, individualized treatment plan, physical restraint.*

independent state of being able to perform a task or to process a thought without needing the direct help of another person or an adaptive device. The *FIM scale* defines "complete independence" as not requiring another person to assist with any of the tasks described as making up the activity and which are typically performed safely without modification, assistive devices, or aids and within a reasonable time. "Modified independence" is the need to have one or more than one of the following: an assistive device, more than reasonable time or there are safely (risk) considerations. See *impaired judgment.*

independent practice association (HCO) an organization that contracts with a *managed care* plan to deliver health services at a single capitation rate. See *capitated.*

indications conditions or circumstances that signify, validate, or provide a rationale for applying a method or plan of *treatment*. Compare with *contraindication.*

indicator a well-defined element that is used to monitor the quality or appropriateness of the services delivered. An indicator could be an activity, a functional *outcome*, an event, or a frequency of occurrences. Examples of indicators might be

1. number of times per month patients used public transportation after discharge (frequency of occurrences)
2. number of readmissions due to *pressure sores* after the patient group has completed a set of protocols (frequency of occurrences)
3. number of patients who are able to return to work (functional outcome)
4. number of patients who followed up with post discharge appointments (activity)
5. number of times the facility received awards or other outside recognition of excellence (event)

The numerical value of the indicator (e.g., the number of times patients ride the bus) are then measured against one of the following: 1. a *benchmark*, 2. prior performance data, or 3. a threshold. In health care there are two different kinds of clinical indicators, an outcome indicator and a process indicator. The first, outcome indicators, are measurable elements that have to do with the degree of health a patient acquires. Types of outcome indicators include: 1. reoccurrence of past drug habit,

2. increased cardiovascular endurance, 3. increased ability to tolerate change, etc. The second, process indicators, are measurable elements that have to do with *standards* of practice and the quality of professional performance. Types of process indicators include: 1. a department's meeting or exceeding all of its professional standards, 2. all staff are appropriately certified, licensed, or registered, or 3. all staff are up to date on their hepatitis B vaccinations.

indicator measurement systems (HCO) a set of performance indicators for inpatient hospitals and other institutional providers maintained by the Joint Commission on Accreditation of Healthcare Organizations.

individualized educational program (IEP) a written, interdisciplinary plan of *intervention* and training for individuals under the age of 24 years and still enrolled in school. IEPs are intended to be written based on the patient's needs — not on the occupation of the professional writing the objective (e.g., there should be no "educational" goal or "recreational therapy" goal). The goals are to be need specific (e.g., increased recognition of coins). For the goal of increased recognition of coins the classroom teacher may work on coin recognition, recreational therapy may work on buying things with coins in a community setting and occupational therapy may work on simple budgeting.

individualized treatment plan (ITP) a written, interdisciplinary plan of *intervention* and training covering medical, vocational, leisure, and other needs of individuals with a disability. Because these ITPs are not just addressing medical needs, the team leader is not required to be a physician. In *intermediate care facilities for the mentally retarded* (ICF-MR federal regulations) the team leader, called a QMRP (*qualified mental retardation professional*) is seldom a physician. It is not unusual for a recreational therapist, occupational therapist, or social worker to be the QMRP for ITPs. ITPs are intended to be written based on the patient's needs —not on the occupation of the professional writing the objective (e.g., there should be no "recreational therapy" goal or "nursing" goal). The goals are to be need specific (e.g., decreased *incontinence* in the community). For the goal of decreased incontinence in the community nursing may work on continence training and techniques, recreational therapy may work on the identification of bathroom signs, and dietary may work on appropriate fluid restriction. See *consumer rights.*

Individuals with Disabilities Education Act (IDEA) (PL 101-476) a federal law, passed in 1991, which re-authorized and amended the *Educa-*

tion for All Handicapped Children Act.

induced demand (FB) increase in the demand and utilization of health care services associated with an increase in the insurance coverage for the services or other non-price factors.

inductive reasoning ability to use past experience to determine general principles. Inductive and *deductive reasoning* are different. If a five year old notices that every time her brother has taken something from her he has a teasing grin and holds his hands behind his back, she could use inductive reasoning to conclude that when she sees him in that posture she should try to figure out what he took. If her Halloween candy is missing and her brother is in the posture, she could use *deductive* reasoning to conclude that he took the candy. See *fluid intelligence.*

industry versus guilt a developmental phase of growth and development referring to the psychosocial aspects of development by Erikson. See the section on Growth and Development (p. 350) for developmental milestones.

indwelling catheter There are two types of urethral catheters; the straight catheter, which is inserted each time the bladder needs to be emptied, and the indwelling, which is placed into the bladder and is secured for multiple uses. The straight catheter, usually has only one tube or "lumen" as part of the catheter. The indwelling catheter has two or three lumens contained in one tube. Indwelling catheters use a balloon type device to prevent the catheter tube from descending (falling out) from the bladder. A catheter with two lumens has one for drainage and one for inflating/deflating the balloon. A catheter with three lumens has one for drainage, one for inflating/deflating the balloon and one for inserting irrigation fluid. The most common type of indwelling catheter is the Foley. The catheter tube is connected to a receptacle to hold the urine. The entire system must closed to prevent infection from entering the tubing and infecting the bladder. Because the catheter is a gravity driven system, the therapist should make sure that the bag is always below the bladder and that the tubing does not have any loops, as urine will flow down but not up over a loop in the tubing. At times it may be necessary for the therapist to catheterize a patient with a cervical level quadriplegia in the community if s/he develops *autonomic dysreflexia.* Autonomic dysreflexia is a life threatening condition and may not allow enough time for the therapist to return to the hospital. Therapists who conduct community integration outings with patients with high levels of quadriplegia need to learn how to catheterize patients. See *incontinence.*

Types of Infections

Arbovirus
- Colorado tick fever

Enteroviruses
- Herpangina
- Poliomyelitis

Gram-Negative Bacilli
- Brucellosis
- Cholera
- Escherichia coli and other enterobacteriaceae infections
- Hemophilus influenza infection
- Plague
- Pseudomonas infections
- Salmonellosis
- Septic shock
- Shigellosis
- Whooping cough

Gram-Negative Cocci
- Meningococcal infection

Gram-Positive Bacilli
- Actinomycosis
- Botulism
- Diphtheria
- Gas gangrene
- Listeriosis
- Nocardiosis
- Tetanus

Gram-Positive Cocci
- Staphylococcal infections
- Streptococcal infections

Helminths
- Ascariasis
- Enterobiasis
- Hookworm disease
- Schistosomiasis
- Strongyloidiasis
- Trichinosis

Miscellaneous Infections
- Ornithosis
- Toxic shock syndrome

Miscellaneous Viruses
- Cytomegalovirus infection
- Infectious mononucleosis
- Lassa fever
- Mumps
- Rabies

Mycoses
- Aspergillosis
- Blastomycosis
- Candidiasis
- Coccidioidomycosis
- Cryptococcosis
- Histoplasmosis
- Sporotrichosis

Protozoa
- Amebiasis
- Giardiasis
- Malaria
- Toxoplasmosis

Rash Producing Viruses
- Herpes simplex
- Herpes zoster
- Roseola infantum
- Rubella
- Rubeola
- Varicella
- Variola

Respiratory Viruses
- Adenovirus infection
- Common cold
- Influenza
- Parainfluenza
- Respiratory syncytial virus infection

Rickettsia
- Rocky Mountain spotted fever

Spirochetes and Mycobacteria
- Leprosy
- Lyme disease
- Relapsing fever

ineffective individual coping an impairment in the patient's *adaptive behaviors* and ability to solve problems related to his/her illness or disability. It is likely that a patient who demonstrates ineffective individual coping related to a newly acquired disability had poor coping skills premorbidly. The professional may want to explore the patient's past coping strategies. This should help the professional identify the specific skills that need to be taught to the patient. A patient with a poor ability to cope with new, distressing situations is not likely to integrate successfully into community-based activities. See *coping mechanisms, problem solving.*

infancy first developmental phase of life which goes from birth until around the age of two years.

infarct an area of tissue that has died because of lack of blood supply.

infection introduction and multiplication of microorganisms that reduce the overall health status of the individual. These microorganisms may grow on the surface or inside the wall of the cell and produce an immunologic response from the individual's body. Microorganisms injure the individual's cells in three ways: 1. they break down the cell walls and introduce toxins into the cells, 2. they multiply to the point of crowding the individual's cells, and 3. they compete with the individual's cells for nutrition. Oddly enough, a higher standard of living may expose the individual to more infections due to greater travel (coming into contact with infections which s/he does not have immunity to), an increased availability of surgery (greater potential for introduction of infection internally), and an increased use of treatments that prolong life but reduce the individual's immune response. The list on this page shows types of infections followed by common examples

Terms Related to Infection

Term	Definition
Asymptomatic Infection	An infection which doesn't present any observable symptoms but which can be measured through lab tests.
Colonization	The multiplication of infection that, despite its multiplication, remains asymptomatic. Individuals with colonization of an infection may be considered to be carriers and spread the infection to others.
Endogenous	An infection whose origin comes from within the individual (e.g., e. coli bacteria from the intestines being introduced into the mouth due to poor handwashing).
Exogenous	An infection whose origin comes from environmental pathogens (e.g., typhoid).
Latent	The eruption (e.g., showing signs of) the infection after a period of time of being asymptomatic. The asymptomatic period may last just a few days to over ten years depending on the type of infection and health status of the individual.
Sub clinical	An infection which doesn't present observable symptoms but which can be measured through lab tests.

of specific infections. The chart above describes some of the terms related to infections. See *bronchitis, endemic disease, endogenous infection, epidemic disease, epidemiology.*

infection control The spread of infection requires three elements: 1. a source of the infectious material, 2. a patient who is susceptible to the infectious material, and 3. a means of transmitting that infectious material to the susceptible patient. Just by the nature of health care facilities, it is not possible to exclude infectious material (patients come in sick), nor is it possible to exclude patients who might be susceptible to infection. The only way to truly control the spread of infection in facilities is to control the transmission. There are four main routes of spreading infections:

1. Contact transmission
    a. Direct Contact (staff to patient or patient to patient)
    b. Indirect Contact (germs transmitted by touching an object, e.g., a tape recorder passed from one patient to another)
    c. Droplet Contact (transmission of germs from a person sneezing, coughing, or talking within a distance of three feet)
2. Vehicle Route Transmission Through Contaminated Items (food, water, drugs, blood)
3. Airborne Transmission (infectious materials which adhere to moisture or dust in the air and are suspended for long periods of time)
4. Vector-borne Transmission (infection spread through an insect or animal as in mosquito-transmitted malaria) (burlingame, 1996)

Terms related to the spread of infectious disease are shown on the next page. See *extended survey, hand-washing, isolation, nosocomial infection.*

inference engine (HCO) a computer routine that co-ordinates the activities of a knowledge- or rule-based decision support system. See *clinical decision support.*

inflection moderation of vocal tone while conversing. In more general terms, a change in course or direction for an action or event.

informed consent permission to perform a medical or research procedure that includes a rational understanding of 1. the proceedings, 2. the foreseeable risks, 3. the expected benefits, 4. the consequences of withholding consent, 5. available alternative procedures, and 6. that *consent* is voluntary. See *intake assessment.*

inhibition ability (or decision) to demonstrate control. Patients who lack inhibition will be unable to repress or terminate behavior appropriately. Contrast with *impulsivity.* See *executive function.*

inhibitory having the influence of stopping an action or event.

initial certification survey (OBRA) a survey for the initial certification of skilled nursing facilities. The surveyors conduct both the *standard survey* and *extended survey.* Special emphasis is given to the structural requirements that relate to qualification standards and patient rights notification, whether or not problems have been identified during the information gathering process. The surveyors are to gather information to verify compliance with every *tag* number (e.g., qualifications of the social worker, dietitian, and activity professional).

initiation starting an action. Individuals with various disabilities, notably *depression* and *mental retardation*, frequently have an impaired ability to initiate purposeful activity. Some impairment of initiation may also be caused by certain medications (usually the medications with *lethargy* as a side effect). Therapists may find that a lack of initiation is one of

Terms Associated with the Spread of Infectious Diseases

Term	Description
endemic	A disease that is continually present in the environment or community even with aggressive efforts to fight the disease.
epidemic	A disease that is affecting a greater number of the population than would be statistically expected.
hyperendemic	A disease which is endemic to the area and which is occurring at a significantly higher rate of infection than would normally be expected.
milieu	The environment in which the infectious agent can be found.
outbreak	A sudden appearance of a disease in clusters of the population but, in number, still a small percentage of the population.
reservoir	The natural environment of the infectious agent; a place where the infectious agent can multiply.
source	The origin of the infectious material.
vehicle	The way the infectious agent is transmitted without direct person-to-person transmission. Examples would be through tainted food or by arthropods (such as mosquitoes).
victim	The individual who has contracted the disease.

the hardest deficits to address. Resolution frequently involves a combination of approaches including patient education, social support, token reward systems, and on-going monitoring. See *executive function, motivation, Parkinson's disease, Parkinsonian gait, post-traumatic stress disorder, Recreation Participation Data Sheet.*

injury See *adolescent injury, falls, head injury, spinal cord injury.*

insane obsolete term for mental disorder.

insanity defense a legal concept that a person cannot be convicted of a crime if s/he lacked criminal responsibility by reason of insanity at the time the crime was committed. The premise is that where an alleged criminal lacks the *mens rea* (evil intent) and the *actus reus* (voluntary conduct) because of insanity or other mental deficiency, such a person lacks criminal responsibility and cannot be convicted. The law specifies that the intent and volition of the defendant is what is measured for determination of a criminal act, not the act itself, no matter how terrible the act. Compare with *competency to stand criminal trial.*

insecticide (HHS) a class of crop protection and specialty chemicals used to control insects on farms and forests, as well as non-agricultural applications such as residential lawn care, golf courses, and public tracts of land.

insight both a cognitive and emotional understanding of a situation. The individual is aware, at least partly, of how a situation may impact him/her and at some emotional level accepts or is resigned to the situation. Individuals who have insight into a situation generally are more able to purposefully change the situation than those with a limited cognitive knowledge and/or a lack of emotional understanding. Individuals with insight into the true status of their physical, mental, emotional, and spiritual health have a greater chance of reaching a cathartic level of functioning. See *catharsis, Dehn's Model of Leisure Health, impaired adjustment, intelligence.*

insoluble fiber See *fiber.*

insomnia (HHS) inability to sleep even in the absence of external impediments, during the period when sleep should normally happen.

instinct probably one of the most controversial terms used in psychology, instinct generally refers to a common reaction to a specific situation with the reaction being a non-learned response. Instinctual behavior can easily be observed — just watch the robin fly south for the winter. However, careful studies of "instincts" have often found that environment plays a larger-than-expected part in shaping the instinctual actions. When a model is finally developed which successfully describes instinct, it will probably refer to a neurological or genetic origin which is somewhat species specific, but which is also impacted by the individual's environment. In humans, many "instincts" are sometimes called "reflexes." (e.g., when a person falls, s/he extends his/her arms to lessen the fall — an action taken without conscious thought).

institutional review board a board that reviews proposals for research when the research has the potential to cause harm. Harm may include the withholding of services as well as the inclusion of experimental services.

institutional settings any program where the patient spends at least five hours a day, five days a week.

instrument a tool used by the professional to obtain

a *measurement* during the *assessment* process. This instrument may be a questionnaire, a machine, or any other device that assists the professional in obtaining the desired measurement.

instrumental activities of daily living tasks that are required to live independently in the community. Instrumental activities of daily living (IADLs) include preparing meals, shopping, managing money, using the telephone, doing housework, and taking medications. See *activities of daily living.*

insulin a secretion by the pancreas of large peptides that act as hormones binding to specific receptors or other cells and function to control blood glucose levels. Insulin is also well known for its growth-factor actions.

intake assessment initial assessment of a patient upon admission to the service. Frequently the intake assessment uses an in-house assessment form or screening tool, saving standardized testing tools for later use. (The therapist conducts the initial intake assessment to determine which standardized tool(s) are indicated for the patient's specific needs.) The intake assessment generally includes information about the patient's name, address, social, and medical history as well as a summary of pertinent information covering abilities and needs within the professional's *scope of practice.* See the chart on the next page. See *risk management.*

integrated delivery system (HCO) an organized system of health care providers spanning a range of health care services.

integrated pest management (IPM) (HHS) the coordinated use of pest and environmental information along with available pest control methods, including cultural, biological, genetic, and chemical methods, to prevent unacceptable levels of pest damage using the most economical means, and with the least possible hazard to people, property, and the environment.

integrated services digital network (ISDN) (HCO) a digital telephony protocol used to provide high-speed connections.

integrated software software modules that have the capability to use data and other information from other modules while maintaining their own databases and files. Integrated software may come from different companies but they are able to integrate functions because they follow pre-set standards for software development.

integration process of uniting two or more entities that are not together, perhaps because of a lack of mutual understanding. Modifying behavior and the environment allows the disparate elements to join. When a therapist works on community integration skills with a patient, s/he uses his/her skills to help the patient modify his/her skills and behaviors and helps the community modify its behavior and environment to allow the patient to become an integral part of the community. See *Community Integration Program.*

integrity 1. a personal attribute that is comprised of characteristics such as: feeling comfortable with oneself, acting in accordance with society's rules, emotional stability, and dependability. Much work has been done around the concept of integrity as it relates to growth and development, employee actions, and psychological well-being. *Employee malfeasance* is frequently measured by using *integrity tests.* In health care, a lack of integrity is frequently associated with an emotional state of despair and hopelessness. *Erik Erikson* constructed an eight-stage model of development of which ego integrity versus despair was the eighth stage of life. 2. an attribute assigned to testing tools that have fairly high to very high reliability and validity.

integrity testing a measurement of a person's inherent integrity vs. dishonesty. Integrity tests are divided into two categories: overt integrity tests and personality-oriented tests. Overt integrity tests, also know as "clear purpose" tests, openly ask questions about the person's past involvement in illegal activities and his/her attitudes toward dishonesty. Overt integrity tests include the Phase II Profile and the Reid Report. Personality-oriented tests, or veiled purpose tests, ask questions which are not obviously related to integrity and therefore do not openly alert the person taking the test that the test taker's level of integrity is being measured. Personality-oriented tests include the Inwald Personality Inventory and the Employee Productivity Inventory.

intelligence an individual's ability to use: 1. adaptability, 2. imagination, 3. *insight,* 4. *judgment,* and 5. *reasoning.* While hundreds of testing tools have been developed to measure intelligence, the basic question of what intelligence is has not really been agreed upon. There are many theories and most intelligence tests are based on one specific theory. The real complaint that intelligence tests are culturally biased may be partly because the theories used to develop the tests are imperfect and fail to measure the underlying cognitive function(s). Intelligence is related to the terms *knowledge* and *executive function* but they are not the same. See *associated features, adaptation, dementia, imagery, intelligence quotient, mental retardation.*

Anatomy of the Intake Assessment Process

Function	Goals	Skills Required of the Professional
To determine the nature of the patient's problem and identify areas, within the scope of practice, which may need to be addressed.	• To establish strengths and areas of need • To establish discharge location to better match up needs with post-discharge resources in the community (See *discharge plan*.) • To determine the likely course of *treatment*	• Solid knowledge base of disabilities, disorders, illness, and dysfunctional behaviors. • Broad understanding of multiple conceptual theories including theories related to the biomedical, sociocultural, psychodynamic, and behavioral models and vocational, community, and leisure involvement. • Ability to obtain information from the patient, patient chart, and other sources in a way which gathers the necessary information and which does not compromise the patient/therapist relationship. • Broad understanding of the resources available for the patient at his/her discharge site and/or the ability to obtain that information in a timely and efficient manner.
To develop an initial relationship with the patient.	• To determine the patient's understanding of his/her strengths and needs • To determine the patient's openness to receiving treatment, ability to understand the situation, and desire to participate in treatment program • To develop a trusting relationship with the patient	• Ability to influence the development of a positive relationship with the patient. • Support the patient by using active *listening skills*. • Ability to cope with the patient's expression of feelings and cope with the situation surrounding the patient's situation without letting (the professional's) emotions or beliefs negatively impact the therapeutic relationship. • Demonstrating appropriate *empathy*, support, and understanding as well as genuine interest in the patient.
To provide the patient with information, including an expectation of the type of treatment and services that will make up the patient's treatment plan.	• To increase the patient's understanding of his/her disability or disease, including impacts, *outcomes*, and the role that his/her behavior may play in the course of the disability or disease • To increase the patient's awareness of options for reducing the impact of the disability or disease • To increase the patient's awareness of treatment options • To obtain a consensus between the patient and therapist for treatment directions • To obtain informed consent for course of treatment	• Ability to describe the nature of the patient's disability or illness in a manner that the patient can understand. • Ability to communicate the patient's needs in a manner that the patient can understand. • Ability to be sensitive to the patient's intended thoughts/behaviors versus the patient's actual thoughts/behaviors. • Ability to articulate the patient's perspective of the situation and understand how the patient's perspective is different from the therapist's. • Ability to describe clearly to the patient his/her choices and the likely consequences of the choices. • Knowledge of what constitutes *informed consent*.

intelligence quotient (IQ) a measure of an individual's relative *intelligence* when compared with others of his/her age. A score of 100 is defined as the average. See *adaptive functioning, learning disability, mental retardation, Slosson Intelligence Test.*

intense sweeteners (HHS) See *low-calorie sweeteners.*

intensity degree to which a force or action is exhibited, experienced, or applied — how much. Intensity may be measured quantitatively (e.g., walk "100 feet quickly" with stand by assist) or qualitatively (e.g., patient to have aide assist until she "feels comfortable and strong enough" to go to the cafeteria by herself). Intensity is an important element to be included in every *prescription* written by the therapist. See *Leisure and Recreation Involvement Measurement.*

intention tremor a neurologically caused, involuntary muscle tremor that increases in frequency when the individual tries to perform a voluntary movement using that muscle. See *tremor.*

interactionalist approach a philosophy that believes that both traits and states are co-determinants of performance. An example of an interactionalist approach would be assuming that an individual with an IQ of 120 (*trait*) and a graduate degree in English (*state*) should be able to write well.

intercity rail transportation (ADA) refers to transportation provided by Amtrak. The ADA accessibility guidelines for intercity rail transportation may be found in the **Buses, Vans, and Systems Technical Assistance Manual** (US Architectural and Transportation Barriers Compliance Board).

interdisciplinary team health care professionals who come from a variety of training backgrounds and who work together as a team to help provide the treatment and services needed by a patient.

intermediary See *fiscal intermediary.*

intermediate care facility for the mentally retarded (ICF-MR) provides health or rehabilitative services for individuals who are mentally retarded or who have related conditions. See *individualized treatment plan, Medicare/Medicaid history, Section 1905 (d).*

intermediate sanction an adverse action taken against a facility due to a significant failure to meet regulatory standards. Intermediate sanctions are actions imposed on the facility to avoid having to close the facility. Sanctions may include stiff fines, forced replacement of administration, or other significant actions against the facility. See *adverse action, nonrenewal, termination.*

intermittent claudication pain caused by a lack of oxygen to the muscles that are being used that feels like cramping muscles. Because of the nature of some types of heart disease, a progressive conditioning program may do little more than increase the patient's *tolerance* of activity and decrease the occurrence of claudication. Patients may be encouraged to exercise through the use of activities multiple times a day to the point of discomfort (and not beyond). *Pain* subsides slowly with rest.

intermittent explosive disorder an inability to exhibit control over one's anger and other aggressive impulses, which results in other people and/or property being injured or damaged. The aggressive behavior is sporadic and of quick onset. This disorder is an official diagnosis found in the **DSM-IV** under impulse control disorders not elsewhere classified.

intermittent mandatory ventilation (IMV) Patients who are placed on respirators and who may still have the physical capability to breathe on their own need to have a period of time when they are slowly weaned off of the ventilator. After long-term use of a respirator the muscles a patient uses to breathe are weak and need to be allowed gradual strengthening through the use of intermittent breathing exercises. This is accomplished by gradually reducing the number of breaths per minute provided by the respirator, allowing the patient to independently breathe between the breaths provided by the respirator. This gradual, independent breathing helps strengthen the patient's breathing muscles while allowing adequate oxygenation.

intermittent tremor See *tremor.*

intermittent tube feedings a type of *feeding tube* feeding which allows a large amount (250 to 400 ml) of liquid nourishment to be dripped (using gravity) into the patient's stomach over a period of 30 to 60 minutes. This slow introduction of fluid reduces the bloated feeling that usually accompanies a faster *bolus tube feeding.* An intermittent tube feeding "normalizes" feeding time, as feeding times usually mimic the frequency and duration of normal meal times.

intern a student who has completed his/her academic training and is completing field placement. Allied health interns are supervised by credentialed professionals in the specific discipline. A medical intern is a physician who has completed all of his/her medical training and is completing his/her field placement. A medical intern is supervised by an attending physician.

internal locus of control See *locus of control.*

internal sensation awareness of sensations to the body not caused by any external event. See *sensation.*

International Classification of Disease, Ninth

Revision, Clinical Modification (HCO) a classification and coding system for health problems and services, maintained by the United States Department of Health and Human Services, used for billing by inpatient hospitals and other institutional *providers*. See *diagnosis*.

International System of Units (SI) (for Système International d'Unités) an internationally agreed upon method of describing distance, mass, and time using centimeters, grams, and seconds. Some other units in the system are hertz, ampere, kelvin, candela, and mole.

internist a physician who specializes in the study of internal medicine. They are experts in the areas of infectious diseases and diseases of the heart, gastrointestinal tract, and other internal organs.

interpersonal skills skills that assist an individual to successfully and mutually interact with others. These skills include: 1. the ability to listen to others, 2. ability to express oneself, 3. the ability to "read" nonverbal communication (*body language*), 4. the ability to mutually arrive at agreements, and 5. an awareness of the rules of social etiquette (including hygiene). Disease or disability that impacts any of the listed skills places the patient at risk of becoming isolated. Especially perplexing is the type of disability experienced with a *traumatic brain injury*. Many individuals who have sustained even a moderate TBI (moderate enough not to require hospitalization) have a decreased ability to read body language. While the individual does not appear disabled, all of a sudden s/he may seem to be "odd" and otherwise socially inappropriate. See *etregenous*.

interpreter a person who translates a message spoken in one language to a different language so that a meaningful conversation can be held. An appropriate interpreter for a health care setting is an adult who is a fluent speaker of both languages in question, not a relative of the patient, who has received professional training as an interpreter. How do you decide if you need to an interpreter? You need an interpreter whenever a patient requests an interpreter or whenever you, as a provider, believe that language or cultural differences may be causing a barrier to clear communication between you and your patient. Legally, you are required to provide language assistance for limited-English speakers if you receive federal funds of any kind. According to Title VI of the 1964 *Civil Rights* Act, no recipient of federal funding may run its programs in such a way as to discriminate on the basis of race, color, or country of national origin. One common form of discrimination on the basis of national origin is ineffective methods of communication between English-speak-

ing staff and limited-English-speaking patients. One method to ensure equal access is to work through trained interpreters. The Office of Civil Rights has taken action in numerous parts of the country against institutions that are out of compliance with Title VI by not providing linguistically appropriate care. How do you choose an interpreter? The quality of interpretive services available in different areas will vary, depending on the sophistication of the local systems and the training available. Contracting certified interpreters is a good idea if certification is available. At the very least, the interpreter should be

- *Fluent in both languages in questions.* Language screening is needed to establish the degree of fluency.

- *Trained as an interpreter.* The fact that a person is bilingual does not make her or him an interpreter; there are special skills involved. While the training available for interpreters will vary by region, some professional training is absolutely necessary. Untrained interpreters are at extremely high risk for adding material, omitting material, changing the message, giving opinions, and entering into long discussions with the patient or provider from which the other is excluded.

- *Not a family member.* Family members have a valid role in providing patient support, however, they are not appropriate interpreters. Family members often edit the patient's message heavily, add their own opinions, answer for the patient, and impede the development of the patient-provider relationship. Patients may be loath to discuss certain problems in front of a family member and confidentiality becomes a concern. Family members are rarely trained interpreters and often are unfamiliar with medical terminology.

- *Never a child.* In addition to the concerns mentioned above, the use of children to interpret creates an inversion of power relations in the family, where parents, not children, are normally in control. Lack of vocabulary in both languages is a serious problem. In addition, children are often traumatized if they are required to pass on bad news or if they are held responsible for negative outcomes.

How can the therapist best work with an interpreter?

- Introduce yourself to the interpreter; establish the interpreter's level of English skills and professional training and request that the interpreter interpret everything into first person (to avoid "he said, she said").

- During the medical interview, speak directly to

the patient, not to the interpreter.

- Speak at an even pace in relatively short segments; pause so the interpreter can interpret.

- Assume that, and insist that, everything you say and that the patient says is interpreted.

- Do not hold the interpreter responsible for what the patient says or doesn't say; the interpreter is the medium, not the source, of the message.

- Be aware that many concepts you express have no linguistic, or often even conceptual, equivalent in other languages. The interpreter may have to paint word pictures of many terms you use; this may take longer than your original speech.

- Avoid highly idiomatic speech, complicated sentence structure, sentence fragments, changing your idea in the middle of a sentence, or asking multiple questions at one time.

- Encourage the interpreter to ask questions and to alert you about potential cultural misunderstandings that may come up. Respect an interpreter's judgment that a particular question is culturally inappropriate and either rephrase the question or ask the interrupter's help in eliciting the information in a more appropriate way.

- Avoid patronizing or infantilizing the patient. A lack of English language skills is not a reflection of low cognitive function or a lack of education. Your patient may be a college professor or a medical doctor in her/his own country, just as easily as s/he may be a farm worker.

- Acknowledge the interpreter as a professional in communication. Respect his or her role.

- Be patient. Providing care across a language barrier takes time. However, the time spent up front will be paid back by good rapport and clear communication that will avoid wasted time and dangerous misunderstandings down the line (Roat, 1996).

interpretive guidelines detailed explanation of the intent of a *regulation* or *standard*.

inter-rater reliability a measure of the agreement between observers on the scoring of an assessment. See the table on the next page.

interscapulothoracic forequarter amputation a procedure that removes the entire arm, the scapula, and part of the upper midsection. Frequently the patient will elect to wear a cosmetic shoulder cap for an increased normalization of appearance instead of a prosthetic device. If the patient chooses to be fitted for a prosthetic device to increase function, a nine-unit device is used.

1. socket

2. cable with modified chest strap
3. waist belt type harness
4. excursion amplifier
5. shoulder joint
6. internal locking elbow
7. forearm lift assist
8. wrist unit
9. terminal device

The socket used is similar to those used for a shoulder disarticulation with an additional extension that goes over the intact shoulder for greater stability.

intervention act of purposely modifying an action or thought to influence the outcome. See *cost-effectiveness analysis, critical pathways, deprivation, individual education program, individual treatment plan.*

intestinal ostomy See *ostomy, intestinal.*

intimacy ability to develop and maintain a very close relationship with another person by sharing common belief systems and a common understanding of the expectations of the relationship itself.

intrinsic literally, from within. Actions taken as the individual's own desire are intrinsic (of the individual's own thoughts and choices). This is opposite to *extrinsic*: actions taken at the urging of others. Participating in a nature walk because you enjoy listening to the sounds and smelling the scents is intrinsic motivation. Participating because you make your partner happy or because you get a positive point for your token economy/*behavior modification program* is extrinsic motivation. Activities undertaken for intrinsic reasons tend to be longer lasting than those undertaken for extrinsic reasons. See *locus of control.*

intrinsic motivation desire to engage in an activity which originates from within oneself; action is not the result of directions or pressure from others.

intrinsic muscles muscles located in the extremities which stay within one part of the limb; whose origin and insertion are both contained in the same part of the extremity.

invariant clauses parts of the thought process which do not rely on one's ability to use logical thinking or to use mathematical calculation.

invasive GAS disease See *group A streptococcus.*

in vitro measured or existing under artificial conditions in the laboratory, e.g., in a Petri dish or test tube; as opposed to *in vivo*.

in vivo (literally, "in life.") 1. something that happens in the body. 2. for sensitivity training, a real time technique that involves assisting a patient to become less sensitive to some fear-provoking stimulus such as heights. In a case where a patient fears an animal, s/he is exposed to the animal at a safe

**The Advantages and Disadvantage of Different Methods of Testing
Inter-rater Reliability of Multidimensional Measures (Kane & Kane, 1981, p. 219)**

	Method	Advantages	Disadvantages
1.	Two or more interviewers administer instrument independently and results on items, scale, and global rating are compared.	Enable comparison of the effect of interviewer difference (such as age, sex, personality, skill) on the responses elicited.	Impossible to distinguish whether incongruence is a result of interviewer or respondent factors. Respondent burden may affect data quality on the second time. A selection bias is created by the limitation to respondents willing or able to have two tests.
2.	Two or more interviewers are present; one conducts the interview while all interviewers record responses and make judgments.	Minimizes respondent burden. Tests ability of more than one interviewer to record items and make judgments congruently when stimulus is held constant.	Interviewer differences in eliciting responses will not be picked up. The group interview may inhibit responses.
3.	The interview is video or audio taped. Additional interviewers record information and make ratings on the basis of the tape.	Same as #2 with the added advantage that many people can be involved in testing their inter-rater reliability. A tangible stimulus remains for use in trying to improve reliability.	Same as #2. Videotaping may be particularly obtrusive and introduces the element of cameraman's focus. Audiotapes provide an incomplete record.
4.	The interview is conducted with one or more observers behind a one-way mirror.	Same as #2 and #3 but less obtrusive than group interviews or tapes.	Same as #2 but depends on interview taking place in a well-equipped office. Does not permit testing of inter-rater reliability in eliciting information or recording it.
5.	One interviewer administers battery, records data, and performs ratings. Additional interviews use that recorded data to do their own ratings.	Minimizes respondent burden. Is less manpower intensive, making larger reliably samples possible.	Does not permit testing of inter-rater reliably in eliciting information or recording it.
6.	Inter-rater reliability of parts of the instrument tested in sections. (This can be done in the method outlined in 1, 2, 3, or 4).	Method is more convenient for interviewer and respondent.	Component parts of a battery may not behave the same way separately as they do when embedded in longer instrument.
7.	Inter-rater reliability as established previously is accepted for component of the battery.	Minimizes startup time.	Same as #6. Also requires assumption that inter-rater reliability achieved with other subjects and other interviewers will pertain.

distance. The animal is then brought closer and closer until the patient can tolerate it. Also known as *reciprocal inhibition decoding.*

involuntary admission admission of a patient to a treatment facility against that patient's wishes. Based on state laws, individuals or representatives of the community (e.g., a mental health worker) may petition the courts to forcibly admit a patient to a psychiatric unit for evaluation. This is done when there is grave concern for the patient's own safety or the safety of the community. The patient keeps the right to appeal his/her institutionalization. See *emergency admission, psychiatric admissions.*

involvement to be part of a process or to include oneself in the actions of a group. The concept of involvement in activities has been studied by psychologists for about 50 years as part of an individual's psychosocial make-up. The idea was to explain why individuals kept on doing or choosing specific actions. More recently (since the 1980's) other fields, including recreation and leisure, have searched for ways to apply the concept of involvement. For recreational therapy this has been especially true in nursing homes. Currently, health care surveyors tend to misunderstand the concept of healthy involvement (quality of life) and attendance (physical presence). Nursing homes have been fined thousands of dollars because some of the residents choose not to attend activities as they feel content with their free time activities (talking to friends, day dreaming about past events, watching television, etc.). This is interpreted by surveyors as the residents not having an appropriate quality of leisure (free time), therefore a lack of quality in their life. Lack of attendance is not the same thing as lack of involvement. Mounir Ragheb (1996) states that "leisure involvement is the degree of commitment to, centrality of, and interest in an individual's leisure and recreation encounters. This state is demonstrated though the reported level of importance of leisure choices made, meanings derived, pleasures obtained, ego-attached, self-expression, and how valuable leisure is to one's life." Ragheb (1996) developed the *Leisure and Recreation Involvement Measurement* to help therapists identify the patient's relative score in each of the six components that make up the construct of involvement: 1. importance (the magnitude to which a person equates a situation or stimulus to either salient-enduring or situation-specific goals), 2. pleasure (the expectation and realization of expressive rewards), 3. interest (preferences for leisure activities), 4. intensity (the depth of engagement in leisure activity or experience, characterized by a mood of high concentration and reflected in the level of immersion or absorption in the designated choice), 5. centrality (the role assigned to a leisure activity relative to other life interests), and 6. meaning (the individual's striving and search for mental, physical, social, and spiritual realization while fulfilling the individual's potential). See *participation (in activities)*.

IPA See *independent practice association*.

ipsilateral pertaining to the same side of the body.

IQ See *intelligence quotient*.

irreversible contracture a condition where soft tissue and connective tissue structures are replaced by tissue such as bone or fibrotic tissue which does not stretch. Irreversible contractures are not amenable to treatment short of surgery. The therapist should take precautions not to stress the irreversible contracture beyond comfort, as serious tearing may result. See *contracture*.

irritability the emotion combined with action when one is dissatisfied or otherwise bothered by an event or thought. The elements of irritability are 1. an overreaction to an event, 2. a heightened degree of sensitivity, and 3. a decreased ability to cope. See *Beck Depression Inventory, lead poisoning, noxious stimulus*.

ischemia a lack of blood flow and a lack of delivery of oxygen to the cells. See *pulse*.

ischial tuberosity the protuberance in the hip bone that humans rest on when they are sitting.

ISDN See *integrated services digital network*.

isokinetic using specialized exercise equipment that involves:
1. contraction of specific muscles through their full range of motion
2. measured resistance provided by the equipment which responds to the strength of the contracting muscles as it moves through the full range of motion.

Compare to *isometric, isotonic*.

isolation to be separated from. In health care there are seven types of isolation precautions. See *strict isolation, contact isolation, respiratory isolation, AFB isolation, enteric precautions, drainage/secretion precautions, blood/body fluid precautions, infection control*.

isologous graft a graft taken from an identical twin (genetically identical). This graft is usually considered a permanent graft.

isometric structured exercises or specified activities which involve:
1. contraction of muscles without moving through its range of motion (without joint movement)
2. increased circulation through muscles due to activity
3. resistance provided by a fixed object (wall, chair, etc.) or by the use of flexors versus extensors.

Compare to *isokinetic, isotonic*.

isotonic structured exercise or specified activities that involve:
1. contraction of muscles with range of motion to joints
2. increased circulation through muscles due to activity
3. a predetermined amount of resistance provided through the use of exercise equipment and or one's own body.

Compare to *isokinetic, isometric*.

ITP See *individualized treatment plan*.

J

Jacksonian seizure due to a localized disease or disorder of the cortex, certain groups of muscles may experience spasmodic contractions or a paroxysmal *paresthesia* may occur over specific sections of the skin. See *seizure.*

jargon words that have meaning to individuals within a specific profession but have little to no meaning for those outside the field. In therapy, some examples of jargon would be "activities of daily living," "leisure barriers" and "phys-dis."

JCAHO See *Joint Commission on Accreditation of Healthcare Organizations.*

J coefficient how much the patient's successful performance on the job (hence "J") correlates with successful performance on vocational performance testing tools. A strong "J" coefficient means that a particular test has a very good ability to predict the patient's future performance on the job.

jejunostomy an ostomy placed in the jejunum section of the intestines. See *ostomy.*

jejunostomy tube a *feeding tube* inserted directly into the mid-portion of the small intestine. A gastrostomy device is required. Jejunostomy tubes reduce the risk of aspiration over *gastric gavage tubes* and are well suited to be used with a pump to provide consistent and slow delivery of formula. Because the small intestine does not usually tolerate the high caloric content of most formulas, the formula must be watered down prior to use.

job description a written description of what the employer expects the employee to accomplish and how the employee is to carry out work tasks. Job descriptions have three primary functions: 1. to match the skills necessary for the job with the *knowledge* and experience required of the applicant, 2. to fairly and precisely represent the job tasks involved in the position, and 3. to provide a basis for evaluation of the employee's performance. The body of a job description usually has seven sections: 1. title of the job, 2. purpose of the position, 3. who the position reports to, 4. minimum and desired qualifications for the position, 5. responsibilities of the position, 6. typical work hours, and frequently, 7. salary range.

job interview the process of screening applicants for positions. To protect an individual's *civil rights* and to decrease the opportunity for discrimination, the United States has established a set of regulations concerning the rights of job applicants. The table on the next two pages outlines some of the regulations concerning questions that may be asked of applicants (D'Antonio-Nocera, DeBolt & Touhey, 1996).

Jobst a brand name for garments used to reduce *scarring.* Also known as elastic stocking. Jobst garments are used to tightly constrict parts of the body that are developing scar tissue, especially after *burns.* The constriction produced by the garments helps: reduce the overall volume of the scar tissue, maintain elastic skin, prevent *hypertrophic scarring* (which may cause *contractures*), and reduce the visual impact of the scar. The garments should be measured carefully to give an appropriate amount of pressure without reducing *range of motion.* Zippers are also important to reduce sheering during the donning or doffing process. Because of the importance of constant pressure on maturing scar tissue, interface molds are required, in addition to the Jobst, for areas that normally develop concavities. Areas that tend to benefit from interface molds include the nose and mouth, anterior chest, feet, and armpit. Patients need to wear the garments 24 hours a day for 12 to 18 months. Patients should have more than one set of garments so that a fresh garment can be put on after activities that causes soiling. See *dressing, edema.*

job stress management a technique to reduce job burnout. Symptoms of burnout include pessimism, slipping productivity, dissatisfaction with the job and an increase in the days taken off from work. Two key techniques of job stress management are obtaining/regaining some control over your job and balancing work with active and interesting leisure outside of, and separate from, work. The first takes cooperation as well as willingness to let some things go and the second takes a concerted effort to enhance active participation in a variety of leisure activities. When control and a healthy leisure lifestyle have been obtained, individuals experience fewer ulcers, better sleep, fewer headaches, and usually a higher resistance to *infections.* To master job stress and integrate it into the job may take six months or more.

Joint Commission on Accreditation of Healthcare Organizations (JCAHO) a private organization (non-governmental) that sets voluntary *standards* of care for many different types of health care settings.

A Guide for Job Application Forms and Interviews

Inquiries Before Hiring	Lawful	Unlawful
Name	Name	Inquiries into any title that indicates race, color, religion, sex, national origin, handicap, age, or ancestry.
Address	Inquiry into place and length at current address.	Inquiry into any foreign addresses that would indicate national origin.
Age	Any inquiry limited to establishing that applicant meets any minimum age requirement that may be established by law.	a. Requiring birth certificate or baptismal record before hiring. b. Any inquiry that may reveal the date of high school graduation. c. Any other inquiry that may reveal whether applicant is at least 40 years of age.
Birthplace, National Origin, or Ancestry		a. Any inquiry into place of birth. b. Any inquiry into place of birth of parents, grandparents, or spouse. c. Any other inquiry into national origin or ancestry.
Race or Color		Any inquiry that would indicate race or color.
Sex		a. Any inquiry that would indicate sex. b. Any inquiry made of members of one sex, but not the other.
Height and Weight	Inquiries as to ability to perform actual job requirements.	Being a certain height or weight will not be considered to be a job requirement unless the employer can show that no employee with the ineligible height or weight could do the work.
Religious Creed		a. Any inquiry that would indicate or identify religious denomination or custom. b. Applicant may not be told any religious identity or preference of the employer. c. Request pastor's recommendation or reference.
Handicap	Inquiries necessary to determine applicant's ability to substantially perform specific job without significant hazard.	a. Any inquiry into past or current medical conditions not related to position applied for. b. Any inquiry into Workers' Compensation or similar claims.
Citizenship	a. Whether a US citizen. b. If not, whether applicant intends to become one. c. If US residence is legal. d. If spouse is citizen. e. Require proof of citizenship after being hired. f. Any other requirements mandated by the Immigration Reform and Control Act of 1986, as amended.	a. If native-born or naturalized. b. Proof of citizenship before hiring. c. Whether parents or spouse are native-born or naturalized.
Photographs	May be required after hiring for identification.	Require photograph before hiring.
Arrest and Convictions	Inquiries into *conviction* of specific crimes related to qualifications for the job applied for.	Any inquiry that would reveal arrests without convictions.

A Guide for Application Forms and Interviews (continued)

Inquiries Before Hiring	Lawful	Unlawful
Education	a. Inquiry into nature and extent of academic, professional, or vocational training. b. Inquiry into language skills, such as reading and writing of foreign languages, if job related.	a. Any inquiry that would reveal the nationality or religious affiliation of a school. b. Inquiry as to what mother tongue is or how foreign language ability was acquired.
Relatives	Inquiry into name, relationship, and address of person to be notified in case of emergency.	Any inquiry about a relative that would be unlawful if made about the applicant.
Organizations	Inquiry into membership in professional organizations and offices held, excluding any organization, the name or character of which indicates the race, color, religion, sex, national origin, handicap, age, or ancestry of its members.	Inquiry into every club and organization where membership is held.
Military Service	a. Inquiry into service in US Armed Forces when such service is a qualification for the job. b. Require military discharge certificate after being hired.	a. Inquiry into military service in armed service of any country but US. b. Request military service records. c. Inquiry into type of discharge.
Work Schedule	Inquiry into willingness or ability to work required work schedule.	Any inquiry into willingness or ability to work any particular religious holidays.
Miscellaneous	Any question required to reveal qualifications for the job applied for.	Any non-job-related inquiry which may elicit or attempt to elicit any information concerning race, color, religion, sex, national origin, handicap, age, or ancestry of an applicant for employment or membership.
References	General personal and work references which do not reveal the race, color, religion, sex, national origin, handicap, age, or ancestry of the applicant.	Request references specifically from clergymen or any other persons who might reflect race, color, religion, sex, national origin, handicap, age, or ancestry of applicant.

1. Employers acting under bona fide Affirmative Action Programs or acting under orders of Equal Employment law enforcement agencies of federal, state, or local governments may make some of the prohibited inquiries listed above to the extent that these inquiries are required by such programs or orders.
2. Employers having federal defense contracts are exempt to the extent that otherwise prohibited inquiries are required by federal law for security purposes.
3. Any inquiry although not specifically listed above, which elicits information as to, or which is not job related and may be used to discriminate on the basis of race, color, religion, sex, national origin, handicap, age, or ancestry is in violation of the law.

JCAHO's surveys are voluntary and usually take place once every three years. They evaluate the performance of approximately 14,000 health care organizations in the areas of behavioral health (including mental health, chemical dependence, developmental disabilities, and case management), ambulatory care, home care, long-term care, and health care networks (including HMOs, PPOs, etc.). Prior to 1994 the standards published by JCAHO were written to reflect the performance of individual departments within the hospital and emphasized structural and process measures. Currently JCAHO's standards reflect an emphasis on interdepartmental performance and functional *outcomes* of the services provided. The 1995 standards address 11 functional areas: *Assessment* of Patients; Care of Patients; Education; *Continuum* of Care; Improving Organizational Performance; Leadership; Management of the *Environment of Care*; Management of Human Resources; Patient Rights, and Organizational *Ethics*;

Management of Information; and Surveillance, Prevention, and Control of Infection. The 1996 *Comprehensive Accreditation Manual for Hospitals* (CAMH) listed the qualifications as[1]:

activities coordinator, qualified: an individual who is licensed or registered, if applicable, in the state in which he or she practices as a therapeutic recreation specialist or as an activities professional and is eligible for certification as such by a recognized accrediting body; or an individual who has had at least two years of experience in a social or recreational program within the last five years, one year of which was full time in a resident or patient activities program in a health care setting; or an individual who is a qualified occupational therapist or occupational therapy assistant; or an individual who has the documented equivalent education, training or experience.

occupational therapist, qualified: An individual who is a graduate of an occupational therapy program accredited by a nationally recognized accreditation body; is currently certified as an occupational therapist by the *American Occupational Therapy Certification Board*; meets any current legal requirements of licensure or registration; or has the documented equivalence in education, training, and experience, and is currently competent in the field, The qualified occupational therapist uses purposeful, goal-oriented activity in assessing, evaluating, or treating persons whose function is impaired by physical illness or injury, emotional disorder, congenital or developmental disability, or the aging process, to achieve optimum functioning, to prevent disability, and to maintain health. (p.717)

physical therapist, qualified: An individual who is a graduate of a physical therapist education program accredited by a nationally recognized accreditation body; meets any current legal requirements of licensure or registration; or has the documented equivalence in training, education, and experience; and is currently competent in the field. Physical therapists assess, evaluate, and treat movement dysfunction and pain resulting from injury, disease, disability, or other health related conditions. Physical therapy includes: 1. performing and interpreting tests and measure-

ments to assess pathophysiological, pathomechanical, electrophysiological, ergonomic, and developmental deficits of bodily systems to determine diagnosis, treatment, prognosis, and prevention; 2. planning, administering, and modifying therapeutic interventions that focus on posture, locomotion, strength, endurance, cardio-pulmonary function, balance, coordination, joint mobility, flexibility, pain, healing, and repair, and functional abilities in daily living skills, including work; and 3. providing consultative, educational, research, and other advisory services. (p. 718)

recreational therapist, qualified: An individual who, at a minimum is a graduate of a baccalaureate degree program in recreational therapy accredited by a nationally recognized accreditation body; is currently a Certified Therapeutic Recreation Specialist (CTRS) by the *National Council for Therapeutic Recreation Certification* (NCTRC); meets any current legal requirements of licensure, registration or certification; or has the documented equivalence in education, training, and experience; and is currently competent in the field. Recreational therapists assess and treat patients individually using interventions to restore, remediate, or rehabilitate to improve functioning and independence in life activities as well as to reduce or eliminate the effects of illness or disability. (pp. 720-721)

recreational therapy assistant/technician, qualified: An individual who, at a minimum, is a graduate of an associate degree program in recreational therapy; meets any current legal requirements of licensure, registration, or certification; or has the documented equivalence in education and experience; and is competent in the field. Recreational therapy assistants or technicians assist recreational therapists to assess and treat patients individually using interventions to restore, remediate, or rehabilitate to improve functioning and independence in life activities as well as to reduce or eliminate the effects of illness or disability. A qualified recreational therapist clinically supervises the work of recreational therapy assistants or technicians. (p. 720)

social worker, qualified: An individual who either has met the requirements of a graduate curriculum (leading to a master's degree) in a school of social work that is accredited by the Council on Social Work Education or has the documented equivalent education, training or experience. (p. 722)

---

[1] From Joint Commission on Accreditation of Healthcare Organizations, **1996 Comprehensive Accreditation Manual for Hospitals**. Copyright © 1995 by Joint Commission on Accreditation of Healthcare Organizations. Reprinted with permission.

speech-language pathologist, qualified: Speech-language pathologists hold either a master's or doctoral degree; the Certificate of Clinical Competence (CCC) of the American Speech-Language-Hearing Association (ASHA); and where applicable, state licensure; or have the documented equivalence in education, training, and experience. These professionals identify, assess, and treat communication and swallowing functions and their disorders. Speech-language pathologists counsel individuals with disorders of communication and swallowing functions, their families, caregivers, and other service providers about the disability and its management. They provide preventive services and consultation and make referrals, the goal of speech-language pathologists is to facilitate the development and maintenance of communication and swallowing functions. (p. 722)

Joint Photographic Experts Group (JPEG) (HCO) a standard for compression of static images.

joule the International System of Units unit of work or energy, equal to the work done by a force of one newton when its point of application moves through a distance of one meter in the direction of the force.

JPEG See *Joint Photographic Experts Group.*

judgment the cognitive ability to make a decision based on a review of various aspects and factors related to the decision as well as being able to reasonably predict the results of an action under consideration. See *associated features, bipolar disorder, cognitive deficits, compulsion, dementia, dressing skills, executive function, Global Assessment of Functioning Scale, intelligence, knowledge, mental retardation, time management.*

judicial review appeal process used by a facility when it disagrees with survey results written up by a state or federal survey team. An additional avenue of appeal, following completion of the administrative appeals process at the appeals council level or departmental appeals board, for *providers* and suppliers denied Medicare/Medicaid participation. Judicial review begins with the US District Court and may proceed to the US Circuit Court of Appeals and to the US Supreme Court. See *survey process.*

K

Kardex the quick reference document on each patient kept at the unit assistant's desk or in the department's office. The Kardex usually includes the basic information on the patient (personal and medical information of significance) and a description of *treatment* and services to be rendered to the patient. Some Kardexes also have space for daily documentation. This information is then summarized in the patient's medical chart on a regular basis. Kardexes are useful when a department uses volunteers. Because of *confidentiality*, the professional staff may not want to include sensitive information in the Kardex but can provide the volunteers with important information. See below for a discussion of what should be included in a Kardex.

General Guidelines for Placing Psychosocial Information in Kardexes

1. The therapist will need to balance the volunteers' need to know how the patient's situation is impacting his/her life with the patient's need for privacy. Patient confidentiality comes first while keeping overall safety in mind.
2. When the patient's injuries are due to abuse, write down the actual injuries and not the kind of abuse.
3. If the patient is experiencing family crises like a pending divorce, a lost child, or other stressful events, ask yourself if the volunteer really needs to know about the stressful events. It is usually best just to write that the patient is under a lot of stress in addition to the injury/disease and suggest that the volunteers be extra sensitive to the patient's need for support.
4. In the case of child abuse or *failure to thrive* of unknown origin, it is best to write "please observe parent-child interaction." This helps take the implied blame off of the parents. (It might not be the parents who are causing the problem.)
5. One of the best rules for determining what to write in the Kardex is to ask yourself if you would feel uncomfortable telling the patient that you are sharing the information with volunteers.

Karnofsky Rating Scale a sliding scale (shown below) that is used to describe the degree to which a patient's functional ability has been impaired by his/her malignant neoplasms. (In Pyle, 1996. p. 250.)

Karnofsky Rating Scale

Score	Description
100	Normal, no complaint or evidence of disease.
90	Normal activity, with minor symptoms.
80	Normal activity, with effort and some symptoms.
70	Cares for self, unable to do normal activity.
60	Requires occasional assistance.
50	Requires considerable assistance and care.
40	Disabled, requires special care and assistance.
30	Severely disabled; requires supportive measures.
20	Very sick.
10	Moribund

keloid scar a scar on the skin formed by an overgrowth of collegenous scar tissue. Keloid scars are raised and rounded with irregular margins. The size of the scar tissue tends to become smaller over the years.

kelvin (k) (named after Lord Kelvin, a British physicist, b. 1824); the *International System of Units* (SI) measurement of temperature. 0 k (zero kelvin) being absolute zero temperature, the lowest temperature possible. To convert a temperature from the Kelvin scale to the Celsius system, add 273.16 to the Kelvin measurement. When you are referring to the unit of measure, the "k" is always used in lower case with no degree sign (°). When referring to the Kelvin scale, the "K" in Kelvin is capitalized. An example of the correct way to write a temperature using the Kelvin scale would be: 285 k.

kineplastic amputation See *cineplastic amputation.*

kinesthesia an individual's conscious awareness of the kinetic *sensations* of his/her body (e.g., position of a body part, perception of movement, perception of weight or pressure).

kinesthetic pertaining to the use of the muscles, ten-

Kolb's Experiential Learning Theory

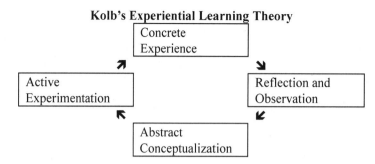

dons, and joints and the corresponding sensations of this movement. *Exercise* programs that encourage integrative movement using the proprioceptors and *equilibrium* (*balance*) are frequently referred to as kinesthetic exercise. See *proprioception.*

Kirshner wire a small wire used for fixation or traction, especially in long bone fractures.

kleptomania an impulse to take articles which one does not need and which one has not purchased or received permission to take. This disorder is characterized by an ongoing problem with impulse control in the area of stealing, not an infrequent act of stealing. Kleptomania is a recognized diagnosis in the **DSM-IV** under the category of *impulse control disorders* not elsewhere classified. See *disability, impulsivity.*

Klinefelter See *chromosomal aberrations.*

knee disarticulation   an amputation through the knee joint. Functional ability is improved through a four-unit device:

1. socket (leather or plastic)
2. fork strap
3. waist belt
4. prosthetic foot

The socket must be fitted to allow weight bearing slightly to the outside (distal) plane. A knee disarticulation is abbreviated "K/B" (knee bearing).

knowledge the collective body of information that an individual (or a community) has available to use. Knowledge is different than *intelligence*, as intelligence is the ability to use knowledge. Executive function is also different from knowledge, as executive function is the application of *judgment* in the use of knowledge and intelligence. See *job description, learning, PEW Health Professions Commission.*

knowledge based systems (HCO) a decision support system based on automated, systematized application of sets of rules or heuristics for analysis of raw data.

knowledge deficit an inability to call upon basic information required to survive in one's environment. A patient who has a knowledge deficit may demon-

strate an inability to: accurately follow through on instructions given, accurately perform skills needed (although physically able to do them), perform within socially accepted norms for behavior and emotional expression, or otherwise function appropriately because of missing information.

Kolb's experiential learning theory a theory about learning that integrates social realities of a student's life with cognitive learning theory. Kolb states that learning is actually a circular continuum as in the figure above. First the learner has a concrete learning experience, as observing a supervisor demonstrate a standing pivot transfer. For the second step, the student thinks about what s/he saw and attempts to develop a framework for understanding and remembering the technique. The third step is when the student takes his/her thoughts about the transfer and compares and contrasts the technique with ones previously learned (similar to Piaget's *accommodation*). The fourth step has the student physically implementing the technique. After the student tries to implement the technique, s/he goes back to the first step; observing his/her own actions (the attempt at implementation) or the actions of the instructor as modifications to the attempted technique are made to improve the technique.

Korotkoff sounds   the sounds heard through a sphygmomanometer that are used to measure blood pressure. These sounds are divided into phases with the first phase and the fifth phase being used to measure systolic and diastolic blood pressure respectively.

Kübler-Ross (Elisabeth)   the author of a theory which states that patients tend to move through five emotional stages on their path to accepting their death. The stages are 1. denial/isolation, 2. anger, 3. bargaining, 4. depression, and 5. acceptance.

Kurtzke Expanded Disability Status Scale an index that is used to measure the functional ability of patients with multiple sclerosis. The first of its two sections produces a score based on the function of different body systems: "pyramidal functions, cerebellar functions, brain stem functions, sensory functions, bowel and bladder functions, visual functions, mental functions, and other functions (Pyle, 1996, p. 257)." The second section, shown to the right, is a ten-point scale to indicate the degree of disability experienced by the patient. The "FS" in the scale refers to the functional scores obtained in the first part of the test. This index is used along with the Ambulation Index (AI).

kyphosis a forward, hump-like curvature of the spine. Compare with *lordosis* and *scoliosis*. See *neurofibromatosis*.

Kurtzke Expanded Disability Status Scale (Kurtzke, 1983)

Score	Criteria
0	Normal neurologic exam.
1.0	No disability, minimal signs on one FS.
1.5	No disability, minimal signs on >1 FS.
2.0	Minimal disability in 1 FS.
2.5	Minimal disability in 2 FS.
3.0	Moderate disability in 1 FS; or mild disability in 3-4 FS, though fully ambulatory.
3.5	Fully ambulatory but with moderate disability in 3-4 FS.
4.0	Fully ambulatory without aid, up and about 12 hours/day despite relatively severe disability. Able to walk without aid 500 meters.
4.5	Fully ambulatory without aid, up and about much of day, able to work a full day, may otherwise have some limitations of full activity or require minimal assistance. Relatively severe disability. Able to walk without aid 300 meters.
5.0	Ambulatory without aid for about 200 m. Disability impairs full daily activities.
5.5	Ambulatory for 100 m, disability precludes full daily activities.
6.0	Intermittent or unilateral constant assistance required to walk 100 m with or without resting.
6.5	Constant bilateral support required to walk 20 m without resting.
7.0	Unable to walk beyond 5 m even with aid, essentially restricted to wheelchair, wheels self, transfers alone.
7.5	Unable to take more than a few steps, restricted to wheelchair, may need aid in transfer, wheels self but may require motorized chair for full day's activities.
8.0	Essentially restricted to bed or chair or perambulated in wheelchair, but may be out of bed much of day, retains self-care functions, generally effective use of arms.
8.5	Essentially restricted to bed much of day, some effective use of arms, some self-care functions.
9.0	Helpless bed patient, can communicate and eat.
9.5	Unable to communicate effectively or eat/swallow.
10.0	Death.

L

lability inability to control inappropriate laughing or crying; extremely variable emotional states. See *impulsivity.*

laboratory observation identifier names and codes (HCO) a set of universal names and codes for identifying laboratory test results in order to facilitate the exchange and polling of clinical laboratory results.

lactate (HHS) an ester of lactic acid produced during non-respiratory glucose combustion. It may accumulate during some disease conditions, leading to lactate acidosis.

lactate dehydrogenase (HHS) an enzyme important to the process of glucose combustion in the body and an important mechanism for cellular energy production.

lactose (HHS) a sugar naturally occurring in milk, also known as "milk sugar," that is the least sweet of all natural sugars and used in baby formulas and candies.

lactose intolerance (HHS) an inherited inability to properly digest dairy products, due to a deficiency in the amount of the enzyme, §-galactosidase in the small intestine. This enzyme is necessary for the hydrolysis of lactose (a disaccharide) into its constituent monosaccharides, glucose and galactose. Symptoms of lactose intolerance, including abdominal cramps, flatulence, and frothy diarrhea, can increase with age.

LADDER approach See *assertiveness training.*

laminectomy surgical removal of the posterior aspect (the arch) of a vertebrae.

lancinating pain a type of pain that is usually described as piercing, tearing, or stabbing.

lanugo the soft hair that covers the body of a newborn child that is almost completely shed by the time the child is nine months old.

laryngitis a hoarseness of the voice (or lack of a voice) due to a swelling of the vocal cords. The swelling is usually caused by an inflammation of the mucous membranes that line the larynx.

laser optical card (HCO) a plastic device of the size of a credit card that can hold large amounts of digital data. Typically, the data cannot be altered once they are written to the card.

late effects the long-term health effects that are a direct result of chemotherapy and radiation after cancer treatment. Over two thirds of children who are diagnosed with cancer now survive past five years. However, approximately 50% have moderate to severe medical problems as a direct result of their cancer treatment decades after they have been considered "cured" of their cancer. The medical problems associated with late effects may include heart, lung, and kidney dysfunction; infertility; memory loss; and, occasionally, second cancers.

latency 1. the time between an exposure to an infection and the clinical manifestation of the infection. See *asymptomatic.* 2. any other inactive time where activity is possible (usually expected) in the future.

latency phase *Freud*'s stage of psychosexual development (around ages five to puberty) when an individual exhibits little or no interest in matters related to sexuality.

latent infection the eruption (e.g., showing signs) of an infection after an asymptomatic period of time. The asymptomatic (latent) period may last just a few days to over ten years depending on the type of infection and health status of the individual. See *infection.*

lateral referring to the side or portion of the body furthest away from the midline of the body. Compare with *medial.*

latex gloves a type of glove worn to protect against contamination from *blood-borne pathogens* and other *OPIMs.* Various state departments of labor and industry (OSHA) have issued hazard alerts for latex gloves due to possibility of staff developing an acquired allergy. The State of Washington's Department of Labor and Industries reports in their November 1997 bulletin that while latex gloves provide protection against blood borne pathogens in a variety of occupations and uses, wearing certain latex gloves can result in allergic reactions for some users. Symptoms of latex allergy can include skin rash and irritation, hives, nasal congestion, *asthma,* and in rare instances, shock, a potentially fatal condition. Individuals who develop an *allergy* to latex may also have some similar cross-reactions to certain foods (avocado, banana, potato, tomato, kiwi fruit, and papaya). Individuals prone to allergies are at greatest risk for developing an allergy to latex products. Because latex gloves provide positive protection against blood borne pathogens, there has been a dramatic increase in the use of these gloves, especially among health care workers, to meet worker protection requirements adopted in the

1980's. With this increased use and changes in glove manufacturing that resulted from the increased demand, there has been a rise in reported allergic reactions by some users. Studies indicate that 8% to 12% of exposed health care workers suffer allergic reactions to latex. In addition to health care, other workers who are at risk but with less frequent glove use include hairdressers, housekeepers, food service workers, and child care workers. These allergic reactions result from exposure to either the proteins or chemicals found in natural rubber latex products. The proteins may also adhere to the cornstarch powder that some manufacturers use to coat the gloves to make them easier to put on and take off. Once on the cornstarch, the protein particles can become dispersed in the air where they are readily deposited on skin and mucous membranes in the eyes, nose, and throat. Regular and repeated use of latex gloves can result in the wearer becoming highly sensitive to the proteins or chemicals found in any latex product. Once sensitized, individuals may react to very small exposures, even products or food handled by someone wearing latex gloves. Common latex products used at work and home in addition to gloves include various medical devices, rubber bands, balloons, and condoms. The State of Washington's Department of Labor and Industry points out that in many instances, depending on the exposure, workers can get the required level of protection from nitrile, vinyl, or other synthetic gloves. When latex gloves are required, powder-free gloves with reduced protein content should be used. Some of this information may be available on the box label. Products that use the term "hypoallergenic" are not lower in protein allergen content and should not be the sole criteria for choosing an acceptable alternative. It is important to keep in mind that the Blood Borne Pathogen Standard states that glove alternatives shall be accessible to those employees who are allergic to the gloves normally provided.

laws a set of expectations, standards, or principles that govern actions or explain relationships between different objects. See *ethics*.

LE lower extremity.

leadership the position of being responsible for a group of people — of making decisions, of providing guidance, of having others follow. Leaders have the ability to have others follow their lead and instructions. Generally leadership requires initiative and the power to direct, drive, instruct, and guide people and/or processes toward the desired *outcome*. There are two different style of leadership prevalent in health care, which are defined by Bradford (1976) in the chart on the next page. See *graciousness*.

lead poisoning a toxic condition caused by ingesting or inhaling lead. Children, especially children living below the poverty line, ingest enough lead from the environment to have over 25,000 children diagnosed with lead poisoning. Lead acts on the body in many different ways including having an impact on the hematologic, renal, and neurologic systems. Lead interferes with the formation of *hemoglobin* causing *anemia*. It also damages the renal system, damaging the cells of the proximal tubules. This damage leads to abnormal excretions of glucose, proteins, and amino acids. The most significant damage, though, takes place in the child's nervous system. Behavioral changes include *hyperactivity*, *aggression*, *irritability*, loss of sensory perception, and impulsiveness paired with a decreased interest in play. With increased ingestion and longer exposure the child may also develop *seizures*, *paralysis*, blindness, *mental retardation*/learning disabilities, and eventually die. Normal levels of lead in children are 0.0 - 30.0 μg. while toxic levels are 110 μg. and up. Treatment involves the removal of lead from the body through the use of chelation therapy (injections of metals which bond with lead to help move the lead out of the body through the urine) and changes in the child's environment to reduce the exposure and access to lead. See *impulsivity*.

learning the process of acquiring *knowledge* and *skills*. There is no one universally accepted definition of learning and, in health care, there tends to be pressure to put learning in very measurable *objectives* and *outcomes*. Generally, when one talks about a patient "learning," one talks about a demonstrated change in behavior and/or skill level.

Learning Disabilities Association of America (LDA) a national organization that advances the education and general welfare of children and adults who have normal (or near normal) intelligence and who have a learning disability. Formerly called the Association of Children with Learning Disabilities.

learning disability a variety of minimum brain dysfunction disorders which interfere with the normal learning process in children with normal to above normal IQs. There are three primary categories of learning disabilities: dyslexia (difficulties with reading), dysgraphia (difficulties with writing), and dyscalculia (difficulties with mathematics). The **DSM-IV** divides learning disabilities (**DSM-IV's** term is "learning disorders") into four categories: reading disorder, mathematics disorder, disorder of written expression, and learning disorder not otherwise specified. No matter how the different types of learning disabilities are divided, the key elements are substantially lower scores on academic and IQ

Leadership Traits

Traditional Leadership	Group - Centered Leadership
The leader directs, controls, polices the members, and leads them to the proper decision. Basically it is his/her group and the leader's authority and responsibility are acknowledged by members.	The group or meeting, is *owned* by the members, including the leader. All members, with the leader's assistance, contribute to its effectiveness.
The leader focuses his/her attention on the task to be accomplished. S/he brings the group back from any diversions. S/he performs all the functions needed to arrive at the proper decision.	The group is responsible, with occasional and appropriate help from the leader, for reaching a decision that includes the participation of all and is the product of all. The leader is a servant and helper to the group.
The leader sets limits and uses rules of order to keep the discussion within strict limits set by the agenda. S/he controls the time spent on each item lest the group wander fruitlessly.	Members of the group are encouraged and helped to take responsibility for its productivity, its methods of working, its assignment of tasks, its plans for the use of the time available.
The leader believes that emotions are disruptive to objective, logical thinking and should be discouraged or suppressed. S/he assumes it is his/her task to make clear to all members the disruptive effect of emotions.	Feelings, emotions, conflict are recognized by the members and the leaders as legitimate facts and situations demanding as much attention as the task agenda.
The leader believes that s/he should handle a member's disruptive behavior by talking to him away from the group; it is his/her task to do so.	The leader believes that any problem in the group must be faced and solved within the group and by the group. As trust develops among members, it is much easier for an individual to discover ways in which his/her behavior is bothering the group.
Because the need to arrive at a task decision is all-important in the eyes of the leader, needs of individual members are considered less important.	With help and encouragement from the leader, the members come to realize that the needs, feelings, and purposes of all members should be met so that an awareness of being a group forms. Then the group can continue to grow.

tests and/or a significant limitation related to written expression. Children, youth, and adults with learning disabilities tend to have a harder time adapting to life in the community. Reading basic informational material (time schedules, current events in the paper, instructions on equipment and games, etc.) may be difficult to nearly impossible. Budgeting, balancing a checkbook, and figuring out how much tip to leave at a restaurant may all be impacted by a learning disability. Often a patient will mask his/her disability by indicting that s/he is not interested in the activity when, in reality, s/he is not able to complete the task due to his/her disability. Learning disabilities generally do not disappear as the individual reaches and goes through adulthood. Many employers and instructors find that they need to adapt their methods of giving information so that an adult with a learning disability can assimilate the material. The chart below, from the National Adult Learning and Literacy Center (1990), is a set of guidelines for working with adults with learning disabilities.

Teaching Adults Who Have Learning Disabilities
Instructors and students should agree on the expected outcomes of a program. They should both be involved in developing work plans on how they expect to reach the student's goals. The following techniques may help to improve student involvement.

- Help set realistic goals.
- Set short-term goals so the student can experience immediate successes.
- Consider meeting goals in variety of ways. Be creative and flexible.
- Involve the student in determining how to evaluate specific goals.
- Involve students in evaluation of their progress.
- Get adult students tested for hearing and vision problems, if necessary.
- Develop a written work plan with learners and make sure they fully understand it.
- Talk with students about what techniques work best for them.
- Discover what truly interests the learner through listening, discussions, and observations.

- Respect the uniqueness of each individual. Encourage risk-taking.
- Help students identify techniques that might be helpful in accommodating their learning disabilities.

Before students begin assignments, they have to understand the instructions. The following techniques may help instructors introduce lessons effectively.

- Tape record or videotape the instructions.
- Make announcements in both oral and written forms — especially changes in the schedule, directions, assignments, or exams.
- Have a model of the finished product available for review.
- Show by example.
- Make directions specific, concrete, and understandable.
- Tell your student what the lesson will be about, and explain what will be done first, second, and so on.
- Give a number of options for completing assignments.
- Review major points of previous sessions. Preview main points to be covered. Outline both in several ways: written on board, presented orally, and outlined in a handout.
- Make clear transitions from one task to another.

The key to effective teaching is to identify and employ techniques and methods that work with students. It is easier for instructors to adjust their teaching methods than it is for students to change the way they learn. The following suggestions may help instructors reach adult learners.

- Build on strengths rather than repeating weaknesses.
- Make eye contact frequently; this helps in maintaining attention and encouraging participation.
- Teach new concepts by relating them to practical applications.
- Be sure reading material is at the right level for the learner.
- Be sure print type is large enough.
- Relate material to everyday situations.
- Use language tied to experience and approaches and reading materials from the home and work environment to stimulate interest.
- Build on what the student already knows; make learning developmental, not remedial.
- Probe "incorrect" responses to discover thought processes.
- Teach students to correct their own mistakes.
- Do not assume that the learner knows something until you ask or teach it.
- Be creative and attempt to vary your teaching style.
- Encourage students to sit in front of the classroom where they can hear well and have a clear view of the chalkboard.
- Keep the learning environment free of visual and auditory distraction.
- Establish a routine; this promotes organization and consistency.
- Use multisensory strategies to present materials; many learners must see, say, hear, and touch before they can develop full mental images that stick and make sense.
- Provide short-term tasks with short breaks between tasks.
- Be flexible with time schedules; work quotas should be adjusted to fit the work speed of each learner.
- Repeat the activity until learning is accomplished, and provide opportunities to review.
- Vary your lessons, reteaching and reviewing in varieties of ways.
- Respect different learning styles.
- Use materials that relate to an individual's experiences.
- Change an activity when it's not working.
- De-emphasize timed tests.
- Incorporate keyboards (word processing or typewriters) into the lesson as much as possible. Studies show that some learners can produce 15 times more writing with a word processor than they can with a pencil or pen.
- Use formulas or rhymes to assist the memory.
- Encourage the use of learning aids and tools (e.g., calculators, highlighter pens, extra worksheets, computerized learning programs, records, tape recorders, films, demonstrations, maps, charts, experiences, figures, rulers).
- Use color wherever possible for visual impact.
- Provide the student opportunities to repeat verbally what has been taught as a check for accuracy.
- Work with other teachers and professionals and ask for ideas or opinions.
- Encourage the learner to find a mentor in addition to the tutor. The mentor can help the learner review information and apply classroom skills to practical situations.
- Suggest reinforcement activities to be used at home, e.g., posting new words on the refrigerator door, repeated listening to a tape of vocabulary words, watching recommend educational television programs.

- Talk with the students about their learning process. Ask them what does and what does not work for them.

The better students feel about their learning experience, the harder they try. A positive environment will foster self-esteem in students, encouraging them to return. Consider the following when working with adult students:

- Pay attention to self-concept enhancement when working with students with learning disabilities.
- Do not embarrass, or insinuate laziness or discourage an individual publicly or privately.
- Reduce emphasis on competition and perfection.
- Praise the learner's accomplishments at the end of every session.
- Communicate to students that you value them through smiling, listening, and eye contact.
- Incorporate a sense of humor into the learning process.
- Praise what you might consider small or minor successes.
- Emphasize students' strengths and make each student a "star" as often as possible.

See *Wide Range Achievement Test*.

learning disorder a specific diagnostic category in the **DSM-IV**, learning disorders include functional problems in reading, mathematics, and writing. The patient's functional ability must be significantly impaired and have a negative impact on his/her day-to-day ability to complete activities of daily living. See *learning disability*.

least restrictive When a patient has artificial limitations placed on him/her, it is his/her right to have the restrictions be as small as possible. An example would be a patient who wanders uninvited into the rooms of others or off the unit. In the past, wanderers were strapped into a wheelchair with its brakes on, even if they did not need a wheelchair to get around. Some facilities have found that placing a wall mural of a set of bookshelves or a fence on the inside of the closed unit doors caused patients who were cognitively impaired and wandering to not attempt to go out the doors. Other facilities have found that the placement of the upper half of cafe curtains over the door (so that the hem is just below the wanderer's eye level) caused the wanderer to stay out of the room. See *Education for All Handicapped Children Act, extended admission, psychiatric admission, Public Law 94-103*.

legionellosis See *Legionnaire's disease*.

Legionnaire's disease (LD) also known as Pontiac fever and legionellosis. (CDC) Legionellosis is an infection caused by the bacterium Legionella pneumophila. The disease has two distinct forms: 1. Legionnaires' disease, the more severe form of infection that includes pneumonia, and 2. Pontiac fever, a milder illness. Legionnaires' disease acquired its name in 1976 when an outbreak of pneumonia occurred among persons attending a convention of the American Legion in Philadelphia. Later, the bacterium causing the illness was named Legionella. An estimated 8,000 to 18,000 people get Legionnaires' disease in the United States each year. Some people can be infected with the Legionella bacterium and have mild symptoms or no illness at all. Outbreaks of Legionnaires' disease receive significant media attention. However, this disease usually occurs as a single, isolated case not associated with any recognized outbreak. When outbreaks do occur, they are usually recognized in the summer and early fall, but cases may occur year-round. About 5% to 30% of people who have Legionnaires' disease die. Patients with Legionnaires' disease usually have fever, chills, and a cough, which may be dry or may produce sputum. Some patients also have muscle aches, headache, tiredness, loss of appetite, and, occasionally, diarrhea. Laboratory tests may show that these patients' kidneys are not functioning properly. Chest X-rays often show pneumonia. It is difficult to distinguish Legionnaires' disease from other types of pneumonia by symptoms alone; other tests are required for diagnosis. Persons with Pontiac fever experience fever and muscle aches and do not have pneumonia. They generally recover in 2 to 5 days without treatment. The time between the patient's exposure to the bacterium and the onset of illness for Legionnaires' disease is 2 to 10 days; for Pontiac fever, it is shorter, generally a few hours to 2 days. The diagnosis of legionellosis requires special tests not routinely performed on persons with fever or pneumonia. Therefore, a physician must consider the possibility of legionellosis in order to obtain the right tests. Several types of tests are available. The most useful tests detect the bacteria in sputum, find Legionella antigens in urine samples, or compare antibody levels to Legionella in two blood samples obtained 3 to 6 weeks apart. People of any age may get Legionnaires' disease, but the illness most often affects middle-aged and older persons, particularly those who smoke cigarettes or have chronic lung disease. Also at increased risk are persons whose immune system is suppressed by diseases such as cancer, kidney failure requiring dialysis, diabetes, or AIDS. Those that take drugs that suppress the immune system are also at higher risk. Pontiac fever most commonly occurs in persons who are otherwise healthy. Erythromycin is the antibiotic currently recommended for treating persons with Legionnaires' disease. In severe cases, a second drug, rifampin, may be used in addition. Other drugs are available for patients unable to tolerate erythromycin. Pontiac fever requires no specific treatment. Outbreaks of legionellosis have occurred after persons have breathed mists that come from a water source (e.g., air conditioning cooling towers, whirlpool spas, showers) contaminated with Legionella bacteria. Persons may be exposed to these mists in homes, workplaces, hospitals, or public places. Legionellosis is not passed from person to person, and there is no evidence of persons becoming infected from auto air conditioners or household window air-conditioning units.

leisure The concept of leisure is not one shared by all cultures and has two different meanings to those that do share that concept. For those who study leisure in the United States and Canada, leisure is generally considered to be a state of mind. Others view leisure as time with an absence of work or commitment. Extensive study has been done in Europe and Northern America concerning all of the aspects of leisure as a state of mind, including the study of interests, *motivations*, attitudes, barriers, *boredom*, satisfaction, etc. Leisure has been described as having many attributes, including "disengagement from matters of the real world, freedom, sense of separation, escape from routine or responsibility, narrowing of attention, and decreased awareness of the passage of time, relaxation, reduction in self-consciousness or evaluation, openness to the present or immediate experience, immersion in the experience, enjoyment, bonding, affection, and spontaneity" (Carruthers 1993). Contrast with *discretionary time*. See *constraints, Leisure Attitude Scale, Leisure Interest Measure, Leisure Satisfaction Scale, premorbid leisure lifestyle.*

leisure ability a model of service delivery developed by Peterson and Gunn in the late 1970's and adapted by the National Therapeutic Recreation Society in 1981. The model was client-oriented and was based on the premise that play, recreation, and leisure are vital components of the human experience. However, not everyone had the basic knowledge and skills required to engage in meaningful leisure activities to promote normal development and to be able to express an appropriate leisure lifestyle. Therefore, the *Therapeutic Recreation Service Model* was developed to conceptualize the degree of involvement required of the recreational therapist or leisure professional. See *Recreation Service Model.*

Leisure and Recreation Involvement Measure-

ment (LRI) (Ragheb, 1996) two measurements to establish how an individual perceives his/her *involvement* in leisure. The LRI has both a short form (24 items, available commercially) and a long form (52 items, available only for research purposes). The table on the next page shows the six components of involvement that are measured by the LRI. It also lists the characteristics of individuals who score either high or low in each of the areas (Ragheb, 1997). See *intensity.*

Leisure Attitude Scale (by Burdge, 1961) an eleven item scale which contrasted work and leisure. Though widely used in research, this Leisure Attitude Scale has many versions, each version having changes that have, in Burdge's opinion, diminished its value. The alpha reliability of this assessment is poor, at only .46. Treatment interventions should not be based solely on the results of this assessment.

Leisure Attitude Scale (by Slivken and Crandall, 1978) This attitudinal scale originally had 20 items, but was reduced to just 10 items that assess the affective component of a person's attitude toward leisure. As its reliability coefficient is only .76, it is not recommended that a therapist base treatment interventions solely on the result of this assessment.

Leisure Attitude Scale (LAS) (by Ragheb and Beard, 1991a) The LAS helps the therapist identify attitudinal barriers to the patient's healthy involvement in leisure activities. This 36-item assessment measures the patient's score on each of 3 subcomponents of attitude: 1. cognitive (general knowledge and beliefs about leisure, beliefs about leisure's relation to other concepts such as health, happiness, and work), 2. affective (perception of his/her leisure experiences and activities), and 3. behavioral (verbalized behavioral intentions toward leisure choices and activities and self-reports of current and past participation). The alpha reliability of the entire assessment is .94 with a range of .89 to .93 for the subscales. Limited normative data is available. Initial studies show that individuals who are in the upper age, education, and income brackets tend to have positive beliefs about leisure activities, but tend to like them less than individuals in the lower level of those categories. Ragheb and Beard report that men tend to have more positive beliefs and feelings toward leisure activities than women. The LAS is one of the subscales of the *Idyll Arbor Leisure Battery.*

Leisure Barriers Inventory (LBI) (Peterson, 1982) This assessment, originally written by Peterson and Dunn, has been passed around and written up in quite a few therapy publications. In its original form, it has not been able to stand up to testing (reliability and validity) and should not be used as an assess-

LRI Categories and Interpretation of High and Low Scores

Component	High Score	Low Score
Importance	Would reserve time for leisure endeavors, rearranges schedule to allow time for these pursuits, has a focus on activities, considers activities as parts of lifestyle, gives them special attention.	Does not allocate time for recreational activities, with no aim or focus toward leisure choices, does not recognize these activities and does not give them attention as parts of daily pursuits.
Pleasure	Claims enjoyment, speedy time passage, feels full after engaging in recreation activities, identifies with activities, able to entertain self, and proud of chosen activities.	Finds no enjoyment in leisure, claims that time is a drag when engaged in recreation activities, reports dissatisfaction with leisure choices, lacks self-entertainment through recreation, has no pride in leisure and recreation pursuits.
Interest	Wants to know details about leisure activities that express person's wishes, considers leisure choices worthwhile, serving certain goals or aims, practices skills needed to improve performance of activities.	Feels that leisure activities are trivial, has no desire to learn details about leisure pursuits, does not practice leisure skills, mostly aimless during free time without goal or orientation.
Intensity	Feels that leisure activities occupy feelings, uses activities to help in discovering things about self, not easily distracted while pursing favorite leisure activities, claims that leisure pursuits give a sense of inner freedom, expects positive outcome from leisure endeavors.	Considers leisure activities peripheral, is easily distracted while doing a leisure activity, claims no discoveries or realization through leisure choices, lacks a sense of inner freedom and intrinsic relatedness, with negative or no expectations from leisure and recreation pursuits.
Centrality	Has a sense of self-responsibility toward choices made to participate in leisure activities, ready to devote effort to master activities, strives to achieve and do well, willing to invest money, time, and energy in leisure pursuits.	Does not intend to put effort into skill acquisition and activity mastery, does not invest to achieve or succeed in recreation pursuits, lacks self-responsibility about leisure outcome.
Meaning	Claims that leisure choices give life meaning and flavor, feels that leisure activities help in expressing self, possesses knowledge of chosen leisure activities greater than the average person, gains a sense of value in life through leisure, feels lost without leisure activities.	Has no self-expression through leisure and recreation activities, shows that these activities do not contribute to the search of meaning in general, has minimum or no knowledge about what is done as leisure choices, lacks sense of value in life derived from leisure.

ment tool to determine treatment objectives for patients.

Leisure Diagnostic Battery (LDB) (Witt and Ellis, 1990) (multiple versions) The LDB helps the therapist measure the patient's perceived freedom as it relates to leisure and other factors that may be barriers to this freedom. Divided into two sections with a total of seven subscales, this assessment measures the following: perceived leisure competence, perceived leisure control, leisure needs, depth of involvement, *playfulness*, barriers to leisure experiences, and leisure preferences. The manual for the LDB provides extensive information on the assessment, as well as information on validity and reliability. The LDB is available in a paper and a computer format.

Leisure Interest Measure (LIM) (Ragheb and Beard 1991b) Therapists have complained about the

common problem of using an activity interest list in which the patient just checks off the activities that s/he likes. Too often the results are questionable. Following Holland's well-respected format of describing the attributes and characteristics of an activity, Ragheb and Beard developed this 29-item assessment. As with the other assessments they developed, Ragheb and Beard used rigorous standards to develop the eight groupings of leisure activities. (Their division of leisure activities into groupings probably is one of the "cleanest" in the field of leisure studies.) The eight categories of leisure activities are 1. physical, 2. outdoor, 3. mechanical, 4. artistic, 5. service, 6. social, 7. cultural, and 8. reading. The therapist is able to obtain a score as to the degree in which the patient is interested in any one of the eight categories. This is helpful when the patient's assessment indicates the need to develop new leisure skills. The therapist is able to determine which activity area(s) would have the greatest interest and, hopefully, the greatest acceptance and success. The alpha internal consistency reliability coefficient for the set of 29 items was .87. This degree of certainty would allow the therapist confidence that the assessment is able to indicate the patient's intensity and breadth of leisure interests. While this assessment is able to stand on its own, it is a subscale of the *Idyll Arbor Leisure Battery*.

leisure models The last few decades have seen the development of a variety of models related to the use of free time and the use of free time activities as therapy. The key models in the field of recreational therapy include the *Therapeutic Recreation Service Model* (also known as the TR Continuum), the Leisure Step Up Model (*Dehn's Model of Leisure Health*), *Health Protection/Health Promotion Model for Therapeutic Recreation Service Delivery,* and the *Recreation Service Model*.

Leisure Motivation Scale (LMS) (Ragheb & Beard, 1990) It is too simplistic to imply that a patient is motivated or not motivated to engage in leisure activities. Motivation is a multi-dimensional attribute and it is important for the therapist to be able to identify which parts of that attribute are of concern if a patient is demonstrating a lack of motivation. If a patient scores moderate to high in all four areas of motivation, it may be that the medication they are taking is the cause of inertia. The four subscales of this assessment are 1. intellectual (the extent to which the patient is motivated to engage in leisure activities that involve mental activities such as learning, exploring, discovering, creating, or imagining), 2. social (the extent to which the patient engages in leisure activities because of the need for friendship and interpersonal relationships and the need to be valued by others), 3. competence-mastery (the extent to which the patient engages in leisure activities in order to achieve, master, challenge, and compete), and 4. stimulus-avoidance (the extent that a patient needs to escape and get away from over-stimulating life situations). The alpha reliabilities for the subscales of this assessment are acceptably large (.90 - .92). Correlations between subscales are also acceptable. The intercorrelation coefficients, viewed with the results of factor analysis, show the components of leisure motivation to be well differentiated. This assessment stands by itself, although it is one of the subscales of the *Idyll Arbor Leisure Battery*. See *scales*.

leisure planning deficit an inability to experience self-initiated leisure activities as a result of a lack of knowledge about leisure opportunities, decreased stimulation from or a lack of interest in leisure activities, poor planning skills, or an inability or unwillingness to use one's leisure time in a manner that is satisfying to the individual.

Leisure Satisfaction Measure (LSM) (Ragheb & Beard, 1991c) The Leisure Satisfaction Measure helps the therapist determine the degree to which a patient perceives his/her general "needs" are being met through leisure. This assessment is one of the four sections of the *Idyll Arbor Leisure Battery* but is able to stand on its own as an assessment. To enhance the therapist's ability to pinpoint the specific area that requires intervention, this assessment divides satisfaction into six subscales: 1. psychological (sense of freedom, enjoyment, involvement, and intellectual challenge), 2. educational (intellectual stimulation to learn about one's self and the world), 3. social (rewarding relationships with other people), 4. relaxation (relief from stress and strain of life), 5. physiological (means to develop physical fitness, stay healthy, control weight, and otherwise promote well being), and 6. aesthetic (perceives that his/her leisure activities are pleasing, interesting, beautiful and generally well designed). The alpha reliability coefficient for the entire scale is quite high, .96, and ranges from .85 to .92 for the six components. Correlation among the subscales was determined by summing scores for the items of each subscale for each of the subjects (N=347) and computing the intercorrelations among the subscales. These correlations ranged from .38 to .66 with a median value of .52.

Leisurescope Plus (Schenk, 1995) a testing tool which uses photographs in collage form to help the patient identify both areas of interest in leisure and his/her attitudes or feelings about each area of interest. See *self-talk*.

Leisure Step Up Model a model of healthy/unhealthy leisure participation outlined by Dave Dehn (1995) in the book **Leisure Step Up**. See *Dehn's Model of Leisure Health, leisure models*.

length of stay (LOS) referring to the length of time a patient is an inpatient in a facility. The average length of stay in facilities across the United States has decreased dramatically over the last decade. An example of the decline can be seen in the table on the next page computed using data from an American Hospital Association Survey of Medical Rehabilitation Hospitals and Programs as reported by Smith (1994).

LENI an acronym (lower extremity noninvasive) used in medical charts to indicate that the patient's legs were checked (visual examination and palpita-

**Average Length of Stay
in Medical Rehabilitation Programs**

Type of Admission	1988	1989	1990
Inpatient Days	38.95	36.24	34.07

tion) for emboli.

leprosy See *Hansen's disease.*

lesion a break in the continuity of an organ or a section of an organ of the body due to disease or trauma.

lethargy an abnormal and undesirable drowsiness or stupor frequently resulting in an increased indifference to one's environment. Lethargy, as a side effect of medication, can place the patient at greater risk of accidents and injury. See *hypothyroidism, initiation.*

leukemia a group of cancers that are a malignancy of blood-forming tissues, involving uncontrolled growth of white blood cells. Leukemias are classified based upon rapidity of course of disease and cell type affected. Over 20,000 adults and 2,500 children develop leukemia every year in the United States. The table below shows some of the types of leukemia. See *bone marrow transplant.*

Types of Leukemia

acute lymphoblastic leukemia (ALL)
acute monoblastic leukemia (AMOL)
acute myeloblastic leukemia (AML)
acute myelomonoblastic leukemia (AMMOL)
acute promyelocytic (APML)
Burkitt's-type acute lymphoblastic
chronic lymphocytic (CLL)
chronic myelocytic (CML)
hairy-cell
monoblastic
null cell lymphoblastic

leukocytes white blood cells. See *lymphocytes.*

Level A requirement — OBRA The 1992 version of OBRA divided the requirements into two levels, Level A and Level B. Level A requirements are major categories of required compliance. Level B requirements are the individual standards, that, when added together with other similar standards, equal a Level A requirement. The 1995 version of OBRA dropped Level A and B requirements. See *OBRA.*

Level B requirement — OBRA the individual standards outlined in the OBRA 1992 regulations. There were almost 300 Level B requirements listed in the OBRA 1992 document. The 1995 version of OBRA dropped Level A and B requirements. See *OBRA.*

libido the basic psychological energy associated with sexual desires or creativity. *Freud* specifically referred to libido as the sexual energy and drive to achieve a pleasurable satisfaction. See *Beck Depression Inventory.*

licensure See *credentialing.*

lid lag an abnormally sluggish movement of the upper eyelid commonly seen in patients with thyroid disease.

Life Safety Code (LSC) a set of fire protection requirements written by the National Fire Protection Association designed to establish minimum requirements that will provide a reasonable degree of safety from fire, smoke, and panic. These requirements cover construction, exiting, protection from hazards and requirements for operational features. The requirements are designed to provide an appropriate level of safety for individuals in health care facilities. LSC surveys are conducted by individual(s) from the office of the state fire marshal or the state health department. See *environment of care.*

Life Satisfaction Scale (LSS) The LSS was developed by Nancy Lohmann (1976) as a result of her research on life satisfaction. This 32-item scale has a reliability coefficient of .89 (.80 is usually considered acceptable). The assessment measures five dimensions of life satisfaction, which provide the therapist with a single score when they are combined. The five dimensions of life satisfaction are 1. pleasure versus apathy, 2. determination, 3. difference between desired and achieved goals, 4. mood at time of assessment, and 5. self-concept. Sainsbury (1993) conducted a study using the LSS and supported the hypothesis that seniors receiving recreational therapy services can improve their perceived life satisfaction in spite of poor or failing health.

light diet a prescribed *diet* that includes most foods; the difference is in how the food is prepared. Raw and fried foods are usually not allowed. Foods that are high in fat, which produce fat, or which are hard to digest are not allowed.

light rail (ADA) refers to a streetcar type vehicle railway operated on city streets, semi-private rights of way, or exclusive private rights of way. Service may be provided by step entry vehicles or by level boarding. The ADA accessibility guidelines for light rail may be found in the **Light Rail Vehicles and Systems Technical Assistance Manual** (US Architectural and Transportation Barriers Compliance Board).

Likert scale a numerical *scale* developed by Rensis Likert which is usually used to measure attitudes and values. The scale, traditionally having five choices, runs from negative (usually "strongly disagree") through neutral ("uncertain") to positive ("strongly agree"). Less traditionally, scales with three, seven, or more choices are offered. The Likert scale allows the results of the individual's attitudes and values to be analyzed mathematically.

limbic system a group of several brain structures associated with emotion and memory. Neurosurgeon Wilder Penfield first observed this association when operating on individuals with unusual seizure activity. Stimulation of the area produced vivid auditory and visual hallucinations of previous experiences. In recent years the amagdala, hypothalamus, and the limbic system have been proposed as the "seat" of emotions.

linkage disequilibrium (HHS/NMDP) an increased frequency of allele associations, more than would be expected based on random distribution.

Lisfranc amputation an amputation of the toes at the metatarsophalangeal joint. Stability for standing and ambulation is achieved through the use of a steel shank in the shoe. This shank provides the patient with a platform to push off from. Cosmetically a toe-filler may also be added to the patient's shoe. A Lisfranc amputation has only minimal impact on most patients' normal lifestyles.

listening skills There are four skills associated with functional listening (McKay, Davis, Fanning 1983). As described in the table on the next page. See *intake assessment*.

Listeria monocytogenes (HHS) a Gram-positive bacterium, found in at least 37 mammalian species, as well as 17 species of birds and possibly some fish and shellfish. The bacteria can be isolated from soil, and is resistant to heat, freezing, and drying. Listeria has been associated with foods such as raw milk, soft-ripened cheeses, ice cream, raw vegetables, raw and cooked poultry, raw meat, and raw and smoked fish. Unlike other pathogenic bacteria, such as salmonella, listeria can survive and grow at temperatures as low as 5°C (41°F). Acute infection with listeria may result in flu-like symptoms including persistent fever, followed by septicemia, *meningitis*, *encephalitis*, and intrauterine or cervical infections in pregnant women. Possible gastrointestinal symptoms include nausea, vomiting, and diarrhea, alone or coupled with other symptoms (mentioned above).

listeriosis (CDC) a serious infection caused by eating food contaminated with the bacterium Listeria monocytogenes, recently recognized as an important public health problem in the United States. The disease affects primarily pregnant women, newborns, and adults with weakened immune systems. It can be avoided by following a few simple recommendations. A person with listeriosis has fever, muscle aches, and, sometimes, gastrointestinal symptoms such as nausea or diarrhea. If infection spreads to the nervous system, symptoms such as headache, stiff neck, confusion, loss of balance, or convulsions can occur. Infected pregnant women may experience only a mild, flu-like illness; however, infections during pregnancy can lead to premature delivery, infection of the newborn, or even stillbirth. In the United States, an estimated 2,500 persons become seriously ill with listeriosis each year. Of these, 500 die. At increased risk are pregnant women — They are about 20 times more likely than other healthy adults to get listeriosis. About one-third of listeriosis cases happen during pregnancy; newborns — newborns rather than the pregnant women themselves suffer the serious effects of infection in pregnancy; persons with weakened immune systems, persons with cancer, diabetes, or kidney disease; persons with AIDS. They are almost 300 times more likely to get listeriosis than people with normal immune systems; persons who take glucocorticosteroid medications; and the elderly. Healthy adults and children occasionally get infected with Listeria, but they rarely become seriously ill. Listeria can get into food. Listeria monocytogenes is found in soil and water. Vegetables can become contaminated from the soil or from manure used as fertilizer. Animals can carry the bacterium without appearing ill and can contaminate foods of animal origin such as meats and dairy products. The bacterium has been found in a variety of raw foods, such as uncooked meats and vegetables, as well as in processed foods that become contaminated after processing, such as soft cheeses and cold cuts at the deli counter. Unpasteurized (raw) milk or foods made from unpasteurized milk may contain the bacterium. Listeria is killed by pasteurization, and heating procedures used to prepare ready-to-eat processed meats should be sufficient to kill the bacterium; however, unless good manufacturing practices are followed, contamination can occur after processing. The general guidelines recommended for the prevention of listeriosis are similar to those used to help prevent other food-borne illnesses, such as salmonellosis. The general recommendations: thoroughly cook raw food from animal sources, such as beef, pork, or poultry; wash raw vegetables thoroughly before eating; keep uncooked meats separate from vegetables and from cooked foods and ready-to-eat foods; avoid raw (unpasteurized) milk or foods made from raw milk; and wash hands, knives, and cutting boards after handling uncooked foods. Recommendations for persons at high risk, such as pregnant women and persons with weakened immune systems, in addition to the recommendations

Summary of Listening Skills

Listening Skill	Description
Basic Total Listening Skills	People want you to listen, so they look for clues to prove that you are. Here's how to be a good listener: 1. Maintain good eye contact. 2. Lean slightly forward. 3. Reinforce the speaker by nodding or paraphrasing. 4. Clarify by asking questions. 5. Actively move away from distractions. 6. Be committed, even if you're angry or upset, to understanding what was said.
Active Listening	1. Paraphrasing: to state in your own words what the other person said. 2. Clarifying: to ask questions until you feel that you correctly understand what the person said. 3. Feedback: after you have paraphrased and clarified what you heard the other person say, you talk about your reactions to what they said — in a non-judgmental manner.
Listening with Empathy	You do not have to agree with the person talking with you, but realize that they have feelings and worth also. Some questions to ask yourself to help develop *empathy*: 1. What need is the [anger, etc.] coming from? 2. What danger is this person experiencing? 3. What is s/he asking for?
Listening with Openness	Your own attitudes and judgment of what the person is saying may get in the way of effective listening. Some of the blocks to listening are 1. Comparing 7. Identifying 2. Mind Reading 8. Advising 3. Rehearsing 9. Sparring 4. Filtering 10. Being Right 5. Judging 11. Derailing 6. Dreaming 12. Placating
Listening with Awareness	Use your own experience and knowledge of history and people and body language to "read" the non-verbal messages being given. Compare what is being said to your own knowledge of history, people, and the way things are. Listen to body language and tone. Does the person's tone of voice, emphasis, facial expression, and posture fit with the content of his or her communication?

listed above: avoid soft cheeses such as feta, Brie, Camembert, blue-veined, and Mexican-style cheese. (Hard cheeses, processed cheeses, cream cheese, cottage cheese, or yogurt need not be avoided.); leftover foods or ready-to-eat foods, such as hot dogs, should be cooked until steaming hot before eating; although the risk of listeriosis associated with foods from deli counters is relatively low, pregnant women and immunosuppressed persons may choose to avoid these foods or thoroughly reheat cold cuts before eating.

listing gait   during ambulation the individual leans toward one side, or "lists." See *gait.*

living wills   legal documents that outline the instructions a patient has for care in the event that the patient is incapable of making health care choices at any time in the future. The primary use of living wills is to describe the patient's choice about using life-prolonging medical care if s/he is terminally ill. The living will is filled out prior to or during the admission process and placed in the patient's chart.

locomotion   the action or ability to move from one location to another. See *ambulatory, extrapyramidal, mobility, physical therapy.*

locus of control   an individual's perception of who or what controls him/her. If an individual thinks s/he is controlled by his/her own thoughts, desires, and actions, then s/he is said to have an *internal* locus of control. If the individual feels that s/he is controlled by outside forces instead of by his/her own thoughts, desires, and actions, then s/he is said to have an *external* locus of control. See *extrinsic, intrinsic.*

Lofstrand crutch . See *Canadian crutch.*

long-term memory   See *memory, memory deficit.*

lordosis   a curvature of the lower back toward the stomach area; an anteroposterior curvature of the spine. Compare with *kyphosis, scoliosis.*

Lou Gehrig's disease   See *amyotrophic lateral sclerosis.*

low air loss bed   commercially known as KinAir, FLEXICAIR, and Mediscus, these beds are made up of multiple independently inflated air sacs that allow an equal distribution of pressure over the body regardless of the position. These beds are used with patients who have *pressure sores* or are at a high risk of developing pressure sores. Implications for treatment include the potential decrease in the ability to transfer self out of bed. It is contraindicated to use equipment or activities that have sharp points for fear of punching an air sac. See *bed.*

low-calorie sweetener   (HHS) non-nutritive sweeteners, also referred to as intense sweeteners. Low-calorie sweeteners can replace nutritive sweeteners in most foods at a caloric savings of approximately 16 calories per teaspoon. Thus, caloric reduction may be achieved when low-calorie sweetened foods and beverages are substituted for their full-calorie counterparts. Examples of low-calorie sweeteners in use in the US food supply are saccharin, aspartame, and acesulfame K.

lower motor neuron lesion (LMN)   a lesion in the cells of the spinal cord (anterior horn cells, nerve roots, or the peripheral nerve system) that impairs the muscles involved, causing them to be *flaccid.*

lower respiratory infection   an infection located in the trachea, bronchi, and/or the lungs. See *upper respiratory infection.*

lumbar   the portion of the lower back which contains the five lumbar vertebrae.

lycopene   (HHS) a carotenoid related to the better-known beta-carotene. Lycopene gives tomatoes and some other fruits and vegetables their distinctive red color. Nutritionally, it functions as an antioxidant. Research shows lycopene is best absorbed by the body when consumed as tomatoes that have been heat-processed using a small amount of oil. This includes products such as tomato sauce and tomato paste. Also see *functional foods.*

Lyme disease   a tick-borne, inflammatory disease which initially causes fever, stiffness, and rash. The distinguishing early symptom is the "bull's eye" rash at the site of the tick bite. Arthritis-like symptoms and cardiac problems appear in later stages. There is a limited chance that dogs (or other animals allowed outside) that are used in pet therapy programs could carry the ticks. All animals used in pet therapy programs should be examined prior to interacting with patients. See *animal facilitated therapy, infection, zoomatology.*

lymph node   (CDC) secondary immune organs distributed at discrete locations throughout the body. These organs play a central role in the activation and trafficking of immune lymphocytes in the body.

lymphocyte   (HHS/NMDP) a type of white blood cell subdivided into T cells and B cells. T cells provide cellular immunity and B cells form antibodies. T cells are responsible for graft-versus-host disease. The majority of leukocytes are lymphocytes or white blood cells, which are important in making antibodies. They are also important in surveying for cells carrying infectious agents as well as for eliminating tumor cells.

lymphokine   cell products that serve as chemical mediators of lymphocyte functions.

lymphoma   (HHS/NMDP) malignant proliferation of lymphocytes, generally within lymph nodes, but sometimes involving other tissues such as the liver and spleen. Lymphoma includes *Hodgkin's* and Non-Hodgkin's diseases.

lymphotrophic   (HHS) denoting a virus that tends to bind to and infects one or more subsets of lymphocytes.

M

macrocephaly a birth defect that has the observable physical characteristic of an enlarged head. This abnormal enlargement of the head does not represent a specific syndrome but is present with a variety of pathological conditions including *hydrocephalus*.

macrophage See *monocyte*.

macrovascular disease See *diabetes*.

mad cow disease (HHS) See *bovine spongiform encephalopathy*.

magical thinking the belief that what one thinks (e.g., that one is a princess) or how one thinks will make events change (omnipotence of thought). Magical thinking is a recognized developmental milestone that usually disappears by around age seven. Magical thinking is different than positive or negative thinking which influences behavior — magical thinking represents the belief in the unlikely. See *defense mechanism, development, medical play*.

magnetic resonance imaging (MRI) The MRI uses a magnetic field instead of radiation to make a three-dimensional image similar to the CAT scan. The MRI produces the clearest and crispest anatomical picture available today. See *computerized axial tomography*.

magnetic strip card (HCO) a plastic card with a magnetic strip on the back that can store about 250 characters, mainly for identification and verification of eligibility for insurance benefits.

mainstreaming a term used in the 1970's and 1980's to mean the placement of individuals with disabilities into groups without disabilities. See *inclusive education, inclusive recreation*.

maintenance program a behaviorally based program that is designed to maintain a desired behavior, weight, or learning level. See *behavior modification program*.

major depressive disorder a diagnostic category in the **DSM-IV** which has six types: mild, moderate, severe (without psychotic features, severe with psychotic features, in partial remission or in full remission); chronic; with catatonic features; with melancholic features; with atypical features; and with postpartum onset. Women have a lifetime risk of major depressive disorder of 10% - 25% and men have a lifetime risk of major depressive disorder of 5% - 12%. The risk of having major depressive disorder as a secondary diagnosis exceeds 20% for general medical conditions such as "diabetes, myocardial infarction, carcinomas, and *cerebrovascular accident*." (**DSM-IV**, p. 341) See *alcohol-induced disorders, depression, substance abuse*.

major life activities (ADA) functions such as caring for oneself, performing manual tasks, walking, seeing, hearing, speaking, breathing, learning, and working. See *activities of daily living, advanced activities of daily living, disability*.

malabsorption syndrome (HHS) syndromes resulting from impaired absorption of nutrients from the bowel.

maladaptive behavior which is used to meet some need but which is not considered to be a positive, productive adaptation to the environment. See *adaptation*.

malaise (CDC) a feeling of general discomfort or uneasiness; an out-of-sorts feeling, often the first indication of an infection or other disease.

malfeasance See *employee malfeasance*.

malignant uncontrolled (or partially controllable) growth or spread of a cancer. Also used to refer to the spread of a negative social influence.

managed care 1. an integrated fiscal and service delivery management system which consists of a review of the patient's health care needs and then the authorization for payment for the required services prior to the services being delivered. The case manager, usually a nurse, takes into account such issues as the *appropriateness* of specific services, the medical necessity of those services and the potential need for particular treatment modalities. Some of the types of managed care are shown in the table on the next page. 2. (HCO) a vaguely defined term referring to various systems of health care delivery that attempt to manage the cost, quality, and accessibility of health care. See *accessibility, availability, capitated, critical pathway, gatekeeper, independent practice association, prior review, rehabilitation centers*.

managed care organization (HCO) an organization, such as a health maintenance organization or preferred provider organization that uses one or more techniques of managed care.

managed competition (FB) an approach to health care reform that combines health insurance market reform with health care delivery system restructuring. The theory of managed competition is that the

Types of Managed Care Models

Type	Discussion
Group	A type of managed care organization which contracts with a single, independent group of health care providers to provide services for its members.
Individual Practice Association	A type of managed care organization that holds contracts predominately with solo or single practice health care providers. These providers may be truly solo practitioners, part of an association of independent practitioners (contract is with the association), and/or multi-specialty group practices.
Mixed	A type of managed care organization which contracts with a combination of individual and group/organizational practices, with no specific type of managed care model predominant.
Network	A type of managed care organization that is primarily made up of multiple contracts with independent group practices. This type of managed care model may use its own staff as well as maintaining contracts with independent practice groups.
Staff	A type of managed care organization in which the organization hires its own health care staff, and directly controls the practice.

quality and economy of health care delivery will improve if independent groups compete with one another for consumers in a government-regulated market.

mandate an action that is required by law. See *CFR*.

maneuver a complex series of specific moves used to measure a patient's *functional ability* or to implement a *treatment*. An example of a maneuver might be opening the fingers of a patient who has a clenched fist. It is easier to open a clenched fist if the patient's palm is facing up instead of down and the thumb is extended away from the palm. This maneuver is useful when the patient has grabbed a staff person or other patient in anger or needs to un-tense his/her arm. Other words for maneuver are "method" or "technique."

mania an abnormally euphoric emotional state which lasts at least a week. The medical criteria for diagnosing mania require that the patient exhibit at least three of the following symptoms (**DSM-IV**): 1. expanded *self-esteem* or grandiosity, 2. reduced need for sleep and frequently feeling rested after just three or four hours of sleep, 3. pressured or excessive speech, 4. racing thought patterns, with little or no insight into his/her degree of limited concentration and brief attention span, 5. easily distracted by insignificant stimuli, 6. increased activity with unrealistic goals being set ("I will run five miles and then visit three different friends before lunch.") or excessive psychomotor *agitation*, and 7. the over-engagement in pleasurable activities without regard for the consequences (going on a shopping spree or engaging in high risk activities without taking the appropriate precautions). The manic episode can be so severe that it interferes with the patient's ability to engage in (and complete) normal *activities of daily living* including self-care, work, and engaging

in healthy leisure activities. A patient may be exhibiting the above symptoms but may not be exhibiting a manic episode if the manic episode is a result of *substance abuse*, medication, or other treatment or hyperthyroidism. A different diagnosis would be given in those situations. *Hypomanic episodes* are episodes of mania that are not severe enough to warrant a manic diagnosis (lasting up to four days and, while behavioral changes are noted, the changes do not cause significant functional problems). See *bipolar disorder, distractibility, pressured speech.*

manual dexterity the ability to coordinate actions and movements of the hands.

manual traction the use of one's hands and muscles to provide the "pull." This type of traction is usually used in first aid or emergency care (e.g., reducing a fracture or relocating a joint). See *traction.*

mapping See *pathfinding.*

marked crosswalk (ADA) a crosswalk or other identified path intended for pedestrian use in crossing a vehicular way. Usually this is denoted by obvious lines that define the path to be used to cross the street. Marked crosswalk does not mean that the crosswalk must have an electric pedestrian crosswalk light.

marketing plan the clearly defined goals (*outcomes*) which define how the business will be presented to the public along with the step-by-step "map" of how each goal is to be achieved.

mask/snorkel/fin a water exercise program developed by Michael Gavin, RPT allowing participants movement in water in a prone position without holding their breath. It is effective for isolated treatment of specific joints as well as allowing mobility for individuals who are not capable of other modes of exercise. See *aquatic therapy.*

mastery ability to demonstrate greater than functional skills for a given task. See *functional ability.*

match (HHS/NMDP) In marrow transplantation, the word "match" relates to how similar the *human leukocyte antigens* (HLA) typing is between the donor and the recipient. The best kind of match is an "identical match." This means that all six of the HLA antigens (2 A antigens, 2 B antigens, and 2 DR antigens) are the same between the donor and the recipient. This type of match is described as a "6 of 6" match. Donors and recipients who are "mismatched" at one antigen are considered a "5 of 6" match, and may be considered suitable for bone marrow transplantation. See *histocompatibility.*

MDS See *Minimum Data Set.*

Meals on Wheels a program which provides up to 14 meals a week for individuals who are over 60 years of age, homebound due to *disease* or *disability,* and have difficulty preparing nutritious meals. The local Meals on Wheels agency in each area delivers the frozen meals right to the individual's home each week. The meals, usually one breakfast and one dinner for each day, include a high quality protein entree, vegetable, and rice or potato, plus a choice of white or whole wheat roll and margarine (dinner) or eggs, pancakes, or French toast, fruit, and a choice of juice (breakfast). The food is prepared with no added salt and contains limited fat and very few spices. While the costs of the meals is minimal and a donation is requested for the food, no eligible participant is denied based on his/her inability to pay.

mean a statistical measure calculated by adding all of the scores together and dividing by the number of people taking the test. Means are used to make logical assumptions about a larger group of people based on the means from a sample group. Knowing that the average (mean) five year old cannot write in cursive allows a teacher to set his/her expectations for writing performance accurately, thus likely reducing stress in a youth. See *standard deviation.*

measurement the process of documenting observed skills and behaviors and/or recording attitudes/feelings. The process of measurement usually measures one of three types of activity: 1. *process measures* (comparing the process of one technique or action to another process, e.g., how are the steps of a new treatment technique different from the steps of another, more established technique), 2. *product measures* (determining "how much" or outcomes of a process, e.g., what is the result of the measured action and how often does the result occur) and, in the arena of measuring impact on consumers 3. *satisfaction measures* (customer perceptions compared to customer expectations). Once it is

determined what is to be measured, the question of how something will be measured needs to be answered. This usually involves defining the scope, criteria, and type of data collection. Measurement, as part of the *evaluation* process has three steps (burlingame, 1996): 1. "scope," which is the identification of the issues and areas to be measured; 2. "*criteria,*" which is the development of a general understanding of the areas to be measured and identifying/developing criteria as to what should be found; and 3. "*data,*" which includes the establishment of the exact method to be used and the actual collection of the information. See *clinical opinion, instrument, scales, test.*

mechanical soft diet similar to the light or convalescent *diet,* this food differs only in that it needs to be prepared for individuals who are not likely to be able to chew the food (e.g., those with no teeth). Whole meats are avoided because they require chewing. See *diet.*

medial referring to the middle portion or the midline of the body; closest to the midpoint. Compare to *lateral.*

Medicaid (Title XIX) (FB) a joint federal/state program that provides health care and health-related services for low-income individuals. Medicaid regulations are established by each state within federal guidelines and the eligibility requirements and services covered vary significantly among the states. In general, Medicaid pays for medical, nursing home, and home health care for individuals who meet the eligibility requirements. In some states, Medicaid also pays for *adult daycare* and in-home services such as personal care and homemaker services. Financial eligibility for Medicaid is determined by a means test, in which a ceiling is placed on the maximum income and assets an individual may have in order to qualify for assistance. The income and asset levels for qualifying vary from state to state. See *Health Care Financing Administration, Medicaid waiver, Medicare/Medicaid history, Section 1905 (d).*

Medicaid waiver an approval from the government to use Medicaid funds in a different manner than outlined by the *Medicaid* law. Medicaid waivers are frequently used to fund demonstration projects.

medical chart See *medical record.*

medical clearance a statement from the patient's physician that s/he is able (cleared) to participate in activities. Medical clearance frequently involves a qualifier that says how much or how strenuous the activity may be. Compare with *medical limitations.*

medical equipment See *environment of care.*

medical information bus (HCO) a hardware and

software standard (IEEE P1073) that enables standardized connections between medical monitoring devices and clinical information systems.

medical limitations the restrictions placed on a patient's activity level by the physician based on the patient's medical status.

medical logic module (MLM) (HCO) a component of the *Arden syntax*.

medically complex a description that indicates that a patient's diagnoses and medical needs fall outside the parameters of most standard *critical pathways* or *protocols*. The patient has enough differences between what is clinically wrong and what is normally seen that the treatment team needs to take a different approach than what would normally be taken. An example might be a patient with a *bipolar disorder* who is also deaf and a diabetic. While most patients with bipolar disorders benefit from medication and participation in various therapeutic groups, a patient who is also deaf and has diabetes requires extra services. The medical team may also need to ensure that the medications prescribed do not have negative interaction patterns with the patient's insulin treatment.

medical management systems systems that are designed to ensure that each patient receives an appropriate quality and quantity of services based on his/her measured need and established *standards* of practice. These systems rely on externally developed standards of practice (standards set by professional organizations), ways to measure the quality of the patient's care as it is taking place, patterns of utilization through the *utilization review* process, *case management*, and effective *customer service*.

medical model The medical model assumes that all illnesses and disabilities originate from specific physical causes and that, once the causes are rooted out and corrected, the patient will experience good health. See *behavioral model, disease model*.

medical play the process of desensitizing the patient to medical treatment by using playful activities. Not every patient is cognitively mature enough to understand a straightforward explanation for what is going to happen or what has happened to him/her. It is normal for us, as adults, to tolerate invasive procedures related to health care (e.g., filling a cavity, pelvic exam, vaccination shot). The ability to tolerate these painful, humiliating affronts to our feelings of *self-esteem* and safety can only be done because we have the cognitive ability to reason through the process. Developmentally, the ability to reason through invasive procedures starts emerging about

Significant Dates in Medicare/Medicaid History

1950	Social Security Act required States to establish programs for licensing nursing homes, but did not specify what the standards or enforcement procedures should be.
1965	Medicare and Medicaid Act passed with responsibility for administration given to the Department of Health, Education, and Welfare (HEW).
1971	Intermediate care facility benefit transferred to the Medicaid program along with *intermediate care facilities for the mentally retarded*. President Nixon also committed the federal government to a program of improvements in nursing homes.
1972	Congress provided full funding for survey and certification activities. Congress also directed HEW to produce a single set of skilled nursing facility requirements.
1974	Final standards for intermediate care facilities and intermediate care facilities for the mentally retarded published.
1975	State of Colorado was sued in federal court on behalf of patients in a Colorado nursing home. Plaintiffs claimed that the Department of Health and Human Services had failed to ensure that patients were receiving quality care.
1982	Institute of Medicine conducted a full-scale study of nursing home regulations, survey and certification process, and enforcement process.
1983	Institute of Medicine study concluded and the Patient Care and Services *Survey Process* was introduced.
1986	New Survey Process implemented.
1987	Omnibus Budget Reconciliation Act (*OBRA*) passed which established a new enforcement system for nursing homes.
1989	Omnibus Budget Reconciliation Act (OBRA) amended the nursing home reform law.
1992	Omnibus Budget Reconciliation Act (OBRA) amended.
1995	Omnibus Budget Reconciliation Act (OBRA) amended.
1998	Medicare starts prospective payment system for nursing homes.

the age of seven years. Many of the patients that a therapist sees will never reach this "age of reasoning." Because they lack the ability to reason through the process, patients react, instead, with increased *stress*, higher levels of *fear*, and possibly higher levels of *acting out*. The therapist working with this category of patient can help ease the *pain* and stress associated with invasive procedures by using age-appropriate methods of preparing patients for what is happening or what has happened as described in the section on developmental stages at the end of the dictionary (p. 350). The terms "dolls" and "puppets" refer to any of the choices available for medical play. These dolls and puppets frequently have "removable" skins that reveal vital organs. Some of the dolls and puppets wear glasses or use a wheelchair. These dolls and puppets are not the ones usually purchased at the local toy store and used by children. See *development.*

medical record the record of the medical care that a patient has received. Medical records are subject to multiple regulations. Also called a "medical chart." See *patient record, Regenstrief Medical Record System.*

medical savings accounts (FB) a trust created or organized exclusively for the purpose of paying the medical expenses of beneficiaries of such a trust.

medical status the degree of illness or wellness that a patient is experiencing.

medical team previously a reference to the entire team of professionals and para-professionals who addressed the patient's health care needs. Now "medical team" refers to the physicians who address the patient's health care needs, while the term "treatment team" refers to the entire team.

Medicare/Medicaid automated certification system (MMACS) a computerized system that collects and maintains *provider* and supplier certification information for program administration and analysis.

Medicare/Medicaid history To many health care practitioners, *Medicare* and *Medicaid* seem to be ageless. In reality, they are fairly new health care funding laws. The chart on the previous page provides a general overview of the historical milestones of the two laws.

Medicare (Title XVIII) (FB) a nationwide, federally administered health insurance program authorized by Title XVIII of the Social Security Act of 1965 to cover the cost of hospitalization, medical care, and some related services for eligible persons over age 65, people receiving Social Security Disability Insurance payments for two years, and persons with *end-stage renal disease*. Medicare consists of two separate but coordinated programs —

hospital insurance (Part A) and supplementary medical insurance (Part B). Health insurance protection is available to insured persons without regard to income and is mainly funded through the US Treasury and the Medicare portion of the payroll tax. See *entitlement programs, Health Care Financing Administration, hospital insurance tax, Medicare/Medicaid history, occupational therapy, Office for Civil Rights Clearance.*

meditation a type of relaxation technique. The purposeful focusing of thoughts on just one thing and attempting to ignore all other stimuli. Many people who meditate position themselves comfortably and then attempt to clear their mind of any thoughts or repeat a word over and over again. Meditation has been helpful in reducing symptoms in patients with high blood pressure, migraine headaches, and heart disease. It has some impact on *anxiety*, *depression*, anger, and obsessive thinking. Relaxation and better breathing happen almost immediately but measurable impact and mastery usually require daily practice over a period of weeks or months. See *hypertension, relaxation techniques.*

medulla See *brainstem.*

melancholia an old-fashioned term for depression.

member in managed care, the covered individual and/or his/her dependents; synonymous with patient and insured.

memory composed of: 1. the physiological process of retaining information (input) as a result of nerve stimulation (retention function), 2. the system that describes how individuals store the input (storage function), and 3. information itself (history function). Memory is also described by how long the input is kept (or where kept) as in short-term and long-term memory. Short-term memory refers to the storage of information that the individual is using or has just used. Thoughts are encoded and organized in *short-term memory*. Because short-term memory has limited ability to store large quantities of information, some of the information is selected, encoded, and shifted to long-term memory. Long-term memory contains past learned information, including information related to concepts and words, rules and

Terms for Memory

Term	Also known As
Long-term Memory	recent memory, recent past memory, remote memory, and secondary memory
Short-term Memory	immediate memory, working memory, primary memory, and buffer memory

social/governmental expectations, organizational strategies, and other memories of past experiences. The table above shows synonyms for the two types of memory. See *alcohol-induced disorder, cognition, dementia, fluid intelligence, memory book, memory deficit, processing deficits, recognition, retrieval.*

memory book a book, usually made by staff and family for a specific patient, to help him/her remember vital information. A memory book is a type of *prosthetic device.* See *graphic output.*

memory deficit inability to recall information stored in one's brain, either short (working) or long-term memory. Depending on the cause of the memory deficit, the individual may exhibit a combination of the following symptoms: poor learning ability, reduced *self-esteem,* short-term *memory* loss, long-term memory loss, *disorientation, confabulation,* and poor safety awareness. Treatment for individuals who have difficulty recalling personal information is provided with a prosthetic device called a *memory book.*

meningitis (CDC) an infection of the fluid of a person's spinal cord and the fluid that surrounds the brain. People sometimes refer to it as spinal meningitis. Meningitis is usually caused by a viral or bacterial infection. Knowing whether meningitis is caused by a virus or bacterium is important because the severity of illness and the treatment differ. Viral meningitis is generally less severe and resolves without specific treatment, while bacterial meningitis can be quite severe and may result in brain damage, hearing loss, or learning disability. For bacterial meningitis, it is also important to know which type of bacteria is causing the meningitis because antibiotics can prevent some types from spreading and infecting other people. Before the 1990's, Haemophilus influenzae type b (Hib) was the leading cause of bacterial meningitis, but new vaccines being given to all children as part of their routine immunizations have reduced the occurrence of invasive disease due to H. influenzae. Today, Streptococcus pneumoniae and Neisseria meningitidis are the leading causes of bacterial meningitis. High fever, headache, and stiff neck are common symptoms of meningitis in anyone over the age of two years. These symptoms can develop over several hours, or they may take one to two days. Other symptoms may include nausea, vomiting, discomfort looking into bright lights, confusion, and sleepiness. In newborns and small infants, the classic symptoms of fever, headache, and neck stiffness may be absent or difficult to detect, and the infant may only appear slow or inactive, or be irritable, have vomiting, or be feeding poorly. As the disease progresses, patients of any age may have

seizures. Early diagnosis and treatment are very important. If symptoms occur, the patient should see a doctor immediately. The diagnosis is usually made by growing bacteria from a sample of spinal fluid. The spinal fluid is obtained by performing a spinal tap, in which a needle is inserted into an area in the lower back where fluid in the spinal canal is readily accessible. Identification of the type of bacteria responsible is important for selection of correct antibiotics. Bacterial meningitis can be treated with a number of effective antibiotics. It is important, however, that treatment be started early in the course of the disease. Appropriate antibiotic treatment of most common types of bacterial meningitis should reduce the risk of dying from meningitis to below 15%, although the risk is higher among the elderly. Some forms of bacterial meningitis are contagious. The bacteria are spread through the exchange of respiratory and throat secretions (e.g., coughing, kissing). Fortunately, none of the bacteria that cause meningitis are as contagious as things like the common cold or the flu, and they are not spread by casual contact or by simply breathing the air where a person with meningitis has been. However, sometimes the bacteria that cause meningitis have spread to other people who have had close or prolonged contact with a patient with meningitis caused by Neisseria meningitidis (also called meningococcal meningitis) or Hib. People in the same household or day-care center, or anyone with direct contact with a patient's oral secretions (such as a boyfriend or girlfriend) would be considered at increased risk of acquiring the infection. People who qualify as close contacts of a person with meningitis caused by N. meningitidis should receive antibiotics to prevent them from getting the disease. Antibiotics for contacts of a person with Hib meningitis disease are no longer recommended if all contacts four years of age or younger are fully vaccinated against Hib disease. There are vaccines against Hib and against some strains of N. meningitidis and many types of Streptococcus pneumoniae. The vaccines against Hib are very safe and highly effective. There is also a vaccine that protects against four strains of N. meningitidis, but it is not routinely used in the United States and is not effective in children under 18 months of age. The vaccine against N. meningitidis is sometimes used to control outbreaks of some types of meningococcal meningitis in the United States. Meningitis cases should be reported to state or local health departments to assure follow-up of close contacts and recognize outbreaks. Although large epidemics of meningococcal meningitis do not occur in the United States, some countries experience large, periodic epidemics.

Overseas travelers should check to see if meningococcal vaccine is recommended for their destination. Travelers should receive the vaccine at least one week before departure, if possible. A vaccine to prevent meningitis due to S. pneumoniae (also called pneumococcal meningitis) can also prevent other forms of infection due to S. pneumoniae. The pneumococcal vaccine is not effective in children under two years of age but is recommended for all persons over 65 years of age and younger persons with certain chronic medical problems.

meningococcal meningitis See *meningitis*.

meningomyelocele See *myelomeningocele*.

mens rea literally "evil intent;" a legal term used to describe one of the components required for a defendant to be found guilty. Lack of mens rea at the time the crime was committed is grounds for a plea of not guilty by reason of insanity. See *actus reus, criminal responsibility, insanity defense*.

mental abuse as defined by federal *Immediate and Serious Threat* regulations in the United States: The failure to prevent mental abuse whereby patients suffer psychological harm or trauma. Conditions/situations that may indicate mental abuse include: 1. patients who appear fearful, suspicious, or timid; shake when approached (jittery) or avoid eye contact; are overly obedient or defensive; who are crying or tearful, withdrawn, and reclusive; and 2. patients who are treated disrespectfully (e.g., laughed at, called names by staff).

mental disorder a psychiatric or behavioral syndrome which significantly impairs the individual's ability to function and is not an expected reaction to events in the environment.

mental retardation (MR) substantial limitations in present functioning characterized by significantly below average intellectual functioning, existing concurrently with related limitations in two or more of the following applicable adaptive skill (*adaptive functioning*) areas: communication, self-care, home

Adaptive Skill Areas for Assessing Mental Retardation

Adaptive Skill Category	Description
Communication	Skills in comprehending and expressing information, thought, symbolic behaviors, or non-symbolic behaviors
Self-Care	Skills in eating, *dressing*, hygiene, *grooming*
Home Living	Skills related to functioning within a home such as clothing care, housekeeping, property maintenance, food preparation, budgeting, safety, and daily scheduling
Social	Skills related to social exchanges with others including initiating, interacting, and terminating interaction with others, receiving and responding to situational cues, recognizing feelings, providing feedback, assisting others, forming and fostering friendships and love, coping with demands from others, making choices, sharing, understanding honesty and fairness, controlling impulses, conforming to laws, displaying appropriate socio-sexual behaviors
Community Use	Skills related to the appropriate use of community resources including shopping, attending religious services, using public transportation and public facilities.
Self-Direction	Skills related to making choices, following a schedule, initiating activities appropriate to the setting and personal interests, completing required tasks, seeking assistance when needed, resolving problems and self-advocacy skills
Health and Safety	Skills related to maintenance of one's health including eating, illness prevention and treatment, interacting with strangers, seeking assistance
Functional Academics	Skills related to learning at school that also have direct application to one's life in terms of independent living
Leisure	Skills in self-entertainment and interaction with others that reflects personal preferences and choices and, if the activity will be conducted in public, age and cultural norms; skills include choosing and self-initiating interests, using and enjoying home and community leisure and recreational activities alone and with others, playing socially with others, taking turns, terminating or refusing leisure or recreational activities, extending one's duration of participation, expanding one's repertoire of interests, awareness, and skills
Work	Skills related to holding a part or full-time job in the community, appropriate social behavior, task completion, awareness of schedules, interactions with co-workers.

Categories of Mental Retardation

Level	IQ Range	% of MR Population	Common Types of Therapy Objectives
Borderline	71-84	75% (combined Borderline and Mild)	community integration skills, independent leisure skills, social skills, basic community safety skills, ADLs
Mild	50-55 to 70		prevocational skills, personal safety skills
Moderate	35-40 to 50-55	20%	social skills, basic community safety, development of leisure skills to be used with staff support/structure, development of understanding of use of basic play/recreation objects, basic sensory stimulation, and environmental awareness
Severe	20-25 to 35-40	5% (combined Severe and Profound)	basic community safety skills, development of leisure skills to be used with staff support/structure, development of understanding of use of basic play/recreation objects, basic sensory stimulation, and environmental awareness
Profound	Below 20-25		development of leisure skills to be used with staff support/structure, development of understanding of use of basic play/recreation objects, basic sensory stimulation, and environmental awareness

living, social skills, community use, self-direction, health and safety, functional academics, leisure, and work. Mental retardation manifests before age 18 (Luckasson, 1992). There is a three-step procedure for diagnosing, classifying, and determining the supports needed by people with mental retardation. The first step, Dimension I (Intellectual Functioning and Adaptive Skills), determines if the person is eligible for supports. A person is eligible if his/her IQ is 70 to 75 or below and if s/he has significant disabilities in two or more adaptive skill areas and if the age of onset was below age 18. The adaptive skill areas that are assessed to determine the supports needed are shown in the chart on the previous page.

The second step includes Dimension II (Psychological/Emotional Considerations), Dimension III (Physical/Health/Etiology Considerations), and Dimension IV (Environmental Considerations). This second step identifies the strengths and weaknesses and the need for supports by describing the person's strengths and weaknesses psychologically and emotionally, by describing the person's overall physical health, and by describing the individual's current environmental placement as well as the optimal environment that would facilitate his/her continued growth and development. The third step identifies the kind and intensity of supports needed for each of the four dimensions. In general, the level of support the person needs parallels the person's limitations. Therefore, this third step requires the interdisciplinary team to determine the general intensities of needed supports across all four dimensions. The four

possible intensities of needed supports are intermittent, limited, extensive, and pervasive. A person classified as needing intermittent support on one or more of the four dimensions does not always need the supports or needs short-term support during lifespan transitions such as an acute medical crisis. A person classified as needing limited supports on one or more of the four dimensions needs time-limited consistent supports, usually requiring fewer staff members than the more intense levels of support, such as supports during the school to community adult transition process. A person classified as needing extensive support on one or more of the four dimensions needs support characterized by regular involvement (for example, daily) in at least some environments (such as work or home) which is not time limited. A person classified as needing pervasive support on one or more of the four dimensions need constant, high-intensity support provided across environments (Fletcher, 1996). Cause: There are many ways in which an individual can acquire an impaired intellectual ability. The table on the next two pages lists a few conditions or events that may lead to mental retardation. In the United States it is not customary to diagnose a child as having mental retardation until s/he has reached the chronological age of three years. This custom is probably because most standardized tests that measure IQ are not written for children younger than 3 1/2 years. Another reason may be that federal and state educational funding for testing and treatment is not available for individuals under the age of 36 months (3 years)

(*Public Law 94-142* and Public Law 101-476). About 10% of the school age population can be considered to be mentally retarded. To help distinguish between the degrees of severity of cognitive impairment, mental retardation is divided into 5 levels as shown in the chart on the previous page.

Impact on functional ability: The primary impacts of mental retardation on an individual's ability to engage in life activities are 1. decreased safety awareness, 2. decreased demonstration of the ability to initiate activity, 3. decreased ability to be independent in ADLs, 4. limited ability to independently achieve a healthy, balanced leisure lifestyle, and 5. increased interest in what might be considered to be age-inappropriate activity (i.e., doll play at age 42). While the cause is unknown, up to 30% of all individuals with mental retardation also have a diag-

nosable psychiatric disorder (compared to 5% of the normal population). The vast majority of individuals who are in the borderline, mild, and moderate levels who still reside in a state institution for the mentally retarded (ICF-MR) are there due to this *dual diagnosis*. For these individuals, the therapist's primary treatment objective may be to decrease the negative impact of the psychiatric disorder on community integration instead of the impact of a sub-normal IQ. See the table on the below for therapy concern. Following that is a list of syndromes and diseases associated with mental retardation. See *cerebral palsy, consumer rights, diabetes, initiation, intermediate care facilities for the mentally retarded, intelligence, intelligence quotient, Recreation Early Development Screening tool, self-injurious behavior.*

Mental Retardation, Concerns for Therapy

Concern	Intervention
decreased safety awareness	Frequently individuals with mental retardation are at increased risk due to vulnerability to neglect and abuse as well as due to a general lack of *judgment*. Specific training programs that replace the need for making a judgment are frequently helpful (e.g., training individuals that the first step to riding a bike is to put on a bike helmet, never cross a road without a "walk" sign).
decreased initiation	Lack of initiation tends to be due to two reasons: 1. lack of knowledge of how to participate in an activity and 2. lack of permission to start an activity. (Many individuals who live facilities are used to being cued to do anything or used to being required to get permission prior to starting an activity.)
decreased ADLs	Lack of ability to tend to one's basic daily living needs significantly impacts one's ability to engage in activities outside of the home. Especially for residents in supportive living situations, emphasis should be considered for skills required for *activities of daily living* (ADLs) in the community, e.g., using public restrooms, washing hands, donning and doffing coats, etc.
limited balance of leisure	Especially for individuals who live in facilities, the opportunity to have leisure opportunities in all domains (fine and gross motor, cognitive and social) tends to be at the whim of the house staff. The therapist can assist in the maintenance of a balanced leisure lifestyle by providing in-services for house staff, providing written instructions, and by monitoring actual participation patterns. The Recreation Participation Data Sheet (RPD) is a good method of monitoring this balance.
age inappropriate behaviors	It takes a long time for an individual with mental retardation to develop appropriate skills. The therapist will need to ensure that any skill that the individual is learning will be appropriate for him/her for the next 15 years.
psychiatric complications	Specific interventions to address the behaviors that negatively impact the individual's ability to integrate into the community should be addressed first, possibly prior to specific skill development. At times there will be individuals who are dangerous to people in the community and should not be integrated. These individuals will need to be taught a balanced set of skills which can be used while residing inside the grounds of the facility.

Syndromes and Diseases Associated with Mental Retardation

Name	Commonly Found Functional Limitations	Commonly Found Physical Attributes
Apert	mental retardation	premature fusion of skull, finger, and toe bones
Bardet-Biedl	mild to moderate mental retardation; loss of night vision which progresses to blindness	obesity; extra or fused fingers or toes

Syndromes and Diseases Associated with Mental Retardation (continued)

Name	Commonly Found Functional Limitations	Commonly Found Physical Attributes
Beckwith-Wiedemann	occasionally mild to moderate mental retardation	large body and tongue; defect in abdominal wall
Cornelia de Lange	mental retardation	small, possibly malformed feet, hands; continuous eyebrows
Cri du Chat	severe mental retardation; degenerating to profound; decreased muscle tone	small head; cries like a catcall when young; wide set eyes, receding chin, bone, joint, and cardiac disorders are common. See *chromosomal aberrations*.
Down Syndrome	mental retardation; decreased muscle tone	small stature, congenital heart disease, atlantoaxial dislocation condition. See *chromosomal aberrations*.
Ehlers-Danlos	increased risk management required during activities	poor healing of wounds; hypertension of joints
Ellis-van Creveld	occasional mental retardation	cardiac defects; short extremities
Erb's Palsy	decreased abduction of arm; decreased flexion of forearm	injury to 5th and 6th cervical nerves due to injury during delivery
Fetal Alcohol Syndrome	delayed development; possible mental retardation; possible hyperactivity	small head, large space between nose and upper lip
Fetal Hydantoin	borderline to mild mental retardation	due to prenatal exposure to anticonvulsants such as phenytoin (dilantin); cleft lip, depressed nasal bridge; widely spaced eyes
Fragile X	possible autistic like behaviors; mental retardation	large head; prominent ears
Goldenhar	possible deafness; occasional mental retardation	ear deficits; lateral cliff-like extension of edge of mouth; cleft palate
Hurler	impaired vision due to cloudy corneas; severe mental retardation; decreased muscle tone	short stature; excessive body hair
Klinefelter	potential osteoporosis; obese trunk with long legs; poor verbal skills and other learning disabilities.	May not develop until adolescence; immature sex organs. See *chromosomal aberrations*.
Lowe	impaired vision due to cataracts; mental retardation; hyperactivity	kidney abnormalities
Menkes	progressive cognitive deterioration; mental retardation	seizures; kinky hair; feeding difficulties
Prader-Willi	borderline to moderate mental retardation; compulsive eating disorder; poor muscle tone	small body stature; rounded face
Riley-Day	decreased sensory awareness; decreased pain awareness; increased risk of choking; emotional lability; mental retardation	
Rubinstein-Taybi	mental retardation	small head; slanted eyes; broad thumb
Sanfilippo	mental retardation with deteriorating cognitive ability; stiffness of joints	coarse facial features
Seckel	moderate to severe mental retardation	short stature; small head
Sjogren-Larrson	difficulty with ambulation due to spasticity in lower extremities; mental retardation	dry, rough, scaly skin
Smith-Lemli-Opitz	irritable; mental retardation; difficulty with eating	droopy eyelids; upturned nose

Syndromes and Diseases Associated with Mental Retardation (continued)

Name	Commonly Found Functional Limitations	Commonly Found Physical Attributes
Trisomy 18	mental retardation; poor fine motor skills due to hand clenched as part of the syndrome	narrow eyes; small head; early death See *chromosomal aberrations*.
Tuberous Sclerosis	seizures; occasional mental retardation	non-malignant tumors of the brain; brownish as well as white patches on skin
Turner	IQ usually low normal with impaired verbal scores; left-right disorientation; difficulty drawing pictures of people; and tendency to remain socially immature.	webbing of neck and short stature. See *chromosomal aberrations*.
Waardenburg	deafness	white hair lock; widely spaced eyes
Williams	mild mental retardation; usually good social skills, poorer motor skills	small stature

menu the options offered the computer user on his/her screen. By offering predetermined selections the computer user has a shortcut to the most frequently used options.

mesencephalon See *midbrain*.

mesh graft When a larger area needs to be covered than donor tissue is available for, the donated skin may be cut to resemble a mesh. This allows the donated skin to be stretched over a larger area. The therapist must take extra caution when working with patients with mesh grafts to ensure the physician's orders related to movement are strictly followed.

messaging standard (HCO) a standard governing the structure of electronic messages between computers.

meta-analysis (HCO) quantitative synthesis of the statistical results of numerous studies on a given topic.

metabolic disorders disorders that result from a loss of metabolic control over one's heartbeat, *blood pressure*, body temperature, electrolyte balance, respiration, or other homeostatic functions. Metabolic disorders can be due to a variety of causes including hepatic failure, renal failure, *hypoglycemia*, diabetic ketoacidosis, and acute intermittent *porphyria*. All of these causes may lead to a metabolic-disorder-caused encephalopathy with symptoms starting out as problems with *memory* (especially most recent memory) and *orientation*. The patient may appear agitated and anxious to the point of being *hyperactive* or just the opposite, appearing quiet and inactive. As the pathology progresses, the patient will become less responsive, eventually leading to a loss of consciousness and potentially death. See *agitation, electroencephalogram*.

metabolic equivalents (MET) a measurement of the amount of energy expended by an adult of average weight while sleeping. It is equivalent (approximately) to one kilocalorie $\bullet$ kg^{-1} $\bullet$ hr^{-1}. METs pro-
vide a measurable way to assess activity and are therefore an important concept for therapists seeking to establish baselines and measure effectiveness of treatments claiming to increase physical fitness. Researchers will also appreciate the advantages of being able to quantify the physical aspects of leisure activity involvement. The table on the next page lists the METs for specific leisure activities at four self-reported intensities.

metastasis the process of *cancer* cells leaving their original site of origin and spreading to other locations in the body. Once in the other location, the cells continue to multiply. Malignant tumors do not have an outer structure or skin, making it relatively easy for cells to separate from the original tumor site and travel through the lymph or blood systems to other parts of the body. Once a tumor has metastasized it tends to be harder to treat.

methicillin-resistant Staphylococcus aureus See *Staphylococcus aureus*.

mezzanine or mezzanine floor (ADA) that portion of a story which is an intermediate floor level placed within the story and having occupiable space above and below its floor.

MIB See *medical information bus*.

micromho one millionth of a mho; a unit of electrical conductance used in galvanic skin response and electrodermal response biofeedback.

microvascular disease See *diabetes*.

microvolt one-millionth of a volt.

midbrain (mesencephalon; middle of the head) the position on top of the brain stem, below the cortex. The brain stem or the medulla, pons, and midbrain, houses the reticulum formation, a complex structure that integrates many sensory and motor functions. This unique formation also influences general levels of consciousness (sleep-awake) and more complex sensory motor functions.

midlife crisis a pop psychology term coined during

Metabolic Equivalents (METs) for Leisure Time Activities
at Four Self-Reported Intensities (Sallis & Owen, 1999).

Activity Type	Type and Intensity Codes	How vigorous was the activity?			
		Very	Fairly	Not Very	Not at all
Athletics	a, vh	8	6	4	2
Table Tennis	m	4	3	2	1
Sailing/boating	m	4	2	2	1
Cricket/football	a, vh	12	8	6	4
Snow Skiing	vh	12	8	6	4
Water Skiing	h	12	8	6	4
Ice Skating	vh	12	8	6	4
Lawn Bowls	m	4	3	2	1
Walking	a, m	7	4	2	1
Jogging	a, vh	13	10	7	4
Calisthenics	a, h	12	9	7	4
Aerobics	a, vh	12	8	6	4
Weight training	m	4	3	2	1
Circuit training	a, vh	12	8	4	3
Swimming	a, h	10	6	3	1
Bicycling	a, m	9	6	3	1
Netball/basketball	a, vh	12	8	4	2
Golf	m	4	3	2	1
Tennis	vh	8	6	4	2
Squash	a, vh	13	10	7	4

Key: a = aerobic activities; vh = very hard activities; h = hard activities; m = low activities

the 1960's to explain personality changes made by individuals in their 40's in response to stress, hormonal changes, failing health, and relationship problems. Midlife itself is considered to span the ages of 40 to 60. Conventional wisdom in the United States assumed that individuals, when reaching the tumultuous age of 40, would stop to re-examine their lives and make major changes. The stereotypical image of a midlife crisis is that men buy red sports cars and enter into affairs with younger women. A study funded by the MacArthur Foundation found that nine out of ten individuals (N=7,800) perceived that they never experienced what they would consider a midlife crisis. Most of the respondents stated that they were relatively content despite challenges such as children (and grandchildren) being born, growing up, and leaving the house; careers changing; parents getting ill and dying; and changes in their physical well-being. As a whole, the respondents indicated that there were only two things that they did not have enough of: money and sex. The trends in popular press have been to drop the age requirement previously associated with midlife crisis and apply it to any group that is experiencing a major change in life patterns. With the crisis seen by dot.com enterprises in the early years of the twenty-

first century, many newspaper and magazine articles are talking about the twenty-something age group experiencing midlife crises because of the downturn in dot.com stock prices. See *empty-nest syndrome.*

milieu environment. In a therapy setting, a therapeutic milieu is an environment that is structured to meet the emotional and survival needs of the patient.

military time using a twenty-four hour clock to measure time instead of the standard twelve-hour clock. With military time, three in the afternoon is 1500 (fifteen hundred) hours.

Mini-Mental State Examination (MMS) This assessment was developed by M. F. Folstein, S. Folstein, and P. R. McHugh (1975). This well-thought-out, easy to use assessment tool measures cognitive functioning. Used by professionals, the interrater reliability is excellent and because of the thorough research that went into its development, the validity is also excellent. See the next page. (The latter part of this assessment may prove difficult for those with visual impairments. It is considered within testing guidelines to use bold, large print where needed.)

Minimum Data Set (MDS) the interdisciplinary assessment tool required for every patient admitted to a nursing home in the United States. Also known as the *Resident Assessment Instrument.*

Mini-Mental State Examination

Maximum Score	
	Orientation
5	What is the (year), (season), (date), (day), (month)?
5	Where are we (state), (county), (hospital), (floor)?
	Registration
3	Name three objects: One second to say each. Then ask the patient to repeat all three after you have said them. Give one point for each correct answer. Repeat them until s/he learns all three. Count trials and record number.
	Number of Trials: _____
	Attention and Calculation
5	Begin with 100 and count backwards by 7 (stop after five answers). Alternatively, spell "world" backwards.
	Recall
3	Ask for the three objects repeated above. Give one point for each correct answer.
	Language
2	Show a pencil and a watch and ask subjects to name them.
1	Repeat the following "No ifs, ands, or buts."
3	A three-stage command "take a paper in your right hand; fold it in half and put it on the floor."
1	Read and obey the following: CLOSE YOUR EYES
1	Write a sentence.
1	Copy a design (complex - a closed shape with more than 4 angles, i.e. ⌂
30	**Total Score Possible**

Minnesota Multiphasic Personality Inventory (MMPI) an objective personality assessment developed in 1937 by Starke Hathaway and J. Charnley McKinley. The MMPI is now in its second edition and is referred to as the MMPI-2. The MMPI-2 has five hundred statements such as "I sometimes tease animals" to which the patient is to respond with "true" or "false" or "I cannot say." The MMPI is scored into ten standardized scales as well as providing feedback on validity [lie scale (to help identify defensiveness or problems with the personality measurement process), infrequency scale (to help identify potential issues of illiteracy or confusion), and suppressor scale (to help mathematically adjust scale to decrease false positives and negatives)] and a "special" category [*anxiety* (which reflects any trends toward psychopathology), repression (reflects the tendency to engage in denial), ego strength (reflects the degree to which the patient is able to function at work and in social situations), and the McAndrews Alcoholism Scale (estimates degree of proneness to addictions)]. The ten clinical scales of the MMPI are *hypochondriasis*, *depression*, hysteria, psychopathic deviance, masculinity-femininity, paranoia, *psychasthenia*, *schizophrenia*, hypomania, and social introversion. See *hypomanic episode*.

minority issues See *consumer rights*.

misogamist an individual who has an aversion to marriage.

misogynist an individual who has an aversion to women.

mission statement a vision statement about what the company does, what it wants to do, and what it values. A mission statement works as a "guiding light," leading the company toward its goal. Every policy, procedure, rule, and aspect of the company's daily operations should create and promote movement toward meeting the company's mission. Mission statements are not static; they need to change as the business/health care environment does.

mitogen substance that induces lymphocyte proliferation.

mixed a term frequently used in the **DSM-IV** to indicate the presence of two or more characteristics associated with a mental disorder.

mixed lymphocyte culture (MLC) (HHS/NMDP) a test that measures the level of reactivity between donor and recipient lymphocytes. See *histocompatibility*.

MMPI-2 See *Minnesota Multiphasic Personality Inventory.*

mobility ability to move from one location to another. For a patient to be considered independent in mobility s/he would need to be able to complete the following tasks without cueing or other assistance:

1. Ability to move from current position (point A) to desired position (point B) including ability to move in bed, with a wheelchair, to transfer, and/or to ambulate with prescribed mobility devices (if any),
2. Ability to use any prescribed mobility techniques and devices in a variety of community settings.

While the patient's initial training in these skills most likely will come from a physical therapist, other therapists will need to supervise, assist, and evaluate the patient in his/her skills related to mobility while on community integration outings. Some specific skills related to mobility are 1. identification of transportation options, 2. demonstration of ability to balance physical (e.g., endurance) and cognitive skills (e.g., map reading) with activity, 3. flexibility in *locomotion* skills/abilities to complement terrain and situation, and 4. ability to plan ahead when necessary to ensure accessibility along the route. See *bed, foam mattress bed, pressure sore, range of motion.*

modality the type of activity used to deliver treatment. A therapy intervention may call for an increased upper extremity active *range of motion* (ROM). The modalities to deliver this treatment could include an exercise program specifically geared toward meeting the goal or a prescriptive set of leisure activities that promote the required range of motion. The *treatment* is range of motion, the goal is increased ROM, and the modality is exercise or leisure activity. See *ethics, multidisciplinary pain center.*

modality-oriented clinic health care settings that provide a specific type of intervention (e.g., biofeedback clinics). The patients referred to this type of clinic generally have already received a comprehensive *evaluation*, so modality-oriented clinics generally do not provide a comprehensive evaluation and seldom offer *case management* services.

MODY maturity onset diabetes of youth. See *diabetes.*

money management the ability to use money as a token system, including the ability to anticipate expenditures, knowledge of mathematics related to money, consumer skills, and skills required to pass and collect money (e.g., checking systems, ATM cards, etc.).

monocyte a large mononuclear leukocyte; an immune cell formed from a precursor to bone marrow. Monocytes circulate in the blood, eventually migrating into tissues throughout the body, including the brain. While in tissue these cells mature and differentiate (activate their immunological functions) into a macrophage or microglial cell. Macrophages respond to trauma, injury, or infections in a matter of hours or days rather than weeks. They also play a significant role in wound repair and healing, ingesting and digesting debris (dead cells).

monosaturated fats See *fatty acids.*

monosodium glutamate (HHS) the sodium salt of glutamic acid. Glutamic acid, or glutamate, is one of the most common amino acids found in nature. In the early part of the century, MSG was extracted from seaweed and other plant sources. Today, MSG is produced in many countries around the world through a fermentation process of molasses from sugar cane or sugar beets, as well as starch and corn

sugar. See *glutamate.*

mood persistent emotional state. Mood is a concern if there are extremes of sustained *emotion* that interfere with *functional ability.* The **DSM-IV** lists four primary categories of mood disorders and two categories of specifiers. The four categories of mood disorders are mood episodes (major depressive episode, manic episode, mixed episode, and hypomanic episode), depressive disorders (major depressive disorder, dysthymic disorder, and depressive disorder not otherwise specified), *bipolar disorders* (bipolar I disorder, bipolar II disorder, cyclothymic disorder, and bipolar disorder not otherwise specified), and other mood disorders (mood disorder due to (name the general medical condition), substance-induced mood disorder, and mood disorder not otherwise specified). Specifiers which are used with mood disorders either describe the most recent episode (mild, moderate, severe without psychotic features, severe with psychotic features, in partial remission, in full remission, chronic, with catatonic features, with melancholic features, with atypical features, and with postpartum onset) or describe the course of recurrent episodes (longitudinal course with or without full interepisode recovery, with seasonal pattern or with *rapid cycling*). While not official diagnostic terms, the therapist may also find the following terms useful in documentation: dysphoric (unpleasant), euthymic (normal, healthy range of moods), expansive (overestimation of importance or without restraint), irritable (annoyed and angry), mood swings (oscillating mood extremes), elevated (confident and cheerful), *euphoria* (intense feelings of grandeur), ecstasy (intense rapture), *anhedonia* (loss of interest in life), grief (appropriate sadness), or alexithymia (inability to describe one's emotions). See *alcohol induced disorders, Beck Depression Inventory, behavioral lability, comorbidity, depression, dual diagnosis, dysthymia, failure to thrive, Global Assessment of Functioning Scale, psychosocial well-being, schizophrenia, schizoaffective disorder.*

mood state (RAPs) about 15% of nursing home patients will have a major depression; about 30% will exhibit noticeable symptomatic signs of a mood state problem. Such signs are often expressed as sad mood, feelings of emptiness, *anxiety*, or uneasiness. They are also manifested in a wide range of bodily complaints and dysfunctions, such as loss of weight, tearfulness, *agitation*, aches, and pains.

morbidity 1. an illness or abnormal condition. 2. the occurrence rate of a disease or abnormal health condition, usually within a specified geography area and time. Examples of morbidity include reports on the occurrence rate of HIV among teenagers within the county over a twelve-month period.

morbid obesity (HHS) a state of adiposity or overweight, in which body weight is 100% above the ideal and a body mass index of 45 or greater.

moribund from the Latin word "moribundus" which means to be in the process of dying; to be very near death.

mortality referring to death, usually referring to the death rate using standardized units of 100, 10,000, or 100,000.

Motion Picture Experts Group (MPEG) (HCO) a video compression standard.

motivation causes for behavior; processes, or internal states that drive a person to action. A person who is demonstrating motivated behavior becomes quickly involved in tasks, is eager to continue with the activity, or can appropriately change the activity as the situation dictates. Patients frequently require motivation to be able to make changes, engage in therapy, or to engage in self-improvement. Conversely, low motivation causes a patient to have a lower *tolerance* for frustration, have difficulty sticking to a task, and limited inclination to initiate activity. Ragheb and Beard (1990) conducted a review of literature for what motivates individuals to engage in free-time activity. The results of their literature review and subsequent field trials, led to four primary factors that motivate an individual to engage in activity. They found that a type of activity, or the perceived benefits of the activity, was a clear and measurable way to describe motivational forces. In the manual of their testing tool, *Leisure Motivation*

Scale, they describe the four factors as intellectual, social, competence-mastery, and stimulus avoidance. See the chart on the next page. See *Freud, leisure, initiation.*

motofacient tremor See *tremor.*

motor skills disorder See *developmental coordination disorder.*

movement referring to motion. Types of movement for the therapist to be familiar with are shown in the chart below. See *Brady kinesia, dyskinesia.*

movement therapy See *dance therapy.*

MRI See *magnetic resonance imaging.*

MRSA See *methicillin-resistant Staphylococcus aureus.*

MS See *multiple sclerosis.*

MSG See *monosodium glutamate.*

multiaxial system To help organize the *assessment* results and problem list of patients receiving psychiatric care, the American Psychiatric Association (APA) developed the multiaxial system. All disorders are placed in one of five axis. The APA's definition of Axis makes it similar to the term "domain." For a complete description of each of the five domains please refer to the **DSM-IV**. A description of the categories within each axis can be found in the table on the next page.

multiculturalism literally meaning many cultures. Cultural pluralism has developed as a result of immigration and a global economy. In the past the United States used the motto of "E pluribus unum" meaning from many to one. As with many of the countries in the world, the United States has shifted

Types of Movement

active	movement voluntarily done through the patient's use of his/her own muscles
angular	movement which changes the angle of two bones joined together by a common joint
associated	movement of body parts which normally would move together, e.g., the eyes
athetoid	movement marked by slow, continuous, writhing movements, especially in the hands
automatic	movement caused by the patient's own muscles, but not a voluntary movement, e.g., blinking of eyes
choreic/choreiform	involuntary jerky and irregular movements of a muscle or group of muscles
contralateral associated	movement of a paralyzed body part which is caused by a voluntary active movement on the non-paralyzed side
dystonic	movement which is a slow, gross motor movement with athetoid characteristics
frenkel's	movement exercises prescribed for patients with ataxia to help restore functional ability
passive	movement of a body part caused by another person or a machine
reflex	movement that is caused by an external stimulus that produces a reliably consistent response. A "knee jerk" is an example of a reflex; patients with spinal cord injuries or nerve damage may have diminished or absent reflexes.
spontaneous	movement which is initiated by the patient without any cueing
synkinetic	small, involuntary movements that naturally accompany larger, voluntary movements. An example might be when a patient pushes hard, his/her facial expression contorts.

Factors Involved in Leisure Motivation

Factor	Description
Intellectual	The intellectual component of leisure motivation is the extent to which individuals are motivated to engage in leisure activities that involve substantial mental activities such as learning, exploring, discovering, creating, or imagining.
Social	The social component is the extent to which individuals engage in leisure activities for social reasons. This component includes two basic needs. The first is the need for friendship and interpersonal relationships, while the second is the need for the esteem of others.
Competence-Mastery	The competence-mastery component is the extent to which individuals engage in leisure activities in order to achieve, master, challenge, and compete. The activities are usually physical in nature.
Stimulus-Avoidance	The stimulus-avoidance component of leisure motivation is the drive to escape and get away from over-stimulating life situations. It is the need for some individuals to avoid social contacts, to seek solitude and calm conditions; for others it is to seek rest and to unwind themselves.

from a cultural expectation of a homogenous population with one language, custom, and tradition into a heterogeneous population accepting many languages, customs, and traditions. This acceptance of a heterogeneous culture is referred to as multiculturalism.

multidisciplinary pain center (MPCs) an interdisciplinary treatment team that includes doctoral level scientists. Generally MPCs provide research and training in addition to patient care for those with either acute or chronic pain syndrome. The types of services provided generally include "comprehensive assessments, diagnoses, nerve blocks, *conditioning*, systematic relaxation training, *biofeedback*, and family therapy" (Scotece, 1993, p. 29). The philosophy and goals of MPCs are generally (Scotece, 1993):

1. to curtail or end narcotic intake where appropriate to avoid potential substance addiction;
2. to encourage increased activity levels by providing graded exercises with education to differentiate hurt from harm;
3. to avoid the use of passive *modalities* such as

heat, massage, or traction, and instead using electrotherapy in conjunction with active exercise, biofeedback and sympathetic and analgesic blocks;

4. to address the psychological and cognitive effects of chronic pain without attempting to infer causes and effects. Cognitive behavioral intervention with group therapy provides insight and operant conditioning principles strengthen healthy behaviors and increase the patient's knowledge of the emotional effects of pain; and
5. to return patients to meaningful work when possible or at least to a more independent, productive lifestyle.

See *multidisciplinary pain clinic, pain, pain clinic.*

multidisciplinary pain clinic a clinically based evaluation and treatment clinic for patients with either acute or chronic pain syndrome. This clinic differs from a *multidisciplinary pain center* as teaching and research activity are not a standard, ongoing functions of the clinic.

multifamily dwelling (ADA) any building containing more than two dwelling units.

Multiaxial System for Reporting Assessment Results

Axis	Areas Which are Usually Placed Under This Axis
Axis I	**Clinical Disorders and Other Conditions That May Be a Focus of Clinical Attention** (e.g., disorders usually diagnosed prior to the age 18 with the notable exception of mental retardation; substance-related disorders, schizophrenia and other psychotic disorders, eating disorders, etc.)
Axis II	**Personality Disorders and Mental Retardation** (e.g., paranoid personality disorder, obsessive-compulsive personality disorder, antisocial personality disorder, schizoid personality disorder, mental retardation, etc.)
Axis III	**General Medical Conditions** (e.g., infectious and parasitic diseases, congenital anomalies, injury and poisoning, diseases of the various body systems, complications of pregnancy, etc.)
Axis IV	**Psychosocial and Environmental Problems** (e.g., problems related to social environment or primary support group, occupational problems, housing or economic problems, difficulty accessing health care services, problems with the legal system, etc.)
Axis V	**Global Assessment of Functioning** (See *Global Assessment of Functioning (GAF) Scale.*)

multi-infarct dementia See *vascular dementia.*

multi-option a type of employee benefit plan that offers its employees a choice of benefit options including an indemnity plan, an indemnity plan tied to a preferred provider agreement, and/or a type of health maintenance organization.

multiple chemical sensitivity disorder (HHS) a controversial diagnosis of an allergy-like sensitivity to an unusually broad range and number of substances. This condition has not been subjected to rigorous scientific scrutiny, and there is considerable doubt as to whether or not it actually exists.

multiple myeloma (HHS/NMDP) a malignant disorder of the plasma cells. Multiple myeloma is frequently associated with bone pain and susceptibility to infection.

multiple personality disorder See **DSM-III-R**.

multiple sclerosis (MS) a chronic disabling disease of the central nervous system. There are two forms of MS: the relapsing/remitting type and the chronic type that progressively gets worse. Most new cases are adults between the ages of 20 and 40, more often women than men. During the course of the disease scattered areas of the myelin covering of the nerves degenerate. The destruction of this myelin covering causes a "short-circuiting" or blocking of the impulses that control a person's actions. The areas that have the degenerated patches are called plaques. As these areas of plaques combine to make larger holes in the myelin covering, the nerve impulses are not able to function correctly and the message that the nerve was carrying is lost in part or whole. If the nerve was carrying information needed for muscle movement, the movement will be weak or absent. If the nerve was carrying information involving sensation, numbness or tingling may be felt. Treatment includes the use of therapy to reduce muscle spasms, contractures of the muscles, and pain. Many patients have noticed that the symptoms get worse when they are under great emotional distress. See *ataxic gait.*

multiplexing (HCO) combination of many low-capacity communications channels into one high-capacity communications channel by interweaving the various channels in discrete time or frequency slices.

multi-step task a task that takes more than one type of action to complete. An example of a multiple step task would be asking a patient to finish up his project, put away his supplies, and go to his room to clean up for dinner. ("Get ready for dinner" is the task.)

Munchausen by proxy real illness in a child secretly caused by the child's caretaker, usually the mother. The caretaker causes the child to become ill so that the caretaker's own psychological needs can be met.

Munchausen's syndrome first identified in the 18th century by the German, Baron von Müchausen; a syndrome classified in the **DSM-IV** as a factitious disorder that presents with complaints of physical illness. Historically it has had a variety of names including "hospital addiction, polysurgical addictions, and professional patient syndrome" (Kaplan, Sadock & Grebb, 1994, p. 634). The current medical term for this disease is *pathomimicry*. This syndrome is better known for a similarly named syndrome, *Munchausen by Proxy*. While Baron von Münchausen's name is correctly spelled with an "ü," the syndrome is correctly spelled with an "u."

muscle strength a standardized rating scale developed by Daniels and Worthingham (1972) to indicate the degree of strength demonstrated by the patient. Shown below. See *spinal cord injury.*

muscle tone also known as *tonus*, the state of a muscle while resting in a partial contraction.

muscular dystrophy a group of genetically based diseases that are all characterized by a progressive atrophy of the muscle tissue (but not the neural tissue). The atrophy of the symmetric groups of skeletal muscle leads to increased weakness, disability, and deformity. The age of onset, the rate of progression, and the groups of muscles affected vary depending on the type of muscular dystrophy. The main course of treatment is physical therapy, modification of activities, and splinting. See *developmental coordination disorder, dystrophic gait.*

music therapy an established health care profession

Manual Muscle Evaluation — Strength

100%	5	N	Normal	Complete range of motion against gravity with full resistance
75%	4	G	Good	Complete range of motion against gravity with some resistance
50%	3	F	Fair	Complete range of motion against gravity
25%	2	P	Poor	Complete range of motion with gravity eliminated
10%	1	T	Trace	Evidence of contractility
0%	0	0	Zero	No evidence of contractility
S			Spasm	If spasm or contracture exists, place S or C after the grade of a move-
C			Contracture	ment incomplete for this reason.

that uses music to address the physical, psychological, cognitive, and/or social functioning of individuals with disabilities or illnesses. See *American Music Therapy Association.*

myalgic encephalomyelitis (CDC) a synonym for *chronic fatigue syndrome* in common usage in the United Kingdom and Canada.

myelodysplastic syndrome (HHS/NMDP) also called pre-leukemia or "smoldering" leukemia; a disease of the marrow in which inadequate platelets, red blood cells, and white blood cells are made. Sometimes a precursor to AML.

myelomeningocele During the first 30 days of development, the fetus may experience an abnormal formation of his/her spinal cord, vertebra, and skin. Myelomeningocele is an abnormal opening in the spinal column, allowing a pouch of membranes containing both the meninges and the spinal cord to balloon out of the bony, protective covering of the spine. Cause: While myelomeningocele is one of the most common neurologically oriented birth defects (1 in 1000 births) there are no clearly identified causes other than a prenatal exposure to the drug Depakene (which accounts for only a small percentage of those with myelomeningocele). Impact on functional ability: For individuals with myelomeningocele, functional limitations will vary depending on the degree of nerve involvement. Manifestations include partial paralysis of the lower extremities with accompanying sensory deficits, bowel and bladder dysfunction, and a significant chance of *hydrocephalus.* See *spina bifida.*

myeloproliferative disorders (HHS/NMDP) a group of disorders characterized by abnormal proliferation by one or more types of marrow cells.

myocardial infarction also known as a "heart attack;" an interruption in the supply of blood to the heart muscle caused by a clot (blockage) or plaque in an artery leading to the heart. The part of the heart that is not receiving blood dies, causing severe pain originating in the chest and radiating down the arms (some variation in the pain pattern can occur) along with sweating and a shortness of breath. Immediate emergency care is required. See *arteriosclerosis.*

myofascial pain See *fibromyalgia.*

myofibril a strand of muscle tissue that is contained within groups of branching threads running in the same direction as the long axis of the muscle cell. See *elasticity.*

myoglobin (HHS) the oxygen-transporting protein of muscle, resembling blood hemoglobin in function.

myopathy referring to a disease of a muscle that causes weakness or wasting. Myopathies are not the result of nerve dysfunction. See *dystrophic gait.*

myostatic contracture a type of contracture where the patient's ROM is decreased through inactivity with no pathological structures evident. A myostatic contracture responds to activities that promote gentle stretching of the affected area multiple times a day. Also referred to as a "tight" muscle.

N

narcolepsy (HHS) a sudden, uncontrollable disposition to sleep occurring at irregular intervals, with or without obvious predisposing or exciting causes.

narrative style of documenting rather than in outline form, this style of documentation is meant to read like a story, employing figures of speech to paint a word picture. This form of documentation is usually very interesting to write and to read. Answer the questions *who, what, when, where, why* to make the documentation complete.

nasal pertaining to the nose.

nasal polyposis the presence of a mass (polyp) located in the nasal cavity, middle metus, or pharyngeal passage that causes nasal obstruction, dry mouth, and snoring. Individuals with nasal polyposis may experience chronic sinusitis and exacerbation of his/her asthma. It is estimated that 7% of the individuals with asthma develop nasal polyposis. This percentage jumps to over 35% with individuals who convert to an *aspirin hypersensitivity triad.*

nasogastric tube (NG tube) a tube that is placed down the patient's nose into the patient's stomach. This tube is used to help provide nutritional supplements for patients who cannot eat because of a jaw injury, neurological damage, or *coma*. See *feeding tube, gastric gavage feeding tube.*

nasotracheal airway See *endotracheal airway.*

National Association for Music Therapy See *American Music Therapy Association.*

National Association of Activity Professionals (NAAP) the nationally recognized membership organization for activity professionals. NAAP's address is PO Box 5530, Sevierville, TN 37864, 423-429-0717, www.thenaap.org.

National Association of Recreation Therapists (NART) an organization formed in 1953 within the United States to help meet the needs of recreational therapists who worked in treatment centers. Charles Cottle, who was the director of Recreation and Education at Mississippi State Hospital, joined 23 other therapists from 19 psychiatric facilities and two state schools (for adults who were mentally retarded) to form NART. NART later joined two other groups to become the *National Therapeutic Recreation Society* under the *National Recreation and Park Association.*

National Certification Council for Activity Professionals (NCCAP) the nationally recognized certification body for activity professionals. NCCAP's address is PO Box 62589, Virginia Beach, VA 23466-2589, 757-552-0653.

National Committee for Quality Assurance (NCQA) the group that develops standards to evaluate the structure and the functioning of quality management systems in managed care organizations. NCQA's address is 2000 L Street, Suite 500, Washington, DC 20036, www.ncqa.org, 800-275-7585.

National Council for Therapeutic Recreation Certification (NCTRC) the nationally recognized certification body for recreational therapists (therapeutic recreation specialists). NCTRC's office mailing address is 7 Elmwood Dr., New City, NY 10956, 845-639-1439, www.nctrc.org. See *Joint Commission.*

National Health and Nutrition Examination Survey (NHANES) (HHS) a series of surveys that include information from medical history, physical measurements, biochemical evaluation, physical examination, and dietary intake of population groups within the United States. The NHANES is conducted by the US Department of Health and Human Services approximately every five years.

national health expenditures (NHE) (FB) an estimate of national spending on health care made up of two broad categories: 1. health services and supplies, which consist of personal health care expenditures (the direct provisions of health care), program administration, and the net cost of private health insurance and government public health activities; and 2. research and construction of medical facilities.

National Institute for Occupational Safety and Health (NIOSH) (CDC) part of the Centers for Disease Control and Prevention within the Department of Health and Human Services. NIOSH is the federal institute responsible for conducting research and making recommendations for the prevention of work-related injuries and illnesses.

National Institute on Disability and Rehabilitation Research (NIDRR) part of the US Department of Education. The Medical Science Division of NIDRR supports research related to the effect of specific interventions on outcomes.

national managed care firm any managed care organization that offers programs in more than one state.

National Recreation and Park Association (NRPA) the United States' largest non-profit service, research, and education organization dedicated to improving the quality of life through effective utilization of natural and human resources. NRPA's address is 22377 Belmont Ridge Rd., Ashburn, VA 20148-4501, 703-858-2153, www.nrpa.org.

National Therapeutic Recreation Society (NTRS) one of the two nationally recognized professional organizations for recreational therapists. NTRS's address is 22377 Belmont Ridge Rd., Ashburn, VA 20148-4501, 703-858-2153. See *American Therapeutic Recreation Association, National Association of Recreational Therapists.*

Nationwide Food Consumption Survey (NFCS) (HHS) a survey conducted by the USDA roughly every ten years that monitors the nutrient intake of a cross-section of the US public.

natural killer cell (NK) thought to provide an important defense against cancer and virus affected cells; (CDC) a lymphocyte that, unlike other lymphocytes, does not require specific activation by foreign antigen. They are considered to play a "front line" role in controlling infection, curbing infection until a specific, coordinated immune response can be mounted.

NCQA See *National Committee for Quality Assurance.*

NCTRC See *National Council for Therapeutic Recreation Certification.*

Necker cube See *reversible figure.*

neck stoma a surgically placed opening in the front of the neck to facilitate breathing. Patients who have a surgically placed stoma (for breathing) require special precautions. For individuals with neck stomas who do not use a respirator, the following stoma care may be followed (per physician's orders):
1. Keep the stoma area clean. Wash hands prior to touching the area.
2. When potential exposure to cold air exists, the use of a stoma bib (made of woven or crocheted cotton) should be used to help warm the air prior to entry into the lungs.
3. Keep the stoma moist by using a thin layer of petrolatum around the edges.

necrotizing fasciitis (CDC) a bacterium (occasionally described by the media as "the flesh-eating bacteria") that destroys muscles, fat, and skin tissue. Early signs and symptoms of necrotizing fasciitis are fever, severe pain, swelling, and redness at the wound site. See *group A streptococcus.*

negative self-evaluation a term used in research that is commonly referred to as "low self-worth."

negative sensation lack of awareness of contact because the contact/stimulation is below the threshold of the nerves involved. See *sensation.*

neglect (patient) as defined by the federal *Immediate and Serious Threat* regulations in the United States: neglect is the failure to provide necessary physical or psychological care, attention, or treatment, resulting in gross neglect. Situations/conditions which may indicate neglect include: patients who are dirty, disheveled, inappropriately clothed for the climate, malnourished, lying in urine and/or feces, exhibiting excessive *pressure sores*/body trauma, incorrect/inappropriate hydration status; and patients who are left alone for excessive amounts of time.

neglect (visual) lack of awareness of one side of the body and space — usually seen in individuals with a right *cerebrovascular accident* (CVA). Individuals with a right CVA show neglect to the left of midline. (Also known as *visuospatial neglect* and *unilateral neglect*.)

negotiated discount a contractual agreement between the health care provider organization/private practice and the insurance company which stipulates how much of a discount *members* of the insurance plan will be granted for a specified service.

nephrosis a kidney disorder where there is a degeneration without any inflammation caused by a number of diseases. The symptoms include *edema* and protein in the urine.

nervous behaviors observable actions that a patient demonstrates when s/he is uncomfortable with a situation. At times these nervous habits become so significant that they reduce a patient's ability to function in his/her environment. Some nervous behaviors include:

body swaying	moistens lips
sits on edge of chair	pacing
can't sit still	leg/arm swinging
nail biting	tapping
clearing throat	flashes of smiles
self-grooming	rocking
clutching hands	repetitive movements
coughing	rigid arms
self-hugging	fidgeting
twitching	scratching
hands restrained or in pockets	

neural tube defect (NTD) (HHS) any malformation of the brain or spinal cord (neurological system) during embryonic development. Infants born with spina bifida, where the spinal cord is exposed, can grow to adulthood but usually suffer from paralysis or other disabilities. Babies born with anencephaly, where most or all of the brain is missing, usually die

Possible Disability Associated with Neurofibromatosis

Concern	Intervention
Cutaneous Lesions: When the skin is affected the patient may have pigmented hairy nevi (frequently on the neck area) and deep furrows of skin over the scalp area.	1. Assist patient in understanding his/her other strengths and help build *self-esteem*. 2. Assist with dressing to cover unsightly tumors and cutaneous lesions when possible.
Endocrine Abnormalities: Depending on the location of the tumors, the individuals may experience: an enlargement of distal parts of the body, especially the nose, ears, jaws, fingers, and toes (acromegaly also known as Marie's disease); arrested physical and metal development (cretinism); precocious puberty; increased risk of kidney stones, *osteoporosis*, spontaneous fractures, and muscular weakness (hyperparathyroidism).	1. Conduct assessment to identify areas of physical and cognitive limitations — adjust activity or equipment to allow maximal involvement in activities of choice. 2. If at risk for spontaneous fractures, educate as to modifications in activity and other precautions to reduce risk of fracture. 3. Assist with dressing to cover unsightly skeletal growth when possible.
Neurologic Impairments: Because some tumors may invade the space normally occupied by the intracranial, spinal, and eighth cranial and orbital nerves, (approx. 10% of patients) the therapist may note developmental delays, cognitive deficiencies, and obstructive *hydrocephalus*. Secondary to these, the patient may also experience blindness and deafness.	1. Maximize development through a good balance of activities that cross all domains. 2. Emphasize development of touch and other sensory skills to prepare patient for possible loss of either vision or hearing.
Peripheral Nerve Involvement: Depending on the location of the tumors, their size, and the space that they have invaded, the patient may experience *pain*, spinal cord compression, *paresis*, and as a result, body disfigurement and limitation in activity.	1. Assist patient in developing pain management techniques and *coping techniques*. 2. Educate patient in options for meaningful activity using adaptive equipment and adaptive techniques.
Skeletal Involvement: Interruption and impairment in the normal spinal development and function possibly leading to *scoliosis*, *kyphoscoliosis*, and disorders related to spinal fusion defects and short stature.	1. Education patient in options for meaningful activity using adaptive equipment and adaptive techniques. 2. Monitor activities to ensure that they do not exacerbate condition. 3. Help patient develop contacts with appropriate resources in the community.

shortly after birth. These NTDs make up about 5% of all US birth defects each year. According to the CDC, the use of sufficient folic acid is enough to eliminate the risk of NTDs. See *folic acid.*

neurasthenia (CDC) nervous exhaustion; a functional neurosis marked by intense nervous irritability and weakness.

neuro-developmental techniques treatment techniques based on the concept that normal movement cannot be superimposed on abnormal *tone.* The techniques aim to inhibit abnormal tone, postures, and patterns and to promote normal movement patterns.

neurofibromatosis an inherited disorder which affects approximately 80,000 Americans; a number which may be under-reported as it frequently goes undiagnosed in individuals who have a mild case of neurofibromatosis. The primary disability is the de-

velopment of soft tumors (neurofibromas) and brown spots on the skin, causing social problems (e.g., unusual looks). These tumors, which affect the individual's nervous system, muscles, bones, and skin also can cause functional limitations and disability depending on the severity and location of the tumors. Also known as the "Elephant Man" disease. The chart above shows possible disability associated with neurofibromatosis, depending on the location of tumors.

neuroleptics See *antipsychotics.*

neurologic sequela neurologic disorders that are secondary, or as a result of an initial disease, treatment, or injury. The neurologic sequela of a severed spinal cord is paralysis below the injury.

neurologist a physician who specializes in the study of the nerves, muscles, brain, and brain dysfunction.

neuromyasthenia (CDC) muscular weakness, usually of emotional origin.

neuron also called a nerve cell. An impulse-conducting cell found in the brain, spinal column, and nerves. Neurons consist of a nucleated cell body with one or more dendrites and a single axon. Traditionally neurons have been associated only with the functioning of the brain but recent research clearly demonstrates that they mediate brain/immune functioning.

neuropathy a measurable disability and/or undesirable change in the peripheral nervous system. Chronic *alcoholism* and *diabetes* are two common causes of neuropathy. There are many different types of neuropathologies. Some are presented in the table below. See *porphyria.*

neuropeptide one of nearly 100 identified small peptides which were originally thought to be secreted only by neurons, hence the name. Recent research shows that both lymphocytes and monocytes secrete and respond to peptides. Immunologists prefer the terms cytokine or chemokine whereas neurologists prefer the term neuropeptide.

neuropsychiatric relating to organic and functional diseases of the nervous system.

neuropsychologist an individual with a PhD in psychology who has additional training and experience in working with patients with *traumatic brain injuries.*

neurotransmitter a chemical substance that transmits or inhibits nerve impulses across a synapse, e.g., serotonin, acetylcholine, dopamine. epinephrine, norepinephrine, and gamma-aminobutyrate.

newton (after Sir Isaac Newton) the International System of Units measure of force; equal to the force that produces an acceleration of one meter per second on a mass of one kilogram.

NG tube See *nasogastric tube.*

nitrite (HHS) a food additive that has been used for centuries to preserve meats, fish, and poultry. It also contributes to the characteristic flavor, color, and texture of processed meats such as hot dogs. Because nitrite safeguards cured meats against the most deadly food-borne bacterium of all, Clostridium botulinum, its use is supported by the public health community. The human body generates much greater nitrite levels than are added to food. Nitrates consumed in foods such as carrots and green vegetables are converted to nitrite during digestion. Nitrite in the body is instrumental in promoting blood clotting, healing wounds and burns, and boosting immune function to kill tumor cells.

nitrosamines (HHS) a digestive reaction product of *nitrite*, a food additive used to preserve meats, fish, and poultry.

no code a medical order, backed up by a legal document signed by the patient or the legal guardian allowing staff to refrain from applying life saving measures to restore breathing or heartbeat. See *do not resuscitate orders.*

nonambulatory referring to an individual who is not able to walk a functional distance. An individual is considered to still be functionally ambulatory if s/he is able to move about with the assistance of a cane, walker, or braces.

Types of Neuropathology

Type	Description
alcoholic	More commonly called alcoholic paralysis, this disorder is a weakening of or paralysis of peripheral nerves because of long-term alcohol abuse.
autonomic	Loss of function because of damage to the nerves that control involuntary actions such as digestion and temperature regulation. Autonomic neuropathy is not a specific disease but a description of symptoms caused by a loss of bodily control over the involuntary or peripheral nervous system.
diabetic	Neurological impairment in many different body systems as a result of the primary diagnosis of diabetes. Diabetic neuropathy is often divided into two categories: somatic and visceral.
peripheral	A general term used to describe numbness of the extremities which may also include paresthesia, burning sensation, and/or lancinating pain
somatic	A common type of peripheral neuropathy affecting the lower extremities, usually bilaterally and most often affecting the sensory nerves more than the other types of nerves. Common symptoms include pain (more often at night, relived to some degree by walking) and paresthesias (tingling, numbness, and sensation of either burning or coldness of the involved limbs). Somatic neuropathy usually involves the absence of knee or ankle jerks.
visceral	A set of disorders that impact the internal organs of the body such as the gastrointestinal tract, the heart, and the genitourinary tract. There are many causes for this type of neuropathy including diabetes.

non-A non-B hepatitis a dated term for hepatitis C.

noncontributory agreement an employee health care benefit package that does not require the employee to contribute to his/her health care insurance policy premium.

nonfluent aphasia speech that is effortful and halting. Auditory comprehension is relatively good but not perfect. Reading comprehension is better than written output. See *aphasia.*

non-Hodgkin's lymphoma a diverse group of cancers that typically originate in T and B lymphocytes and are generally first noticed by the patient because of "lumps" in the neck, groin, or axilla (armpit). Many patients with non-Hodgkin's lymphoma remain relatively symptom free for years allowing fairly normal, unlimited activity. During periods of radiation or chemotherapy some patients may experience hair loss and nausea. Other patients can be quite ill with CNS involvement (especially patients with HIV infection). Patients may experience numerous interruptions in their normal lifestyle due to multiple hospitalizations. Partly because of the diverse nature of this group of lymphomas a variety of classification systems are used. One of the classification systems developed in Ann Arbor, Michigan (the Working Formulation) divides Non-Hodgkin's Lymphoma into three grades (see below).

nonrenewal the decision not to renew a time-limited-agreement following expiration. The decision whether to terminate or not renew a Medicare or Medicaid *provider* agreement depends on the timing of an onsite survey, i.e., how close in time the survey is to the expiration date or *automatic cancellation clause* balanced with the seriousness of the *deficiencies* cited and/or the possibility of instituting an intermediate sanction. Nonrenewal and cancellation

are preferred to termination, if termination would be effective after the projected renewal or automatic cancellation date. See *adverse actions, intermediate sanction, reconsideration, termination.*

nonscheduled injury an injury not specifically listed on workman's compensation tables because the level of disability must be determined on a case-by-case basis. The United States has developed a system to compensate workers who suffer permanent injuries on the job. Nonscheduled injuries are those to the torso, head, abdomen, and thorax and are described as affecting a certain percentage of the body (the whole body being 100%). Each state provides its own guidelines to physicians for the determination of permanent *disability* resulting from these injuries. See *scheduled injury.*

normalization the process of modifying the environment or the person's skills to allow the person to "fit in" better in his/her community. See *consumer rights, inclusive education, inclusive recreation.*

normative groups/norms Professionals frequently want to determine if the behaviors or attitudes demonstrated by one specific individual can be considered within a "normal" range (e.g., whether the behaviors or attitudes are typical for a specific group). To help determine what is "normal" (norms) a sample group of individuals who, by definition, fit into the group is selected (normative group). Some examples of normative groups include 1. male/female, 2. fourth graders/fifth graders, 3. white/African-American/Hispanic-American, and 4. eight year olds/nine year olds. The testing tool is administered to this sample group and the results are scored. The pattern(s) of the scores obtained allow a professional to determine if the individual's behaviors or attitudes fall within the "norm," or typical pattern, for

Grades of Non-Hodgkin's Lymphoma

Grade	Discussion
Low Grade Non-Hodgkin's Lymphoma	A non-aggressive lymphoma that is difficult to bring into remission. Radiation and/or chemotherapy may be indicated. Five years after diagnosis, approximately 70% of patients are still living but may not have achieved remission. Most patients with low-grade non-Hodgkin's lymphoma will not survive the disease in the long run.
Intermediate Grade Non-Hodgkin's Lymphoma	Usually treated aggressively with chemotherapy and radiation therapy. The five year survival rate is high, approximately 85%, depending on the stage of cancer when treatment first started. Myelosuppression may be a problem.
High Grade Non-Hodgkin's Lymphoma	Very aggressive lymphomas (including lymphoblastic and Burkitt's) typically seen with both bone marrow and CNS involvement. Treatment involves leukemia-type chemotherapy, possibly a bone marrow transplant. Long periods of inpatient hospitalization in protective isolation cause significant interruption in vocational, social, and leisure involvement. Periods of myelosuppression should be anticipated as a side effect of treatment.

his/her normative group. Having one's scores fall into the typical range for one's normative group may or may not be a significant and meaningful event and does not imply good or bad. In fact, not every behavior or attitude would be expected to have a "norm," as logical choices create too much of a spread. A good example is leisure interest. It is expected that, while there may be some similarities in leisure preferences for each normative group, there are just too many choices to make one or two activities a typical choice. And while there clearly are undesirable choices made by some individuals as to their leisure preferences (drugs being one such choice), there does not exist a list of the best leisure preferences.

nosocomial infection *infections* that the patient contracts because of exposure after admission to a treatment or other health care center. This exposure is usually due to poor *infection control* technique used by staff. Approximately 5% of all patients develop a nosocomial infection usually caused by group A Streptococcus pyogenes, Staphylococcus, Escherichia coli, Klebsiella, Proteus, Pseudomonas, Hemophilus influenza, hepatitis viruses, Candida albicans, and aspergillus. See *handwashing, immediate and serious threat.*

noxious stimulus item or action that irritates. A noxious stimulus response is a nerve reaction to something that is not healthy or produces an undesirable or even damaging result. See *irritability.*

NRPA See *National Recreation and Park Association.*

Nursing Home Case Mix and Quality Demonstration a project used to gather information from a multi-state mix of nursing homes that was used to provide a framework for HCFA's *Prospective Payment System.* This project had two objectives: 1. develop and help implement two systems (a case-mix classification system to be the basis for Medicare and Medicaid payment and a quality monitoring system to measure the impact of this classification system on the quality of services provided the resident and 2. provide information to help with the survey process.

nursing supervisor the person who is the supervisor of the nursing staff. Nursing supervisor usually indicates an individual who holds a management position in a health care setting. This individual usually supervises other nurses, nurse's aides, and frequently, therapists and non-nursing para-professionals. When the Administrator of a long-term care facility is out of the building, the next in charge is usually the nursing supervisor. A nursing supervisor usually has a bachelor's or master's degree in nursing.

nutraceuticals (HHS) substances in or parts of a food that may be considered to provide medical or health benefits beyond basic nutrition, including disease prevention. Research indicates this term might not appeal to consumers. See *functional foods.*

nutrition in relationship to *relaxation techniques,* eating healthy foods that give the body better energy levels and reduced vulnerability to illness. Eating well and avoiding fast foods or convenience foods, will help support the other efforts for reducing stress.

nystagmus a rhythmic jerking or movement of the eyes.

O

obesity Although precise definitions vary among experts, overweight has traditionally been defined as 10% to 20% above an optimal weight for height. Some scientists argue that the amount and distribution of an individual's body fat is a significant indicator of health risk and therefore should be considered in defining obesity. Abdominal fat has been linked to more adverse health consequences than fat in the hips or thighs. Thus, calculations of waist-to-hip ratio are preferred by some health experts to help determine if an individual is overweight or obese.

objective 1. pertaining to that which can be seen and measured without, necessarily, any interpretation as to why. An objective measurement might be the number of times a patient presses the nursing call light in a two-hour period. 2. a measurable written statement which defines who will do what, when, how long, and how an observer can tell when the written statement has been met. Example: The patient (who) will attend to task (what) for ten minutes (how long) by November 8 (when) as evidenced by good eye contact and non-interruption of activity during group (how to measure). Objectives are usually one of a number of measurable statements grouped together which help meet a generally stated, overall desire called a *goal*. In therapy, objectives are frequently divided into therapy objectives and service objectives. Therapy objectives are objectives which outline expected patient behaviors (e.g., will ambulate twenty five feet without assistance within a reasonable amount of time by November 11, 2002). Service objectives are objectives which outline expected staff behaviors (e.g., will provide patient with AFO orthosis by November 11, 2002). See *diagnosis, learning, quantitative research, risk management, socialization.*

objective sensation a cognitive awareness of an event through the use of multiple senses. See *sensation.*

oblique rotation (non-orthogonal factoring) a type of mathematical number crunching of test scores to help "cluster" items on a test into groups. As with other types of factor analysis, oblique rotation can accommodate over a hundred variables, compensate for random error and simplify complex interrelationships between questions on the testing tool. However, many find oblique rotation results more diffi-

cult to interpret than other types of factors rotations. See *orthogonal rotation.*

OBRA the name of the federal legislation that outlines the minimum requirements for facilities licensed as skilled nursing facilities in the United States. The full title of the legislation is the **Nursing Home Reform Provisions of the Omnibus Budget Reconciliation Act of 1987**. This act was passed in 1987 and modified in 1992 and 1995. See *CFR, Medicare/Medicaid history, resident council.*

obsession an internally driven thought or action which is repetitive, non-productive, and pathological in nature. See *compulsion, psychasthenia, refuting irrational ideas, thought stopping.*

occlusion closure of a blood vessel, closing off. See *embolus.*

Occupational Exposure to Blood-Borne Pathogens Standard a federal law in the United States which outlines regulations to reduce the incidence of employee's exposure to blood-borne pathogens while at work. These requirements are found in the Occupational Safety and Health Act (OSHA) and enforced by the Occupational Safety and Health Administration. OSHA requires that each workplace has a set of written policies and a set of procedures to ensure that all employees are protected from exposure to *blood-borne pathogens*. These policies are to be contained in an *exposure control plan*. The exposure control plan includes an exposure determination, which details the extent of occupational exposure of the employees as well as the plan to control exposure to blood-borne pathogens. See *personal protective equipment.*

occupational therapist an individual who has completed all of the training and exams required by the American Occupational Therapy Certification Board (AOTCB) or who has met state requirements to be called an "Occupational Therapist." See *Joint Commission.*

occupational therapy a clinical specialty which uses "purposeful activity with individuals who are limited by physical injury or illness, psychosocial dysfunction, developmental or learning disabilities, poverty, and cultural differences, or the aging process to maximize independence, prevent disability, and maintain health. The practice encompasses evaluation, treatment, and consultation." (American Occupational Therapy Association).

occupiable (ADA) a room or enclosed space designed for human occupancy in which individuals congregate for amusement, educational, or similar purposes or in which occupants are engaged at labor and which is equipped with a means of egress, light, and ventilation.

occurrence screen the use of a predetermined indicator to signal the need for a quality assurance review of a specific aspect of patient care. An example might be the determination that a sibling with head lice spent five hours in the pediatric playroom before his/her condition was discovered (predetermined indicator which initiated the occurrence screen — infectious event in pediatric playroom). Occurrence screens help determine whether events are structural in nature (e.g., availability of information and resources) or process in nature (e.g., the degree of skills and timeliness in the delivery of health care services).

office enrollment the period of time in which the employees of an organization may choose to switch health insurance programs or options. This occurs when the employees have a *dual option*.

Office for Civil Rights (OCR) clearance a determination that a new facility is complying with all civil rights regulations. Determination of compliance with *civil rights* requirements, obtained from the regional office for Civil Rights is required before a facility may have its first state or federal survey from the *Department of Health and Human Services* (DHHS). Compliance with OCR requirements is a pre-requisite for participation in the *Medicare* program. OCR clearance involves a review of the provider's record regarding discrimination based on race, color, or disability under Section 504 of the *Rehabilitation Act of 1973* and other non-discrimination requirements prescribed by the DHHS.

Older American's Act a program that funds a variety of services which help elderly stay in their homes. As with all federal programs, the Older American's Act must be renewed every three to five years (*sunsetting*). Congress failed to formally renew the Older American's Act in 1992 but continued to fund some of its programs on a year-to-year basis. The issue causing the lack of renewal is not that the programs don't work, but the struggle the United States Congress is having over federal vs. state control of funds. Also at issue is language in the law that gives preferential funding to minority elderly. As affirmative action programs continue to come under increased scrutiny and disfavor, this language in the Older American's Act has proven to be a stumbling block.

olfactory pertaining to the sense of smell.

olfactory hallucination See *hallucination.*

oligonucleotide (HHS/NMDP) sequence of nucleic acids used as a probe in DNA-based human leukocyte antigen tissue typing.

ombudsman a representative of a government (usually state) program who is appointed to receive and investigate complaints of *abuse* made by individuals in licensed and certified facilities. The ombudsman program was mandated and funded by the Older Americans Act amendments of 1975. Acting as an advocate for the patient, s/he assesses and verifies each complaint and then seeks a way to resolve it. An ombudsman must report findings to the appropriate agencies (law enforcement and Department of Health Services) and help to achieve equitable settlements to issues. The concept of ombudsman programs originated in Scandinavia in the 1800's.

Omnibus Budget Reconciliation Act See *OBRA.*

omnisexual a descriptive word for an individual who has no distinct sexual preference and who engages in sexual activity of many kinds, varieties, and forms.

on-line analytical processing (OLAP) (HCO) a database architecture that supports querying of complex, multidimensional *databases*.

open amputation an amputation where the surgical site is left open to drain.

open-ended health maintenance organization members individuals who are members of an HMO but who also have the additional benefit of being able to self-refer to providers outside of the HMO network. See *point of service.*

open head injury See *traumatic brain injury.*

operant conditioning causing behavior modification by rewarding desired behaviors and punishing undesired behaviors. See *behavior modification program, conditioning.*

operational definition a definition created to serve as a theoretical foundation from which test items may be written. Producing an operational definition allows the creator of a testing tool to decrease the ambiguity of what would otherwise be an abstract or hypothetical concept. An operational definition will (hopefully) be solidified into a formal definition once the property(ies) and relationship(s) are tested and found to be true.

operational part (ADA) a part of a piece of equipment or appliance used to insert or withdraw objects or to activate, deactivate, or adjust the equipment or appliance (for example, coin slot, push button, handle).

opiates drugs derived from opium that cause sleep or

Organizational Performance

Dimension of Performance	Description of Performance
Doing the Right Thing	The **efficacy** of the procedure or treatment in relation to the individual's condition. (The degree to which the care of the individual has been shown to accomplish the desired or projected outcomes.)
	The **appropriateness** of a specific test, procedure, or service to meet the individual's needs. (The degree to which appropriate care is available to meet the individual's clinical needs, given the current state of knowledge.)
Doing the Right Thing Well	The **availability** of a needed test, procedure, treatment, or service to the individual who needs it. (The degree to which appropriate care is available to meet the individual's needs.)
	The **timeliness** with which a needed test, procedure, treatment, or service is provided to the individual. (The degree to which the care is provided to the individual at the most beneficial or necessary time.)
	The **effectiveness** with which tests, procedures, treatment, or service is provided to the individual. (The degree to which the care is provided in the correct manner, given the current state of knowledge, to achieve the desired or projected outcomes for the individual.)
	The **continuity** of the services provided to the individual with respect to other services, practitioners, and providers and over time. (The degree to which the care for the individual is coordinated among practitioners, among organizations, and over time.)
	The **safety** of the individual (and others) to whom the services are provided. (The degree to which the risk of an intervention and risk in the care environment are reduced for the individual and others, including the health care provider.)
	The **efficiency** with which services are provided. (The relationship between the outcomes — results of care — and the resources used to deliver individual care.)
	The **respect** and caring with which services are provided. (The degree to which the individual or a designee is involved in his or her own care decisions and to which those providing services do so with sensitivity and respect for the individual's needs, expectations, and individual differences.)

relief from pain, including codeine and morphine. See *comorbidity*.

OPIMs Other Potentially Infectious Materials. OPIMs is the term given to body fluids (other than blood) that can carry the *HIV* or *hepatitis* viruses. See *exposure control plan*.

opioids natural and synthetic chemicals that have opiate-like effects including endorphins and synthetic methadone. See *comorbidity*.

optical character recognition (OCR) (HCO) automated scanning and conversion of printed characters to computer-based text.

organic brain syndrome a general category of disorders of cognitive functioning including dementia, delirium, amnesiac syndrome, organic anxiety syndrome, intoxication, and withdrawal. While this term was commonly used prior to 1994, its use should decline. Originally called *organic mental syndrome* in the **DSM-III-R**, it is not found in the **DSM-IV**. The types of organically caused brain syndromes once grouped under organic mental syndrome are now re-grouped into different categories.

organic food agricultural products that are grown without using synthetic, non-agricultural substances to control pests, improve soil quality and/or enhance processing. Techniques that may be used include crop rotation, cultivation, mulching, soil enrichment, and the "encouragement" of predators and microorganisms that naturally keep pests away. The now widely accepted definition allows farmers to use natural pesticides, but nothing synthetic. Genetically engineered products are also not considered organic.

organization a group of two or more individuals who are working toward a common goal and who mutually agree to coordinate efforts. The basis of the goals and mutually agreed upon coordination requires a defined structure which provides a description of acceptable behaviors and processes. The *organizational manual* (policy and procedure manual) is usually the location where the defined structure and processes are written down.

organizational deficit the inability to mentally process information in an organized manner. This includes an inability to sequence, classify, prioritize, and/or identify relevant features of objects or events. Compare with *processing deficits*. See *sequencing skills*.

organizational manual the document which outlines the defined structure and processes of an organization. The organizational manual usually has two parts: the first which defines the organization's mission and how the mission causes them to relate to other organizations and the second which defines the organizational structure and the lines of authority within the organization.

organizational performance Professional standards call for the ongoing improvement of an organization's performance. A good quality assurance program will help the organization identify which dimensions of performance are functioning well and which ones need improvement. There are two main dimensions of performance: 1. doing the right thing and 2. doing the right thing well as shown in the table on the previous page.

orientation the ability to be cognitively aware of and express time, place, personal data, relationship(s) of significant others to self, one's own condition and purpose (identity/role). Compare with *confusion, validation*. See *contextual orientation, delirium, dementia, dementia syndrome of depression, metabolic disorders, psychosis, temporal orientation*.

orotracheal airway See *endotracheal airway*.

orthogonal rotation In fields associated with social sciences, it is hard to connect a variable such as self-esteem with levels of stress. The two variables (self-esteem/stress) are not lineal in nature (they are not an equal distance from each other as the numbers 3, 6, and 9 are). Orthogonal rotation is one of the various rotational strategies used to help obtain a clearer pattern of variables that share something in common. Using the numerical scores achieved through orthogonal rotation, the developer of the test can see how successful s/he was in grouping or classifying the variables. The closer to +1.00 or -1.00, the better the grouping or classification match.

orthosis a type of brace which is applied externally to a deformed or compromised body part to provide control, correction, and support. When an orthosis provides control or provides correction, it does so by either putting extra stress or pressure on a body part or by reducing stress or pressure on a body part. To provide support the orthosis functions by reducing the *weight bearing* load of the body part and pro-

vides rigidity to reduce destabilizing motion. Three organizations have worked together to unify the terminology associated with orthosis. They are the American Orthotic and Prosthetic Association (AOPA), the Task Force on Standardization of Prosthetic-Orthotic Terminology of the Committee on Prosthetic-Orthotic Education (CPOE), and the National Research Council. These organizations based the standardization of terminology on the joint and region that the orthosis covers or controls. Abbreviations for orthoses are shown in the accompanying table. The material that the orthosis is made of is usually left up to the discretion of the orthotist unless the *prescription* specifically states the material to be used. Each prescription should include the type of orthosis to be made along with the type of control that is to be allowed by the orthosis. The three primary types of control provided by the orthosis are 1. free motion, 2. assisted motion, or 3. resisted motion. Compare with *dynamic splint*. See *FIM, immediate and serious threat*.

Abbreviations for Orthosis

Abbreviation	Description
AFO	ankle-foot orthosis
AO	ankle orthosis
CO	cervical orthosis
CTLSO	cervicothoracolumbosacral orthosis
EO	elbow orthosis
EWHO	elbow-wrist-hand orthosis
FO	foot orthosis
HKAFO	hip-knee-ankle-foot orthosis
HO	hand orthosis, hip orthosis
KAFO	knee-ankle-foot orthosis
KO	knee orthosis
SEWHO	shoulder-elbow-wrist-hand orthosis
SIO	sacroiliac orthosis
SO	shoulder orthosis
TLSO	thoracolumbosacral orthosis
TO	thoracic orthosis
WHO	wrist-hand orthosis

oscillating support bed commercially known as "Roto-Rest," "Tilt and Turn," and "Paragon 9000," these beds "rock" the patient in a 124° arc from side to side, oscillating continuously like an oscillating fan. This movement relieves pressure on any one part of the body. The patient is "wedged" into position in the bed with foam wedges and supports. The bed is used with patients who are at high risk of developing pneumonia due to bed rest or at risk for developing *pressure sores*. Implications for treatment include an increased risk for lost *range of motion*, increased risk for isolation due to visual blockage (wedges blocking view) and due to noise of machinery and the wedges covering the ears and increased frustration level from difficulties having a conversation with the patient as the bed moves. See *bed.*

osmolality (HHS) osmotic concentration; an indicator of fluid balance in the body's tissues.

ossification development of bone.

osteoarthritis a type of arthritis that leads to degenerative changes and deformities in the joints. Osteoarthritis has numerous causes that impact the patient's condition. Some of the conditions that may be factors in the development and progression of osteoarthritis include disease process (including hyperparathyroidism, metabolic disorders, or endocrine disorders), trauma (including previous joint disease or damage or occupational repetitive use trauma), genetic disorders (including type II collagen abnormalities and epiphyseal dysplasia), and obesity. See *degenerative joint disease.*

osteopetrosis (HHS/NMDP) a disorder of the bones in which hardening of tissue obliterates the marrow, leading to severe anemia, deformities of the skull, and compression of the cranial nerves, all of which may cause early death.

osteoporosis a reduction in the mineral content and internal structure of bone mass that causes a reduction in stature. Osteoporosis is caused by the aging process (post menopausal women, the primary cause) or by immobility (casting, paralysis, etc., the secondary cause). Patients with osteoporosis have an increased risk for bone fractures and can experience chronic pain. Osteoporosis has a large impact on health care in the United States with costs from osteoporotic fractures totaling $14 billion a year. Os

teoporosis is a disease that primarily affects women, with a disproportionate number of hip fractures (75%) occurring in women. One third of women with osteoporosis will experience a vertebral fracture after they reach 65 years of age; one third will experience a hip fracture after they reach 80 years of age. Research has shown that in addition to regular exercise, calcium intake during childhood, adolescence, and early adulthood helps build a "bone bank" of calcium stores. While bone length is established by age 20, bone strength and density continue to develop through age 30. See *neurofibromatosis.*

ostomy, intestinal surgical placement of an artificial opening from the intestines to the surface of the abdomen. An ostomy may either be a permanent or temporary solution to abnormalities or diseases of the intestine and anus. The bowel movements bypass part of the intestines, allowing the waste products to be collected in a self-adhesive bag (a pouching system). The stoma is the portion of the intestine that is pulled out and placed outside of the surface of the skin forming the ostomy opening. The stoma has a raw, red to pink appearance though it is not painful. (Intestinal tissue does not sense pain due to the lack of pain receptors.) Causes: A variety of anatomical and neurological disorders require the placement of an ostomy. The most common reasons for an ostomy to be placed in children and youth is either a congenital (from birth) malformation of the anal/rectal structure or *Hirschsprung's disease* (lack of nerves in the intestine to help push along waste). The combined occurrence of Hirschsprung's disease or anatomical malformation is approximately one in five thousands live births. Placement in older adults may be due to intestinal cancer. Impact on functional ability: Wearing of a pouching system seldom limits physical activity. Swimming is even possible as long as the pouching system is leak free and se

Therapy Considerations with Ostomies

Concerns	Intervention
leakage/smell	The a bag may leak due to poor technique in applying the bag or due to activity-induced dislodgment. Since the smell has obvious social isolation potential, the professional should start to solve the problem by assessing the type of activity and movement which compromises the integrity of the seal and then either work with nursing to modify the system (preferable) or work with the patient to modify the activity.
skin integrity	The small intestines have three primary sections: the duodenum, the jejunum (jejunostomy), and the ileum (ileostomy). An ostomy placed in the large intestines is called a colostomy. The higher up in the intestinal system the ostomy is, the more erosive and fluid the bowel movement is. A leaking ileostomy is at the greatest risk of causing a skin breakdown. Therapy intervention is the same as dealing with leakage.
poor self-esteem	Develop self-esteem through successful completion of activity and through self-esteem programs.

cured with waterproof tape. The collection of gas is common and the patient should be taught how to release gas if s/he is cognitively and physically able. Adolescents are somewhat put off by having an ostomy and pouching system as the wearing of tight clothing is contraindicated. Tight pants cause the stoma to become irritated and bleed. Adolescents or adults with poor *self-esteem* tend to sabotage their pouching system, allowing it to leak and smell, increasing the alienation of their peers. Therapy concerns related to ostomies are shown in the table on the previous page.

OT See *occupational therapy.*

other or unknown substance-related disorders pathological use of drugs of abuse that are not specified under their own categories in the **DSM-IV** under *substance-related disorders.* Example of the drugs within this category are anabolic steroids, nitrite inhalants ("poppers"), nitrous oxide, over-the-counter and prescription medications not otherwise covered by the eleven categories (e.g., cortisol, antihistamines, benztropine), and other substances that have psychoactive effects. An example of a pathological use of an unknown substance would be taking a drug that is unknown (e.g., swallowing a bottle of pills when you do not know what the pills are for). Within this **DSM-IV** disorder are twelve categories of use patterns (all start out with "Other or Unknown Substance"): intoxication, withdrawal, induced delirium, induced persisting dementia, induced psychotic disorder with delusions, induced psychotic disorder with hallucinations, induced mood disorder, induced anxiety disorder, induced sexual dysfunction, induced sleep disorder, and related disorder.

outbreak a sudden appearance of a disease in clusters of the population but, in number, still a small percentage of the population. See *infection.*

outcome the results of an action. In health care "outcome" refers to the anticipated and/or actual result expected as a direct result of a treatment intervention or staff action. In the 1970's the quality of health care services was frequently measured by evaluating whether a facility had the appropriate policies, procedures, and equipment in place (systems approach). It quickly become apparent that a facility could have all appropriate systems in place and not be able to make a meaningful change in a

patient's status. During the late 1980's and well into the 1990's the trend in measuring the quality of services shifted away from the systems approach to the outcomes approach. Facilities are now expected to have functional, workable systems in place that produce meaningful outcomes. A sketch of the outcome process is shown below. See *care conference, confounding variable, coordination, critical pathway, decision making, disease management, efficiency, hypothesis, indicator, intake assessment, Joint Commission, leadership, learning, marketing plan, narrative style, pragmatic, problem solving, prognosis, quality improvement, randomized controlled trial, rehabilitation centers, risk adjustment, risk factors, standard.*

outcome indicator See *indicator.*

outcome research (HHS) a type of research increasingly used by the health industry which provides information about the results of a specific procedure or treatment regimen: the subject (clinical safety and efficacy), the subject's physical functioning and lifestyle, and economic considerations such as saving/prolonging life and avoiding costly complications.

out of area benefits health care benefits which are provided outside of the managed care enrollee's *service area.*

outpatient care services received which are delivered outside of a licensed hospital or nursing home. Care provided through a home health care agency, while technically outpatient care, is still usually referred to as home health care and not outpatient services. Day treatment programs which have a duration of no more then a few months are usually outpatient programs, where longer term, maintenance programs are usually not considered to be outpatient care.

oversight the process of reviewing the work being done or services being provided to determine how well the work or service meets performance expectations. The job of oversight evaluation is usually completed by individuals who are not providing the work or service that is being evaluated (e.g., outside evaluators).

over-stimulation excitement to the point that the stimulation produces a decreased ability to function. Since each individual has a different threshold where they are overstimulated and because the

Outcome Process

problem identified	→	solution defined	→	intervention to solve problem	→	problem corrected
(assessment)		*(goal/objective)*		*(care plan/tx)*		*(outcome)*

amount of sleep or food or illness can affect an individual's threshold, it is hard to indicate the amount of stimulation required before over-stimulation is achieved. See *boredom.*

overstretch the excessive lengthening of soft muscle tissue that allows range of movement beyond the normal limits. This overstretching is beneficial in some activities (i.e., gymnastics and yoga), but for patients with mobility and/or balance problems, overstretch can be a hazard. Stability is compromised with overstretched tissue.

overutilization the use of health care services which are 1. not based on assessed need, 2. in excessive amounts, or 3. provided in a higher-level setting than is needed by the patient. The provision of a vocational skill session when the patient's prescription is for a leg cast is an example of overutilization related to services not based on assessed need. Providing the patient with seven therapy sessions related to the use of public transportation when four sessions would normally be indicated based on the patient's skill and needs is an example of overutilization related to excessive amounts of treatment. Admitting a patient to an inpatient rehabilitation unit for a back strengthening program is an example of overutilization related to services provided in a higher-level setting than is needed.

overweight See *obesity.*

P

pain   a generally localized feeling of discomfort brought about by the stimulation of special nerve endings. It is thought that pain is an adapted state to help the individual protect the area that is uncomfortable. The degree of pain that a person "feels" is influenced by three factors.

1.   biologic factors
2.   psychological factors
3.   social factors

The professional can have a significant impact on the patient's *tolerance* for pain (or lack thereof) and change the degree to which the patient's lifestyle is limited because of pain. Both the prevention of further movement which will actually cause biological damage as well as psychological training to increase tolerance are suitable areas for the professional to work. Also, increasing the patient's social skills to minimize the negative impact of pain is often addressed by the professional. The professional can decrease the patient's need to talk about his/her pain by increasing awareness and interest in other things and by helping the patient redefine his/her role from "victim" to a healthier role. These changes will increase the patient's tolerance for pain. A person may also experience psychological pain as a result of distressing events or thoughts. The charts below show some of the types of pain and other terms related to pain. See *biofeedback, chronic inflammation, endorphins, euphoria, intermittent claudication, medical play, neurofibromatosis, pain at rest, phantom pain, progressive relaxation, reflex sympathetic dystrophy,*

pain at rest   a burning, tingling feeling which results from decreased oxygen flow to the affected limb. This decreased flow may be, in part, caused by positioning (the limb placed above the level of the heart and/or pressure over the arteries leading to the muscles) and/or caused by long periods of rest. (The heart tends to be less productive during sleep and/or during events that lead to *deconditioning*.) Encouraging the patient to engage in activities which allow the affected limb(s) to be positioned below the heart will help decrease the pain at rest. See *pain.*

pain clinic   a facility that focuses on the diagnosis

Types of Pain

Type of Pain	Conditions
cancer pain	bony metastases, nerve, and organ infiltration, spinal cord involvement
neurogenic pain	peripheral neuropathy, reflex sympathetic dystrophy, shingles, spinal stenosis
skeletal pain	osteoarthritis, rheumatoid arthritis, spondylosis deformans
soft tissue pain	"pulled" muscles
vascular disease pain	ischemic ulcers, peripheral vascular disease with claudication

Terms Related to Pain

Term	Description
acute	pain which is expected to resolve in six months or less
at rest	pain due to lack of blood flow to the affected extremity
chronic	pain which is expected to take longer then six months to resolve
gate control therapy	the concept that the sensation of pain can be interrupted before it reaches the brain, thus decreasing or eliminating the sensation of pain
intractable	pain or discomfort that cannot be relieved
intermittent	pain that comes and goes
phantom limb	the sensation of pain in an absent limb due to neurological processes
psychogenic	pain which originates from the mental/thought process instead of having a physiological origin
referred	pain in a part of the body other than the injured or diseased part
threshold	the point that the sensation of pain becomes noticeable
tolerance	the individual's ability to tolerate or endure the sensation of pain

and management of patients with chronic pain. A pain clinic differs from a multidisciplinary pain clinic in two ways: 1. it may not use a full multidisciplinary approach to the assessment and treatment of pain and 2. many pain clinics specialize in the a particular type of pain or location of pain (e.g., back pain or headache pain). See *multidisciplinary pain center, multidisciplinary pain clinic, modality-oriented clinic.*

palliative care the type of care provided for patients who have active, progressive diseases (who have reached the far-advanced stage of the disease process) for whom cure or restoration has been ruled out. Patients receiving palliative care have a focus on quality of life which includes: the ability to receive adequate pain and symptom management; ability to still exercise reasonable control over their own life; chances to strengthen relationships with those close to them, while lessening ties with others; avoiding the prolonging of life with heath care interventions; and having others help ease their burdens. Palliative care is a shift from standard health care in that the treatment team works on what best satisfies the wishes and needs of the patient and his/her family instead of following the typical medical intervention for the specific disease process.

palpation the use of one's hand to determine the physical characteristics of a body part: how firm the part is, the shape the parts take on, and the range of movement of the part.

panic attack the primary symptom of *anxiety* disorders, which may occur without an obvious pattern or cause. Typically these attacks are short in duration and cause a severe sense of dread, sweating, heart *dysarthymias*, and a feeling of not being connected with the world around them. See *applied relaxation, biofeedback, breathing, Global Assessment of Functioning Scale.*

panic disorder a disorder where the patient has spontaneous and unexpected occurrenceS of panic attacks. Panic disorder is a relatively new diagnosis being formally recognized in 1980. See *dual diagnosis, panic attack.*

paralysis complete loss of voluntary movement. See *developmental coordination disorder, Guillain-Barré syndrome.*

paraphasia condition characterized by fluent utterance of speech sounds in which unintended syllables, words, or phrases are prominent during speech. See *aphasia.*

paraphilia sexual actions and thoughts that are considered by society to be perversions or deviations from acceptable sexual behavior. Types of paraphilias include exhibitionism, fetishism, pedo-philia, transvestism, voyeurism, and zoophilia.

paraphrasing See *listening skills.*

paraplegia a paralysis of the lower portion of the body. See *swing-through gait.*

parasympathetic nervous system part of the autonomic nervous system which activates to slow down the heart rate; causes the coordinated, rhythmic, and sequential contraction of the smooth muscles of the digestive tract (to digest food), ureters (to urinate), and bile duct (to move bile); and relaxes sphincter muscles. See *autonomic nervous system.*

paraxial deficiencies a weakness or other disabling condition which affects only one side of the limb along the axis, versus a *transverse deficiency* which affects the entire width of the limb.

paresis weakness; partial or incomplete paralysis. See *neurofibromatosis.*

paresthesia an abnormal and frequently intense feeling of burning and prickling ("biting ants") felt by the patient even though there is little or no pressure on the affected spot. See *Jacksonian seizure.*

Parkinsonian gait a highly stereotypical gait in which the patient has impoverished movement of the lower limbs. There is generalized lack of extension at the ankle, knee, hip, and trunk. Diminished step length and a loss of reciprocal arm swing are noted. Patients have trouble initiating movement and this results in a slow and shuffling gait characterized by small steps. Because patients with Parkinsonian gait often exhibit flexed postures, their center of gravity projects forward, and they keep moving faster and faster to keep their *balance.* The patient, in an attempt to regain his balance, takes many small steps rapidly. The rapid stepping causes the patients to increase his walking speed. In some cases patients will break into a run and can only stop their forward progress when they run into an object. Less common than the forward propulsive gait pattern is a retropulsive pattern that occurs when patients lose their balance in a backward direction (retropulsion is more common in patients with cerebellar lesions) (Rothstein et. al., 1991, p. 728). See *festination gait, initiation, cerebellum.*

Parkinsonian movements a group of physical side effects of psychotropic medications characterized by uncontrolled tremors and muscular rigidity. This is actually more common than Parkinson's disease, which it is not related to. Compare to *tardive dyskinesia.*

Parkinson's disease a chronic disease which causes neurological damage. Usually developing later in life, Parkinson's disease is most commonly known by the muscular tremors and peculiar gait. It was first described by an English physician named James

Parkinson. Those with the disease progressively loose sensory-motor coordination and have difficulty initiating activity. Activity requires excessive energy causing individuals to tire quickly. See *Parkinsonian gait, fatigue, initiation.*

partial extended survey a survey conducted by Health Care Financing Administration if substandard care is found during an *abbreviated standard survey.* Surveyors are directed to review the facility's policy and procedure manuals, staffing patterns, inservice training records, and infection control program. The surveyors are also to review staff qualifications and all contractual agreements with outside providers. If the problem was found to originate in a quality of care *tag,* the surveyors are directed to review the accuracy of the patient's *assessments.* See *CFR.*

partial hand amputation an amputation through one or more phalanges or metacarpals of the hand or a partial amputation of the thumb. Therapy include retraining in fine motor skills for enjoyed activities and the use of adapted equipment when needed. Cosmetically, the use of wired finger fillers in gloves assists the patient who is concerned about appearance.

partial hospitalization outpatient psychiatric *day treatment programs* that serve as a transitional program for previously hospitalized psychiatric patients.

participation (in activities) to take part. Participation is used in many different, and often conflicting, ways by professionals. Some use the word participation to mean "attendance in an activity" while others view participation as involvement. Participation is not the same as attendance. Participation is appropriately used to describe the patient's performance in all phases of the activity. The five categories that define the concept of "participation" are patient-controlled behaviors, so any and all patients have the opportunity to be fully successful, regardless of their ability level. (See the chart on the next page.) For information on the components of participation as involvement, see *involvement. Dehn's Model of Leisure Health* uses the concept of attendance versus participation as a means to measure health. See *Recreation Participation Data Sheet, risk management.*

participation (in federal health care funding) to be eligible to receive federal health care dollars for services provided. See *effective date of participation.*

passive the act of not taking action; of letting others or events in one's life control what happens. It is normal for people to choose to be passive in large group situations.

passive movement movement of a body part caused by another person or a machine. See *movement, range of motion.*

passive stretching the action of someone else (besides the patient) gently applying force to stretch tight tissue. Passive stretching is usually done by the PT, OT, or certified nursing assistant using prescribed range of motion exercises. See *plasticity.*

passive surveillance See *surveillance.*

passive tremor See *tremor.*

patent ductus arteriosus (PDA) Prior to birth, the fetus' heart has an opening between the aorta artery (oxygen enriched) and the pulmonary artery (oxygen depleted). This opening is used by the fetus to bypass the lungs and closes prior to birth. Patent ductus arteriosus describes the failure of the fetus' heart to mature prior to birth and seal this opening. The child's heart with this defect must work harder to successfully circulate oxygen-enriched blood.

pathfinding the ability to determine the route one needs to take to reach one's destination based on previously learned information. One of the basic skills for living independently in the community is pathfinding. A person uses visual, auditory, and cognitive memory to find where s/he wants to be. To understand pathfinding as a multi-sensory process, close your eyes and "walk" the path between your office and your parked car or the bus stop. What did you "see" as you mentally walked to your car (or bus stop)? Therapists may test a patient's pathfinding skills by writing out instructions for the patient to follow. These instructions include five turns (some left and some right) to a location the patient has not been before. After reaching the desired location, the therapists asks for the written instructions back and has the patient retrace his/her steps. Patients without significant cognitive impairment should be able to retrace their path without *cueing* and without the written instructions. See *associated features, directionality.*

pathognomonic (of a sign or symptom) characteristic or indicative of a disease, denoting especially one or more typical symptoms.

pathological referring to a disease or disorder process that is abnormal and undesired.

pathological gambling an ongoing pattern of unhealthy and excessive gambling regardless of the consequences of the gambling losses. Pathological gamblers go beyond what most people would find acceptable, seeming to be driven to continue in this maladaptive behavior. Pathological gambling is a recognized diagnosis in the **DSM-IV** under the category of impulse control disorders not elsewhere classified.

pathomimicry a false disorder in which an individ-

Categories of Patient-Controlled Behaviors in Participation

Category	Description
Attention	The level of concentration demonstrated by the participant. Good listening is the main component of attention although the participant's degree of effort to understand and clarify what is being heard, as well as the degree of appropriate physical body posture to help facilitate good listening is important. The participant who is demonstrating good attentiveness will be listening to others in the group and expects to be listened to when it's his/her turn to speak. This participant is also able to demonstrate the ability to take advantage of the opportunity to learn from watching others when s/he is idle. Generalized to solo activities, the ability to observe and understand the environment which is part of the activity.
Attitude	The outward demonstration of attitude. The participant with a good attitude will show a positive approach to others, the activity, and himself/herself. S/he may make positive comments to others and/or to find a creative way to share his/her concerns with others. A participant's attitude not only affects his/her performance but that of the whole group. Generalized to solo activities, the participant demonstrates inquisitiveness. Anger, hostility, and irritability are not present.
Camaraderie	The participant's ability to demonstrate camaraderie toward the group, to be able to be inclusive to others, to be cooperative, to accept loss or input about substandard performance, and to allow others to take the lead when appropriate. The ability to demonstrate camaraderie tends to be contagious. Generalized to solo activities, the ability to feel a oneness with individuals who have had the same experience or a oneness with the environment.
Effort	The level of effort that the participant exerts as s/he engages in the activity. The participant with good participation skills demonstrates a consistently high level of effort regardless of the situation, activity, disability, or his/her skill level.
Preparedness	The participant's ability to come to the activity ready to participate, including having a positive attitude, willingness to make an effort, all necessary supplies, and ability to pay attention. The quality and fullness of participation depends on how prepared the participant is when s/he come to the activity. The participant who is able to demonstrate a consistently good level of participation comes to the activity in the appropriate mental frame of mind so that s/he will be able to gain from the activity. On the occasional times that the participant is able to identify that s/he would not be able to come prepared to participate in a positive sense, s/he is able to excuse himself/herself from the activity, recognizing that his/her frame of mind, and lack of preparedness may negatively influence the others in the group.

ual logically and convincingly presents himself/herself as having a physical illness when none exists. Also known as *Munchausen syndrome*.

pathophysiology the study of the correlation between the physical manifestations of a disease and the underlying disease process. Treatment of disease is not considered to be a primary purpose for the study.

patient See *client*.

patient record (HCO) the repository of information about an individual patient, usually stored on paper, but more recently in electronic form in a computer system. See *medical record*.

patient satisfaction a vital aspect of the effectiveness and appropriateness of the *treatment* provided is the patient's perception of the quality of the services. In a study completed by Press, Ganey Associates, Inc. of 139,830 former patients in 225 hospitals the top 14 factors that influenced patient satisfaction

were 1. staff's concern for patient privacy, 2. staff's sensitivity to the inconvenience of sickness and hospitalization, 3. adequacy of information given to family members concerning the patient's condition and treatment, 4. overall cheerfulness of the hospital's environment, 5. promptness and attitudes of the nursing staff when called by patient, 6. extent that nurses took patient problems seriously, 7. nurse's attention to the personal and special needs of the patient, 8. courtesy of the technician who took blood, 9. technician's explanation of tests and treatments, 10. likelihood that the patient will recommend the hospital to others, 11. friendliness of the nursing staff, 12. information available from the nursing staff about tests and treatments, 13. technical skill of the nurses, and 14. skill level of the technician who took the patient's blood (Kreitner, Hartz & Pflum, 1994). Patient satisfaction is an important *quality assurance* measure.

Patient Self-Determination Act a federal regulation which is part of the original OBRA Act of 1987 which required that all health care facilities must provide their patients with information on *advanced directives*. See *living wills*.

payer person, company, or government entity that will be paying all or part of the patient's bill.

PC card (HCO) a credit card-sized computer peripheral or peripheral interface used with portable and desktop computers. Also known as a PCMCIA card.

PCMCIA card See *PC card*.

pedagogy typical teaching strategies used with children. This teaching strategy assumes that the student is like an empty vessel to be filled by the teacher. The emphasis is on the teacher being in charge of the teaching with the students assuming a more passive role. This is different than *andragogy*, a *teaching* strategy used with adults. See *learning disabilities*.

pedicle graft To ensure adequate nourishment to the autogenous graft, part of the graft will remain connected to the donor site while the rest is attached to the recipient site. Usually the donor site is a piece of skin next to the injured site, but at times the pedicle graft will come from a different part of the body causing the individual to be placed in an awkward, uncomfortable position for a period of time. In addition to the trauma that caused the need for a graft, the patient usually experiences pain due to the muscle and joint strain of being immobilized in an unnatural position.

pedophilia a clinically recognized mental disorder where the adult (over age 16) has ongoing fantasies, sexual urges, or behaviors associated with prepubescent children that have lasted at least six months. These sexual thoughts, urges, and behaviors are significant enough to impact the individual's *functional ability*. The majority of pedophiles engage in genital fondling or oral sex with children under the age of thirteen years with the exception of pedophiles who engage in incest. Incest frequently involves vaginal or anal penetration by the perpetrator. See *disability*.

peer review the review of services provided by professionals who hold the same credentials as the individual or group providing the service. This term and concept are key components of both utilization management activities and *quality assurance* programs.

peer review organization (PRO) Legislation created in 1972 which mandated the development and use of organizations to ensure that medical care was of high quality, reflecting the most current *standards* of care (Public Law No. 92-603 of the Social Security Amendments and modified with Public Law 94-182 of the Social Security Act of 1975). These

physician organizations, under contract with the *Health Care Financing Administration*, ensure that Medicare beneficiaries and Medicaid recipients receive care which is medically necessary, reasonable, provided in the appropriate setting, and which meets professionally accepted standards of quality. PROs are to intervene when quality problems are identified. The PRO must give the attending physician an opportunity to discuss questioned care with a physician reviewer before the PRO utilizes interventions which are available to them such as education, intensified review, alternate timing review, etc. (and ultimately sanctions), to effect changes in behavior. See *Health Care Quality Improvement Act of 1986*.

pelvic inflammatory disease See *chlamydial infection*.

penetration 1. entering or breaking through a barrier. 2. the percentage of employees within a given employment group that a managed care organization is able to enroll. See *saturation*. 3. the percentage of an X-ray that passes through an object.

people first language a concept related to the use of language to reduce negative attitudes toward individuals with disabilities. Instead of referring to individuals with disabilities as "the quadriplegic" or "the retarded child," the concept of people first language encourages using the phrases "the man who has quadriplegia" or "the child who is mentally retarded." Using the disability as a modifier to the person is considered to be more sensitive, placing more emphasis on the person and less on the disability.

people movers See *automated guideway transit*.

peptide natural or synthetic compounds containing two or more amino acids where the carboxyl group of one amino acid is linked to the amino group of another amino acid. The larger peptides (called polypeptides) have in excess of 100 amino acids while proteins have 200 or more.

perceived competence in leisure the perception that one has the ability to engage in leisure activity. There are two distinct aspects to perceived competence in leisure: external competence (an individual's evaluation of his/her abilities compared to the others in the same age group and gender) and internal competence (an individual's evaluation of his/her abilities compared to his/her own expectations of performance).

perceived freedom (of leisure) a proposed precondition of leisure involvement and satisfaction, perceived freedom in leisure is a perception that one has the opportunity to voluntarily make choices about one's leisure. See *Comprehensive Leisure Rating Scale*.

perception deficit an inability to recognize objects

or to misjudge one object's relationship to another object due to an inability to distinguish:
1. context (figure-ground),
2. significance of an object,
3. intensity of an object, and/or
4. the identity of a previously familiar object.

percussion a technique used to mechanically dislodge mucus from the lungs. Using a slightly cupped hand, the therapist alternately strikes ("claps") the patient's chest over the segment of the lung being treated. The clapping is carried out in a rhythmic fashion. The therapist works on one location for a few minutes or until the patient feels the need to cough. Percussion (and associated *vibration*) should not be painful or cause irritation to patients with sensitive skin. Percussion is contraindicated for patients with low platelet counts or anti-coagulation therapy, unstable angina or chest pain due to recent surgery. Percussion should also be avoided over areas of tumor, over bony prominences, over breast tissue in women or over fractures or osteoporotic bone.

per diem staffing an on-call worker who is used to cover when the regular staff person is not working his/her "normal" hours or when the patient census and/or load is above what the regular staff are able to cover. In the United States many therapists receive two weeks of vacation time each year. Many departments feel that they can "make do" for the two weeks a therapist is on vacation. However, the typical employee also misses five working days a year due to illness, has an average of ten days holiday leave a year and five days continuing education leave a year, creating a six week yearly absence instead of just the two weeks for vacation. Because of the ongoing efforts to cut health care costs, many facilities run lean when it comes to staffing. The pay

rate for per diem staff is 20-40% higher than regular staff. This extra hourly rate is to make up for not being part of the usual benefits package and to compensate the worker for an irregular schedule. Per diem workers need to have the same employee orientation and on-the-job training as regular employees.

perfectionism the unhealthy and irrational pursuit of excellence. The pursuit of perfection instead of the attainment of a rational, yet high standard of performance, is a maladaptive trait that can be seen in some psychiatric disorders such as *anorexia nervosa*. A perfectionist acts on the belief that mistakes in performance are unacceptable. This failure to meet unobtainable standards of performance often leads to self-doubts and fears of rejections from others. Individuals who work toward excellence tend to generally enjoy the process and events that lead up to their achievements. While perfectionism is not considered to be a psychiatric disorder, it is recognized as a vulnerability factor for other recognized disorders. The construct for perfectionism recognizes three different subcategories of perfectionism: 1. self-oriented perfectionism, 2. other-oriented perfectionism, and 3. socially prescribed perfectionism. Self-oriented perfectionism is the expectation by the individual that s/he will be perfect. Typical problems associated with this type of perfectionism include exacerbated and prolonged clinical depression, anorexia nervosa, prolonged elevations in cardiovascular responses, and interpersonal conflicts with others related to over-committing and not following through. Other-oriented perfectionism is the expectation that others (such as one's co-workers, family members, government employees, or others) should be perfect. Typical problems associated with this type of perfectionism include excessive anger

Perfectionism: Myths and Realities
(University of Texas at Austin Counseling and Mental Health Center, 1999)

Myths	Realities
I wouldn't be the success I am today if I weren't such a perfectionist.	Perfectionism does not lead to success and fulfillment. Although some perfectionists are remarkably successful, what they fail to realize is that their success has been achieved despite, not because of, their compulsive striving.
Perfectionists get things done and they do things right.	Perfectionists often have problems with procrastination, missed deadlines, and low productivity.
Perfectionists are determined to overcome all obstacles to success.	Although perfectionists follow an "I'll keep trying until it's perfect" credo, they are especially vulnerable to potentially serious difficulties such as depression, writer's block, and performance and social anxiety.
Perfectionists just have this enormous desire to please others and to be the very best they can.	Perfectionistic tendencies often begin as an attempt to win love, acceptance, and approval.

with others, relationship problems related to dissatisfaction with the other person. Expecting others to be perfect tends to cause an individual to be rigid/inflexible and non-spontaneous. Socially prescribed perfectionism is the belief that others (such as one's co-workers, family members, government employees, or others) expect oneself to be perfect. Hewitt (1999) states: "Socially prescribed perfectionism has been associated with a variety of symptoms including, anxiety, depression, eating disorder symptoms, and hostility. Most importantly, this dimension of perfectionism has been found to predict not only suicide thoughts and behaviors in adults and adolescents, but also serious suicide attempts. Furthermore, there are a variety of achievement-related problems that arise from this kind of perfectionism, such as procrastination and self-handicapping (i.e., where individuals spend time finding excuses for poor performance rather than preparing for a performance). Finally, perfectionistic self-presentation involves a variety of difficulties such as precluding one from seeking appropriate help for difficulties and not benefiting fully from treatment due to great difficulties in self-disclosing personal information." Some of the myths and realities of perfectionism are shown on the previous page.

performance See *organizational performance.*

performance goals statements about the desired level of quality and quantity of services provided. Performance goals tend to be of three types: thresholds, benchmarks, and permitted variance. Thresholds are the desired minimum performance levels allowed within the practice group or agency. Thresholds may be greater or lesser than benchmarks, which are industry performance standards (accepted standards of practice). Permitted variance goals are performance goals that differ from accepted standards of practice as conditions dictate a reasonable variance. Examples of permitted variances which differ from standards of practice may relate to the number of patients a therapist is expected to see (therapists who see patients with extremely complex *dual diagnoses* may have a lower therapist to patient ratio) or to the outcomes expected (doctors who see patients with both AIDS and cancer may have a higher death rate among their patients than doctors who do not see very many patients with AIDS).

period prevalence (HHS) the number of existing cases of an illness during a period or interval, divided by the average population.

peripheral blood stem cells (PBSC) (HHS/NMDP) a cell with the potential to produce all the components of blood that is obtained from peripheral blood rather than from bone marrow.

peripheral nervous system the system of nerves outside of the brain and the spinal cord. The peripheral nerves consist of the spinal nerves (31 pairs), the autonomic nervous system nerves (sympathetic and parasympathetic), and the cranial nerves.

PERRLA (pupils equal, round, react to light, accommodation) an abbreviation used to document that the patient's eyes have been examined and found to be within normal expectations. If problems are found with the eyes during an exam, PERRLA is not written in the chart note. Instead, the health care professional documents the abnormal findings.

perseveration getting "stuck" on a response. This can be either a verbal or a motor response.

persistent tremor See *tremor.*

persistent vegetative state a coma-like state of the body and mind. Legally, persistent vegetative state was defined by the New Jersey Superior Court as being "the body functions entirely in terms of its internal controls. It maintains temperature. It maintains digestive activity. It maintains heartbeat and pulmonary ventilation. It maintains reflex activity of muscles and nerves for low-level conditioned responses. But there is no behavioral evidence of either self-awareness or awareness of the surroundings in a learned manner." (Jobes, 529 A. 2d 434 NJ 1987) See *coma.*

personal digital assistant (PDA) (HCO) a hand held computer, usually with no keyboard, that is used for communications or data collection and analysis.

personal protective equipment (PPE) equipment provided to employees to control the exposure to blood-borne pathogens and *OPIMs.* While personal protective equipment can be many different items, it generally is considered to be gowns (used to protect clothing from possible soiling), facemasks and safety goggles (used to protect the eyes, mouth, or face from splashes), waterproof gloves (to protect hands), boots (to protect shoes), and earplugs (to protect ears from loud noises). See *blood-borne pathogens, occupational exposure to blood-borne pathogens standard.*

personal safety (aquatic) the awareness of risk and danger associated with activity within and around a water environment and performance of behavior necessary for safety. Personal safety refers more to a cognitive capacity as opposed to physical skill. The ability to perform functional aquatic activities does not determine an individual's actual safety around a body of water. See *aquatic therapy.*

pertussis (CDC) a highly communicable, vaccine-preventable disease that lasts for many weeks and is typically manifested in children with paroxysmal spasms of severe coughing, whooping, and post-tussive vomiting. This disease results in high morbidity and mortality in many countries every year. In the United States, 5000-7000 cases are reported each year. Incidence of pertussis has increased steadily since the 1980's. The highest incidence since 1967 (2.9/100,000) was reported in 1996, when 7796 cases of pertussis were reported. Major complications are most common among infants and young children and include hypoxia, apnea, pneumonia, seizures, encephalopathy, and malnutrition. Young children can die from pertussis; in the United States 5-10 children die every year. Most deaths occur among unvaccinated children or children too young to be vaccinated. Transmission occurs through direct contact with discharges from respiratory mucous membranes of infected persons. Risk groups include children who are too young to be fully vaccinated and those who have not completed the primary vaccination series. Like measles, pertussis is highly contagious with up to 90% of susceptible household contacts developing clinical disease following exposure to an index case. Adolescents and adults become susceptible when immunity wanes.

pervasive developmental disorders a specific diagnostic category in the **DSM-IV**, pervasive developmental disorders include sub-functional ability in social interaction, communication skills, and the presence of *stereotyped behaviors*, activities, and interests. Included in this grouping of disorders is autistic disorder, Rett's disorder, childhood disintegrative disorder, and Asperger's disorder. See *autism, schizophrenia.*

pesticide (HHS) a broad class of crop protection chemicals including four major types: insecticides used to control insects; herbicides used to control weeds; rodenticides used to control rodents; and fungicides used to control mold, mildew, and fungi. In addition, consumers use pesticides in the home or yard to control termites and roaches, clean mold from shower curtains, stave off crab grass, kill fleas and ticks on pets, and disinfect swimming pools, to name just a few "specialty" pesticide uses.

pet therapy See *animal facilitated therapy, zoomatology.*

PEW Charitable Trusts a national philanthropy group based in Philadelphia that established the *PEW Health Professions Commission* in 1989. The purpose of the PEW Commission is to determine approaches to help reform state educational programs, workforce planning, and licensure systems. This commission will have long-range impact on the formal training and continuing education training re-

quirements of all health care professionals within the United States. See *PEW Health Professions Commission.*

PEW Health Professions Commission The PEW Health Professions Commission Taskforce on Health Care Workforce Regulation reviewed the current state of professional training of health care professionals, of health care *credentialing* and aspects of consumer safety and protection. What they found was a lack of consistency within each professional group's training requirements nationally, significant variation of what each state required for health care professionals, inconsistent definitions of the *scope of practice* for professionals, inconsistent *reimbursement* practices within and across regions, impairment of the delivery of health care services due to territoriality of each professional group (to the detriment of good services to the public), and overall, a confusing set of messages sent to the public who used the health care services. The taskforce published ten recommendations shown below to address these problems. One of the most controversial recommendations of the PEW Taskforce is to eliminate some of the licensure laws that restrict certain practices to just one or two disciplines. For example, this would open up the workplace for recreational therapists to do more ADLs and occupational therapists to engage in more leisure education. It would also allow the use of para-professionals like nurses aides in place of registered nurses for some duties. Another aspect of the recommendations would be the establishment of a core *knowledge* base for all therapists, with each specialty group taking coursework specific to their field after they have completed the core courses. This would require a restructuring of many university departments, espe-

PEW Taskforce Recommendations

1. standardizing regulatory terms
2. standardizing entry-to-practice requirements
3. removing barriers to the full use of competent health professionals
4. redesigning regulatory board structure and function
5. informing the public about practitioner practices
6. collecting data on the health professions
7. assessing practitioner competence and assuring continuing competence
8. reforming the professional disciplinary process
9. evaluating regulatory effectiveness
10. understanding the organizational context of health professions regulation

cially in the field of recreational therapy, as most of the core courses are now offered in medical colleges. See *SAFE.*

phantom pain either a dull or sharp *pain* felt by a patient that seems to originate from a limb that is no longer present (has been amputated). This pain is very real and frequently limits the patient's ability to concentrate on activities. The professional may want to note the patient's description of the pain (burning, electrical, or throbbing) and the duration of the pain. Eventually the patient learns to localize the pain to the stump.

pharmacy benefit management (PBM) (HCO) a method of managing pharmaceutical benefits for insurers and employers that uses disease management, pharmacy networks, negotiated discounts and rebates, lists of preferred drugs, and online *utilization review.* Also, an organization (pharmacy benefit manager) that performs PBM services.

phenotype (HHS/NMDP) the physical expression of genes inherited for a particular characteristic. For example, a person who inherited a brown eye color gene (Br) and a blue eye color gene (Bl) has a phenotype of brown eyes. Contrast with *genotype.*

phlebitis See *thrombophlebitis.*

phobia a fear not based on logic or the reality of the situation that is persistent, intense, and causes the individual to run away from the object of fear. See *applied relaxation, dual diagnosis.*

phocomelia a birth defect in which the arms and/or the legs are absent at birth. The hands and feet are attached to the trunk.

photoplethysmograph See *plethysmograph.*

photoplethysmography (PPG) a method to measure and monitor vasoconstriction and dilation. PPG provides an accurate and reliable measurement of autonomic nervous system involvement. Recall vasoconstriction is often a sympathetic nervous system reaction. The technology for photoplethysmography was developed in the 1960's by physiology researchers and is used for assessment and monitoring of peripheral blood flow, e.g., to the hands and feet.

photosensitivity the abnormal and undesirable response of the skin to sunlight. This response is a direct result of medications taken by the patient or due to a disorder. The typical response is a heightened risk of sunburn. See *baclofen, porphyria, side effect.*

physiatrist a medical doctor who specializes in physical medicine.

physical abuse bodily harm one individual inflicts on another individual. It is emotionally hard for the therapist to work with individuals, especially children, who are physically abused. At times it seems unexplainable that an abused individual would want to stay with the abusing other and may even lead the therapist to call into question his/her feelings as to whether the situation is bad enough to warrant a change. However, study after study, both with animals and with humans, has shown that severe mistreatment increases the emotional attachment to the abuser. The reality of this goes against "logic." We assume that individuals want to get away from pain and broken trust. However, since research has shown (Sanderson, 1995) that an unusually strong (and unhealthy) bond occurs with physical abuse, the therapist will need to help the patient make decisions about safety first. *Cognitive therapy* and other interventions should be undertaken after the patient is safe whenever possible and practical. Physical abuse in health care facilities is defined by federal *Immediate and Serious Threat* regulations in the United States as the failure to protect patients from bodily harm or trauma. Conditions/situations that may indicate patient abuse include: 1. patients who have bruises, cuts, burns (cigarettes, etc.); 2. patients who state that they have been abused; 3. staff, family, or others who state that abuse has occurred; and 4. fractures without adequate explanation or corroborating evidence to support them.

physical activities (as outlined by the US Department of Labor) The US Department of Labor lists twenty physical activities as part of an *evaluation* for work hardiness. Assessment for return to work after a labor and industry claim should include information on the individual's *functional ability* to perform each of the twenty activities shown below. See *ergonomics, work hardening.*

physicalization a term used in Viola Spolin's book *Improvisation for the Theater.* Different from taking an intellectual or psychological approach to communication during theater games, the individual takes a physical, non-verbal approach. The purpose is to encourage the freedom of physical expression, hopefully opening the door for greater insight.

Physical Activities

balancing	crouching	hearing	pushing	standing
carrying	feeling	kneeling	reaching	stooping
climbing	fingering	lifting	seeing	talking
crawling	handling	pulling	sitting	walking

physical medicine and rehabilitation (PM & R) a specialty in health care which is based on the bodies of knowledge in 1. cognition, 2. functional anatomy, 3. neuromuscular physiology, and 4. exercise physiology. The accrediting body for this specialty is *CARF: the Rehabilitation Accreditation Commission.*

physical restraints any mechanical means of restricting a patient's movement, including geri-chairs, seatbelts on wheelchairs (when used to restrict standing), and gates across doors. (RAPs) Studies of nursing homes show that between 30% and 40% of patients are physically restrained. This is quite serious since negative effects of restraint use include declines in patients' physical functioning (e.g., ability to ambulate) and muscle condition, *contractures*, increased incidence of *infections* and development of *pressure sores*, *delirium*, *agitation*, and *incontinence*. Moreover, restraints have been found in some cases to increase the incidence of *falls* and other accidents (e.g., strangulation). Finally, patients who are restrained face the loss of autonomy, *dignity*, and self-respect. In effect, the use of physical restraints undercuts the major goals of care — to maximize independence, functional capacity, and *quality of life*. Thus, the goal of minimizing or eliminating restraint use has become central to both clinical practice and federal law. The primary reason given for applying restraints is to protect patients from falls and accidents. Facilities are also concerned about potential lawsuits and malpractice claims that might result if patients should fall. Other reasons cited for restraint use include: to provide postural support or positioning for patients, to facilitate treatment (e.g., preventing patients from pulling out IV lines or NG tubes), and to manage behaviors such as wandering or physical aggressiveness. The experience of many health care providers suggests that facility goals can often be met without the use of physical restraints and their negative side effects. In part, this involves identifying and treating health, functional, or psychosocial problems that may be causing the condition for which restraints were ordered (e.g., falls, wandering, agitation). Minimizing use of restraints also involves care management alternatives such as: modifying the environment to make it safer; maintaining an individual's customary routine; using less intrusive methods of administering medications and nourishment; and recognizing and responding to patients' needs for psychosocial support, responsive health care, meaningful activities, and regular exercise.

physical therapist an individual who has completed the required education, training, and experience and is accredited by a nationally recognized accreditation body. See *Joint Commission.*

physical therapy treatment provided by qualified individuals to remediate and restore posture, *locomotion*, *strength*, endurance, cardiopulmonary function, balance, coordination, joint mobility, flexibility, healing, and repair to improve functional ability. See *Joint Commission.*

Physician Data Query (PDQ) (HCO) a system of online (Internet) information regarding various cancers, ongoing clinical trials, and individuals and organizations involved in cancer care, maintained by the National Cancer Institute.

physician hospital organization the group representing physicians and the hospitals in which they work. The group is responsible for negotiating contractual agreements with third party payers.

physician services health care services that are provided directly by a physician.

phytochemical (HHS) substances found in edible fruits and vegetables that may be ingested by humans daily in gram quantities and that exhibit a potential for modulating the human metabolism in a manner favorable for reducing risk of cancer. See *functional foods.*

pica the unnatural mouthing and chewing or eating of objects in a developmentally inappropriate manner. Causes for pica include a severe nutritional deficit, some types of mental disorders, and some levels of mental retardation. See *childhood psychiatric disorders, feeding and eating disorders of early infancy.*

Pick's disease a type of *dementia* that frequently develops before the age of 65. This type of dementia affects the cerebral cortex and the frontal lobes. The loss of function in this part of the brain causes the patient to lose intellectual functioning and to lose an awareness of social "rules." Both because this disease frequently strikes its victims at an early age and because awareness of social skills and norms vanishes, this is a particularly challenging disability to treat. See *dementia.*

picture archiving and communications system (PACS) (HCO) a computer-based system of storing and retrieving radiographic and other images in digital form.

PID pelvic inflammatory disease. See *chlamydial infections.*

PIE charting a style of writing in the medical chart using the following format: patient's problem, intervention taken, and an evaluation of the outcome.

pink eye See *conjunctivitis.*

pituitary (HHS) also known as the hypophysis; a gland at the base of the brain with two functionally distinct lobes involved in regulating growth, metabolism, and maturation.

pixel (HCO) the smallest displayable area on a computer screen.

PL See *public law.*

placebo (HHS) sometimes casually referred to as a "sugar pill." A placebo is a "fake" treatment that seems identical to the real treatment. Placebo treatments are used to eliminate bias that may arise from the expectation that a treatment should produce an effect.

plan administration the management of a managed care program including all business functions separate from the direct provision of health care. This includes accounting and billing, personnel, marketing, purchasing, and legal affairs.

plan of correction *provider*/supplier's written plan on the statement of deficiencies and plan of correction (HCFA 2567), stating what corrective actions will be made and the completion date for correction. A provider will ordinarily be expected to achieve compliance within 60 days of the survey, however, more time may be permissible for certain types of deficiencies. It is vital that the therapist work directly with the administrator to outline any plan of correction for deficiencies found in the delivery of therapy services. The correction of deficiencies takes staff time, time that is already stretched to meet the needs of the patient load. Be realistic in what your department or team can achieve in 60 days. Work with the administrator to ensure that the deficiencies cited by the surveyors can be corrected with the plan of correction that outlined. See *acceptable plan of correction, automatic cancellation clause, survey process.*

plaque a deposit of fatty material in the lining of a blood vessel. Build up of plaque in or near the brain can lead to the blockage of the blood vessel, resulting in a *cerebrovascular accident.*

plasma the fluid portion of the blood, rich in soluble proteins with a wide range of functions.

plasticity the tendency for soft tissue to resume a slightly longer length after a period of gentle *passive stretching.* Muscles are made up of bundles of fibers called myofibril. Each myofibril is made up of shorter, overlapping fibers called sarcomere that are made up of actin and myosin filaments. During contraction the actin and myosin filaments slide closer together (overlap more) causing the muscle fibers to contract. When the myofibrils experience repeated, prolonged periods of gentle stretching, the amount of sarcomeres are increased, allowing an actual lengthening of the muscle. See *myofibril, sarcomere.*

platelet a component of the blood important in clot-

ting. Inadequate amounts of platelets will lead to bleeding and bruising easily. These are the smallest cells in blood and contain no hemoglobin.

platform crutch crutches that have a horizontal support or trough for the patient's arm which bears the weight of the patient's body (instead of having the palm bear the weight as in the Canadian or the auxiliary crutch). See *crutch.*

playfulness (elements of) a complex skill that goes through many different developmental stages. In general, playfulness requires the ability to be spontaneous, creative, aware of one's environment, and imaginative. Playful interactions require a balance of positive exchanges with one's environment, with one's self (body, thoughts, and feelings), and with others. Being playful is healthy. See *Leisure Diagnostic Battery.*

playground injuries injuries suffered on a playground. See the table on the next page for information on playground injuries.

plethysmograph a device for measuring changes in the volume of organs or other body parts. It is often used to measure the sexual response pattern of a male or female client. It is called a penile plethysmograph for males and photoplethysmograph for females.

PMS See *premenstrual dysphoric disorder.*

pneumonia inflammation and swelling of the lungs due to infection. The patient experiences chest pain, fatigue, and chills. Full recovery may take several months, even with antibiotics. See *bed, oscillating support bed, respiratory isolation.*

poetry therapy a term used by J. Leedy who suggested using poetry (either by writing it or reading it) to allow the patient to express his/her thoughts and to find greater awareness of self. By reading poetry written by others a patient may find someone to identify with and a springboard for opportunity to share thoughts or concerns with others. By writing poetry the patient may find a means to release his/her emotions of fear, doubt, anxiety, and internal conflict.

point of service a type of health benefit plan in which the individual has the right to select providers outside of managed care organizations, although this choice frequently results in a reduced percentage of the bill being covered. This type of service is also known as an *open-ended health maintenance organization.*

policy a formal statement which defines how a facility views a specific topic or event. For example, "The Professional will conduct an assessment of each patient's activity needs within 7 days of admission." The policy statement is then followed by a

Playground Injuries (CDC)

Topic	Discussion
How large is the problem of playground-related injuries?	Each year in the United States, 200,000 preschool and elementary school children visit emergency departments for care of injuries sustained on playground equipment (about 1 injury every 2½ minutes). About 35% of all playground-related injuries are severe (e.g., fractures, internal injuries, concussions, dislocations, amputations, crushes). Public playgrounds account for about 70% of injuries related to playground equipment. In schools, most injuries to students between the ages of 5 and 14 years occur on playgrounds.
Which playground equipment causes the most injury?	Most injuries occur when children fall off swings, monkey bars, climbers, or slides. Falls off of playground equipment to the ground account for more than 60% of all playground-related injuries. Slightly less than 3% of all playground injuries require hospitalization.
How many children die each year because of playground-related injuries?	Each year, nearly 20 children die from playground-related injuries. More than half of these deaths result from strangulation and about one-third result from falls.
What costs are associated with playground-related injury?	In 1995, the costs were $1.2 billion for children younger than 15 years old.
What is CDC doing to prevent playground-related injuries?	The National Center for Injury Prevention and Control, CDC, funds the National Program for Playground Safety (NPPS), which works to prevent playground-related injuries and the attendant suffering and costs. This program is based at the University of Northern Iowa in Cedar Falls, Iowa. 800/554-PLAY; www.uni.edu/playground.
What are the goals of NPPS?	To implement a national plan for the prevention of playground-related injuries. To maintain a clearinghouse of materials on playground safety and make those materials available to anyone who requests them. To provide an information hotline on preventing playground-related injury. To hold training programs for teachers and playground safety inspectors. To research the impact attenuation characteristics of playground surfaces under a variety of conditions.

procedure that outlines how that policy will be implemented.

policyholder the individual to whom the health care insurance policy is issued. Family members are frequently also covered under the benefit program but they are not considered to be the policyholder.

poliomyelitis an infection of the nervous system, caused by one of three polioviruses, which may cause paralysis. Also known as "polio."

polyincestuous sexual abuse between family members that spans more than two generations.

polysubstance dependence the use of three or more drugs of abuse over a 12 month (or longer) period of time. The three or more drugs of abuse must come from the list in *substance-related disorders* with the exception of caffeine and nicotine, which do not count as polysubstance dependence drugs. Generally, an individual with a polysubstance dependence meets the criteria for *substance dependence* with a variety of drugs, not just one primary drug with occasional use of two or more other drugs. See *comorbidity.*

Pontiac fever See *Legionnaire's disease.*

population-based study a study of all the population group (not just those who receive services in the treatment center). An example would be the evaluation of the percentage of all individuals with spina bifida who use the local parks and recreation program instead of evaluating only the percentage from the public schools. (In the latter case you would be missing individuals who are in private schools or who do not attend school at all.)

porphyria inherited disorders that result in increased production of porphyrins. Common symptoms are abdominal pains, *photosensitivity*, and *neuropathy*. Acute intermittent porphyria is more common in women and can be caused by changes in hormone balance or starvation and crash dieting, among other things. See *metabolic disorders.*

positron emission tomography (PET scan) (CDC) an imaging technique that relies on the detection of gamma rays emitted from tissues after administration of a natural biochemical substance into which positron-emitting isotopes have been incorporated.

post traumatic amnesia See *amnesia.*

post-traumatic stress disorder (PTSD) an individ-

Warning Signs Associated with PTSD (Matsakis, 1994, p. 208).

As you work to heal from your trauma, both in sessions and outside, you need to monitor your reactions. This work includes talking to your counselor, doing writing or other exercises about the traumatic events you experienced or the aftereffects, emotional effects, or subsequent related events. If you experience any of the following symptoms while doing such work (or at any other time) stop what you are doing immediately and talk to your counselor or another mental health professional.

- Hyperventilation (uncontrollable gasping for air or rapid breathing), uncontrollable shaking, or irregular heartbeat
- Feelings that you are losing touch with reality, even temporarily, for instance, having hallucinations or extreme flashbacks of the event
- Feeling disoriented, spaced out, unreal, or as if you might be losing control
- Extreme nausea, diarrhea, hemorrhaging, or other physical problems, including intense, new, or unexplainable pains, or an increase in symptoms of a preexisting medical problem, for example, blood sugar problems if you are diabetic
- A desire to hurt yourself
- Self-destructive behavior such as alcohol or drug abuse, self-induced vomiting, or overspending
- Suicidal or homicidal thoughts
- Memory problems

Also call for help if you are having so much emotional pain, anxiety, or anger that you fear you are going to die. Mild anxiety is a normal reaction, but extreme anxiety or despair needs professional attention as soon as possible.

If you are unable to contact your counselor and are truly frightened, go to the emergency room of a local hospital. Meanwhile, do the following:

- Focus on something besides the trauma
- Touch a physical object (a wall, a chair, whatever is near by)
- Talk to someone right away
- Avoid isolating yourself or taking alcohol, drugs, or other mood-altering substances
- If you are angry, try expressing it in a safe way, such as talking to a trusted friend, punching a pillow, or tearing up a telephone directory.

Even if you feel certain you do not need professional help, if you experience any of the reactions listed above, take a break from trauma work and follow one of these suggestions. Keep in mind that having a strong reaction to thinking about the trauma or otherwise working on healing doesn't make you a failure. Developing symptoms as a result of being in therapy doesn't reflect an inability to heal or a hidden unwillingness to heal. Instead, your reactions probably reflect the degree of traumatization you endured, which was not under your control. Your reactions have nothing to do with your strength of character.

ual's response to an unexpected, extraordinary life event that produces a sustained painful response. The patient may experience an interruption in his/her normal sleep patterns, inability to concentrate, increased likelihood of being startled, and decreased ability to initiate activity. PTSD is an anxiety disorder that was first recognized by the American Psychiatric Association in 1980. Chronic PTSD may actually be mistakenly diagnosed as a major *depression* or take on the form of psychosomatic symptoms. Symptoms frequently seen in patients with PTSD:
- overwhelming feeling of not being safe
- alteration in thinking patterns (due to fear)

- alteration in emotional equilibrium (deficit in ability to temper emotions)
- decreased ability to internally calm oneself and to utilize *relaxation techniques*
- decreased ability to follow through on social commitments and relationships
- negative self-talk, impairing realistic view of actual attributes

Symptoms that the therapist is likely to see include
1. the re-experiencing of the trauma through flashbacks, intrusive memories, and nightmares;
2. increased arousal when coping mechanisms fail exhibited by difficulty concentrating, hypervigilance, increased startle response, outbursts of anger,

and problems sleeping; and 3. a general avoiding of things associated with the trauma, developing an emotional numbing. The primary goal for patients with PTSD is to increase their ability to cope and/or to increase their *self-esteem* and self-confidence. This is generally achieved only through the mastery of specific skills related to their ADLs or their leisure. The *cognitive therapy* aspect of the patient's treatment will probably alternative between dealing with feelings and finding relief from the feelings (e.g., temporarily ignoring/hiding feelings and learning to enjoy life). The key attributes of the therapist should be consistency, predictability, and supportiveness. Warning signs associated with PTSD are shown on the previous page. See *initiation.*

posterior referring to the back part of a structure; the dorsal surface of the body.

post-test See *pre-test.*

postural drainage the use of gravity to help remove unwanted secretions from the airway. Patients frequently show a resistance to postural drainage because of *boredom, agitation, pain,* etc. The development of enjoyable activities to be engaged in during drainage helps increase compliance.

postural dysfunction the patient's decreased ability to engage in activities caused by a shortening of soft tissue and muscle weakness. The patient experiences *fatigue* and a limiting *range of motion* that can frequently be overcome through the prescriptive use of activities. Compare with *postural fault.*

postural fault an abnormal alignment of the body caused by *pain,* not caused by structural defects or *postural dysfunction.*

potential the maximum degree of skill or wellness that a patient is judged capable of reaching given the right interventions and environment.

poverty of content See *alogia.*

poverty of speech See *alogia.*

power-assisted door (ADA) a door used for human passage with a mechanism that helps to open the door or relieves the opening resistance of a door, upon the activation of a switch or a continued force applied to the door itself. See *automatic door.*

powerlessness a perception that one is unable to influence one's own life, that one is not able to significantly affect an outcome, or a perceived lack of control over a current situation. A patient who feels powerless to control the events of his/her life will be less likely to initiate activity. See *helplessness.*

PPE See *personal protective equipment.*

practice guidelines based on both clinical literature and expert consensus, practice guidelines are statements about the provision of appropriate services (type, quality, and quantity) based on the patient's

specific clinical circumstances. In some situations the term is used interchangeably with "*protocols.*" See *appropriateness, clinical practice guidelines.*

pragmatic the belief that actions are valuable only if their *outcomes* are positive; making choices based on actual results.

preadmission review the *assessment* process to determine that an admission to treatment is appropriate. This assessment takes place before admission.

pre-certification Many insurance companies help manage their costs by requiring a patient to get pre-approval of insurance coverage before undergoing treatment. Without this "pre-certification" for insurance coverage, neither the patient nor the provider can be sure that the fees will be covered.

precipitating factors an event or action that directly causes something else to happen. If an adult in her late 80's falls at home and breaks a hip, the fall and resulting hip fracture are considered to be the precipitating factors to her being admitted to a nursing home.

predictor a specific skill or health status that, based on past experience, means that something else can be expected to happen. An activity *assessment* which shows that a new patient chose to be isolated in his home for two years since his wife's death is usually a predictor of difficulty in getting the patient to join in activities.

preexisting condition a health care condition that existed prior to the individual's enrolling in a health care benefit/insurance program. Depending on state law and the insurance contract, preexisting conditions may or may not be covered and, if covered, are frequently subject to a period of months before the new policy will cover expenses related to the preexisting condition.

preferred provider agreement (PPA) an agreement between a provider and an indemnity styled health care program in which the provider agrees to discount his/her services for individuals who are covered by that health care plan. In turn, the individuals covered tend to have lower co-payments when they use professionals who have signed the preferred provider agreement.

premenstrual dysphoric disorder a cycle of mood changes and feelings of physical and psychological discomfort triggered by a woman's menstrual cycle. The "downward" mood swing starts soon after ovulation and resolves approximately five days prior to menstrual flow. Over 70% of women report some symptoms. Previously known as premenstrual syndrome (PMS).

Determining Patients at Risk for Pressure Sores

This table (from Shannon, 1984) will to help determine a patient's risk for developing pressure sores. Patients with a score of 16 or less on this assessment scale are at significant risk for developing pressure sores. To obtain a score, evaluate the patient's appropriate level in each of the eight risk categories that are listed across the top of the table. Add the values of the patient's level in each of the eight categories to obtain the patient's score for risk of developing a pressure sore.

Risk for Pressure Sore Assessment Scale

Mental Status	Continence	Mobility	Activity	Nutrition	Circulation	Temperature	Medications
4 Alert	**4** Continent	**4** Fully mobile	**4** Ambulatory	**4** Good	**4** Immediate capillary refill	**4** 98°-99° (36.6°-37.2°)	**4** No analgesics, tranquilizers, or steroids
3 Apathetic	**3** Incontinent of urine (without catheter)	**3** Slightly limited	**3** Walks with assistance	**3** Fair	**3** Delayed capillary refill	**3** 99°-100° (37.2°-37.7° C)	**3** One of the above
2 Confused	**2** Incontinent of feces	**2** Very limited	**2** Confined to wheelchair	**2** Poor	**2** Mild edema	**2** 100°-101° (37.7°-38.3° C)	**2** Two of the above
1 Stuporous or co-matose	**1** Incontinent of urine and feces	**1** Immobile	**1** Bedridden	**1** Cachectic (malnourished)	**1** Moderate to se-vere edema	**1** >101° (>38.3° c)	**1** All of the above

245

premenstrual syndrome (PMS) See *premenstrual dysphoric disorder*.

premorbid leisure lifestyle the combination of activities that the patient participated in prior to his/her injury or illness.

prescription a course of action (including giving medication) that is made up of four parts:

1. the mode of treatment (e.g., type of activity (movement, cognition, etc.) or type of medication required)
2. duration of treatment program (e.g., 14 days)
3. frequency of treatment (e.g., two times a day)
4. intensity of treatment (e.g., maintenance of 120% resting heart rate for 15 minutes or one 50-mg capsule)

See *orthosis*.

pressured speech speech that is too fast, too intense; a symptom of various psychiatric disorders. See *bipolar disorder*.

pressure garment See *Jobst*.

pressure release lifting or moving the body to relieve pressure on areas compressed by gravity, constricting garments, or appliances.

pressure sore (also known as "skin breakdown," "bedsore," "pressure ulcer," or "decubitus ulcer.") a breakdown in the normally healthy condition of the skin due to pressure or sheer. A Stage One pressure sore is a red mark that does not fade in 30 minutes after pressure has been relieved. A Stage Two pressure sore is a blister or an open sore which is just skin deep and caused, at least in part, by pressure or sheer. A Stage Three pressure sore is an opening in the skin and into the muscle caused, at least in part, by pressure or sheer. A Stage Four pressure sore is an opening in the skin and muscle down to the bone caused, at least in part, by pressure or sheer. Risk factors for developing pressure sores are shown on the previous page. (RAP) Between 3% and 5% of patients in nursing facilities have pressure sores. Sixty percent or more of patients will typically be at risk of pressure sore development. Pressure sores can have serious consequences for the elderly and are costly and time consuming to treat. However, they are one of the most common, preventable, and treatable conditions among elderly who have restricted *mobility*. Successful outcomes can be expected with preventative and treatment programs. See *activities of daily living, bed, crutch, epicondyle, exacerbate, incontinence, indicator, low air loss bed, neglect, physical restraint, significant change, space boot, ulcer*.

pre-test a functional or intelligence test given before any treatment or instruction is given. A second test called a post-test, is usually given after the treatment or instruction to measure change. The **Community Integration Program** by Armstrong and Lauzen uses pre-test/post-test procedures.

prevalence (HHS) the number of existing cases of a disease in a defined population at a specified time.

pricing strategies the ability to "name a price" for the services provided by the therapist is complex. The provider must take into account many aspects including the actual cost of labor and supplies, the cost of running a business, the cost of meeting regulations and standards, and much more. The chart on the next page (Klein, 1994) lists some of the questions the provider may need to ask prior to "naming a price."

primary database (HCO) data collected directly from individuals (e.g., surgery, observation) or documents (e.g., medical record review). See *database*.

prion a protein particle without nucleic acid; appears to be responsible for several infectious diseases of the nervous system including Creutzfeldt-Jakob disease and bovine spongiform encephalopathy (BSE).

prior review the process of determining that a proposed treatment or admission to services is indicated based on the information already gathered on the patient and his/her needs. In *managed care* systems, prior review and approval is frequently a requirement for the services and admission to be covered financially by the third party payer. Also known as prior authorization, prior certification and prior determination.

Privacy Act (HCO) the Federal Privacy Act of 1974 (5 USC Section 552a, 1988), which protects individuals from nonconsensual disclosure of confidential information by government agencies. See *confidentiality*.

private branch exchange (PBX) (HCO) an institution's internal phone system, which may include voice-messaging capabilities.

problem list a numbered list that contains the problems that interfere with the patient's health and functional ability. A problem list is part of a *problem-oriented record*. Almost all health care documentation has some kind of problem-oriented recording.

problem-oriented record (POR) a system of charting in the patient's medical chart in which only events that are problematic are documented. By using the POR method of *documentation* the assumption is that everything that should be done was done and would be evident by a positive outcome. This method of documentation does not work well in today's health care environment because it doesn't meet standards for quality assurance. See *problem list*.

Pricing Strategies

Factors	Considerations
General Concerns	• What type of business environment do you operate in? Is it highly competitive? • What will it be like in the future? • What is the level of managed care activity? • Are you defending a high private insurance or injured worker mix?
Competitor Facts	• Who are they? • What are their operating characteristics, facilities, strengths, and weaknesses? • What is their current pricing? • What is their market share? • What is their relative market image? • How do they compare against you, item for item? • Can and do they compete on price, service, and quality?
Operating Costs	• What are the real costs associated with delivering your services? • What are the sales and management costs? • What are the fixed cost burdens attributable to the delivery of specific services? • What are the costs of serving different contracts? • What profit margin is necessary to provide a reasonable return on the investment of resources?
Competitive and Customer Markets	• What are the current pricing levels for your competitors? • What is the recent price trend? • Where is the market going? • What are the changes in delivery of services? • How price sensitive is the market? • How service sensitive is it? • How results sensitive? • Who has won the most contracts recently and with what configuration of services and pricing?

problem solving the process that takes place when an individual is not able to reach a desired goal directly. Some of the skills associated with problem solving include: 1. the ability to identify the desired *outcome*, 2. the ability to gather and consider relevant information, 3. anticipating potential solutions, and 4. the selection of the action(s) that are most likely to get the desired outcome. See *cognition, cognitive deficits, cognitive retraining, cognitive therapy, counselor, ego, executive function, generalization, imagery, ineffective individual coping, processing deficits, time management skills.*

procedure 1. a pre-determined set of actions taken to achieve a desired health goal. 2. the step-by-step description of how staff are to complete the intent of a policy. Procedures are best stated with action verbs such as the ones shown below.

process indicator See *indicator.*

processing deficits Processing deficits tend to fall into three categories: 1. the inability to regulate the information being received (e.g., not being able to handle in a productive manner: the rate of reception, the amount being received, the type of information being received, other noises and input, and information overload); 2. the inability to organize the information being received (e.g., not being able to maintain information in *memory*, group the information with similar information to allow analysis and *prob-*

List of Action Words to Use in Procedures

accepts	analyzes	approves	arranges	avoids	carries through
collects	completes	concludes	conducts	confers	decides
delivers	denies	describes	distributes	endorses	engages
executes	files	fills	forwards	informs	keeps
notifies	observes	obtains	performs	plans	presents
prevents	processes	promotes	purchases	reports	requests
returns	runs	secures	sends	sets	supervises
takes	terminates	upholds	uses	visits	writes

lem solving and use internal conversations to help retrieve information (Which way is it to the recreation center?)); and 3. the inability to regulate the manner in which information is expressed (e.g., not being able to monitor one's responses to ensure correctness and sequencing that make sense, plan the response to ensure that it is presented in an organized manner and know when one needs more information before a response is appropriate (asking for clarification)). Compare with *organizational deficit*. See *sequencing skills*.

professional an individual who has attained a high degree of skill and extensive specialized training to be able to perform the tasks of his/her occupational group. A professional has knowledge of the standardized techniques, philosophical base and ethical code of his/her occupation and adheres to them to produce an excellence in service and product. Membership in one's professional organization and regular communication with one's occupational peers is vital for professional growth and development. Professionals and professional groups are dynamic (always changing) and change with as the environment in which they practice change. See *credentialing*.

professional misconduct actions that are considered unprofessional and unethical. These actions include obtaining a professional credential fraudulently; practicing fraudulently including practicing beyond the field's authorized *scope of practice*; demonstrating gross incompetence during any one therapy session; outright negligence or ongoing incompetence; refusing to provide treatment to any patient because of the patient's race, religion, color, or national origin; assisting, in any manner, an unqualified individual to perform activities requiring a credential; practicing while under the influence of alcohol, drugs, or mental disability; and being found guilty of committing a crime while working. See *credentialing*.

prognosis a well thought out guess about an *outcome*, based on clinical experience and clinical opinion, which predicts how the patient's health and/or skill level will change over a specific period of time.

progressive relaxation a type of relaxation technique. The purposeful tensing then relaxing of body parts in a prescribed fashion. The technique, first developed by Edmund Jacobson in 1929, usually progresses through hands, forearms, biceps, head, face (forehead, cheeks, nose, jaw, tongue), shoulders, neck, chest, stomach, lower back, thighs, buttocks, calves, and feet. This type of relaxation technique has been helpful in the treatment of muscle tension and *pain* (including neck and back pain), muscle spasms, *fatigue*, high blood pressure, *depression*, in-

somnia, and *anxiety*. With practice twice a day for about fifteen minutes, mastery and noticeable change should be seen in about two weeks. See *coping skills training, hypertension, relaxation techniques*.

progress notes the section of a patient's medical chart where information about the patient's ongoing needs and treatment is written. It is used as the main communication system for the interdisciplinary team. The most successful *progress notes* tend to be interdisciplinary — each member of the team writes pertinent information as it develops. An often-used statement in health care states, "If it isn't written down, it didn't happen." While this is obviously not true, it does emphasize the importance of writing key information in the progress notes. See *care conference, care plan*.

prompt 1. a timely delivery or timely action. 2. the cue given to an individual to assist him/her in taking the next step of a task or action. See *cueing*.

proprietary standard (HCO) a technological standard developed by a single vendor or vendor group. The standard's specifications may be publicized or held confidential.

proprioception the integrated action of all the *senses* that helps a person know his/her position, location, orientation, and to sense when and how much his/her body parts have moved. See *ataxia, kinesthetic*.

proprioceptive neuromuscular facilitation (PNF) methods of promoting or hastening the response of the neuromuscular mechanism through stimulation of sensory receptors. This stimulation is accomplished through spiral and diagonal mass movement patterns. The water medium accommodates movement in more planes than on land, allowing participants more freedom to perform these patterns. See *aquatic therapy*.

proprioceptive testing any test that measures the patient's ability to sense the location and position of a body part while his/her eyes are closed.

prospective payment system (PPS) a system under which Medicare payment is made at a predetermined, specific rate for each hospital admission. All admissions are classified according to a set of specific *diagnostic related groups*. For hospitals/hospital units excluded under PPS, see *exclusion*.

prospective research (HCO) *research* in which patients are observed as they receive health services. See *retrospective research*.

prospective study (HHS) epidemiological or other kinds of research that follows a group of people over a period of time to observe the effects of diet, behavior, and other factors on health or the incidence of disease. In general, this is considered a more valid research design than *retrospective* research.

prostate cancer cancer of the prostate, the second most common type of cancer in males. Prostate cancers are usually a "primary" cancer, meaning that the cancer originated in the prostate and did not metastasize from another location.

prosthetic/prosthesis 1. an artificial replacement for a body part that is missing. 2. an external device which helps improve function, such as a *memory book* or *hearing aid*. See *dressing*.

Protection and Advocacy for the Mentally Ill Individual Act 1986 (Public Law 99-319) allows states to establish and operate a protection and advocacy system for persons labeled mentally ill. These services protect and advocate the rights of such individuals through activities to ensure enforcement of the Constitution and statutes and through investigating reports or incidents of *abuse* and neglect of persons labeled mentally ill. A person eligible for services under this law is an individual who has a significant mental illness or emotional impairment, as determined by a mental health professional qualified under state law and who is an inpatient or patient in a facility rendering care or treatment and for the period of ninety days following discharge from such a facility. (100 Stat. 478) See *Public Law 94-103.*

protein (HHS) a complex nitrogenous compound made up of amino acids in peptide linkages. Dietary proteins are involved in the synthesis of tissue protein and other special metabolic functions. In anabolic processes they furnish the amino acids required to build and maintain body tissues. As an energy source, proteins are equivalent to carbohydrates in providing four calories per gram. Proteins perform a major structural role in all body tissues and in the formation of enzymes, hormones, and various body fluids and secretions. Proteins participate in the transport of some lipids, vitamins, and minerals and help maintain the body's homeostasis.

protocol a defined (written) *treatment* or set of treatments which have a clearly defined format, length of intervention, and stated expected results when used with a specific group of patients who all share common clinical conditions. Foto and Swanson (1993) list five elements of a practice protocol:

1. Expected results stated at admission
2. Comparison of patient's function with group norms
3. Relationship of treatment strategy to test findings
4. Personalized functional attributes

5. Use of tests with known predictive and corrective value

See *clinical decision making, clinical protocol, day treatment program, eclectic approach, medically complex, practice guidelines, rehabilitation centers.*

provider individuals or businesses who hold the appropriate license, certification, registration, or who are authorized by law to deliver specific professional or health services. The term "provider" usually also implies that there is a contractual agreement between the payer (e.g., Blue Cross) and the provider (e.g., therapist or facility) to provide services which meet practice guidelines and which are within the scope of coverage. See *due process, entrance conference, exit conference, federal jurisdictional survey, fiscal intermediary, judicial review, Medicare/Medicaid Authorized Certification System, nonrenewal, plan of correction, reasonable assurance.*

proximal referring to the nearest point to a person's midline.

pseudodementia See *dementia syndrome of depression.*

pseudomyostatic contracture With certain kinds of neurological disorders (e.g., hypertonicity due to cerebral palsy), the muscle may be held in contraction without any tissue damage evident. The decrease of hypertonicity may be achieved through various types of activities, most notably therapeutic swimming in a pool with the correct water temperature.

psoriasis a chronic skin disorder that varies in severity from person-to-person and is subject to "flair-ups." Psoriasis is caused by the over-production of epithelial cells. Psoriasis patches are reddish on the outside with white, dry scales making up the center of the patch.

psychasthenia anxiety and obsessive-compulsive traits. The *MMPI-2* uses psychasthenia as one of its ten clinical scales and includes within this scale the tendency for fearfulness, demonstrating obsessive-compulsive symptoms, holding interpersonal hostility, feeling tension, holding specific phobias, and demonstrating impaired *concentration.*

psychiatric admissions There are a variety of classifications related to how and why a patient is admitted to a psychiatric unit. The table on the next page outlines the primary routes taken for admission to a psychiatric unit. See *consumer rights.*

psychiatric hospital an institution primarily engaged in providing to inpatients, by or under the supervision of a physician, specialized psychiatric services for the diagnosis and treatment of mental illness and emotional disturbances. A psychiatric hos-

Psychiatric Admission Routes

Type	Description
involuntary admission	Based on state laws, individuals or representatives of the community (e.g., a mental health worker) may petition the courts to forcibly admit a patient to a psychiatric unit for evaluation. This is done when there is grave concern for the patient's own safety or the safety of the community. The patient keeps the right to appeal his/her institutionalization.
emergency admission (involuntary)	Due to perceived danger to self or others a person may be institutionalized for 48-72 hours (the length of time depends on state law).
temporary admission (involuntary)	The patient is currently an inpatient and has a trial where the psychiatrist presents compelling arguments as to the need to continue involuntary institutionalization for up to 60 days longer. The patient may be represented by himself/herself and/or a lawyer.
extended admission (involuntary)	After the emergency and/or temporary admission, the patient and psychiatrist reconvene with the court. Depending on the state, the psychiatrist may ask for an extension of the involuntary admission for 60-120 days. Federal law requires that individuals be confined in the *least restrictive* treatment setting possible.
voluntary	The patient admits himself/herself to a treatment program and is free to leave at any time.

pital must maintain clinical records on all patients to determine the degree and intensity of the *treatment* provided as prescribed in regulations at 42 CFR 482.61. The hospital must also meet staffing requirements necessary for the institution to carry out an active program of treatment for mentally ill persons prescribed in regulation 42 CFR 482.62. See *active treatment for inpatient psychiatric services*.

psychiatric rehabilitation the recovery of social, vocational, and personal functioning to the fullest extent possible through education, medications, and environmental supports. Rehabilitation efforts aim at helping the individual: acquire skills; find supportive and functional living and working environments that compensate for the deficits in personal functioning; and adjust to the level of functioning that is realistically attainable. Comprehensive rehabilitation involves *assessment*, training, and modification of natural environments in areas important to personal and community life, self-care including medications and symptom self-management and consumerism, patient living, recreational activities, transportation, food preparation, choice, and use of public agencies. Specific goal setting, within these generic areas, should be conducted with the active involvement of the patient and his/her family and significant others. (Kuehnel, Liberman, Storzbach, Rose, 1990)

psychiatric seclusion — inappropriate as defined by the federal *Immediate and Serious Threat* regulation in the United States: a failure to ensure that the removal of patients from their normal environment to an area from which their egress is prevented is done appropriately and/or failure to ensure that there is adequate and appropriate monitoring of patients while in seclusion. Situations/conditions that may indicate inappropriate psychiatric seclusion include:

1. use of a seclusion room that is unsafe (temperature is too hot/cold, patients cannot be observed at all times, exposed pipes, breakable glass, or other harmful materials), 2. incidents of bodily trauma/injury while in seclusion, 3. clinical records reflecting either absence of justification or inappropriate justification for seclusion, 4. incident reports reflecting injuries during *restraint* process, 5. seclusion that is used as a punishment, 6. *incident reports* that reflect an increase in suicide attempts by patients who are in seclusion.

psychoactive drugs See *psychotropic medications*.

psychodrama a counseling technique developed by Jacob Moreno, MD, in the 1920's. Psychodrama focuses on understanding and resolving internal conflicts by acting out the conflict.

psychomotor agitation nonproductive, excessive, motor, and cognitive behaviors in response to personal tension or neurological impairment. See *agitation*.

psychoneuroimmunology (PNI) a term that evolved during the 1980's to create an awareness and promote interdisciplinary focus to ascertain how emotional and cognitive functioning could affect immunological responses through traditional neurological connections.

psychosis an inability to tell the difference between real life and fantasy. A patient with psychosis will have a difficult time with reality *orientation* and reality awareness while creating his/her own "reality." This is different from an neurosis in which the patient can be based in and recognize basic realities but places a different "twist" to them. See *dopamine, self-hypnosis*.

psychosocial referring to both psychological and social elements and the interplay between them. The

DSM-IV combines psychosocial and environmental factors that significantly impact the development or the exacerbation of psychiatric disorders. Psychosocial problems are recorded under Axis IV of the *multiaxial system* used to diagnosis psychiatric disorders. See *psychosocial and environmental problems*.

psychosocial and environmental problems This is a formal term used in the **DSM-IV**. Psychosocial and environmental problems (also referred to as Axis IV) are problems in the patient's community and environment that affect the patient's treatment outcome. The **DSM-IV** lists nine specific psychosocial and environmental areas of concern: problems with primary support group, problems related to the social environment, educational problems, occupational problems, housing problems, economic problems, problems with access to health care services, problems related to interaction with the legal system/crime, and other psychosocial and environmental problems.

psychosocial well-being (RAPs) Well-being refers to feelings about self and social relationships. Positive attributes include initiative and involvement in life; negative attributes include distressing relationships and concern about loss of status. On average, 30% of the patients in a typical nursing facility will experience problems in this area, two-thirds of whom will also have serious behavior and/or mood problems. When such problems coexist, initial treatment is often focused on *mood* and behavior manifestations. In such situations, treatment for psychological distress is dependent on how the patient responds to the primary mood/behavior treatment regimen.

psychotropic medications (OBRA) (also known as psychoactive drugs.) a medication that is given to a patient to modify the patient's behavior or thought patterns. If a patient is receiving a psychotropic medication to modify his/her behavior, the facility should be able to show that less invasive behavioral interventions were tried first and failed. The chart below lists some of the psychotropic drugs. When surveyors come into the facility, they ask for a list of all the patients currently receiving psychotropic drugs. Using this list, they pay special attention to these patients to ensure that they are receiving the necessary care and not being over medicated. (**State Operations Manual Provider Certification**, Department of Health and Human Services, p. 5-358) (RAPs) Psychotropic drugs are among the most frequently prescribed agents for elderly nursing home patients. Studies in nursing facilities suggest that 35% - 65% of patients receive psychotropic medications. When used appropriately and judiciously, these medications can enhance the *quality of life* of patients who need them. However, all psychotropic drugs have the potential for producing undesirable side effects or aggravating problematic signs and symptoms of existing conditions. An important example is postural hypotension, a condition associated with serious and life-threatening side effects. Severity of *delirium* side effects is dependent on the class and dosage of drug, interactions with other drugs, and the age and health status of the patient.

public accommodations (ADA) The following pri-

Psychotropic Medications

Anti-depressants	Anti-anxiety, sedative/hypnotic	Anti-psychotics
Asendin (Amoxapine)	Ativan (Lorazepam)	Haldol (Haloperidol)
Aventyl, Pamelor (Nortiptyline)	Halcion (Triazolam)	Haldol Deconate (Haloperidol Deconate)
Prozac (Fluoxitene)	Centrax (Prazepam)	Inapsine (Droperidol)
Desyrel (Traxodone)	Librium (Cholrdiazepoxide)	Loxitane (Lorapine)
Elavil (Amitriptiline)	Paxipam (Halazepam)	Mellaril (Thioridazine)
Lithonate, Lithane (Lithium)	Restoril (Tamazepan)	Moban (Molindone)
Ludiomil (Maprotiline)	Serax (Oxazepam)	Navane (Thiothixene)
Nardil (Phinelzine)	Valium (Diazepam)	Orap (Pimozide)
Norpramin (Desipramine)	Vistaril, Atarax (Hydrozyzine)	Serentil (Mesoridazine)
Parnate (Tranylcypromine)	Xanax (Alprazolam)	Sparine (Promazine)
Sinequan (Doxepin)	Dalmane (Flurazepam)	Stelazine (Trifluoperazine)
Tofranil (Imipramine)	Klonapin (Clonazepam)	Taractan (Thlorprothiexene)
Marplan (Isocarboxazid)		Thorazine (Chlorpromazine)
Vivactil (Protiptyline)		Tindel (Acetophenazine)
		Trilafon (Perphenazine)
		Prolixin, Permitil (Fluphenazine)
		Prolixin, Deconate (Fluphenazine Deconate)

vate entities are considered public accommodations for the purposes of the ADA, if the operations of such entities affect commerce: a) an inn, hotel, motel, or other place of lodging, except for an establishment located within a building that contains not more than five rooms for rent or hire and that is actually occupied by the proprietor of such establishment as the residence of such proprietor; b) a restaurant, bar, or other establishment serving food or drink; c) a motion picture house, theater, concert hall, stadium, or other place of exhibition or entertainment; d) an auditorium, convention center, lecture hall, or other place of public gathering; e) a bakery, grocery store, clothing store, hardware store, shopping center, or other sales or retail establishment; f) a laundromat, dry cleaner, bank, barber shop, beauty shop, travel service, shoe repair service, funeral parlor, gas station, office of an accountant or lawyer, pharmacy, insurance office, professional office of a health care provider, hospital, or other service establishment; g) a terminal, depot, or other station used for specified public transportation; h) a museum, library, gallery, or other place of public display or collection; i) a park, zoo, amusement park, or other place of recreation; j) a nursery, elementary, secondary, undergraduate or postgraduate private school, or other place of education; k) a daycare center, senior citizen center, homeless shelter, food bank, adoption agency, or other social services center establishment; and l) a gymnasium, health spa, bowling alley, golf course, or other place of exercise or recreation.

public health agency an official agency established by state or local government to promote the public health of the population.

Public Law 93-112 (1973) Section 504 of the Rehabilitation Act of 1973. This act prohibits discrimination by any entity that receives federal funds and specifies affirmative action programs as well as nondiscrimination requirements. See *Rehabilitation Act of 1973*.

Public Law 94-103 and **Public Law 95-602** (1978) The Developmental Disabilities Assistance and Bill of Rights Act. These two funding acts provided individuals with *developmental disabilities* with a federal funding program to provide training services in the *least restrictive* environment. The Bill of Rights Act added individuals who were disabled prior to their twenty-second birthday to the list of those who could qualify for funding through developmental disability programs. These acts also mandated (and funded) state programs for *protection and advocacy* for individuals covered by these two laws.

Public Law 94-142 (1975) The Education for All Handicapped Children Act. This act mandates the provision of appropriate educational programs for all children between the ages of three years and twenty-one years who are developmentally disabled. These programs must be made available to qualified individuals at no cost. See *mental retardation, The Education for All Handicapped Children Act*.

Public Law 96-247 (1980) The Civil Rights of Institutionalized Persons Act (CRIPA). This act provides the Attorney General of the United States the power to prosecute individuals and organizations that violate the Civil Rights of individuals who are institutionalized.

Public Law 99-319 See *Protection and Advocacy for the Mentally Ill Individual Act of 1986*.

Public Law 99-457 See *Education of the Handi-*

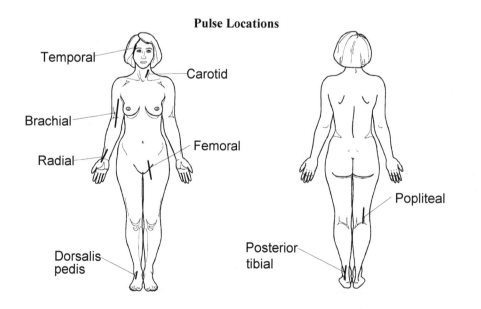

Pulse Locations

capped Amendments of 1986.

Public Law 101-336 Americans with Disabilities Act. This law mandates that public and private facilities, transportation systems, and organizations do not discriminate against an individual because of a disability. Unlike Public Law 93-112 (Rehabilitation Act of 1973), this law does not mandate affirmative action, but may require the employer or facility to pick up the cost of accessibility. See *Americans with Disabilities Act.*

Public Law 101-476 See *Individuals with Disabilities Education Act.*

public use (ADA) describes interior or exterior rooms or spaces that are made available to the general public. Public use may be provided at a building or facility that is privately or publicly owned.

pulmonary relating to the lungs.

pulmonary stenosis a narrowing in the proximity of the pulmonary valve causing a decreased amount of blood to reach the lungs to be oxygenated.

pulse the measurable surge of blood through the arteries and veins. Therapists should be skilled in the techniques associated with taking a patient's pulse (palpation of pulses). The patient may already be experiencing a decreased pulse to various body parts due to physiological reasons or may experience *ischemia* (lack of blood flow and lack of delivery of oxygen) due to poorly fitted equipment and/or exposure to cold. Pulses are usually recorded as the number of beats per minute. In addition, the therapist

will need to indicate whether the pulse was

1. normal,
2. diminished or
3. absent.

An absent pulse is obviously an emergency situation. Pulses are taken at eight locations on the body as shown on the previous page. See *autonomic hyperactivity, escharotomy, tachycardia, vital signs.*

pulse wave velocity (PWV) the speed of propagation for the local change in blood pressure as the blood passes from the left ventricle to the aorta. Increases in pulse wave velocity represent increased sympathetic tone in the cardiovascular system.

purchaser (HCO) an organization (usually a large employer) that purchases health insurance (usually for its own employees).

purulent referring to the production of pus or to having pus. See *drainage/secretion precaution isolation.*

pyelonephritis a kidney disorder which is caused by an infection of the ducts that carry urine.

pyramidal tracts a group of nerve cells going from the brain down the spinal cord to control voluntary and reflex activity of muscles.

pyromania an impulse control disorder that is exhibited by the act of setting fires to achieve pleasure, gratification, or to relieve built up tension. Pyromania is a recognized diagnosis in the **DSM-IV** under the category of impulse control disorders not elsewhere classified. See *disability.*

Q

quadriplegia a paralysis of all four of the individual's limb; a loss of movement below the shoulders/head.

qualified interpreter (ADA) an individual who is able to interpret effectively, accurately, and impartially both receptively and expressively, using any necessary specialized vocabulary. See *interpreter*.

qualified mental retardation professional (QMRP) The federal government of the United States identifies minimum qualifications for individuals who may assume the lead position on the treatment team in institutions and group homes for individuals who are mentally retarded or developmentally delayed. The federal law that regulates intermediate *care facilities for the mentally retarded* (ICF-MRs) also stipulates that *professionals* who conduct the assessments and who write the training programs must have QMRP status. burlingame and Blaschko (1991) summarize the QMRP requirements in the chart below. See *individualized treatment plan*.

qualitative research a method of *research* which is based on the use of subjective information, information based on an individual's opinion about his/her own feelings, or a report on the perception of someone else's feelings or attitudes. This type of research does not typically record information using numerical symbols and analyzes the information using non-statistical analysis methods (e.g., narrative discussions for evaluation of the results instead of graphs and charts). The method of information collection uses an open-ended method of collection instead of a tightly controlled system. Contrast with *quantitative research*.

quality assessment the measurement of the *appropriateness* of the care and services and of the quality and usefulness of the management systems used to deliver the care and services. Many different testing tools and measurement techniques are used to assess the quality of care. Just as in patient care, the staff identify the area(s) assessed that need improvement or that are at risk of degeneration.

quality assurance the way in which a facility 1. identifies (potential) problems, 2. determines a systematic way to decrease the problems, and 3. monitors the success of the facility in decreasing the problems. The purpose of a quality assurance program is to safeguard and improve the quality of care each patient receives. Over the last two decades the concept of quality assurance has seemed to spin out of control in terms of the vocabulary used to describe the concept. Every year or so there was a new "in" term used when talking about quality assurance. (Some are shown in the accompanying table.) Part of the reason for this is that theories and research on quality assurance concepts have exploded, because this is one of the most frequently financed programs in terms of staff effort and continuing education programs. This is due, in part, to regulatory agencies re-

Minimum Qualifications for QMRP

Occupational Title	Credentialing	Requires Licensing by State if Applicable	Tag #
Occupational Therapist	Eligible for Certification by AOTA	Yes	W171
Occupational Therapy Assistant	Eligible for COTA by AOTA	Yes	W172
Physical Therapist	Eligible for Certification by APTA	Yes	W173
Physical Therapy Assistant	Eligible for certification by the American Physical Therapy Association	Yes	W174
Psychologist	Master's degree in psychology from accredited school	Yes	W175
Recreation Staff	Bachelor's degree in recreation, art, dance, music, or physical education	No	W178
Speech-Language Pathologist	Eligible for CCC in Speech-Language Pathology or Audiology by ASLHA or meet educational requirements and accumulated experience	Yes	W177

quiring that each facility have an effective and up-to-date quality assurance program. In many ways, the explosion of terms related to quality assurance is just the process of further defining the term and dividing all of the concepts that used to be grouped under the term "quality assurance" into multiple separate terms and meanings. It is still appropriate to use the term "quality assurance" when one is referring to the global concept of making sure that one's work meets standards of excellence. When talking about the various aspects of determining what the areas of need (or substandard quality) are or when talking about the mechanisms to address the areas of need, it is best to use the specific term(s) that apply to that aspect of quality assurance. There are many models describing the steps necessary for the implementation of a quality assurance program. The chart on the following page from Cunninghis and Best Martini (1996) is one example of the steps taken. For a quality assurance program to work, it must have the active involvement of all of the facility's staff. The facility should empower the employees by allowing them authority and autonomy which is equal to their required duties and responsibilities related to quality programming. To do this, the facility should train every employee about the organization's mission and vision statements. Part of these statements should reflect that change will be a normal part of the facility's growth, not the exception. This change is a result of identified customer requirements, identified through continuous evaluation, measurement, and improvement. This process requires an uninterrupted flow of communication and dissemination of information along with continual self-assessment. See *volume indicators, clinical indicators, continuous quality improvement, occurrence screens, focused reviews, important aspects of care, Health Care Quality Improvement Act of 1986, benchmark, complaint, critical pathways, peer review, quality improvement.*

Words Related to QA

Terms	Abbr.
Continuous Quality Improvement	CQI
Improving Organization Performance	IOP
Management by Objectives	MBO
Performance Improvement	PI
Participative Management	PM
Quality Circles	QC
Total Quality Improvement	TQI
Total Quality Management	TQM

quality improvement improving the level of performance or quality of outcomes of a key process within the facility or department. To be able to identify a process that could be improved, the facility staff need to assess the current performance and measure that performance against benchmarks and thresholds. This assessment generally emphasizes a critical look at the systems and processes involved. See *benchmark, threshold, quality assurance, continuous quality improvement, incident report.*

quality improvement program description the formally written document which identifies the area(s) that require an improvement of quality, the specific mechanisms for that improvement, how improvement will be measured, who will hold the accountability, and the desired outcomes. This document is reviewed and approved by the facility's governing body and reviewed periodically. See *accountability, important aspects of care.*

quality improvement work plan the written plan which outlines the specific actions and the time line for those actions over a year's time.

quality indicator a term specifically used with the nursing home prospective payment system. The data used to calculate the quality indicators comes directly from the *Minimum Data Set* (MDS).

quality of care the degree to which the patient's health care outcomes meet or exceed *standards* based on current medical knowledge and standards of practice.

quality of life (measurements of/components of) the degree to which the patient perceives that his/her life has meaning and comfort. Quality of life is considered very important for patients living in a nursing home, residential facility, or involved with hospice services. *OBRA* states (Tag 240): A facility must care for its patients in a manner and in an environment that promotes maintenance or enhancement of each patient's quality of life. See *dementia, physical restraints, psychotropic drugs.*

quantitative research a method of *research* that is based on collecting *objective* (observable and measurable) data that can be recorded numerically. This conversion of data allows the researcher to conduct statistical analyses on the numbers, usually gathered from a large number of subjects. The exception to quantitative research using large numbers is the single-subject research design that employs its own special methods of analysis. The collection of data in quantitative research relies on a structured system of data collection and uses tables and graphs to depict the results. See *qualitative research.*

Steps of Quality Assurance Programs

Step 1	Identifying Issues and Selecting Study Topics	Obviously it is essential to begin with a determination of what service needs to be improved to provide quality service. This first step has you look closely at the problem to specifically identify what is not right. Unfortunately, many quality assurance programs concern themselves with issues that are not important, or with procedural items that can be easily remedied, rather than those that justify being part of long-range planning.
Step 2a	Establishing Indicators	Identifying elements that can be monitored to measure changes made. The elements or characteristics of the service you select to measure should be a general statement about what the service would look like if there was not a problem.
Step 2b	Developing Criteria	Developing criteria for each indicator. Writing a plan that spells out exactly what should be found and ideally in what quantity and in what time frame.
Step 3a	Determining Methodology	Establishing the exact method to be used to collect information: from which sources, by whom, how often, how long, and how the results are going to be used.
Step 3b	Collecting Data	Implementing the chosen methods of data collection.
Step 4a	Understanding the Problem	Reviewing and assessing collected data to see what, where, and how serious the problems are. Deciding which problem areas should be the focus of further study.
Step 4b	Setting Standards	Standards are set to describe the desired outcomes in a measurable way.
Step 4c	Finding Solutions	Searching for possible ways to reach the standards set.
Step 4d	Writing an Action Plan	The methodology for implementing a change is determined along with decisions about who is to have the responsibility and what the time frames will be.
Step 4e	Implementing the Plan	Putting into action the strategies that have been developed.
Step 5a	Assessing the Outcomes	Did the plan work? Do the problems still remain? Has there been some improvement? This procedure often entails a repeat of steps 3 and 4: going back and re-collecting the data and then analyzing the results to see if the standards have been reached.
Step 5b	Identifying New Issues or Continuing to Work on the Old	If the problems are not solved, new strategies must be planned. If, however, the process has been successful, a new plan should be developed for the next area of focus. As stated earlier, quality assurance is an ongoing process and does not stop once a particular problem is corrected. It is also necessary to periodically go back and monitor earlier plans and see if the goals are continuing to be met. Two or three past issues may be chosen at random for an on-going audit in addition to the main topic of study. These could be changed periodically on a rotating basis to assure that new problems have not arisen in any of these areas.

quarterly notes information placed in the progress notes of a patient's medical chart which summarizes the patient's treatment and status over the past 90 days. See *documentation*.

R

radiation therapy treatment that uses radiation to destroy a specific area of a neoplasty or a specific type of cell. May be used to help destroy a patient's diseased bone marrow and immunosuppress the rejection mechanism in preparation for a marrow transplant.

radionuclide scans (CDC) any of a variety of medical imaging methods that rely on atomic isotopes that decay and emit radiation.

RAI See *resident assessment instrument, minimum data set.*

ramp (ADA) a walking surface that has a running slope greater than 1:20.

Rancho Los Amigos scale an eight-point *scale* that is used to indicate the degree to which cognitive functioning is impaired, usually in adults with brain injury. The table below is from burlingame and Blaschko (1997).

Rancho Los Amigos Scale

Level	Description
Level One	No response to stimuli (coma)
Level Two	Generalized response to stimuli (inconsistent and non-purposeful)
Level Three	Localized response (specific but inconsistent response to stimuli)
Level Four	Confused — agitated (heightened state of activity with decreased ability to process information)
Level Five	Confused — inappropriate, non-agitated
Level Six	Confused — appropriate
Level Seven	Automatic — appropriate
Level Eight	Purposeful and appropriate (normal)

random assignment See *randomization.*

randomization (HHS) a process of assigning subjects to experimental or control groups so the subjects have an equal chance of being assigned to each group. Randomization is used to control for known, unknown, and difficult-to-control-for *variables.*

randomized controlled trial (HCO) a form of prospective *research* in which patients are randomly assigned to groups that receive different health services and are then observed for differences in *outcome.*

random sample (HHS) a procedure to select subjects for a study in which all individuals in a population being studied have an equal chance of being selected. Using a random sample allows the results of the study to be generalized to the entire population. The term random also applies to assignments within controlled studies, or the division of subjects into groups. Random assignment ensures that all subjects have an equal chance of being in the experimental and control groups, and increases the probability that any unidentified variable will systematically occur in both groups with the same frequency. Randomization is crucial to control for variables that researchers may not be aware of or cannot adequately control, but which could affect the outcome of an experimental study.

range of motion (ROM) degree of motion (*flexion* and *extension*) of a joint. ROM exercises work to increase or maintain the maximum degree of *movement.* **PROM**—passive range of motion is when a joint is moved by some other person. In nursing homes, PROM is usually done by aides and nursing staff. **AROM**—active range of motion is when the patient moves the joint by his/her own efforts. In many states, occupational therapists, physical therapists, physicians, nurses, and aides are licensed to perform ROM exercises. However, most regulatory agencies expect all therapists to know enough about range of motion to be able to implement the appropriate type and use the appropriate precautions while interacting with the patient. Other professionals may work with the physical therapist or occupational therapist to develop a set of activities that promote the appropriate range of motion activity for a patient. The professional would then supervise the patient during these activities. There are five primary causes for a loss of ROM (Kisner and Colby, 1990, p. 109): 1. prolonged immobilization, 2. restricted *mobility*, 3. connective tissue or neuromuscular disease, 4. tissue pathology due to trauma and 5. congenital or acquired deformities. There is not a singly agreed upon, "normal" ROM. The ROM in degrees listed on the next page is from Daniels and Worthingham (1972). In parentheses next to the ROM degree is the range of "normal" ROM according to the 12 other primary ROM tables (Rothstein et al 1991, p. 62-66). See *bed, burn, cerebral palsy, dance therapy, isokinetic exercises, isometric, isotonic, Jobst, modality, passive movement, passive*

Range of Motion

Shoulder				
Flexion	--- (130-180)		Extension	50 (30-80)
Abduction	--- (150-184)		Internal Rotation	90 (55-95)
External Rotation	90 (40-104)		Horizontal Abduction	--- (30-45)
Horizontal Adduction	--- (135-140)			
Elbow				
Flexion	160 (143-160)			
Radioulnar				
Pronation	90 (75-90)		Supination	90 (70-90)
Wrist				
Flexion	90 (60-85)		Extension	90 (60-85)
Radial Deviation	25 (15-35)		Ulnar Deviation	65 (30-75)
Hip				
Flexion	125 (100-130)		Extension	15 (10-45)
Abduction	45 (30-55)		Adduction	0 (0-45)
Internal Rotation	45 (20-47)		External Rotation	45 (36-60)
Knee				
Flexion	130 (135-160)			
Ankle				
Plantar Flexion	45 (45-65)		Dorsiflexion	--- (10-30)
Subtalar Joint				
Inversion	--- (30-52)		Eversion	--- (15-30)

*Three other systems that are used to record ROM are 1. 180 to 0 system by Clark (1920), 2. the 360 Degree system by West (1945), and 3. the SFTR System of Recording ROM Values by Gerhardt and Russe (1975).

stretching, postural dysfunction, scar, sensorimotor, strain, stretching.

RAP See *resident assessment protocol.*

rape the attempted or actual sexual intercourse forced on an non-consenting individual. A victim of rape requires both medical and emotional support. While it is estimated that only 10% of all rapes are reported, one is reported every seven minutes on the average in the United States. While individuals of any age (male or female) may be attacked, the average age of a victim of rape is 13½ with one out of every seven victims being prepubertal. See *post traumatic stress disorder, trust.*

rapid assays (HHS) methods of checking for pathogens on or in food products. These diagnostic tests use emerging technology to identify and remove impurities from foods before they reach the consumer. There are two major types of rapid assays. Antibody-based assays link a "familiar" characteristic on a pathogen's surface (the antigen) to a substance known as an antibody. When this connection is made, the test registers "success." Similarly, nucleic acid-based assays use the unique genetic materials of the cells to detect a pathogen.

rapid cycling a feature of either Bipolar I disorder or Bipolar II disorder. Rapid cycling refers to the presence of at least four major *mood* swings within the past twelve months. To be counted as rapid cycling, the mood must have been at least one week in duration with total *remission* between episodes. See *bipolar disorder.*

rating system See *scales and rating systems.*

rational decision making the process of taking something that was confusing and obscure and making it clear and rational. This is usually used to discuss behavioral choices made when an individual is faced with more information than s/he can reasonably take in. The individual copes by grouping information or simplifying information to make decision making easier. See *coping skills.*

rational emotive therapy See *refuting irrational ideas.*

rationalization justifying one's actions or feelings with reasons or explanations that seem acceptable, without looking at the true reasons. It is the most common defense mechanism. See *coping mechanisms.*

Raynaud's disease a peripheral vascular disorder found mostly in females 18 to 30 years old. Raynaud's disease presents as abnormal vasoconstriction of the extremities upon exposure to cold or emotional stress. To be considered a disease the symptoms must have been present for two years. Otherwise the symptoms are classified as Raynaud's phenomenon.

rBST See *recombinant bovine somatotropin.*

reading See *graphic input.*

reality orientation a formal or informal program to assist the patient in knowing who they are, where they are, why they are there and when it is. This program includes both verbal and non-verbal cues. See *quality of life.*

reasonable assurance *Providers* or suppliers seeking to participate in Medicare or Medicaid, who were previously terminated for those programs based on a HCFA finding of noncompliance, must convince HCFA that they have resumed and can maintain compliance. Reasonable assurance requires a provider/supplier to operate for a certain period of time (as establish by HCFA) without recurrence of the *deficiencies* that were the basis for the *termination*. Participation can only resume following this reasonable assurance period.

reasoning the ability to consider information presented and then to create inferences and/or conclusions. The skill of reasoning requires that the individual is able to draw upon past experiences and is able to be flexible in the possible interpretations of why an event occurred. See *cognition, concrete thinking, ego, intelligence.*

receptive communication See *communication.*

receptor a specialized neural cell which is sensitive to stimulation. Once it receives enough stimulation to make it fire, it will pass the information on to the next neural cell.

recipient an individual who is eligible for Medicaid or other health care programs.

reciprocal inhibition decoding See *in vivo.*

recognition the ability to correctly tell if one has seen, experienced, or heard an object or event previously. This requires an individual to 1. store information in long/short-term *memory*, 2. recognize the shape and/or patterns associated with the object or event, 3. recall past events that may be similar, 4. mentally review the possible choices from memory and select the one that matches, and 5. feel confident that one's recognition process is accurate.

recombinant bovine somatotropin (rBST) (HHS) a synthetic hormone virtually identical to a cow's natural somatotropin, a hormone produced in its pituitary gland that stimulates milk production. Treatment with rBST can increase a cow's milk production by 10% to 15%.

recombinant DNA (rDNA) (HHS) the DNA formed by combining segments of DNA from different organisms.

reconsideration the initial action in the administrative review process for any Medicare provider or supplier dissatisfied with a *denial* or *nonrenewal*. The facility must submit a request for reconsideration within 60 days following the determination.

recreational therapist a clinician who is professionally trained and credentialed to provide services to restore, remediate, or rehabilitate the patient's functional ability while using leisure and activities as *modalities*. It is a term frequently used instead of the term "therapeutic recreation specialist." See *Joint Commission, National Council for Therapeutic Recreation Certification.*

recreational therapy a clinical specialty which uses leisure activities as the *modality* to restore, remediate, or rehabilitate the patient's functional ability and level of independence and/or to reduce or eliminate the effects of illness and disability.

recreational therapy diagnosis Unlike the biomedical diagnoses made by a physician, the recreational therapy diagnosis considers the patient's reaction to a disease or injury. These problems can be physical (decreased activity), emotional (depression), social (social isolation), cognitive (confusion, disorientation), and/or spiritual. The identification of these problems is essential in the assessment of baseline levels and treatment planning.

Recreation Early Development Screening Tool (REDS) a screening tool that helps the therapist estimate the patient's functional ability in five areas related to leisure: play, fine motor, gross motor, sensory, and social/cognition. The tool looks at developmental milestones between birth and one year of age. The tool is usually used by a recreational therapist who then selects a second tool to obtain more specific functional ability. The REDS is usually used with adults with severe *mental retardation* or learning disabilities and not infants. See *General Recreation Screening Tool, Denver Developmental Screening Test.*

Recreation Participation Data Sheet (RPD) a standardized *data* collection sheet that provides descriptions of activities allowing the therapist to analyze the patient's balance of free-time activities. Data is collected in seven areas 1. *participation* level, 2. *initiation* level, 3. independence level, 4. physical level, 5. satisfaction level, 6. group size, and 7. total time in activity.

Recreation Service Model a continuum for the delivery of recreation and recreational therapy services developed by burlingame (1997). The model was modified in 2001 to reflect terminology changes made by the World Health Organization. See the diagram on the next page.

Recreation Service Model

Recreational Therapy	Organized Recreation	Independent Recreation

Micro   Mezzo   Macro

ADA Compliance Where Appropriate to Accommodate Individuals with Disabilities

Assistance Provided by a CTRS, CLP, or Other Qualified Individuals

Specific Levels of Intervention Provided by a Certified Therapeutic Recreation Specialist

Body Structure	Function	Activities	Participation	Leisure Education Level	Organized Recreation Programs	Leisure Activities
	Maximizing the Body's Own Ability	Development of Skills, Techniques, or Use of Adapted Equipment	Application of Skills, Techniques & Abilities in Community			
Scope of Service: To reduce or prevent the interruption of (or interference with) normal physiological & developmental process. Most often associated with acute medical or psychiatric events. Therapists may also address issues of infection control and disease prevention.	**Scope of Service:** To enhance cognitive, physiological, or emotional function. Therapist addresses changes on a system level (cardiovascular, cognition, coordination, communication). Therapist may also monitor side effects of medication or address issues of edema and skin integrity through positioning.	**Scope of Service:** To enhance perform-ance of component (basic) skills required of an activity in a manner considered within the normal range. Therapist addresses the need to modify or enhance the individual's functional ability through adaptive techniques or equipment.	**Scope of Service:** To facilitate the use of component (basic) skills within a community setting. Therapist addresses the application of component (basic) skills and techniques along with the use of adaptive equipment to integrate into the community.	**Scope of Service:** To facilitate the acquisition of new skills, techniques, and/or knowledge to engage in leisure of choice. Little to no additional modification is needed due to physiological or psychological impairment, disability, or handicap.	**Scope of Service:** Facilitating recreation through the provision of facilities, staff, and other resources. Learning new skills is not the emphasis of the service, although the further development of skills may be.	**Scope of Service:** No direct service provided by recreation professionals.
Examples: • seizure • acute psych. crisis • catheter displacement • autonomic dysreflexia	**Examples:** • strength/endurance • cognitive retraining • coordination, ROM • executive function • anhedonia • tardive dyskinesia	**Examples:** • social skills • leisure counseling • anger management • relaxation training • advanced ADLs	**Examples:** • identifying & using community resources • combining multiple tasks (plans/lists, transportation, shopping, meal prep.)	**Examples:** • Instruction on: • Internet use • swimming • foreign language • skiing • painting	**Examples:** • attend concert • golf course • baseball • hiking in state park • summer camp	**Examples:** • writing poetry • walking along beach • talking with friends • painting

The continuum starts at the disease level where maximum services are required and extends to look at recreation where an individual is able to recreate without services from anyone else. On the service-intense side of the model, clinical intervention (recreational therapy) is divided into four levels: body structure, function, activities, and participation. (These had previously been disease level, impairment level, disability level, and handicap level). The model then has two levels of recreation service: leisure education and organized recreation programs. The final level of service is actually self-service, recognizing that individuals can and should be able to recreate without assistance. The model follows and expands the division of clinical services developed by the World Health Organization's in its International Classification of Function and Disability (ICIDH-2). By following an existing model, the field benefits from established standards for testing, protocol development, and reimbursement practices. See *leisure models*.

Red Book a reference book of testing tools formally titled **Assessment Tools for Recreational Therapy, Second Edition** by burlingame and Blaschko (1997).

redundant array of independent disks (RAID) (HCO) multiple computer disks configured as a single disk to provide either data redundancy or enhanced access speed.

re-feeding syndrome a medical risk associated with the recovery process of long-term anorexia. The heart may be damaged by long-lasting anorexia. Heart failure occurs because of the added demands of the digestive system when the patient starts eating more normally again.

referral the request to add a patient to one's case load. This request may come from a physician, a member of the treatment team, a family member, or anyone else who has a legitimate, legal right to make decisions concerning the patient's care. Deborah Wieder-Singer (1994) lists ten important elements in the development and maintenance of a good referral network. See *discharge summary.*

1. Diversify your referral sources

2. Be active in the local community
3. Know what your physician wants
4. Be convenient
5. "Mackay 66" your physicians (Mackay, 1995)
6. Let physicians know what you know
7. Be conscientious
8. Increase your referral sources' business
9. Keep patients happy
10. Perform quality therapy

reflex movement movement that is caused by an external stimulus, which produces a reliably consistent response. A "knee jerk" is an example of a reflex; patients with spinal cord injuries or nerve damage may have diminished or absent reflexes. See the table below for a rating system for deep tendon reflexes. See *movement*.

reflex sympathetic dystrophy Seen frequently in individuals with *hemiplegia* caused by a *cerebrovascular accident*, reflex sympathetic dystrophy is a painful condition caused by partial damage to the nerves in the shoulder area. Symptoms include severe *pain*, hypersensitivity, and *paresthesia*s.

refuting irrational ideas the process of using self-talk to stop obsessive or *compulsive* thought patterns that are non-productive and *stress* producing. People normally engage in internal dialogs with themselves. This internal dialog is called *self-talk*. Refuting irrational ideas is a relaxation technique developed by Albert Ellis in 1961 (also known as rational emotive therapy). Ellis reasoned that emotions felt do not necessarily have a direct connection to what is actually happening. He felt that the problem lay someplace between the actual event and the emotions, or in unrealistic self-talk. Ellis felt that emotions arose out of the self-talk and interpretation of the event resulting from the internal dialog. By learning how to refute irrational ideas, the patient may be able to reduce his/her psychological arousal, reduce body tensions, and reduce stress due to *anxiety*, guilt, anger, low *self-esteem*, and *depression*. Mastery of this technique usually takes twenty minutes of practice each day for a few weeks. See *relaxation techniques.*

Regenstrief Medical Record System (RMRS)

Rating System for Deep Tendon Reflexes

Numeric Rating	Description of Function
4+	brisk, hyperactive, clonus
3+	is more brisk than normal, but does not necessarily indicate a pathologic process, gross functional ability not usually impaired
2+	normal
1+	low normal, with slight diminution in response, having minor impact on functional ability
0	no response

(HCO) a *clinical information system* at the Regenstrief Institute, Indiana University, Indianapolis, Indiana. See *medical record.*

regression the temporary or permanent loss of ability to demonstrate skills that one previously had the ability to perform. See *diminished.*

regular diet a *diet* which allows most kinds of foods, provides a balanced nutritional intake, allows the patient some selection, and which totals 1400 calories in every 24-hour period.

regulation a specific standard that is part of a law; a legal requirement to meet or exceed. See *CFR, interpretive guidelines.*

regulatory agency the agency or department which, by law, is responsible to ensure that specific legal *standards* are being met. Regulatory agencies have individuals called "surveyors" who go to each facility to evaluate the quality of care being delivered. The Health Standards and Quality Bureau (HSQB) (the survey branch of the *Department of Health and Human Services* in the United States) is an example of a regulatory agency. See *survey process.*

rehabilitation the process of restoring one's health and functional status after disabling disease, injury, or addiction through purposeful intervention.

Rehabilitation Act of 1973 federal legislation establishing programs aimed at promoting the employment and independent living of people with disabilities. A precursor to the *Americans with Disabilities Act.* See *civil rights, consumer rights, Office for Civil Rights Compliance.*

rehabilitation agency an agency which provides an integrated, multidisciplinary program designed to upgrade the physical functions of individuals who are handicapped or disabled by bringing together a team of specialized rehabilitation personnel. At minimum, a rehabilitation agency must provide physical therapy, speech pathology, recreational therapy or occupational therapy, and social or vocational adjustment services to patients, based on their assessed need.

rehabilitation centers a facility providing rehabilitation services. The growth in the number of rehabilitation centers across the United States has increased significantly over the last two decades. The table below (Smith, 1994) gives an example of the growth. This growth will probably slow in the

next decade due to a variety of factors. Coile (1994) identified ten leading trends in rehabilitation medicine:

1. Slowdown of growth
2. Consolidation
3. *Managed care* contracting
4. HMO rehab programs
5. *Outcomes* management
6. *Case management*
7. *Databases* (measure clinical effectiveness)
8. Treatment *protocols*
9. *Subacute* rehabilitation
10. Fraud and self-referral regulation

See *health maintenance organizations.*

reimbursement the money paid by third party payers for professional services rendered. See *adjudication, adjusted historical payment base, allowed coverage, appropriations, assignment, authorization of services, average adjusted per capita cost, balance of bill, beneficiary, capitated, common procedural terminology (CPT), cost sharing, delegation, denial, diversional program, federal financial participation, fee-for-service, fiscal intermediary, flexible spending account, function related groups, HCPCS, hospital insurance, induced demand, Medicaid, Medicare, payer, PEW Health Professions Commission, precertification, pricing strategies, prospective payment system, recipient, retrospective review, scrip, single payer system, uncompensated care, utilization review.*

relapse recurrence of illness after apparent recovery.

relational database (HCO) a collection of computer-based information that is organized or accessed according to relationships between data items. See *database.*

relaxation the purposeful effort to release tension in one or more muscles. A patient's ability to decrease tension in muscles usually becomes more efficient with practice. While some patients may be able to increase this skill through self-directed efforts, most will require some direct training from the professional. See *relaxation techniques.*

relaxation response a concept that is used to describe the body's "relaxation" from sympathetic dominance. The relaxation response is facilitated through mental focusing and abdominal breathing techniques.

Yearly Estimates of the Number of Rehabilitation Centers in the US

Type of Facility	1985	1987	1989	1991	1993	1994
Hospitals which only do rehabilitation medicine	68	88	125	152	180	187
Hospitals with rehabilitation units	386	539	642	672	783	804
Comprehensive Outpatient Rehabilitation Facilities (CORFs)	86	141	184	201	229	237

relaxation techniques a group of actions that an individual can take to reduce stress and anxiety. There are seventeen primary relaxation techniques: *breathing, progressive relaxation, meditation, visualization, applied relaxation, self-hypnosis, autogenics, brief combination techniques, biofeedback, thought stopping, refuting irrational ideas, coping skills training, goal setting and time management, assertiveness training, job stress management, nutrition, and exercise.* Each individual will want to develop a combination of these techniques that best meets his/her needs. See *conflict, deprivation, post traumatic stress disorder.*

reliability the degree to which the quality and quantity of something being measured will remain stable and the degree that your ability to measure the something was close to being a true measurement (accurate). The therapist must have a good description of the exact action or event that is going to be measured and be able to have others duplicate or come up with exactly what the therapist came up with. In 1990, Julie Dunn presented a workshop on client assessment validation procedures. The table below is from that presentation. A "perfect" reliability, represented as a reliability coefficient of 1.00, is never achieved. However, the closer the reliability correlation coefficient is to +1, the more perfect the relationship. See the following table for guidelines

Methods of Estimating Reliability

Type	Meaning	Procedure
test-retest method	measure of stability	Give the same test twice to the same group with any time interval between tests from several minutes to several years. Compute a correlation coefficient to relate the scores of first and second testing.
equivalent-forms method	measure of equivalence	Give two forms of the test to the same group in close succession. Compute a correlation coefficient to relate the scores on the two forms.
test-retest with equivalent forms	measure of stability and equivalence	Give two forms of the test to the same group with increased time interval between forms. Compute a correlations coefficient to relate the scores on the two forms.
split-half method	measure of internal consistency	Give test once. Score two equivalent halves of test (e.g., odd items and even items); correct reliability coefficient to fit whole test by Spearman-Brown formula.
Kuder-Richardson	measure of internal consistency	Give test once. Score total test and apply Kuder-Richardson formula.
alpha	measure of internal consistency	Give test once. Score total test and apply formula to compute alpha.
inter-rater	measure of consistency of raters	Have more than one rater observe the same situation. Compute percent agreement of rater's score.

Interpreting the Quality of a Testing Tool's Reliability

Reliability Correlation Coefficient	Discussion
.85 - .99	High to very high. Tests with a reliability coefficient above .85 can comfortably be used for individual measurement and diagnosis.
.80 - .84	Fairly high. Tests with a reliability coefficient between .80 and .84 hold some value when used for measuring an individual's attributes. Reliability coefficients with scores in this range are highly satisfactory for group measurement.
.70 - .79	Moderately low. Tests with a reliability coefficient in this range are of doubtful value when used with individuals. This range is still adequate for use in measuring group attributes.
.50 - .69	Low. Tests with reliability coefficients in this range should not be used to determine individual treatment or educational goals. Tests in this range have limited but some value when used in group measurement.
Below .50	Very low. Not adequate for use with individuals or groups.
*It is also possible to have reliability correlation coefficients that are expressed by negative numbers, with "-1" meaning a perfect opposite, or negative, relationship.	

on interpreting the quality of reported reliability. See *test-retest reliability*.

reminiscence the process of recalling events in a patient's past; a normal process as one ages.

remission the absence of a disease or disability which was present before. Remission is not the same as a cure. The term is most frequently associated with *cancer* or psychiatric disorders.

remotivation the *treatment* program which helps bridge the time a patient is concerned only about his/her own problems and the time when s/he is ready once again to help others in the community.

renal relating to the kidneys.

report card (HCO) a summary set of indicators of the performance of health care providers or insurance plans in delivering health services to patients.

repression See *coping mechanisms*.

research the purposeful and systematic process of gathering information on a specific subject following prescribed methods of information (*data*) collection. There are two general categories of research: *quantitative* and *qualitative*. See *institutional review board, meta-analysis, prospective research, retrospective research, randomized control trial, statistical control, systematic review*.

research design (HHS) how a study is set up to collect information or data. For valid results, the design must be appropriate to answer the question or hypothesis being studied.

reservoir a natural environment for an infectious agent; a place where an infectious agent can multiply. See *infection*.

resident 1. an individual who receives health care services. See *client*. 2. an physician completing post-medical school training beyond the first (internship) year.

Resident Assessment Instrument (RAI) an interdisciplinary assessment tool developed by the Health Care Financing Administration to be administered to every patient admitted to a nursing home in the United States. Also known as the *Minimum Data Set*.

Resident Assessment Protocols (RAPs) outline for organizing MDS (Minimum Data Set) elements, including clinically relevant information concerning the long-term care population, to be used in the development of *care plans*.

resident care plan the overall plan of action and treatment that the treatment team develops with the resident's input, based on the assessment of the resident's needs and standards of practice. The resident *care plan* is reviewed on a regular basis, whenever the resident's condition changes, and at least once a year under US laws.

resident council the governing body made up of residents who discuss concerns about their living environment, propose changes, and work with the administrator and staff of a long-term care facility or an inpatient psychiatric unit to resolve problems. By federal law (*OBRA*), long-term care facilities are required to have resident councils.

residual confounding (HHS) the effect that remains after one has attempted to statistically control for variables that cannot be measured perfectly. A particularly important concept in epidemiological studies because knowledge of human biology is still developing. Unknown variables could exist that could significantly change conclusions made on the basis of epidemiological research.

residual limb the portion of a limb that remains after an *amputation*.

resistance the act of opposing a force. When applied to movement, resistance is the use of one's muscles to move in a direction that is fighting gravity, cohesion, viscosity, turbulence, or friction. When an individual moves from a sitting position to a standing position s/he experiences resistance from gravity.

resocialization regaining the ability to interact socially. As a result of some illnesses and disabilities, the patient may experience a period of time when s/he has lost interest or the ability to interact with others socially. When a patient is emotionally and/or physically ready to return to social interactions, s/he may need a supportive environment and/or adaptive equipment to build upon the social skills s/he still has. The program and structured environment that promotes this is called a resocialization program. See *socialization*.

resource identification skills the ability to find resources within the community. Some resource identification skills include the ability to find the location of a desired destination and having knowledge of where to find what one wants (e.g., swimming/lake, baseball/park, food/restaurant, etc.).

respiratory isolation an isolation procedure for patients with epiglottis, measles, *meningitis*, meningococcal *pneumonia*, meningococcemia, mumps, pertussis (whooping cough), and some types of pneumonia. The isolation procedure includes: 1. masks are indicated for those who come close to patient, 2. gowns are not indicated, 3. gloves are not indicated, 4. hands must be washed after touching the patient or potentially contaminated articles and before taking care of another patient, 5. articles contaminated with infective material should be discarded or bagged and labeled before being sent for decontamination and reprocessing. The signs for respiratory isolation are always blue.

respite care a temporary vacation or break given to those who care for one or more individuals who are ill or disabled. The respite care workers usually have the same level of training as the regular caregivers. Frequently respite care is provided at the home or the facility of the respite workers. In many states, respite care homes or centers are required to be licensed.

resting tremors a jerking or shaking of the muscles when the muscle is not actively being used but is being supported, as in Parkinsonism. See *tremor.*

restraints objects or systems of limiting a patient's movement. Medications to control a patient's activity level and behavioral patterns are legally considered restraints. At times restraints may be medically indicated but too often they are overused and abused. It is the patient's right not to be restrained unless all other options have been tried and have failed. See *consumer rights, falls, medical play, physical restraints, psychiatric seclusion, show of force.*

restraints — inappropriate as defined by the federal *Immediate and Serious Threat* regulation in the United States: Inappropriate restraints are any form of restraint (physical devices, drugs, or procedures) that in some way restricts a patient's physical and/or mental independence/autonomy, the use of which cannot be justified by appropriate assessment or which are not monitored properly. Situations/conditions that warrant investigation of inappropriate restraints include: 1. clinical records which reflect either an absence of justification or incorrect justification for use of restraints, 2. restraints that are applied as punishment, 3. serious or unexplained injures during the restraint process, 4. restraints that are improperly applied, 5. patients who appear unusually drowsy and/or apathetic, and 6. a failure to monitor patients exhibiting symptoms of *tardive dyskinesia.*

retrieval 1. a cognitive process of locating information previously entered into long-term *memory* in such a manner that it is usable and contextual. 2. accessing information stored in an archive (e.g., a computer database, historical files, or other storage area).

retrograde amnesia See *amnesia.*

retrospective research (HCO) *research* in which patients are observed after they have received health services. See *prospective research.*

retrospective review a review of the services provided to the patient performed during the course of a *utilization review.* Funding may be denied retrospectively as a result of a utilization review finding that the services delivered were unnecessary.

retrospective study (HHS) research that relies on recall of past data, or on previously recorded information. Often this type of research is considered to have limitations, because of the number of variables that cannot be controlled and because memory is not infallible.

retrovirus (CDC) a family of RNA viruses that have the unique characteristic of producing an enzyme that makes a DNA copy of its genetic information from an RNA template (the opposite of what normally takes place). The most widely recognized of these viruses is HIV, the causative agent in AIDS. Another virus from this family (HTLV-1) has been associated with T cell leukemia.

reversible figure any figure that appears to reverse itself through spontaneous reversal of perspective. The Necker cube at the right is an example of a reversible figure.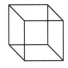

rheumatic fever an infectious disease that is often the result of inadequately treated streptococcal infection of the upper respiratory system, also known as "strep throat." Rheumatic fever usually develops suddenly a few weeks after the apparent recovery from strep throat or scarlet fever. Joint pain, fever, vomiting, and abdominal pain are symptoms initially seen. Damage may be caused to the heart, brain, joints, and skin.

ribonucleic acid See *RNA.*

RICE an abbreviation for rest, ice, compression, and elevation. An order usually written as part of the treatment for *sprains* or *strains.*

rickets abnormal bone formation because of a lack of vitamin D. See *vitamin D deficiency.*

right to appeal (OBRA) A transfer or discharge from the long-term care facility that has not been initiated by the patient may be appealed by the patient or his/her responsible party. The intent of this right to appeal is that no one is discharged from a facility without the party's *consent.* The appeal is filed with the Department of Health Services within ten days of notification of a proposed transfer/*discharge* and the decision will be made by DHS within thirty days from the date the notice was issued.

right to refuse treatment legal doctrine holding that a person, even when involuntarily committed to a hospital, may not be forced to submit to any form of treatment against his/her will unless a life and death emergency exists. See *civil rights, consent, informed consent.*

rigidity the act of being cognitively, perceptually, or socially unbending/inflexible. A muscle is said to have rigidity when it is in a strong contraction.

risk 1. taking an action even though there may be a possibility of injury or loss. In management, a risk is accepting the possibility of a loss in a given situation because it is expected that the action will improve the ongoing success of the business. See *risk management.* 2. (HHS) a term encompassing a variety of measures of the probability of an outcome. It's usually used in reference to unfavorable outcomes such as illness or death.

risk adjustment (HCO) statistical control of patient risk factors in the analysis of the utilization and *outcomes* of health services; also, control of financial risk factors faced by insurance companies.

risk factor 1. anything statistically shown to have a relationship with the incidence of a disease; cause and effect are not implied. 2. (HCO) key health problems and background characteristics that affect the patient's *outcome*, independent of the specific kinds of services received.

risk management in business, the identification of potential losses and then the controlled management of the situation that may cause the loss. The level of risk is identified to determine which risks are great enough that they need to be addressed. Frequently, the degree or level of risk for activities is divided into three levels: 1. high risk, 2. medium risk, and 3. low risk. High risk are activities that require instruction, lengthy training, and practice to perform safely (to control the level of risk). An example of a high-risk activity is ocean kayaking. Medium-risk activities are activities that require instruction, some supervision, and practice prior to engaging in the activity. An example of a medium-risk activity is cross-country skiing. Low-risk activities are activities which require little to no instruction and practice to reduce risk. An example of a low-risk activity is watching television. To decrease the risk to practitioners, complete documentation of services and therapy provided should be maintained for each patient. Head (1993) listed the following nine principles of good risk management related to practice and documentation as:

1. the initial *assessment* of the patient is complete (See *intake assessment.*)
2. patient goals and *objectives* correspond to the initial assessment
3. *treatments* are realistic, measurable, and consistent with patient goals and objectives
4. the evaluation documents timely progress toward meeting stated goals and *objectives*
5. patient education and *participation* is clearly documented
6. records are kept safe and confidential (See *confidentiality.*)
7. personnel are scheduled in a way that provides sufficient time for complete *documentation*

8. authorized personnel have appropriate access to records in order to provide the necessary *continuity of care*
9. policies and procedures are established in writing

See *falls, incident reports.*

risk taking the degree to which an individual is willing to engage in an activity that involves a significant degree of risk.

ritualistic behaviors behaviors that are performed time after time in the same manner. Many ritualistic behaviors tend to be relatively healthy, normal behaviors that help people cope with *stress* and the multitude of choices given to them every day. Ritualistic behaviors are usually developed because they helped an individual achieve a satisfactory solution to a need. Ritualistic behavior tend to become unhealthy in two primary ways: 1. the behavior originally developed did not achieve a healthy and satisfactory solution to the need being presented and yet the individual still ritualized the behavior and/or 2. the behavior was originally developed to solve a need but it did not change to adjust to a new situation.

RNA (HHS) also known as ribonucleic acid. RNA is a molecule similar to DNA that functions primarily to decode the instructions carried by genes for protein synthesis.

role the behavior pattern expected for a particular situation and/or in a particular social group. Many types of roles are learned through the socialization process. The chart on the next page lists four means of assimilating roles through a social process.

role-playing a counseling technique that has the patient act out a role to help problem solve. This type of therapeutic drama technique (along with *sociodrama* and *psychodrama*) is based on the premise that acting out situations can help induce a behavioral and/or psychological change in the patient. Through role-playing the patient can practice social skills, replay upsetting interactions with others, or experiment with new behaviors. Role-playing helps decrease the patient's anxiety concerning a new behavior. Part of this reduction is from supportive feedback on the effectiveness of the behavior(s) being practiced.

rollator See *walker.*

ROM See *range of motion.*

roomrate the amount of reimbursement an insurance company or entitlement program is willing to pay for the patient's stay and the associated treatment and services. Associated treatment and services includes nursing services, housekeeping services, dietary services, and depending on the unit or coverage

Assimilated Roles (Whaley and Wong, 1991, p. 75)

Type of Role	Description
Achieved Role	Roles acquired through effort, and children must do something to attain them. Achieved roles include educational, occupational, religious, and recreational roles. These are based on performance and are acquired through satisfaction of specific requirements. The direction of these role achievements is strongly influenced by values conveyed to the children by their parents. For example, some parents believe that a college education is essential; others encourage children to seek occupational gratification.
Adopted Role	Roles that are sometimes transient, such as the role of patient or traveler. More often, adopted behavior patterns become fixed into what are known as character roles and apply to the unique behaviors that the child displays in a given situation. Such roles as the leader, the followers, the clown, or the show-off are examples of adopted roles. They are frequently adopted when playing the role meets a need or is the response to a complementary role in another.
Ascribed Roles	Roles that are strictly defined by the culture and very little deviation is allowed in modifying them. Ascribed roles apply to general traits such as sex, age, kinship, social class, and ethnic origin. There are culturally determined behaviors that must be adhered to regarding these roles, and they are expected to be learned in the home. For example, a child who attempts to change an ascribed role (such as sex) will be confronted with serious problems.
Assumed Roles	Roles related to fantasy that are especially important in childhood. This is one of the dominant means for children's adjustment and socialization. Children continually assume roles of persons they observe in their environment. The environment is a primary resource for learning the conduct that befits their position or status. Assumed roles only become a problem if they persist into the world of reality. For example, a child who persistently plays an infantile role is severely hampered in relationships with peers.

type, therapy services. Compare with *fee-for-service*.

Rosenthal effect a type of deliberate and/or unintentional behavior on the part of the researcher that influences the *outcome* of research. Typically this behavior causes some of the test subjects to react differently. Some of the cases include the researcher's tone of voice being different with different individuals, a perception of closeness or comfort created by the researcher with some individuals but not others, or rating similar behaviors differently due to the researcher's own biases.

roseola also known as roseola infantum, exanthem subitem, and pseudorubella; an acute disease of infants or very young children caused by HHV-6 and characterized by high fever lasting 4-5 days. When the fever ends, a faint, pink rash appears on the neck, trunk, and thighs. The rash may last from a few hours to two days.

rounds the short *care conference* or patient update that usually takes place right on the unit and involves the members of the patient's treatment team. Rounds usually take place daily or weekly, depending on the patient's progress and unit schedule.

rubella (HHS) also known as German measles, an acute disease marked by skin rash and swollen lymph nodes, symptoms of a mild respiratory disease, but generally without fever. It is caused by an RNA virus of the togavirus family.

rubor the normal coloring of the skin. A deep purple color in the extremities caused by poor venous return and dilated capillaries is called "dependent rubor." When treating patients with dependent rubor, the therapist should try to encourage activities that allow the raised positioning of the affected limb. Such simple solutions as having the patient sit in a Lazyboy type chair with the foot rest up allow a patient's legs to be raised and yet a card table (or similar table) may be used over the foot rest to allow a game of cards or other activities.

rule-based expert system (HCO) a decision support system based on large numbers of heuristics, or rules of thumb, derived from analysis of action patterns of experts or from published literature.

rule of nines a formula used to determine the percentage of body surface burned. The head is considered to be 9%, each arm 9%, each leg 18% (2x9), the anterior trunk and posterior trunk are each 18%. The perineum area is the only area not assigned a value of 9%, but instead is assigned a value of 1%.

rule out a phrase used as part of a preliminary diagnosis. The health care provider may have several possible diagnoses that fit the presenting symptoms. Usually one seems most likely, but it may be necessary to perform additional tests to eliminate (rule out) the other possible diagnoses.

run-length encoding (HCO) a *data* compression scheme in which extended series of repetitive data are replaced by the first item in the series and a token indicating the length of the data run.

running slope (ADA) the slope that is parallel to the direction of travel. See *cross slope*.

rural health clinic (RHC) a clinic which provides primary health care services located in a rural area designated as either an area with a shortage of personal health services or primary medical care manpower. The RHC must have a physician, a physician assistant, and/or a nurse practitioner on staff.

S

saccharin (HHS) the oldest of the non-nutritive sweeteners; currently produced from purified, manufactured methyl anthranilate, a substance occurring naturally in grapes. It is 300 times sweeter than sucrose, heat stable, and does not promote dental caries. Saccharin has a long shelf life, but a slightly bitter aftertaste. It is not metabolized in the human digestive system, is excreted rapidly in the urine, and does not accumulate in the body.

sadism a psychiatric disorder involving cruelty, usually of a sexual nature, first described by Marquis de Sade in 1740. The perpetrator receives sexual excitement or gratification through inflicting pain or humiliation on another person who may or may not be a consenting partner. See *algolagnia*.

sadomasochism a psychiatric disorder that combines two disorders first described by Marquis de Sade and Leopold von Sacher-Masoch. de Sade described a disorder in which an individual derives pleasure by physically or psychologically hurting another (*sadism*). von Sacher-Masoch described a disorder in which an individual derives pleasure by being personally physically or psychologically hurt by himself/herself or by another person (masochism). See *algolagnia*.

S.A.F.E. an acronym from the *PEW Commission* used to describe the attributes of a quality health care system. S.A.F.E. stands for: Standardized where appropriate, Accountable to the public, Flexible to support optimal access to a safe and competent health care workforce and Effective and efficient in protecting and promoting the public's health, safety, and welfare.

safety management See *environment of care*.

salmonella (HHS) a Gram-negative bacterium, occurring in many animals, especially poultry and swine. In the environment, salmonella can be found in water, soil, insects, factory and kitchen surfaces, animal fecal matter, raw meats, poultry (including eggs), and seafood. Acute symptoms of the illness caused by the salmonella species include nausea, vomiting, diarrhea, abdominal cramps, headache, and fever.

SAP note a type of chart note that includes a summary of the patient's situation, an assessment of the interventions indicated, and a description of a plan to carry out the indicated interventions. See also *SOAPIER notes, SOAP notes*.

sarcoidosis (HHS) a systemic disease involving the lungs, lymph nodes, skin, liver, spleen, eyes, phalangeal bones, and parotid glands, characterized by granular nodules. Its cause is not known.

sarcoma (HHS/NMDP) a malignant solid tumor most frequently found in muscle.

sarcomere the smallest unit of *myofibril* in muscles. See *elasticity*.

saturated fats See *fatty acids*.

scales and rating systems *measurements* (tools) with defined intervals which helps arrange objects or events into groups. Scales play a major role in testing and defining *functional ability*. There are many different types (structures) of scales, as well as scales that measure specific functional abilities. The type of scale that should be used varies depending on the population served. The FIM Scale is used in rehab medicine, the Global Assessment of Functioning is used in psychiatry, and "intermittent-limited-extensive-pervasive" is used in developmental disabilities. Some terms related to scales are shown on the next page. See *FIM Scale, Global Assessment of Functioning Scale, Glasgow Coma Scale, Likert Scale, Rancho Los Amigos Scale, Frankel neurological assessment, mental retardation, spinal cord injury.*

scar the tissue that replaces skin or other cells after the healing of a wound. Scar tissue lacks oil glands and lacks elastic tissue. As a scar ages, it usually contracts, causing a reduction in *range of motion* to the affected area. A *keloid scar* is a scar with excess fibrous growth. Medical intervention is important during the healing process to reduce the development of keloid tissue. Keloid tissue, especially from untreated third-degree burns, is at increased risk of malignancy. See *hypertrophic scarring, Jobst, malignant.*

scar tissue adhesions contracture The presence of scar tissue between healthy tissue will decrease ROM through adherence of the scar tissue to surrounding healthy tissue. The types of tissues that may be involved are skin, muscles, tendons, and/or the joint capsules themselves. The primary intervention for scar tissue adhesions is prevention. The adhesions may be prevented or reduced through enjoyable activities that promote the use of the affected area through its complete range of motion. Some "burning" or "stretching" may be experienced by the

Terms Related to Scales

Type	Description
Attitude	Any scale that helps identify attitudes that individuals hold. Examples include the *Leisure Motivation Scale* and the *Free Time Boredom Scale*.
Difficulty Scale	Any scale or test that is developed so that items are developed with different degrees of difficulty to help measure degree of competence.
Interval Scale	Any scale with each level or interval clearly defined by equal "steps." Examples of interval scales include the thermometer and IQ tests.
Nominal Scale	Any scale that names the categories it measures. Examples include gender, title, state, and athletic uniform numbers.
Ordinal Scale	Any scale that groups using generalized units. A hospital playroom may be for "preschoolers" while the recreation room on the adolescent floor is for "adolescents." Each room groups activities based on a generalized idea of what children of that age would enjoy, but is not specified by an interval scale (e.g., 9 months through 36 months).
Psychological Scale	Any scale that uses some kind of system to measure a psychological characteristic or variable. The *Global Assessment of Functioning* is a psychological scale.

patient; discourage painful ranging during activities.

scheduled injury The United States has developed a system to compensate workers who suffer permanent injuries on the job. Scheduled injures are those to extremities, vision, or hearing and are usually assessed at a fixed percentage (for example, the loss of a particular body part results in the awarding of a certain number of weeks of pay). See *disability, nonscheduled injury*.

schizoaffective disorder a mental disorder which is marked by a combination of a *mood disorder* (major depressive, manic, or mixed episode) and *schizophrenia*. There are two subtypes for schizoaffective disorder: bipolar type and depressive type.

schizophrenia an organically-based set of mental disorders in which the patient demonstrates at least two of the following: *delusions, hallucinations*, disorganized speech, disorganized or catatonic behaviors, and/or negative symptoms such as a flattening of *affect*, a lack of speech, or inability or lack of desire to make choices. If the patient is experiencing bizarre active auditory hallucinations or bizarre delusions, the patient is not required to have at least two of the listed symptoms. The symptoms must also be significantly and negatively impacting the patient's ability to function socially and/or vocationally, have lasted at least six months (with symptoms possibly controlled during that time) and not related to a *schizoaffective* or *mood* disorder, as a result of substance use or general medical conditions, and not related to *pervasive developmental disorder*. Schizophrenia has four subtypes: paranoid type (delusions or frequent auditory hallucinations), disorganized type (disorganized speech, behavior, and/or affect), catatonic, or undifferentiated (not fitting into the other three categories). Schizophrenia affects about 1% of the population of the United States, affecting males and females equally. Men usually have an earlier onset than women, with the peak age of onset for men being between 15 and 25 years of age and women between 25 and 35 years of age. The etiology of schizophrenia is not known but some interesting data has been gathered, leading some to wonder if there is a viral component or an environmental component to the cause of schizophrenia. To give an example, children born between the months of January and April in the northern hemisphere are more likely to have schizophrenia while children born between the months of July and September in the southern hemisphere are more likely to have schizophrenia (Kaplan et al, 1994). As research continues, our knowledge of the causes and treatment have improved greatly. The introduction of atypical antipsychotic medications has greatly reduced the bizarre behaviors with minimal neurological side effects. This has now allowed mental health professionals to better evaluate the impact that the environment has on acute schizophrenic crisis and how to modify the environment to decrease the incidence. See *catatonia, dissociation, Minnesota Multiphasic Personality Inventory*.

science the study of how things work, relate to each other, or evolve; practiced by systematic recording, evaluation, and interpretation. Theories are developed through study to explain why something happens. Science is divided into two different types: pure science which is the study and recording of phenomena to gain more knowledge and applied science which is the study of how to use the knowledge gained through pure science in practical, day-to-day applications. See *ethics*.

scoliosis a lateral curvature of the spine. See *Harrington rod, kyphosis, lordosis, neurofibromatosis*.

scope of practice the set of skills and techniques

generally accepted as being part of a professional group's area of expertise. See *body of knowledge, credentialing, intake assessment, PEW Health Professions Commission, professional misconduct.*

scree plot a graphical representation of plotted *eigenvalues*. The term "scree" comes from the field of geology and refers to the broken rock debris that collects at the bottom of a steep slop. A scree plot has a line that shows a rapid drop down on the graph, then a leveling off to a gradual slope. Generally, in statistics, this type of scree (the gradual slope) is also considered to be debris and would not be retained as being significant.

scrip Medical scrip is part of an endowment program. The scrip can be used in place of money to pay for services rendered and equipment received.

script a formally written out dialog and a mapping of activity and movement used by all staff in a center when training patients. The purpose is to ensure that all staff present the training in a consistent manner, enhancing the patient's ability to learn.

seasonal affective disorder (SAD) a disorder in which individuals become depressed at the end of fall or early winter. This disorder tends to resolve itself after a few months, only to reappear again the next fall. The most common symptoms include fatigue and lethargy. Overeating and carbohydrate cravings are also common. A minority of individual who suffer from seasonal affective disorder show almost opposite symptoms including eating less, sleeping less, and losing weight along with their lethargy. Women tend to be affected more than men, with the most likely onset is just before menstruation or menopause. In addition, higher latitudes also seem to play a part, probably because the light level changes are greater there. Typical treatment involves the use of light therapy. The individual engages in activities such as reading or other work which allows him/her to sit in front of a light box which contains very intense fluorescent lights for about 30 minutes a day. Seasonal affective disorder (SAD) is not listed as an independent diagnose in the **DSM-IV** but can be found as a pattern of *depression* with either a major depressive disorder, bipolar I disorder or bipolar II disorder. One of the diagnostic criteria is that the episodic depression cannot be better explained by psychosocial stressors (e.g., memory of the death of a loved one during that time of year).

secondary brain injury injury to the brain caused by subsequent physiological or pathophysiological response to the initial injury. Some secondary brain injury causes include a re-bleed from a hemorrhage, increased pressure, cerebral edema, hydrocephalus, *anoxia*, or cerebral infections. See *traumatic brain injury.*

secondary data (HCO) *data* originally collected for one purpose (e.g., program administration) and then analyzed for a different purpose (usually research or evaluation). Data reported by other than the original researcher.

second impact syndrome a second concussion received some time after a severe *traumatic brain injury*, which the patient experiences prior to the complete clearing of the first injury. The second injury tends to multiply the damage for the first injury instead of just adding to the original damage.

Section 1905(d) of the Social Security Act, 42 USC 1396d(d) *Medicaid* Program. This Act provides the states with grants to help provide the mandated services for individuals with developmental disabilities. In most cases this grant covers 55% of the cost of care for an individual in an ICF-MR. The allocation per individual is referred to as "FFP" or *Federal Financial Participation*. See *intermediate care facility for the mentally retarded.*

securement devices (ADA) a mechanical object which ties a wheelchair or a mobility device to a vehicle. A securement device is not a seatbelt and should never be used to tie the passenger to his/her mobility device.

security management See *environment of care.*

seizure an abnormal release of electrical impulses in the brain. When these electrical impulses are released at a normal rate, an individual is able to think, move, and experience "normal" activity. An abnormal release causes one or more of these three areas to malfunction. The word "seizure" is a generic term, with many different sub-classifications. An individual who has a tendency to have seizures frequently is considered to have *epilepsy*. Many of the individuals who have seizures can successfully integrate into the community without any obvious symptoms. However, this stability is usually brought about by the use of medications. The therapist should evaluate the potential increased risk of injury during activity due to the side effects of medications. Individuals who do not have their seizures successfully controlled by medications may have a diminished level of alertness. Some individuals with a seizure disorder may be more likely to experience a seizure when exposed to strobe lights and video games. The therapist may want to be acutely observant while the individual is engaged in these activities to note if they are susceptible to seizures due to this kind of stimulation. The chart on the next page shows some terms related to seizures. See *autism (chart), electroconvulsive treatment, electroencephalogram, epilepsy.*

Seizures

Seizure Types	Frequency	Observable Aspects	Duration	Comments
Akinetic Seizures		loss of tone and muscle movement	short duration, multiple times a day, more frequently in a.m. than p.m.	individual is unable to break fall during seizure and significant injury may result
Focal		depends on part of brain experiencing the abnormal electrical impulses	varies	isolated to one part of brain
Grand Mal	accounts for 60% of all seizure disorders	two phase seizure: 1. tonic with loss of consciousness, stiffening of body, irregular breathing, drooling, possible incontinence, 2. clonic with jerking caused by alternating rigidity and relaxation of muscles	tonic 10-20 seconds; clonic about 30 seconds, may last up to 30 minutes	just prior to seizure individual may feel pre-warning signs called "aura"
Infantile	rare — but 85% with this type also have mental retardation	dropping head, flexion of arms	may be short in duration but occur hundreds of times a day	also known as infantile myoclonic seizure or jackknife epilepsy; poor prognosis
Myoclonic		brief, involuntary jerking of extremities with or without loss of consciousness	May be short.	
Petit Mal		hard to recognize, loss of consciousness without loss of muscle tone, may stare absentmindedly, may rapidly blink eyes	5-20 seconds; 20 or more seizures a day common	usually occurs between 4 to 12 years; about one third of individuals with petit mal develop grand mal
Psychomotor	more common in adults	involuntary repetitive actions — as simple as rubbing of hands, lip smacking	usually 10-60 seconds; rarely occur over 1 or 2 times per day	also known as temporal lobe seizure; caused by abnormal electrical activity in the temporal lobe; may experience emotional changes after seizure
Post traumatic	depending on degree of damage — age — concern with individuals with significant subdural injury due to traumatic brain injury	usually evident within one year of traumatic brain injury		four specific groups with TBI are at greater risk and should be watched closely on community integration outings: 1. diffuse cerebral edema, 2. open depressed skull fracture, 3. acute subdural hematoma, or 4. an original GCS (Glasgow Coma Scale) score of 8 or less.
Simple Febrile	5-10% of all children under 6 years	loss of consciousness, generalized jerking	less than 10 minutes	associated with fever

self-control the ability to: 1. know what is expected, 2. monitor one's own behavior, 3. have adequate coping skills to deal with beyond normal stress, and 4. regulate responses to maintain reasonable behavior.

self-esteem the feeling that one is of worth or value to others and to self. Self-esteem is earned, not just learned through books and lectures. Actual accomplishment leads to good self-esteem. See *conduct disorder, Culture-Free Self-Esteem Inventories, dance therapy, dependent personality disorder, dysthymia, empowerment, imagery, mania, medical play, memory deficit, post traumatic stress disorder, refuting irrational ideas.*

Self-Esteem Index a multi-disciplinary assessment that is used to identify youth between the ages of 7.0 through 18.11 who may have problems related to low self-esteem, socially inappropriate behavior, and/or problems with adjustment. This assessment tool is norm referenced and measures the way the patient perceives his/her value. The patient is asked to answer 80 question using a four-point scale ("Always True" to "Always False"). The Self-Esteem Index has four scales: 1. Academic Competence, which measures self-esteem in school, education, academic competence, intelligence, learning, and other scholarly pursuits, 2. Family Acceptance, which measures self-esteem at home and within the family unit, 3. Peer Popularity, which measures the quality, importance, and nature of relationships and interactions with individuals outside the family unit, and 4. Personal Security, which measures perception about one's physical appearance and personal attributes such as distinctive traits of body, character, conduct, temperament, and emotions. This assessment may be administered to individuals or in a group setting and usually takes less than 30 minutes to administer.

self-hypnosis a type of relaxation technique. The process of restricting your thought process to a very limited scope, practicing inertia, and responding passively at the most to stimuli in the environment. A type of "zoning out." Practicing twice a day for one to two weeks should help establish mastery. Patients with headaches, insomnia, or minor anxiety can benefit from this technique. This technique is contraindicated for patients with *dementia, delirium,* intoxication and withdrawal, *psychosis,* paranoia, or severe *mental retardation.* See *relaxation techniques.*

self-injurious behavior (SIB) the *compulsive* damage to tissue that an individual self-inflicts. SIB includes biting, scratching, hair pulling, and head banging. The at-risk populations include individuals with *autism, mental retardation* (especially individuals who function at the "severe" level) as well as some children and adults who were placed on stimulant medications (for *attention deficit hyperactivity disorder*). In the case of the medicine-induced SIB, the incidence of SIB ceases when the medication is discontinued. See *associated features, behavioral therapy.*

self-management the ability to control one's actions and thoughts. The ability to self-manage one's thoughts and actions includes multiple skills such as self-assessment, self-detachment, self-feedback, self-motivation, self-expression, and self-care.

Self-Perception Profile of Children This assessment is a self-reported assessment for children and youth. The Self-Perception Profile of Children has five specific competency/adequacy domains (scholastic competence, social acceptance, athletic competence, physical appearance, and conduct/behavior/morality). A score is given in each of the five domains, as well as a general self-worth score. Structured so that half of the choices are on the left side of the statement and the other half of the choices are on the right, the child first decides which kind of "kid" s/he is and then indicates whether the statement is really true or sort of true for him/her. The items are scored on a four-point scale with six items for each subscale. The score sheet that the child sees for the Self-Perception Profile of Children is titled "What I Am Like." A sample is shown on the next page. This assessment is available through its author, Susan Harter, PhD, at the University of Denver (Colorado), sharter@nova.psy.du.edu, 303-871-3790.

self-stimulation the stimulation of one's own nerves, frequently as a result of being in an environment deprived of normal stimulation. Some types of developmental disabilities will decrease the individual's ability to receive or understand stimulation from the environment. These individuals also tend to engage in a high level of self-stimulation. Self-stimulation, in most cases, is not considered to be socially acceptable in public.

self-talk the internal dialog that an individual has with himself/herself. This is the discussion that an individual uses to arrive at a decision. An example would be "Wow, I really like that dress. Ugh! It's $75. I have just enough money to get the new tires my car needs. But still, I've got to have that dress. Maybe my car can go one more month without new tires..." Allowing time for self-talk can reduce the therapist's level of confidence with testing results, especially with tests like the *Leisurescope Plus*. In most cases, the therapist will receive better test re-

What I Am Like (Self-Perception Profile of Children)

	Really True for Me	Sort of True for Me				Sort of True for Me	Really True for Me
1.	☐	☐	Some kids feel that they are very *good* at their school work	**BUT**	Other kids *worry* about whether they can do the schoolwork assigned to them.	☐	☐
2.	☐	☐	Some kids find it *hard* to make friends	**BUT**	For other kids it's pretty *easy*.	☐	☐
3.	☐	☐	Some kids do very *well* at all kinds of sports	**BUT**	Others *don't* feel that they are very good when it comes to sports.	☐	☐

sults if s/he limits the time a patient has for self-talk during testing. See *coping techniques, refuting irrational ideas.*

senile obsolete term, replaced by "dementia."

sensation a message carried by the nerves as a result of some action or event. Terms associated with sensation are shown below. See *causalgia, diabetes, dysesthesia, hyperesthesia, hypoesthesia, kinesthesia, threshold of sensation on two-point discrimination test.*

senses Traditionally, there are five senses: sight, hearing, smell, taste, and touch. Other senses include pressure, proprioception, pain, temperature, hunger, thirst, and spatial, time, and visceral sensations. See *astereognosis, extrasensory perception, hallucination, thalamic pain.*

sensorimotor referring to the coordination of one's senses with one's movement (motor behavior). Some of the functional skills that require a fair degree of sensorimotor skill are gross and fine motor coordination, muscle control, dexterity, strength and endurance, tactile awareness, and *range of motion.*

sensory deprivation See *deprivation.*

sensory integration the body's ability to take in stimulation from its environment using a variety of sensory organs all at the same time. This information is then interpreted and integrated into a coherent view of the world.

sensory overload the state in which the body is receiving more sensory input than it can handle (or comfortably ignore).

sensory stimulation a type of *treatment* intervention used with patients who have a significant cognitive loss and are not able to initiate and produce purposeful interaction with the environment. This intervention involves the frequent (multiple times a day, 5 or more minutes at a time) introduction of objects to stimulate the senses. Sensory stimulation is usually more productive if more than one sense is being stimulated at a time. See *bed rest.*

sentinel surveillance (CDC) a monitoring method that employs a surrogate indicator for a public health problem, allowing estimation of the magnitude of the problem in the general population.

Terms of Sensation

absent	lack of awareness of contact
articular	awareness of the contact and movement of joints
cutaneous	awareness of contact with the dermis (skin)
delayed	awareness which happens some time after the initial contact
diminished	a subnormal awareness of contact
epigastric	referring to "that sinking feeling" produced by worry or fear; felt in the stomach
hyper	an abnormally increased awareness of contact
internal	awareness of sensations to the body not caused by any external event
negative	lack of awareness of contact because the contact/stimulation is below the threshold of the nerves involved
objective	a cognitive awareness of an event through the use of multiple senses
vascular	awareness of a change in the tone of the surface capillaries (e.g., blushing)

sequela *pl.* **sequelae** (HHS) any abnormal condition following as a consequence of a disease, injury, or treatment.

sequencing skills   the ability to place objects or events in a logical order: by time, by number or other recognized pattern. See *organizational deficit, processing deficit.*

service entrance   (ADA) an entrance intended primarily for delivery of goods or services.

severe combined immunodeficiency disease (SCID) (HHS/NMDP) congenital defect of the immune system leading to frequent life threatening infections. Marrow transplantation is the current treatment of choice. Most patients have an early onset of SCID detected due to infection, usually by three months of age.

sexual abuse in young children   the sexual mistreatment of a child or youth by fondling, forced participation in unnatural sexual acts, rape, or other behavior considered to be "perverted." Young children seldom (if ever) come right out and tell the therapist that they have been sexually abused. Developmentally, young children are not normally exposed to the vocabulary and actions associated with intercourse. It is therefore important that the therapist become familiar with the developmentally appropriate terms used and actions typically used by children who have been abused. In young children, but also to some extent in AMACs (Adults Molested As Children), the non-verbal signals such as the behaviors listed below (adapted from Lamers-Winhelman,

1988) can be seen. Not all child victims will exhibit every one of these signs. On the other hand, some non-abused children may have one or more of these signs. A single such sign is insufficient to conclude that sexual abuse has occurred. If sexual abuse is suspected, further diagnostic work and confirmation is indicated. By law, all health care and education professionals are required to report suspected child abuse, usually within 24 hours of having a reasonable suspicion.

sexually transmitted diseases (STD)   diseases that primarily spread through sexual intercourse or genital contact. The primary STDs are AIDS, *gonorrhea*, syphilis, scabies, herpes genitalis, anorectal herpes and warts, genital candidiasis, non-specific urethritis, *chlamydial infections*, cytomegalovirus, chancroid, granuloma inguinale and lymphogranuloma venereum, pediculosis, and trichomoniasis.

shared decision support systems   (HCO) designed to inform patient/provider about decisions regarding prevention, diagnosis, management, and treatment.

Shared Medical Systems (SMS)   (HCO) a vendor of hospital information services and products.

short-term memory   a temporary memory system that will pass information to be remembered on to the long-term memory. Short-term memory will usually hold about six to eight items or short ideas for a few seconds to up to a minute or so. The information stored in the short-term memory can either be forgotten or transmitted to the long-term memory. For this transfer to happen the information needs to

Recognition of Child Sexual Abuse In Young Children

- Reluctance to undress in front of others (doctor, school nurse, gym class).
- Dislike of their own body. They often think that bodies are dirty and ugly.
- Movement that is stiff and inhibited in nature, fearful or repulsed with body contact.
- When walking or running, upper legs are pressed together, as well as buttocks. (It seems as if their pelvic areas are locked.)
- Fear of body contact initiated by others — especially adults. (When touched they stiffen, especially when on upper legs, buttocks, or abdomen.)
- They have a lack of potential to enjoy themselves or to enjoy "playing around" with other children.
- They are uncomfortable sitting on adult's laps. (If asked to come and sit on an adult's lap, the child will obey but not sit comfortably.)
- They are reluctant to touch other children and adults. They will not join in rough and tumble play. In fact, they are afraid of it.
- They are extremely anxious when asked to lay down on their back (such as in gym class). For the young, diapering can be terrifying with corresponding reactions of fright and panic.
- When lifted up or caught, these young children don't react with a normal "reflex" (e.g., arms and legs encircling the person catching them.) They hold their legs stiff together and straight down.
- Non-spontaneous movement in play. (For instance, when entering gym class, such children look for a bench and sit down, legs neatly pressed next to each other, backs stretched out, with blank looking faces. However exciting the physical education materials may be, however exciting the play of the other children, they do not join the group by themselves.)

be coded and organized prior to the transfer. See *memory.*

shoulder disarticulation an amputation through the glenohumeral joint. Functional ability is improved through the use of a seven unit prosthesis:

1. socket
2. cable and modified chest strap harness
3. shoulder joint
4. internal locking elbow
5. forearm lift assist
6. wrist unit
7. terminal device

The socket for this prosthesis device extends from the patient's spine posteriorly, fitting snugly against the neck and extends to the xiphoid process anteriorly. The shoulder joint, also called a bulkhead spacer, allows some abduction, adduction, flexion, and extension. A shoulder disarticulation is abbreviated "SD."

showering the debriding of a wound or burn through the use of a high pressure, hand-held showerhead to irrigate the injured area.

show of force the planned actions taken by staff when a patient is out of control and a danger to himself/herself or others. A show of force is called on the unit and all staff assigned to respond in a crisis meet in the proximity of the patient who is out of control. A team leader is identified and each staff person is assigned a body part to hold. Other staff are assigned to the task of applying any restraint (physical and/or medications) that are to be used. The team leader informs the patient that s/he is going to be taken down and restrained for his/her own protection. On the command of the leader, all staff execute their roles, whether it is to grab and hold a body part or to apply a restraint. It cannot be overstated how overwhelming taking part or observing a show of force can be, or how dangerous it can be to both staff and patient. A show of force will frequently use as many as eight staff people to take down one patient. This is an extremely frightening event for others patients to watch. Many patients are already afraid that they will "lose it," but then to see someone else taken down in such a fashion only adds to the other patients' anxiety. Loss of control and safety are big issues. Safety of the staff should also be considered throughout the entire process. Staff will need to glove up (in case of bleeding) and staff at the patient's head risk the chance of being bitten. A patient who is extremely strong and violent can hurt staff as they try to hold and take him/her down. Show of force practice should be a regular event for all staff just like fire drills and other emergency training. See *assault cycle, restraints.*

shunt a tube surgically placed within the body to help redirect the flow of body fluids. See *hydrocephalus.*

SIB See *self-injurious behavior.*

sickle cell anemia See *anemia.*

side effect the secondary effect of a treatment. Many medications have side effects — most of them undesirable. An example would be antibiotics that frequently cause *photosensitivity.* Non-medication based treatment may also have side effects. For example, the variety of wheelchairs available to the consumer today is far greater than ten to twenty years ago. The therapist is now able to prescribe a wheelchair that maximizes the patient's ability to self-propel with maximum results using limited energy. However, a potential side effect of such precise positioning and scientifically developed movement patterns may be a repetitive use injury. *Ergonomics* is an important factor to build into all adapted movements and equipment.

SIDS See *sudden infant death syndrome.*

sign (in testing) a characteristic that has been previously identified as having significance related to a *diagnosis* or *treatment.* A fever is one sign of an infection. Signs may be identified through testing, through maneuvers or through the clinical observation of the therapist. Some examples of signs are shown on the next page.

signage (ADA) displayed verbal, symbolic, tactile, and pictorial information.

significant change in a patient's status (RAP/OBRA) a significant change means any of the following:

*   Deterioration in two or more *activities of daily living*, communication, and/or cognitive abilities that appears permanent. For example, simultaneous functional *and* cognitive decline often experienced by patients with chronic, degenerative illnesses such as Alzheimer's disease or pronounced functional changes following a *cerebrovascular accident.*
*   Loss of ability to freely ambulate or to use hands to grasp small objects to feed or groom oneself, such as sponge, toothbrush, or comb. Such losses must be permanent and not attributable to identifiable, reversible causes such as drug toxicity from introducing a new medication or an episode of acute illness such as influenza.
*   Deterioration in behavior, mood, and/or relationships that has not been reversed by current staff interventions.
*   Deterioration in a patient's health status, where this change: places the patient's life in danger,

Types of Signs

Sign	Description
Amoss's Sign	A sign that a patient has suffered a painful spinal injury is when the patient places his/her arms far behind himself/herself for support as s/he goes from a flat position to a sitting position on the bed.
Antecedent Sign	Any type of sign that gives the patient and/or staff an indication that a disease event is about to happen.
Baillarger's Sign	Uneven pupils in patients with dementia, indicating a paralysis versus a lack of compliance with a command.
Barré's Sign	The iris's ability to contract is slowed in individuals with mental deterioration.
Barré's Pyramidal Sign	A sign that there is a disease process in the pyramidal tract occurs when the patient is asked to lie face down, bend his/her knees, and keep them in this position and the patient cannot keep his/her legs up (bent at the knees).
Linder Sign	To check to see if the patient's leg pain originates in the spine. With the patient sitting on the floor or table with his/her legs out straight and arms behind him/her the patient is to move his/her chin to chest. If this movement causes upper posterior leg pain, the pain is sciatic (pain running down the back of the leg caused by nerve irritation in the lower spine).
Vital Signs	The measurement of a patient's blood pressure, pulse, respiration, and temperature. Variation from "normal" in any of the four vital sign measurements can indicate a medical problem.

e.g., cerebrovascular accident, heart condition, or diagnosis of metastatic cancer; is associated with a serious clinical complications, e.g., initial development of a Stage III or Stage IV *pressure sore*, the initial onset of non-relieved delirium or recurrent loss of consciousness; or is associated with an initial new diagnosis of a condition that is likely to affect the patient's physical, mental, or psychosocial well-being over a prolonged period of time, e.g., Alzheimer's disease or diabetes.

- A serious clinical complication.
- A new diagnosis of a condition that is likely to affect the patient's physical, mental, or psychosocial well-being over a prolonged period of time.
- Onset of significant weight loss (5% in last 30 days or 10% in last 180 days).
- A marked and sudden improvement in the patient's status, for example, a comatose patient regaining consciousness.

single payer system   a fiscal system in which all health care insurance moneys are funneled into one fund. An example of a single payer system is the health care system in Canada.

single photon emission computed tomography (SPECT scan) (CDC) an imaging technique that measures the emission of photons of a given energy from radioactive tracers introduced into the body. As with other forms of computer-assisted tomography, the technique produces a series of cross-sectional images of internal anatomy.

sinusitis   an inflammation of the paranasal sinuses. The inflammation may be from an infection, from air pollution, allergies, or a structural defect of the sinuses.

site   (ADA) a parcel of land bounded by a property line or a designated portion of a public right-of-way.

site improvement   (ADA) landscaping, paving for pedestrian and vehicular ways, outdoor lighting, recreational facilities, and the like, added to a site.

skeletal traction   the use of pins surgically inserted into one or more bones. A weight or other means of pull is then attached to these pins to achieve traction. See *traction.*

skill   the ability to demonstrate a refined pattern of movements or tasks. A skill is the result of specific, learned neural, physiological processes whereas an *ability* is a more generalized motor planning and/or cognitive process. Motor skill requires competence in five areas: 1. coordination, 2. agility, 3. balance, 4. timing, and 5. speed. See *debilitation, learning.*

skilled nursing facility   a subacute health care facility with licensed nurses 24 hours a day but without a physician 24 hours a day.

skin breakdown   See *pressure sore.*

skin conductance activity (SCA)   a measure of electrical current flow, which is a correlate of sweat gland activity. Measured in micromhos (a unit of electrical conductance), SCA is used in the treatment of anxiety and depression. Galvanized skin response (GSR) and electrodermal response (EDR) are two biofeedback techniques that utilize this process.

skin integrity See *pressure sore.*

skin traction the use of equipment to provide a pulling force on the skin surface indirectly causing a pull on the skeletal system itself. Because the counter-pull is frequently achieved by the patient's weight on the mattress, activities that involve rolling or other movement may reduce the effectiveness of the treatment and are therefore contraindicated. See *traction.*

sleep apnea a group of potentially lethal disorders in which breathing recurrently stops during sleep for long enough to cause measurable blood deoxygenation. It may be caused by an inability to move respiratory muscles or by a blockage of the airway.

sleeping accommodations (ADA) rooms in which people sleep; for example, dormitory and hotel or motel guest rooms or suites.

Slosson Intelligence Test — Revised (SIT-R) one of the more commonly used IQ tests. This IQ test measures the patient's norm-based ability in six cognitive domains: information, comprehension, arithmetic, similarities and differences, vocabulary, and auditory memory. The SIT-R uses contemporary language and is free of significant demographic, racial, or sex biases for ages 4 years and up. Some individuals with traumatic brain injuries may score within "normal" range on IQ tests. The therapist may want to review the sub-scores to see if there are indications that a specific cognitive skill is impaired enough that it may impact the patient's ability to successfully re-integrate into past and future activities. See *intelligence quotient.*

smart card (HCO) a plastic device the size of a credit card with an embedded computer processor and memory.

SOAPIER note a style of writing in the medical chart which follows a specific format: subjective information, objective information, assessment, plan of care, intervention(s), evaluation of effectiveness of intervention, and revision to plan of care. See *SOAP note.*

SOAP note a style of writing in the medical chart that follows a specific format: subjective complaints, objective (observable) description of the problem, assessment of the problem, and the plan for intervention. See the example.

social acceptance the act of being favorably taken into a social group; the process of achieving equal status with one's peers; to be equally valued by one's peers; to be received and acknowledged as being a part of the social give and take of a group. Achieving social acceptance within one's community is an important aspect of *inclusion* for individu-

als with disabilities. Therapists who help their clients focus on developing skills necessary to achieve social acceptance work toward increasing the client's active *participation* in his/her community and increasing the beneficial use of *leisure* and free time. Basic *social skills* are critical to begin the process of gaining social acceptance in the community. However, achieving equal status/value also requires advanced skills related to social acceptance. Some of these include risk taking, initiation, and negotiation. Risk taking includes the ability to go beyond one's comfort zone to take actions that may lead to failure and to develop interests and skills in multiple arenas previously unexplored. Initiation of interactions includes the initiation of deliberate and subtle actions to influence social acceptance and to actively engage in formal and informal mutually satisfying interactions with others. Negotiation for social acceptance includes the ability to suggest various options to resolve conflict, offer compromises, and to bargain with others to nurture social acceptance. Initiation of social acceptance usually occurs in the absence of obstacles to social acceptance. Negotiation skills occur when there are obstacles to social acceptance. (Devine, 2000)

social history (elements of) one of the essential parts of a patient *assessment.* The social history presents a biography of the patient beginning with birth and includes number of siblings, important situations from childhood (orphaned, often uprooted, secure and loving), education, religious background, occupation, military experience, marriage(s), children and other important family and friends, retirement, and events leading up to hospitalization. See *intake assessment.*

social interaction skill learned skill that helps facili-

SOAP Note

S	Patient states that he has to go to the bathroom to empty his urine bag too often, that it interrupts his participation in activities.
O	Patient left activity at 6:15 p.m., 6:39 p.m., and 7:10 p.m. to empty bag. Bag was less than ¼ full each time patient left activity to empty bag. Patient came back with empty bag.
A	Patient is leaving activity for some reason and using the urine bag as an excuse. Bag does not require emptying.
P	1. have nursing evaluate potential pathology associated with catheter and incontinence program. 2. meet with patient privately to confront about behavior.

tate interactions with others. Some social interaction skills are 1. ability to listen, 2. ability to initiate conversation, 3. ability to respond logically to something another said, 4. awareness of the personal space of others, 5. demonstration of appropriate body language congruent with situation and discussion, and 6. appropriate volume of voice. See *graciousness*.

social interface (HCO) a human-computer interface design approach in which users interact with representations of physical objects or, in some cases, anthropomorphic agents displayed by their computer.

socialization the process of learning the social expectations of one's culture, developing the skills to successfully interact with others, and using both the knowledge and skills on a regular basis. Prior to the development of a greater understanding of the affective and cognitive aspects of "socialization," many therapists wrote the patient's objective as "to increase socialization." It is now felt that using this objective is the same as a nursing objective stating "maintain health." This objective is far too vague and gives the impression that the professional did not complete an assessment that was detailed enough to delineate the patient's specific needs. See *acculturation, resocialization*.

Social Security See *entitlement programs*.

social services director an individual hired by a long-term care facility to assist the patient and his/her family adjust to changing health status and functional ability and to assist the patient/family in the application for ancillary services and financial support to receive necessary services. In the United States, the federal legislation that regulates long-term care facilities is called OBRA. The qualifications for social services directors is defined as an individual with a bachelor's degree in social work or similar professional qualifications.

social worker an individual who has completed the required education, training, and experience to provide social work services. See *Joint Commission*.

sociodrama a counseling technique that uses role-playing activities to problem solve a group issue instead of focusing on one individual's issues. The purpose of sociodrama is to explore solutions to problems that the group members have in common. Instead of role modeling a specific person, the protagonist(s) act out a character type (e.g., over-protective father).

socket refers to the cavity of a prosthetic device in which the stump is placed.

soft diet See *mechanical diet*.

software accessibility Not all software is easily used by individuals with disabilities. The Checklist for

User-Friendly Software on the next page is from burlingame (1998b, pp. 478-479).

soluble fiber See *fiber*.

somatization disorder a disorder in which an individual has recurrent and multiple health complaints of a physical nature for which an organic cause cannot be found.

space (ADA) a definable area, e.g., room, toilet room, hall, assembly area, entrance, storage room, alcove, courtyard, or lobby.

space boots specially cushioned boots which help maintain the normal angle of the foot and ankle and prevent *pressure sores* on the heal and foot.

spasm a sudden involuntary contraction of the muscles.

spastic having a varying stiffness or tightness of a limb caused by spasms.

spasticity See *cerebral palsy, baclofen*.

spatial orientation to be orientated to where one is in relation to the environment. The ability to distinguish between and use both visual and non-visual input (e.g., proprioception, a mental map of where one is in relationship to room, etc.) to understand the layout of one's world.

Spearman-Brown formula a statistical procedure which helps determine the consistency with which a testing tool measures what it says it is measuring. The Spearman-Brown formula provides the researcher with better and more detailed information than basic *split-half reliability*.

special cause variation See *variation*.

special education See *Education for all Handicapped Children Act*.

special therapeutic diet a *diet* which is selected to meet the patient's specific needs due to allergies, caloric intake (high or low), diabetes, or for patients needing particular amounts of specific types of food (e.g., salt, fat, fiber, or protein).

speech-language pathologist an individual who has completed the required education, training, and experience to hold a Certificate of Clinical Competence from the American Speech-Language-Hearing Association. See *Joint Commission*.

speech recognition (HCO) automated conversion of spoken words into computer-based text. Some speech recognition systems recognize only one person's voice; others are speaker-independent but recognize a more limited vocabulary. They may recognize continuous speech or, more commonly, require that slight pauses be inserted between words.

speech therapist See *speech-language pathologist*.

speech therapy interventions to reduce communication and swallowing disorders. See *Joint Commission*.

Checklist for User-Friendly Software

Feature	Description	Issues of Accessibility
Easy-to-Read Screens	Key components of easy-to-read screens are uncluttered screens, simple text, and menu items in both graphics and text.	Option to make text larger on screen for individuals with visual impairments. Text in single columns with no asterisks, dashes, or other non-alphabetical characters used (not readable by voice-synthesis software).
Consistency	Predictable placement of menus and objects within the window. Predictable response of objects and menus throughout the program.	Consistently placed menu items are especially important for individuals who use programs which enlarge the screens, as the menu item may not always be on the screen in such situations. Consistency in the use of key commands helps adapt shortcuts.
Intuitive Characteristics	Clear and logical options for using the program increase the user's comfort level.	Some intuitive programs adjust their speed and other characteristics by learning the user's interactive patterns. This makes the program easier to use.
Logical Labels	The use of graphics and terms that are self-explanatory.	Logical labels are especially important for individuals using a screen reading program.
Instructional Choices	For educational software, a program which allows a variety of levels of difficulty and personalization.	Allows adjustment of the program to the client's functional level. Many allow adjustment to reaction time.
Graphics	If well presented and used logically, graphics expand the usability and understandability of the program.	Graphics support reading skills, especially for individuals with graphic input disorders. With scanning ability, can help personalize memory book.
Friendly Documentation	The documentation written to support the program should be clear and easy to read.	The written document should help the user understand how to modify the usage/speed/control of the functions of the program to allow for greater adaptation.
On-Screen Instructions	Steve Job of Apple Computers once said there are only two rules that apply to on-screen instructions: 1. assume that the user lost the written manual and 2. assume that s/he lost the manual before s/he read it.	Following logical sequencing and allowing the reader to advance the screens at his/her own pace is important. On-screen instructions should follow the guidelines under "easy-to-read screens" for use with screen readers.
Auditory Cues	Using either a voice synthesizer and/or a sound card, many programs can make sounds to alert the user to problems or as part of the entertainment.	Best when the auditory cues can be modified to meet the individual's specific needs. Tends to increase attention span of those using the program.
Visual Cues	Program that uses graphics and hidden text to cue the user for everything from spell check to prompts to help use the program.	Visual cue programs may not function as well with screen-enlargement programs, as the visual cue may be in another location on the screen.
Built-In Access Methods	The ability to use devices other than the keyboard or mouse to run program.	Allows the client to use the adaptive device with which s/he is familiar.
Built-In Utilities	Multiple programs packaged into one unit.	Reduces amount of system conflict and increases ease of navigation between features.
Alternatives to a Mouse	Allows more than one way to make menu choices.	Increases options for individuals with disabilities who have trouble using a mouse.
Optional Cursors	A program that allows changes to the shape and size of the cursor.	Allows option of a cursor that is easier to see with a visual impairment.
Creation of Custom Programs	A program that helps you use its elements to create your own customized software program.	Opens up many options for the therapist to customize programs to help the client improve function at his/her own pace.

spider-web profile a type of diagram used to display change. This type of diagram is very useful in displaying outcome changes due to intervention as it is very easy to read. The example below displays a patient's FIM score upon admission to a rehabilitation unit and upon discharge (from Niemeyer and burlingame, 1998, p. 242).

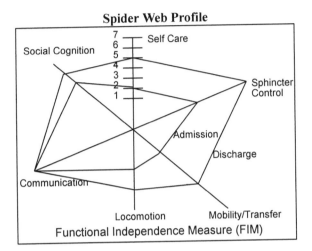

Spider Web Profile

Functional Independence Measure (FIM)

spina bifida a group of birth defects in which the posterior bony covering of the spinal cord fails to develop. In some cases the opening allows the contents of the spinal canal to protrude, forming hernial cysts. Spina bifida may occur in up to 25% of younger children and still be found 5% to 10% of adults. If there is no hernia, it is usually detected only by accident. The table below describes the most common types of spina bifida. See *myelomeningocele*.

spinal ataxia See *ataxic gait*.

spinal cord injury (SCI) injury to the nerves in the *spine*. After a spinal cord injury the loss of function is determined by the level of the spinal cord where the injury occurred, the severity of the injury, and the anatomical portion of the cord body involved. The "level" of the spinal cord injury is determined by the nerve(s) injured (not the vertebra involved). These nerves are classified according to the level of the cord at which they emerge (e.g., C-5 refers to an injury of the spinal cord at the fifth nerve of the cervical segment). The American Spinal Injury Association has developed a method for defining spinal cord injury that describes 28 locations on the body to test for sensation and ten locations to test for motor function. It is much easier to test the sensory function than the motor function because the sensory nerves go to specific locations in the body. Muscles, especially in the thorax, tend to be controlled by more than one nerve from the spinal cord. The muscles selected were chosen because most have only two levels of innervation. The "severity" of a spinal cord injury is usually measured by the American Spinal Injury Association Impairment Scale (AIS), which is a modification of the *Frankel Neurological Assessment for Spinal Injury*. This classification system has five levels of completeness (A through E) and describes the degree of motor and sensory function lost, as shown in the following table. The test for completeness is made in the sacral segments (S4-S5) because it provides a consistent measure of completeness during the healing process, which is not possible by measuring the completeness at higher levels on the spine. The "anatomical portion" of the spinal cord body injured also determines functional loss. The body of the spinal cord is divided into three columns (funiculi): the anterior

Levels of Spinal Cord Injury

A:	**Complete.** No motor or sensory function is preserved in the sacral segments S4-S5.
B:	**Incomplete.** Sensory but not motor function is preserved below the neurological level and includes the sacral segments S4-S5.
C:	**Incomplete.** Motor function is preserved below the neurological level, and more than half of key muscles below the neurological level have a muscle grade less than 3.
D:	**Incomplete.** Motor function is preserved below the neurological level, and at least half of key muscles below the neurological level have a muscle grade of 3 or more.
E:	**Normal.** Motor and sensory function is normal.

Common Types of Spina Bifida

Type	Contents of Hernial Cyst
spina bifida occulta	failure of the vertebral column to close with no herniation
spina bifida cystica	failure of the vertebral column to close with herniation, also referred to by the three names below, depending on the contents of the hernial cyst
meningocele	protrusion of the meninges through the vertebral column
myelocele	protrusion of the spinal cord through the vertebral column
myelomeningocele	protrusion of both the meninges and spinal cord through the vertebral column

(primary functions include motor function, posture reflexes, light touch, and pressure), the lateral (primary functions include subconscious *proprioception* for control of *locomotion*, temperature, and motor function), and the posterior (primary functions include proprioception, two-point discrimination, deep pressure, touch, and vibration). When the sensory testing for spinal cord injury is done, both pinprick and light touch are used to help determine which of the three columns are affected. Spinal cord injuries impact more than just motor and sensory function. Patients with spinal cord injuries also frequently experience neurogenic symptoms (*hypotension*, bradycardia, and impairment of reflexes), *bowel and bladder disorders* (urinary retention and paralysis of the bowel), and loss of perspiration below the level of a complete spinal injury. To help standardize reporting, funding, and research, many facilities use a *FIM* score sheet to summarize patients functional ability at admission and then again at discharge. The FIM score sheet for spinal cord injury is shown in the column to the right. See *autonomic dysreflexia.*

spine a flexible column made up of 31 pairs of spinal nerves protected by 33 vertebrae that are separated by intervertebral disks, located in the posterior aspect of the trunk. The column has five segments: cervical (seven vertebrae and eight pairs of nerves), thoracic (twelve vertebrae and twelve pairs of spinal nerves), lumbar (five vertebrae and five pairs of spinal nerves), sacral (five vertebrae and five pairs of spinal nerves), and coccygeal (four fused vertebrae and 1 pair of spinal nerves). The spine is a series of curves starting with the anteriorly convex cervical curve, followed by the concave thoracic curve, the convex lumbar curve and the concave pelvic curve. In adults, the spinal cord ends at the upper aspect of the second lumbar vertebra with a meningeal sheath continuing on to anchor the cord to the dorsal surface of the coccyx.

split-half reliability a method of determining the internal consistency of a testing tool. There are several methods used to determine a testing tool's split-half reliability. The most common is to create two tests out of the one testing tool. This is frequently done by placing all of the even numbered items in one of the subtests and the odd numbered items in the second subtest. This technique should work as long as this division creates two similar tests and the two tests are administered to the sample group of subjects. The closer the findings match between the two subtests, the greater the internal consistency of the testing tool. See *Spearman-Brown formula.*

Spinal Injury FIM

L	7	Complete Independence (Time, Safety)	**No**
	6	Modified Independence (Device)	**Helper**
E	**Modified Dependence**		
V	5	Supervision	
E	4	Minimal Assist (Subject = 75% +)	**Helper**
L	3	Moderate Assist (Subject = 50% +)	
S	**Complete Dependence**		
	2	Maximal Assist (Subject = 25% +)	
	1	Total Assist (Subject = 0% +)	

	Admit	Discharge
Self-Care		
A. Eating	☐	☐
B. Grooming		
C. Bathing		
D. Dressing - Upper Body		
E. Dressing - Lower Body		
F. Toileting		
Sphincter Control		
G. Bladder Management	☐	☐
H. Bowel Management		
Mobility		
Transfer:		
I. Bed, Chair, Wheelchair	☐	☐
J. Toilet		
K. Tub, Shower		
Locomotion		
L. Walk/Wheelchair	W☐ ☐	W☐ ☐
M. Stairs		
Communication		
N. Comprehension	A☐ ☐	A☐ ☐
O. Expression	V☐ ☐	V☐ ☐
Social Cognition		
P. Social Interaction	☐	☐
Q. Problem Solving		
R. Memory		
Total FIM	☐	☐

Note: Leave no blanks: enter 1 if patient not testable due to risk.

split-thickness graft a shallow graft that contains only part of the superficial layers of the dermis.

spontaneity involvement initiated by oneself; a feeling of making a choice without being unduly influenced by others. A voluntary action. Spontaneity is a major characteristic of leisure.

spontaneous movement movement that is initiated by the patient without any cueing. See *movement*.

sprain movements that result in severe stress, stretching, and/or tears of the soft tissues around a joint capsule, in a muscle or the associated connecting ligaments or tendons. Also the resulting injury. Sprains are classified into three levels called degrees. See *RICE, tissue injury, degrees of.*

staffing people who perform work at a facility. Facilities have many different categories of employees to draw from to fill their staffing needs. The table on the following page from D'Antonio-Nocera, DeBolt, and Touhey (1996) outlines some of the choices and pros and cons of each choice.

standard statements of minimal levels of acceptable performance or *outcomes* (quality) and the expected range of acceptable performance or outcomes (scope and quantity) set by groups which have the authority to set standards (e.g., professional groups, credentialing organizations). See *delegation, indicator, interpretive guidelines, Joint Commission, medical management, Peer Review Organization, quality of care, regulatory agency, utilization review.*

standard deviation a measure of how much a score deviates from the mean (or outside the spread of scores considered to still be within a normal, or "average," range). To determine the standard deviation of a test you would determine the normal spread of "average" scores, called a *variance*, then take the square root of the variance. The first standard deviation (from the mean score on the test) contains around 68% of the scores (with around 32% of the test takers falling either above or below the test takers in the first standard deviation). The second standard deviation contains around 95% of all the test takers (the 68% of the test takers whose scores fell closest to the mean score plus the next 27% of the test takers who scores fell immediately above or below the first standard deviation). The third standard deviation contains the next 4% of the individuals with scores either significantly above or below the mean. We use standard deviations to let us understand the results of a test which we are not familiar with or to compare the individual's scores on two different tests. Let's say that the psychologist informed the team that a child's IQ was 25 points below normal, or two standard deviations below normal. Next, the occupational therapist reported that

the child's functional performance on a kitchen skills test was 35 points below normal, or one standard deviation below normal. While the actual scores on the two tests had little meaning when compared, the comparison of the standard deviations was not only comparable, but also significant. Comparing standard deviations, the team could surmise that the youth had difficulty processing information cognitively but had learned specific ways of completing kitchen tasks to make up for some of his/her cognitive deficit. The child's performance was not as delayed as his/her intelligence.

standardized testing tools an assessment that was developed using at least the minimum professional standards associated with the development and testing of a measuring device. This usually involves baseline reliability and validity. Also, the exact wording and order of test questions must always remain the same on a standardized test. When the same questions, or similar questions, are used for the same test, each different form is called a "version." Copies of standardized testing tools that are shared between different facilities may lead to changes in the standardization of the testing tool which invalidates the results, as well as having a strong chance of violating copyright law and violating professional ethics.

standard survey in the United States under the OBRA legislation for long-term care facilities, a patient-centered, outcome-oriented inspection which relies on a case-mix stratified sample of patients to gather information about the facility's compliance with OBRA requirements. Based on the specific procedures, the Standard Survey assesses: 1. compliance with patients' rights; 2. the accuracy of patients' comprehensive assessments and the adequacy of care plans based on these assessments; 3. the quality of services furnished, as measured by indicators of medical, nursing, rehabilitative care, drug therapy, dietary and nutrition services, activities and social participation, sanitation, and infection control; and 4. the effectiveness of the physical environment to empower patients, accommodate patient needs, and maintain patient safety. If a surveyor, in conducting the information gathering tasks of the standard survey, identifies a possible noncompliant situation related to any requirement, investigation of the situation is done to determine whether the facility is in full compliance with the requirements. There are three other types of survey in addition to the standard survey. They are 1. *extended survey*, 2. *partial extended survey*, and 3. *initial certification survey*. See *survey process.*

Types of Staff

Category	Primary Characteristics	Pro's	Con's
Salaried — Exempt	Workers who are paid a pre-determined amount regardless of how many hours they work. The worker's hours are defined by tasks and responsibilities instead of a time clock.	• Workers tend to work as many hours as needed to get the job done — usually over 40 hours a week. • Most workers appreciate the ability to use their own judgment about how long to work.	• Workers may work too many hours increasing the chance of "burn out." • Some employees may feel that they work too many hours but do so because of peer pressure.
Hourly — Non-exempt	Workers who are paid a pre-determined amount for each hour they work. In most cases these workers get paid time and a half for any work exceeding 40 hours in one week. The worker's hours are defined by a time clock and not necessarily by tasks and responsibilities.	• Employees understand that they must get their assigned tasks done within their normal schedule and use good time management skills to achieve that expectation.	• Employers must set (and enforce) strict rules concerning the use of overtime or else the facility's budget will be thrown out of whack.
On-Call — Per Diem	Workers who do not have regularly scheduled hours but are called in to work to cover another staff's absence or when a facility is experiencing a shortage of staff. The worker's hours are defined by the absence of other employees or an unusually large number of residents.	• Ensure continuation of programming in staff's absence. • Can fill in as a "temporary" employee if the regular employee suddenly ends his/her employment with the facility.	• Employees may be oriented to the facility's policies and procedures but tend to have difficulty learning about all the residents at once — potentially having a negative impact on resident care.
Leased	Workers who are employees of another company are leased to a facility on a long-term basis. The worker's hours may be based on a salaried or hourly basis.	• Facility does not have to address human resources and payroll. • Employees may be able to receive a better benefits package.	• Potentially increases personnel costs for the facility. • Some loss of control over the employees.
Temporary Agency Staff	Workers who are employees of another company and are leased to a facility on a short-term basis. The worker's hours are almost always defined by a time clock and not necessarily by tasks and responsibilities.	• Can help fill in to ensure minimum compliance with number of staff required by law. • Can help provide minimum programming coverage when the facility experiences a temporary shortage of staff.	• Usually not familiar with facility's policies and procedures. • Hourly cost of using temporary staff may be double what a facility would pay for its own staff.
Minors	Workers under 18 years (age varies by state). Most states have stringent rules concerning the working conditions and hours of this classification of employees.	• In the long-term, helps mold the younger generation into the type of employees the facility will want to hire. • Provides work experience. • Inexpensive hourly staff to perform simple tasks.	• Worker usually lacks maturity level desired in the workplace. • "Work-ethic" not fully developed yet. • Extra paperwork required by most states.

staph See *Staphylococcus aureus*.

Staphylococcus aureus (CDC) Staphylococcus aureus, often referred to simply as staph; a bacteria commonly found on the skin of healthy people. Staph can be found on the skin, in the nose, and in blood and urine. Occasionally, staph can get into the body and cause an infection. This infection can be minor (such as pimples, boils, and other skin conditions) or serious (such as blood infections or pneumonia). Healthy people rarely get staph infections. Methicillin is an antibiotic commonly used to treat staph infections. Although methicillin is very effective in treating most staph infections, some staph bacteria have developed resistance to methicillin and can no longer be killed by this antibiotic. These resistant bacteria are called methicillin-resistant Staphylococcus aureus, or MRSA. An individual may carry MRSA either as a colonization or as an infection. Colonization means that MRSA is present on or in the body without causing illness. Infection means that MRSA is making the person sick. MRSA infection usually develops in hospital patients who are elderly or very sick, or who have an open wound (such as a bedsore) or a tube (such as a urinary catheter) going into their body. A precise number is not known, but according to some estimates as many as 80,000 patients a year get an MRSA infection after they enter the hospital. The number who become colonized is not known. Although MRSA is resistant to many antibiotics and often difficult to treat, a few antibiotics can still successfully cure MRSA infections. Patients who are only colonized with MRSA usually do not need treatment. MRSA can spread among other patients, who are often very sick with weak immune systems that may not be able to fight off infections. MRSA is almost always spread by physical contact and not through the air. Hospitals usually take special steps to prevent the spread of MRSA. One of these steps may be to isolate a patient with MRSA from other patients. Procedures vary from one hospital to another, but the following often occurs: 1. The patient is placed in a private room, or in a room with one or more patients who also have MRSA. 2. The patient's movement from the room is limited to essential purposes only, such as for medical procedures or emergencies. 3. Health care workers usually put on gloves (and sometimes hospital gowns) before entering the patient's room, remove their gloves (and gowns) before leaving the room, and then immediately wash their hands. 4. Visitors also may be asked to put on gloves (and sometimes gowns), especially if they are helping to take care of the patient and likely to come in contact with the patient's skin, blood, urine, wound, or other body substances. Visitors should always wash their hands before leaving the patient's room to make sure they don't take MRSA out of the room with them. The length of time an individual needs to remain in isolation varies. The hospital staff will determine when it is safe for a person with MRSA to come out of isolation. In hospitals, the most important reservoirs of MRSA are infected or colonized patients. Although hospital personnel can serve as reservoirs for MRSA and may harbor the organism for many months, they have been more commonly identified as a link for transmission between colonized or infected patients. The main mode of transmission of MRSA is via hands (especially health care workers' hands) which may become contaminated by contact with a) colonized or infected patients, b) colonized or infected body sites of the personnel themselves, or c) devices, items, or environmental surfaces contaminated with body fluids containing MRSA. Standard precautions, as described in the "Guideline for Isolation Precautions in Hospitals" (*Infection Control Hospital Epidemiology, 17*:53-80), should control the spread of MRSA in most instances. Standard precautions are included in the chart on the following page, "Standard Precautions Used with Methicillin-resistant Staphylococcus."

state an attribute that is changeable and is a direct result of the situation or environment. When the situation or environment changes, the attribute would also expect to be changed. A student who was not ready to give his report in front of class may become suddenly anxious (state) if the teacher were to call on him. See *trait*.

State Technical Institute Leisure Activities Project (STILAP) The STILAP is a leisure interest survey originally developed by Nancy Navar and Carol Ann Peterson in 1974 and updated by Navar in 1990. The patient is presented with a check list of 123+ activities and is asked to indicate one of four answers: "M" (much: for those activities that s/he participates in regularly during appropriate seasons), "S" (sometimes: for those activities that s/he has done but not on a regular basis), "I" (interested: for those activities that s/he would like to learn), and no answer (blank: for activities where none of the other 3 answers apply). The purpose of the assessment is to help the patient achieve a balanced leisure lifestyle by 1. assessing the patient's leisure skill and participation patterns, 2. categorizing the patterns (and thus, assumed skills) into leisure competency areas, and 3. providing a systematic way for the therapist to measure the degree to which the patient's leisure lifestyle is balanced. The assessment

Standard Precautions Used with Methicillin-Resistant Staphylococcus

Topic	Discussion
Room Selection	Placing a patient with MRSA in a private room. When a private room is not available, the patient may be placed in a room with a patient(s) who has active infection with MRSA, but with no other infection. Ensuring that patient-care items, bedside equipment, and frequently touched surfaces receive daily cleaning.
Handwashing	Wash hands after touching blood, body fluids, secretions, excretions, and contaminated items, whether or not gloves are worn. Wash hands immediately after gloves are removed, between patient contacts, and when otherwise indicated to avoid transfer of microorganisms to other patients or environments. It may be necessary to wash hands between tasks and procedures on the same patient to prevent cross-contamination of different body sites.
Gloving	Wear gloves (clean non-sterile gloves are adequate) when touching blood, body fluids, secretions, excretions, and contaminated items; put on clean gloves just before touching mucous membranes and non-intact skin. Remove gloves promptly after use, before touching non-contaminated items and environmental surfaces, and before going to another patient, and wash hands immediately to avoid transfer of microorganisms to other patients or environments.
Masking	Wear a mask and eye protection or a face shield to protect mucous membranes of the eyes, nose, and mouth during procedures and patient-care activities that are likely to generate splashes or sprays of blood, body fluids, secretions, and excretions.
Gowning	Wearing a gown when entering the room if you anticipate that your clothing will have substantial contact with the patient, environmental surfaces, or items in the patient's room, or if the patient is incontinent, or has diarrhea, an ileostomy, a colostomy, or wound drainage not contained by a dressing. Remove the gown before leaving the patient's room. After gown removal, ensure that clothing does not contact potentially contaminated environmental surfaces to avoid transfer of microorganisms to other patients and environments.
Appropriate Device Handling	Handle used patient-care equipment soiled with blood, body fluids, secretions, and excretions in a manner that prevents skin and mucous membrane exposures, contamination of clothing, and transfer of microorganisms to other patients and environments. When possible, dedicating the use of noncritical patient-care equipment and items such as stethoscope, sphygmomanometer, bedside commode, or electronic rectal thermometer to a single patient (or cohort of patients infected or colonized with MRSA) to avoid sharing between patients. Ensure that reusable equipment is not used for the care of another patient until it has been appropriately cleaned and reprocessed and that single-use items are properly discarded. Periodically clean the person's room and personal items with a commercial disinfectant or a fresh solution of one part bleach and 100 parts water (for example, one tablespoon of bleach in one quart of water).
Patient Transportation	Limiting the movement and transport of the patient from the room to essential purposes only. If the patient is transported out of the room, ensure that precautions are maintained to minimize the risk of transmission of microorganisms to other patients and contamination of environmental surfaces or equipment.
Appropriate Handling of Laundry	Handle, transport, and process used linen soiled with blood, body fluids, secretions, and excretions in a manner that prevents skin and mucous membrane exposures, contamination of clothing, and transfer of microorganisms to other patients and environments. If MRSA is judged by the hospital's infection control program to be of special clinical or epidemiologic significance, then Contact Precautions should be considered.

takes about 30 minutes for the patient to fill out and an additional 15 minutes for the therapist to score.

static air bed   commercially known as *TENDER Cloud, Soft-Care, Pulsair*, and *Lotus*, these beds have compartments for air or water which either allow the gradual movement between cells or mechanically force the movement between cells (like a wave action), to reduce pressure on the skin.

Implications for treatment include a potentially decreased ability to transfer self out of bed and an increased risk for sweating due to plastic covers on the mattresses. Equipment or activities that have sharp points are contraindicated for fear of puncturing an air sac. Also known as alternating air bed or water mattress bed. See *bed*.

static balance   the ability to remain upright while

sitting or standing with little or no challenge to *balance*. See *crutch, dynamic balance*.

statistical control (HCO) control of confounding variables in retrospective *research*, either by classifying patients into groups that are homogeneous with respect to those variables, or by adjusting for the variation in the outcome variable that is accounted for by those confounding variables.

stereotyped behavior a behavior that the individual persistently engages in without having the internal flexibility to change the behavior as the situation changes. These behaviors may be simple postural, gestural, or verbal movements that have little or no apparent meaning or may be repetitive behaviors that recur at inappropriate times. In fact, the stereotypic motor movements seem almost driven, interfering with normal activities of daily living and may lead to injuries if preventative measures are not taken. Stereotypic behaviors include compulsive handwashing, compulsive straightening of objects on the table, or *echolalia*. Stereotypic movements include rocking, picking, self-biting, head banging, and waving. Dopamine appears to be associated with stereotypic movement. See *pervasive developmental disorders, tic disorder.*

story (ADA) that portion of a building included between the upper surface of a floor and the upper surface of the floor or roof next above. If such portion of a building does not include occupiable space, it is not considered a story for purposes of ADA guidelines. There may be more than one floor level within a story as in the case of a mezzanine or mezzanines.

strain When a patient participates in activities which involve a *range of motion* in excess of the patient's normal range or involve repetitious movements in excess of the patient's accustomed level of activity, slight trauma occurs. This trauma usually occurs in the musculotendinous unit. Good assessment of the patient's current level of activity combined with moderation and warm-up activities should decrease the chance of injury. See *fatigue, RICE.*

strength the measurable amount of force produced by a single muscle or a set of muscles. See *muscle strength.*

streptococcal toxic shock syndrome (STSS) (CDC) Streptococcal toxic shock syndrome causes blood pressure to drop rapidly and organs (e.g., kidney, liver, lungs) to fail. STSS is not the same as the "toxic shock syndrome" frequently associated with tampon usage. Early signs and symptoms of STSS include: fever, dizziness, confusion, and a flat red rash over large areas of the body.

stress the nonspecific response of a person to demands in the environment. The degree to which the individual is unable to cope with stress is equal to the amount of wear and tear on the individual's body. As the body engages defenses against demands in the environment, it produces measurable structural and chemical changes. These changes can be measured accurately, although some of the measures gauge the amount of damage as a result of the demands, while other measures gauge the individual's ability to adapt to the demands. Selye (1978) reported that the combined damage and adaptation was called the "stress syndrome" or the "general adaptation syndrome" (GAS). The general adaptation syndrome has three stages: 1. the alarm reactions; 2. the stage of resistance, and 3. the stage of exhaustion. One common treatment intervention for therapists is teaching mechanisms for coping with stress. Some of the signs of stress are listed in the table on the next page. See *brief combination techniques, coping techniques, emotion, euphoria, flexibility, goal setting and time management, hypochondriasis, imagery, job stress management, medical play, refuting irrational ideas, ritualistic behaviors, tic disorders.*

stress inoculation See *coping skills training.*

stressors circumstances that exist or events that occur in the environment which are a psychological and/or physiological threat to the well-being of an individual or individuals.

stretching a prescribed activity designed to lengthen soft tissue that has been pathologically shortened.

- **passive stretching** the action of someone else (besides the patient) gently applying force to stretch tight tissue. Passive stretching is usually done by the PT, OT, or certified nursing assistant using prescribed range of motion exercises.

- **active stretching** patient initiated movement designed to increase *range of motion* in affected soft tissue and joints. This is usually carried out in physical therapy using a prescribed *exercise* program or in therapy/activity programs using a prescribed set of activities designed to achieve the desired outcome.

The professional should encourage activities that involve the slow static stretching of muscles lasting between 10 to 30 seconds. Activities that involve bouncing stretches or ballistic stretches increase the patient's chance of injury, especially after a period of immobility (Karam, 1989, p. 1). See *elasticity.*

stretching, selective Decreased *range of motion* for selected muscle groups can greatly increase the level of independence for patients with thoracic and cervical spinal injuries. After a full examination the physician or the physical therapist will determine the amount of tightness for the extensor muscles of the lower back that will enhance the patient's balance. A slight tightness will allow greater balance while leaning forward in a wheelchair for patients with no active control of the back extensors. The professional should note the degree of tightness desired and ensure that the patient's activities do not jeopardize that stability.

strict isolation   an isolation procedure used with patients with diphtheria, Lassa fever and other viral hemorrhagic fevers, plague, smallpox, varicella (chicken pox), and zoster. The procedure for strict isolation is 1. masks are indicated for all persons entering room, 2. gowns are indicated for all persons entering room, 3. gloves are indicated for all persons entering the room, 4. hands must be washed after touching the patient or potentially contaminated articles and before taking care of another patient, 5. articles contaminated with infective material should be discarded or bagged and labeled before being sent for decontamination and reprocessing. The sign for strict isolation is always yellow.

stroke   See *cerebral vascular accident.*

structural frame   (ADA) The structural frame shall be considered to be the columns and the girders, beams, trusses, and spandrels having direct connections to the columns and all other members that are essential to the stability of the building as a whole.

structured data entry   (HCO) a *data* collection technique that constrains the language and format of clinical descriptions for the purpose of ensuring uniform, unambiguous, interchangeable messages.

stump revision   the revision of a stump or the scar tissue, to increase function or improve cosmetic appearance.

stupor   being close to unconsciousness. The patient exhibits minimal response to stimuli, including pain. Stupor may be caused by neurological or psychological disorders.

subacute   a level of medical and rehabilitative care that is less intense than what is expected as a patient in an acute hospital but more intense than what is expected as a resident in a nursing home. Patients on subacute care units are medically frail, often requiring one to three hours of therapy services a day before they are able to be discharged. Generally, patients transferred to subacute care units no longer require high-technology monitoring or complex medical procedures. Instead, their medical needs are better met with the coordinated efforts of an interdisciplinary team of nurses, therapists, and physicians. There is a trend to alternately use the term "subacute" to refer to a two-level inpatient rehabilitation designation. The first level is for patients who require both extensive medical and rehabilita-

The Signs of Stress (Selye, 1976)

1. General irritability, hyper-excitation, or depression
2. Pounding of the heart
3. Dryness of the throat and mouth
4. Impulsive behavior, emotional instability
5. The overpowering urge to cry or run and hide
6. Inability to concentrate
7. Feelings of unreality, weakness, or dizziness
8. Predilection to become fatigued
9. Floating *anxiety* (fear without knowing exactly what is causing the fear)
10. Emotional tension and alertness ("keyed-up")
11. Trembling, nervous tics
12. Tendency to be easily startled
13. High-pitched, nervous laughter
14. Stuttering and other speech difficulties
15. *Bruxism*
16. Insomnia
17. Hyper motility (hyperkinesia)
18. Sweating
19. The frequent need to urinate
20. Diarrhea, indigestion, queasiness in the stomach, and sometimes even vomiting
21. Migraine headaches
22. Premenstrual tension or missed menstrual cycles
23. Pain in the neck or lower back
24. Loss of or excessive appetite
25. Increased smoking
26. Increased use of legally prescribed drugs
27. Alcohol and drug addiction
28. Nightmares
29. Neurotic behavior
30. Psychoses
31. Accident proneness

tive services while the second level is for patients who require more rehabilitative services and minimal medical services. See *rehabilitation centers.*

subacute stage   the second of three stages of the healing and maturation of an illness or injury. The subacute stage usually begins about the 4th day after an injury is marked by noted repair of the injured area. The subacute stage usually is over by the 21st day after the onset of an injury, but may last as long as six weeks (Kisner & Colby, 1990). During this time, the remaining blood clots are absorbed and replaced by fibroblastic activity (which produces *collagen*). Immature connective tissue and granulation tissue form (to speed up the delivery of oxygen to the injured site). These tissues are very susceptible to damage by overstretching, overuse, or by being pulled/sheered in the wrong direction. Pain may be experienced by the patient as the immature tissue is stretched just past its normal limit. Some gentle stretching (in consultation with the physical therapist) is recommended to reduce the adherence to surrounding tissues during the healing process. See *acute stage, chronic stage.*

subclavian artery a branch of the innominate artery on the right and a branch of the aortic arch on the left that supplies blood to the neck, upper limbs, thoracic wall, spinal cord, brain, and meninges.

sub-clinical infection an infection which doesn't present in observable symptoms but which can be measured through lab tests. See *infection.*

subcutaneous tissue the fatty and fibrous tissues which are situated just under the skin.

substance abuse the maladaptive use of drugs in such a way as to impact other parts of the individual's life. The **DSM-IV** lists four behavioral and observable indications that someone is abusing a substance. The first is that the use of the substance is causing problems in a major area of the individual's life, whether it be work, family, friends, or free time activities. The abuser is not able to fulfill basic responsibilities, e.g., taking care of kids, finishing homework, getting to work. The second is a pattern of using which endangers the user's life and possibly the well-being of others, e.g., driving under the influence, getting stoned while taking care of young children. The third is problems with the law over the use or possession of drugs of abuse. The fourth is the continuance of using the substance even though the individual is aware that the use is impacting his/her life, e.g., losing his/her job due to a failed drug test, being aware that s/he beats his/her spouse only when under the influence. See *bipolar disorder, comorbidity, drug abuse, dual diagnosis, mania, substance dependence, substance-related disorder.*

substance dependence a continued used of a drug of abuse even though there are obvious negative consequences to the continued use. The **DSM-IV** sites a group of behavioral, cognitive, and physiological symptoms as well as a pattern of repeated self-administration of the drug of abuse. Substance dependence leads to *tolerance, withdrawal,* and *compulsive drug-taking behavior.* Individuals who have a substance dependence usually have a craving for the drug of abuse. To identify that an individual has a substance dependence, the individual must exhibit at least three behavioral, cognitive, or physiological symptoms listed under tolerance, withdrawal, and/or compulsive drug-taking behavior. Additionally, individuals who have a substance dependence disorder tend to spend more time (or take more) of the substance than they originally intended to, tend to have tried (unsuccessfully) to stop usage, and have most,

if not all, of their time taken up with substance use patterns or "socializing" with others who also use. Individuals with substance dependence have pathologically reduced meaningful leisure time skills, activities, and experiences. Of all groups who need and receive leisure counseling, this population is one of the most impaired in the healthy use of free time. Knowledge of resources, peers to recreate with, and even which activities to engage in are frequently severely diminished. The *Leisure Step Up Model* and associated program developed by Dehn (1995) helps the therapist and patient address this severe deficit. See *substance abuse, substance-related disorder.*

substance-related disorder a large category of disorders all related to the use and abuse of a drug that is recognized as a drug of abuse (including alcohol). The **DSM-IV** divides substance-related disorders into two groups and eleven classes. The two groups are substance use disorders (substance dependence and substance abuse) and substance-induced disorders (substance intoxication, substance withdrawal, substance-induced delirium, substance-induced persisting dementia, substance-induced persisting amnestic disorder, substance-induced psychotic disorder, substance-induced mood disorder, substance-induced anxiety disorder, substance-induced sexual dysfunction and substance-induced sleep disorder). The eleven classes of substances which are involved in substance-related disorders are alcohol; amphetamine or similarly acting sympathomimetics; caffeine; cannabis; cocaine; hallucinogens; inhalants; nicotine; opioids; phencyclidine (PCP) or similarly acting arylcyclohexylamines; and sedatives, hypnotics or anxiolytics. There are two additional categories listed in addition to the eleven substance-specific categories. The two additional categories are *polysubstance dependence* and *other or unknown substance-related disorders.* An additional type of drug listed under substance-related disorders is actually not a drug of abuse but toxins. The **DSM-IV** places the following toxins in this category: "heavy metals (e.g., lead or aluminum), rat poisons containing strychnine, pesticides containing acetylcholinesterase inhibitors, nerve gases, ethylene glycol (antifreeze), carbon monoxide, and carbon dioxide (p. 175)." Inhalants that are used for the purpose of becoming intoxicated are also included in the category of toxins. This group of toxins includes fuel and paint. See *comorbidity, substance abuse, substance dependence.*

sucralose (HHS) the only low-calorie sweetener that is made from sugar. It is approximately 600 times sweeter and does not contain calories. Sucralose is highly stable under a wide variety of processing conditions. Thus, it can be used virtually anywhere sugar can, including cooking and baking, without losing any of its sugar-like sweetness. Currently, sucralose is approved in over 25 countries around the world for use in food and beverages. In the US, the FDA has been petitioned to approve the use of sucralose in 15 different food and beverage categories.

sucrose table sugar; a diglyceride composed of glucose and fructose. See *carbohydrates*.

sudden infant death syndrome (SIDS) the sudden and unexpected death of an infant during sleep. SIDS strikes children between the ages of two months and twelve months who otherwise seem normal and healthy. SIDS is the most common cause of death in children under one year of age in the US.

sugar soluble carbohydrates responsible for the sweetness of food. The two principal categories of sugar are monosaccharides (a single sugar such as glucose or fructose) and disaccharides (a double sugar such as sucrose or lactose).

suicide the taking of one's own life; purposely causing one's own death. See *dual diagnosis, bipolar disorder, depression, delirium tremens, Global Assessment of Functioning Scale.*

sundown syndrome a combination of symptoms that tend to become more pronounced in the evenings. The primary symptoms of sundown syndrome are *agitation, disorientation,* and emotional stress. The physiological trigger to the increased symptoms is unknown but the three leading hypothesis are decreased sensory input from the light, progressive *fatigue,* and dehydration. Given that these symptoms occur in adults with *dementia* who have difficulty taking care of themselves, all three causes may be mutually contributing to the problem. The eyes' ability to take in light decreases as one ages, so a decrease in light, as during the sunset, would be compounded by the physiological *visual impairment.* Being unable to initiate how much liquid or rest one needs could lead to a chronic state of *dehydration* or fatigue. Therapists should strive to avoid using the slang term "sundowner," as it is a pejorative term.

sunsetting a component of many health care licensing laws which require that the licensing legislation be renewed by the state legislature every five or so years or else the law authorizing the licensing expires (sunsets).

superego *Freud* described three elements of a person's psyche that constantly battle to influence the individual's behavior. Superego is the term given to those "messages" ingrained in the person's conscious about what is "right" and what is "wrong" as taught by his/her parents, teachers, and society as a whole. The other two elements are *id* and *ego.*

supervisor an individual whose job includes overseeing the work of other employees. The eight practices of a good supervisor are listed below (Caruso, 1982).

1. Good supervisors think of themselves as supervisors.
2. Good supervisors strive to establish positive relationships between themselves and supervisees within a collaborative framework.
3. Good supervisors foster open communication among all parties in an interactive supervisory process.
4. Good supervisors recognize the personal and professional developmental levels of their supervisees and plan accordingly.
5. Good supervisors recognize that self-supervision is an ultimate goal for the supervisee.
6. Good supervisors think of supervision as an activity that is planned and systematic and one that takes a variety of forms.
7. Good supervisors design a process of evaluation that has as its primary focus the improvement of the quality of the experience and care that patients in health care settings receive.
8. Good supervisors recognize the importance of supervisory self-assessment and reflection.

Supplemental Security Income (SSI) See *entitlement programs.*

support surface a type of surface prescribed for patients with skin integrity problems. The primary purpose of a prescribed support surface is to prevent skin breakdown. This is done by selecting a surface that can relieve pressure and shear forces that produce pressure ulcers. Jay (1997) discusses three types of issues to be considered when patients use support system beds and surfaces: patient care; psychosocial; and safety, reliability, and service issues. Patient care: The first table on the next page describes patient care issues beyond the primary role of reducing pressure, shear, and maceration. Psychosocial: Unless the patient is comfortable and the clinician satisfied, the support surface is not doing its job completely. Fortunately, most support surfaces are inherently comfortable, as they conform well to the human body and help reduce the excessive pressure points that are a primary cause of discomfort. However, there are other areas of comfort that can be improved. The second table looks at these psychosocial issues. Safety, reliability, and service: Obviously, products have to be reliable in use. The simplest way to approach this is to ask the supplier or manufacture what might go wrong. The third table describes some of the questions a therapist needs to ask. See *bed.*

Patient Care Issues in a Support Surface (Jay, 1997)

Issue	Description
Transfers	Can the patient independently transfer on and off the surface? How easy are caregiver-assisted transfers? This is especially important in the home.
Movement from room to room	When necessary, can the bed be easily moved from room to room (e.g., radiology, surgical suite, physical therapy)? Can a patient be placed directly from the operating table onto this surface after a flap procedure and moved to his or her room, eliminating the need for a stretcher?
Reduction of shear from spasticity	Patients with high tone or spasticity can develop ulcers, particularly at the heels. How effectively does the surface reduce this repetitive shear?
Physical therapy, traction, continuous passive motion	Is the surface stable enough to allow for these treatments? Can a family member or clinician sit on the edge of the bed to be closer to the patient?
Cardiopulmonary resuscitation (CPR)	Is there a foolproof mechanism that permits CPR, or is the surface automatically compatible with a crash board?
Positioning deformities and contractures	Patients with deformities and/or contractures can be difficult to position properly. How easily does the surface conform to the deformity? Can the patient be held in the position desired by the clinician?
Patient sliding	Has the surface been designed to help prevent the patient from sliding to the foot of the bed (with potential shearing of the heels)? Does the patient tend to slide into the bed rails (with increased risk of extubation or trauma to the extremities)?
30-degree side-lying position	Because the patient lies on neither the sacrum nor the trochanter (two primary sites at risk for pressure ulcer development), the 30-degree side-lying position is considered safe. Can a patient be positioned effectively without sliding back on the sacrum or forward on the trochanter?
Patient turning	How easy is it for the patient to turn or for the clinician to do the turning?
Heavy patients	Can the surface handle a patient weighing more than 400 pounds? Can it handle a 200-pound patient without bottoming out when the head of the bed is raised or the patient is lying on his or her trochanter?

Psychosocial Issues in a Support Surface (Jay, 1997)

Issue	Description
Perspiration or clamminess	A breathable, urine-proof cover that permits vapor transmission will help to prevent discomfort from perspiration and clamminess. A true low-air-loss system also can help by delivering airflow to the patient's skin.
Excessive heat or dryness	Air-fluidized beds have been criticized for generating too much heat, despite excellent wound healing properties. However, any motorized system will add heat to a room, particularly if two such beds are in the same room or if a room is not air-conditioned (as may be the case in the home).
Noise	The noise level of a product should be evaluated. Motors can be annoying to the person on the bed for long periods. Clinicians should be aware that the patient hears this noise much more loudly than s/he does because his or her head is immersed in the system.
Patient disorientation	As far back as 1968, patients reported experiencing hallucinations while on powered air systems. This disorientation seems to be more of a problem on powered air systems that produce noise and/or a floating feeling.
Appearance	Although not an issue of comfort, the appearance of a patient in bed is important to both the patient and family members. The bed should resemble a standard home or hospital bed as much as possible to decrease the look of morbidity or acuity that could intimidate family members at a time when the patient needs more contact.

Psychosocial Issues in a Support Surface (Jay, 1997) (continued)

Issue	Description
How much training is involved?	Although clinician satisfaction is related primarily to resultant wound healing on a specialized surface, ease of use is an important secondary parameter. Clinicians are busy people. The simpler the solution, the easier it is to use properly. Are special adjustments required? What happens when an alarm goes off? Will the support surface interact with standard hospital equipment (beds, linens. incontinence pads)? Does it utilize the standard hospital bed, or is retraining required for a new bed frame?
How complicated is it to use?	Ease of use is especially important in the home, where caregivers have less preparation and are more likely to be under heavy psychological pressure when treating a loved one. How user-friendly is the support surface? How much clinician time is it going to require? Do computer modules, technological displays, or electronic equipment enhance or detract from the clinician's ability to care for the patient? Is the product intuitive or is it complex?

Safety, Reliability and Service in a Support Surface (Jay, 1997)

Issue	Description
What happens during a power failure?	Will the product deflate? Is the patient put at risk? How long will the backup battery work? This is especially important in the home, where lightening strikes or floods can cause lengthy power outages.
What happens if the support surface is punctured?	Hypodermic needles and other sharp objects are sometimes pushed into the surface. Will it deflate? Is it self-sealing?
Will the added support surface compromise bed-rail height?	Patients pulling themselves over bedrails and onto the floor can be a problem when an overlay sits on top of a standard mattress. This is particularly true with the taller powered air overlays. In this case, the bed's mattress should be removed and replaced with a lower profile supplemental mattress provided by the support surface supplier.
Quality of the supplier	No product is completely foolproof. What are guaranteed delivery, pickup, and service turnaround times? (Two hours is a common standard in metropolitan areas.) Is service available 24 hours per day, 7 days per week? What are the supplier's accreditations?
Warranty and service contracts	These should be explored when a support surface is purchased for long-term home use for a specific patient or for the institution itself. How long is the warranty? Is it for full replacement or do costs of replacement increase over time? Are there costly service fees?
Weight of the bed	Can the floor or elevator of the institute or home support the bed weight? This is a particular problem with air-fluidized beds, which generally weight more than 1,600 pounds.
Infection control	Does the bed pass institutional infection control standards? Can it be cleaned easily between regular supplier maintenance intervals? Can blowers spread infection to other rooms?
Regulatory approvals	Does the support surface meet all local and national fire safety codes? Is it UL approved? Is it approved by the Food and Drug Administration?
Biomedical engineering approvals	The Joint Commission on the Accreditation of Healthcare Organizations requires biomechanical engineering to check every piece of equipment before use in acute care facilities. How much time does this take?
Continuity of care	Can the same or similar equipment follow the patient from hospital to subacute care to long-term care to home care? This is increasingly important in today's managed care environment, in which patient transfers are becoming the rule, not the exception. Some suppliers do not provide the same model of the product during these changes, causing inconvenience or dissatisfaction on the part of the patient and clinician. Some of the newest technologies are not funded in all patient care environments. Individualized patient care plans should be implemented.

surveillance the ongoing monitoring of events in a manner that can achieve results (the reporting of information) in a uniform manner relatively quickly. The emphasis on surveillance is the ability to gather information in a practical manner, allowing for some error, versus a more time consuming and fully accurate manner. Surveillance is a technique used to detect changes in trends or distributions that may require further (more accurate) evaluation of what may be causing *variances*. Changes in policies, procedures, and protocols may be indicated through findings during surveillance and further investigation. Active surveillance is the systematic review of each event or case following a pre-set time limit for completion of the review. An example would be a standard review of all charts to ensure that a discharge summary was written or that every patient has a signed (or refused) photo release form. Passive surveillance is more random in nature. Examples would be a review of only the records for patients who had complaints called in to HCFA, a review of missing laundry for only those residents in a nursing home who complained about missing items, or a review of care for every patient mentioned on an incident report.

survey process evaluation by an outside agency to measure the quality of services being provided. This evaluation, called a "survey," is usually done by the government and/or a private credentialing agency (e.g., Joint Commission or CARF). A survey team is sent to the facility for a short period of time (usually 2 days to 2 weeks) to evaluate service delivery by sampling approximately 10% of the patient records. The surveyors will frequently evaluate patient records back 6 - 12 months or more to be able to identify trends in patient care. Surveyors obtain information from many sources as they evaluate the organization's compliance with standards. One of the methods they use is to interview staff. Being asked questions by a surveyor can be very stressful for staff. Staff will find that they can reduce their stress level if they follow a standard format for answering a surveyor's question and practice until they feel comfortable with the process. The two basic steps in answering a surveyor's question are shown in the table below. Just before the survey team leaves the facility, they will have an informational "exit" meeting with the administration to give a gen-

How to Answer a Surveyor's Question

Step	Discussion	Example
1. Restate the intent.	Make sure that you understood what the surveyor asked. Restate the questions that you heard the surveyor ask you.	"How does our department ensure that we are providing a good environment of care?"
2. Identify the structures that support the intent of the question.	The structures which support an intent of a questions (e.g., environment of care) would include any policies and procedures the department follows, any committee (and committee minutes) which the staff attend or support, any forms used to help meet the intent, specific orientation and on-going education provided for staff, aspects of the department's quality assurance program which address the intent of the question, and any questionnaires used to identify patient degree of satisfaction.	"Our department enhances the environment of care for our patients through compliance with our policies and procedures. Some examples include our policies concerning staff preparedness for a disaster situation, marking and handling of hazardous materials and waste, life safety, security management, and other aspects of environment of care." "Two of our staff are members of the Therapeutic Environment Committee and I sit on the Medical Equipment Utilization Committee as well as the Patient Care Quality Assurance Committee." "We have a manual of forms which we use in our department, including employee orientation and continuing education forms and material safety data sheets. They are located right next to our policy and procedure manual. All staff are required to review this manual at least annually." "Our last two patient satisfaction surveys included questions about the environment of care. The results have been summarized and changes implemented. That information is in the Quality Assurance Manual in the main staff office."

eral overview of their findings. The survey team will then meet after they leave the facility to write up the formal survey document. The time period just before and during a survey tends to produce extreme stress among staff. This is a normal response, however, not a very productive one. The surveyors will be evaluating the services delivered over a long period of time as well as the current treatment environment in the facility; they will be able to tell if the facility has brought in extra staff just for the time of the survey. One element of a survey that tends to produce excessive stress is the fact that most surveys just list areas that need to be improved. (Surveys done by state and federal agencies are not allowed to put positive comments in the survey document — only citations of substandard care.) There are usually over 300 areas evaluated during a survey. See *extended survey, initial certification survey, partial extended survey, standard survey, entrance conference, exit conference, federal monitoring survey, Health Care Financing Administration, judicial review, Medicare/Medicaid history, plan of correction, regulatory agency.*

swing bed hospital a hospital located in a rural area with fewer than 50 beds approved to provide long-term care services.

swing-through gait This gait involves the movement of the crutches toward the direction that the patient is moving. The crutches are placed and then the patient swings his/her lower body to the point where the crutches are anchored and continues through beyond that point. The swing-through gait is most often used by patients who have difficulty with alternate leg movements either due to balance difficulties or due to paralysis. See *paraplegia.*

swing-to gait gait where the patient places both crutches in front of him/her and swings the legs to the position directly between the two crutches.

Syme's amputation an amputation through the ankle joint. Functional ability is improved with a three unit prosthetic device.
1. a patellar tendon bearing orthosis
2. a distal weight bearing socket
3. a partial foot replacement
The therapist may want to evaluate the condition of the skin under the orthosis after a strenuous activity to ensure that the integrity of the skin is not compromised. Red marks should fade 100% in 30 minutes and skin abrasions should be absent. (Red skin after 30 minutes is a first-degree *pressure sore*, abrasion is a second-degree *pressure sore.*)

symmetric encryption (HCO) encryption of a message with a key derived from a password that must be known by both the sending and receiving parties.

sympathetic nervous system part of the autonomic nervous system; activates the heart to increase the heart rate, causes blood vessels to constrict and raises *blood pressure*. See *autonomic nervous system.*

synapse the region between one nerve cell and another nerve, muscle, or gland. The transmitted signal from the first nerve is passed to the second cell by the chemical action of a *neurotransmitter.*

syncope a feeling of being light headed followed by a short loss of consciousness; also known as "fainting." Syncope can be alleviated or avoided by placing one's head between the knees at the first sign of light-headedness.

syndrome a group of symptoms, behaviors, or disabilities that are interrelated and cause somewhat predictable problems for the person with the syndrome.

syngeneic bone marrow transplant (HHS/NMDP) transplant of bone marrow cells from an identical twin in which immunosuppression drugs are not required.

synkinetic movement small, involuntary movements that naturally accompany larger, voluntary movements. An example might be when a patient pushes hard, his/her facial expression contorts. See *movement.*

syphilis (HHS) an acute and chronic disease caused by the bacteria Treponema pallidum, transmitted by direct contact, usually through sexual intercourse.

systematic desensitization a technique combining relaxation and imagery to decrease sensitivity to fear-provoking stimuli. Instead of exposing the person to the real fear-provoking stimulus, the person imagines the stressor and uses relaxation exercises to decrease sensitivity.

systematic review (HCO) extraction of specific items of information from numerous *research* works on a given topic and comparison of those items across those works using structured methods.

systematized nomenclature of medicine (SNOMED) (HCO) a system for classifying and coding health problems, symptoms, and services.

systemic cause variation See *variation.*

systemic lupus erythematosus an inflammatory disease of connective tissue occurring predominantly in women (90%). It is usually considered to be an autoimmune disease although some people suggest the involvement of a mycobacterium.

T

tablet computer (HCO) a computer with an integrated display and digitizer, rather than a keyboard. Also known as a clipboard or pentop computer.

tachycardia a heartbeat over 100 beats per minute. Pathological tachycardia is the body's attempt to delivery more oxygen to its cells by pumping more oxygenated blood. See *pulse*.

tactile referring to the sense of touch.

tactile defensiveness the reaction from a patient who is hyper-sensitive to touch — the withdrawing of a body part when it is touched because the touch is irritating and uncomfortable due to excessive neurological reaction. See *hypersensation*.

tag the number assigned to each measurable element of a regulation (law). See *CFR, initial certification survey*.

tanking the total immersion of a patient's body into a whirlpool or Hubbard Tank to facilitate debridement.

tardive dyskinesia a movement disorder brought about by long-term use of antipsychotic medications. Prolonged use of antipsychotic medications triggers a heightened sensitivity in the dopamine receptors. This heightened sensitivity causes the individual to demonstrate abnormal movement patterns. Not only are these abnormal movement patterns a disability in themselves, they also tend to make other people uncomfortable around the individual. Possible early indications of tardive dyskinesia include: 1. involuntary repetitious facial movements, 2. lip smacking, 3. tics or spasms, 4. chewing motions with mouth, 5. ocular movements (eyes rolled up and fixed in position), 6. difficulty swallowing (many of these medications suppress the cough reflex), and 7. rocking or swaying. It is important for all staff working with individuals taking antipsychotic medications to continually watch for the onset of these side effects. Discontinuing the use of the medications may stop the process of tardive dyskinesia. However, in many cases the individual will continue to exhibit the symptoms at the same level indefinitely. The earlier the syndrome is identified, the better the chances are that the symptoms will subside. In some cases muscle relaxants are prescribed, usually only for short-term use during the early stages of the syndrome. It is not unusual for all of the symptoms to subside during sleep. Women, the elderly, and individuals who have had a long history of taking antipsychotic medications are the three groups most likely to demonstrate the symptoms. However, each individual seems to have his/her own threshold level, so the symptoms may occur in men and women at any age regardless of the dosage taken or the length of time administered. Compare to *Parkinsonian movements*. See *restraints — inappropriate*.

target heart rate the desired heart rate to be achieved during cardiovascular activity. The target heart rate is always determined before the patient is involved in a prescribed program that increases a patient's cardiovascular endurance. The professional may want to consult the patient's physician when determining the target heart rate. Some medications may modify the patient's responsive heart rate, making the use of standardized target heart rate scales undesirable.

task analysis See *activity analysis*.

Tay-Sachs disease (amaurotic familial idiocy) a rare birth defect that strikes those of Ashkenazic Jewish ancestry about 100 times more often than the rest of the population in the United States. The primary disabling trait of this disease is the lack of enzyme hexosaminidase A, causing a progressive demyelination (breakdown of the protective covering) of the central nervous system cells. By the age of one and a half years most children with Tay-Sachs disease are blind, by age 2 years the child is susceptible to numerous infections, including bronchopneumonia. Death usually occurs before age 5.

T cell See *T lymphocyte*.

teaching providing information in a way that it can be learned. Often the therapist must teach a patient new ideas and/or skills to further the therapeutic process. Timby and Lewis (1992) list the following techniques for effective teaching. The patient is likely to learn best when s/he has an interest in the subject. Spark the patient's interest, provide just enough information each time to let it "sink in," and remember that the judicious use of repetition helps increase the likelihood that the information will be remembered. See *andragogy, learning disability, pedagogy*.

Techniques for Effective Teaching
(Timby and Lewis, 1992, p. 29)
- Collaborate with the patient on content, goals,

and a realistic time for accomplishing the task.

- Develop a written plan that builds from a. familiar to unfamiliar, b. simple to complex, and c. normal to abnormal.
- Select teaching methods and resources that are compatible with the patient's preferred style for learning.
- Arrange an appropriate location for the learning to take place that will be comfortable and free from distractions.
- Make sure the patient is wearing sensory aids, such as a hearing aid, glasses, or contact lenses, if s/he has need of them.
- Review information covered during earlier teaching sessions.
- Assess the patient's interest and level of comfort at periodic intervals during the teaching session.
- Postpone or discontinue a teaching session if the patient is not physically or emotionally ready.
- Inform the patient as to when and how his/her learning will be evaluated.
- Use vocabulary that is within the patient's level of understanding, neither beneath nor above it.
- Build on the patient's prior knowledge and experiences.
- Involve the patient actively through sharing ideas and handling equipment.
- Stimulate a variety and as many of the senses as possible.
- Use sophisticated language or vocabulary unless it leads to misunderstanding and a potential for harm.
- Allow time for questions and answers.
- Use equipment similar to the equipment the patient will need to use.
- Arrange an opportunity for the patient to use or apply the new information as soon as possible after it is taught.
- Provide written information or sample equipment that the patient can use for practice or review.
- Summarize the key points that were covered during the current period of teaching.
- Review the progress toward reaching goals.
- Evaluate the need for further teaching.
- Establish the time, place, and content for the next teaching session.

telemedicine (HCO) the use of information technology to deliver medical services and information from one location to another.

temporal orientation the ability to tell and use time (time of day, time of year, time of life, etc.). See *ori-*

entation.

temporary admission admission of a patient to a facility against his/her wishes. The patient is currently an inpatient and has a trial where the psychiatrist presents compelling arguments as to the need to continue involuntary institutionalization for up to 60 days longer. The patient may be represented by himself/herself and/or a lawyer. See *psychiatric admissions.*

tendon reflex examination a non-standardized test that measures the degree of reactive movement of a tendon when it is hit in a brisk manner. While tendon reflexes are generally graded from 1 (low) to 4 (high), there tends to be a large variation between one therapist and another. Treatment protocols and therapy interventions/precautions should not rely heavily on a patient's tendon reflex grade unless the therapist is comfortable that s/he knows how the specific tester grades reflexes.

terminal care intervention for patients who are approaching death. Most often these care needs are addressed by a signed *advanced directive* and usually strive to provide comfort for the body (freedom from pain if possible) and provide solace for the mind/soul (religious intervention when requested).

termination (of Medicare/Medicaid funding) the loss of qualification to received federal health care funds for services due to a determination of noncompliance with health care standards or due to the closure of the business. See *adverse actions, intermediate sanctions, nonrenewal, reasonable assurance.*

test *measurement* of specific skills or knowledge using a predetermined set of questions or tasks; a trial or *evaluation.*

test-retest reliability a way to test the internal stability (reliability) of a testing tool across time. The way to determine test-retest *reliability* is to give a specific test to a group of people and then give the same test to the same group of people at a later time. The purpose of this procedure is to determine how much an individuals' score will change from the first to the second administration of the tool, being careful to assure that no intervention is used between the two administrations of the test. (Giving the test twice with an intervention between the two administrations is a measurement of outcome or impact of the intervention and not the reliability of the testing tool.) If the scores are very similar in a test-re-test situation, then the test is said to have a "high and positive correlation." A perfect correlation would be a 1.0 correlation. However, just because of the nature of human beings, the tester would anticipate some variation to be normal, so a correlation of

.85 would still indicate a good stability (reliability) of the testing tool.

tetralogy of Fallot (TOF) a group of four birth defects of the heart which cause a mixture of oxygenated and non-oxygenated blood to be pumped throughout the body. After a series of surgeries to correct TOF, the individual should require no restrictions for physical activity.

text telephones (TTs) (ADA) machinery or equipment that employs interactive graphic (i.e., typed) communications through the transmission of coded signals across a standard telephone network. Text telephones can include devices known as TDDs (telecommunication display devices or telecommunication devices for individuals who are deaf) or computers.

thalamic pain a spontaneous pain or change so that a normal sensation feels painful.

thalassemia (HHS/NMDP) a group of chronic, inherited anemias. Particularly common in persons of Mediterranean, African, and Southeast Asian ancestry.

thanatology the study of how people cope with death.

The ARC See *Association of Retarded Citizens.*

theory a set of explanations for why something happens or exists.

therapeutic blood level the level of medication in the blood that proves to be therapeutic; not sub-therapeutic or toxic.

therapeutic community a unit, facility, or other structured environment which strives to meet the patient's needs in a holistic manner (physical, social, emotional, and psychological). Not all facilities provide a therapeutic community. See *milieu.*

Therapeutic Recreation Service Model a service model developed by C. A. Peterson and S. L. Gunn in 1979 that represents a way to conceptualize the deliver of recreational therapy services. The continuum consists of three levels: treatment as a necessary antecedent to leisure involvement (therapy), acquisition of leisure related knowledge and skills (education), and acquired leisure ability participated in voluntarily (participation). A diagram of the model is shown on the next page. See *leisure ability, Recreation Service Model.*

therapeutic recreation specialist See *recreational therapist.*

therapy process a method of identifying patient needs and of problem solving that has the following steps: 1. *assessment*, 2. *diagnosis*, 3. plans, 4. implementation, and 5. *evaluation.*

third-party reimbursement reimbursement for services paid by an entity besides the person who re-

ceived the services. An insurance company is responsible for third-party reimbursement to pay for medical services received by its subscribers. The four most prevalent errors in billing which resulted in improper payments were insufficient or no documentation (45%), lack of medical necessity (37%), incorrect coding, and non-covered/allowable services.

thoracic pertaining to the thorax (chest).

thoracic lumbar sacral orthosis (TLSO) a body support made of plastic that fits over the chest, abdomen, and lower back that is also called a "body jacket." A TLSO is designed to support an unstable or recently fused spine. See *orthosis.*

thought stopping a technique used to stop compulsive or obsessive thoughts which are counterproductive in nature. The training usually involves the use of a key word (e.g., "Stop") commanded by the patient followed by a time period of meditative thoughts, or an absence of thought. This technique was introduced by Bain in 1928 and adapted by J. Wolpe in the late 1950's. Mastery of this technique usually requires the patient to use the technique every time a counterproductive thought arises over a week's period of time. This technique has had success with patients who have exhibited problems with sexual preoccupation, obsessive thoughts, obsessive memories, overreaction to fear, and hypochondria. See *relaxation techniques, obsession, compulsive.*

three-point gait When the patient is unable to ambulate due to intolerance of weight bearing on one of the legs, two crutches are used to bear the weight instead of the limb.

threshold for evaluation the point at which an individual or organization has met minimum quality or quantity expectations to allow an initial evaluation to begin. An example would be for a student to provide documentation that s/he has the minimum education and experience to sit for a professional credentialing exam or for a facility to provide documentation that it qualifies for its first accreditation review.

threshold of sensation the point at which a nerve has received enough stimulation to be able to "fire" and send a signal to the next nerve. See *sensation.*

thromboangiitis obliterans inflammation of the small arteries caused by decreased circulation in the extremities. This disease is a direct result of the patient's use of nicotine and/or smoking and will be resolved after the patient gives up the use of nicotine and/or smoking. The hands and feet are the most affected, causing increased concern for frostbite when the patients are engaging in winter sporting events. This disease is sometimes referred to as

Therapeutic Recreation Service Model

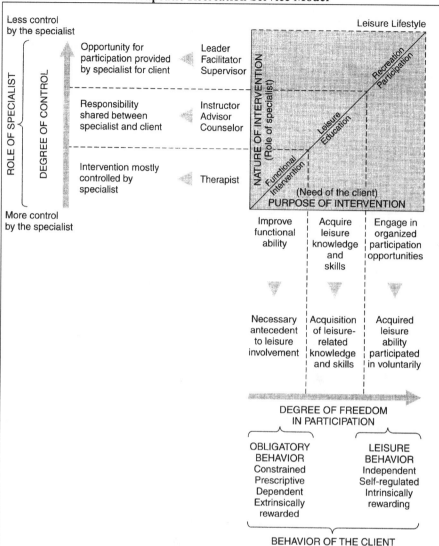

From Carol Ann Peterson & Norma J. Stumbo, **Therapeutic Recreation Program Design: Principles and Procedures, 3rd Edition**. Copyright © 2000 by Allyn and Bacon. Reprinted with permission.

Buerger's disease.

thrombophlebitis an inflammation of the wall of a vein.

thrombus a clot within the heart or a blood vessel that may lead to obstruction. See *cerebrovascular accident, myocardial infarction.*

thyroid (HHS) a two-lobed structure located in front of and on either side of the trachea, producing the hormone thyroxin; of or relating to the thyroid gland.

thyroid-stimulating hormone (HHS) a hormone of the anterior pituitary gland that stimulates and regulates the development and secretory activity of the thyroid gland.

thyrotoxicosis (HHS) poisoning from hyperthyroid-

ism.

tic disorders the presence of a sudden, rapid, non-rhythmic motor movement or vocalization that is stereotypic in nature. Tic behavior can be somewhat controlled and tends to become diminished when the individual is engaged in an enjoyable, relaxed activity. *Stress* increases tic activity. Tic behaviors are classified as either simple or complex. The **DSM-IV** lists three primary types of tic disorders: Tourette's disorder (multiple motor and one or more vocal tics present multiple times a day), chronic motor or vocal tic disorder (single or multiple tics either motor or vocal in nature, but not both types), and transient tic disorder (single or multiple tics which last for less than one year). See *childhood psychiatric disor-*

Severity of Tissue Injury

Degree or Grade	Description
First Degree, Grade 1	The onset of mild pain within 24 hours of an impact with another object or excessive pulling of tissue. Some tissue damage is evidenced by mild swelling and local tenderness. Pain may be evident with direct pressure or when the tissue is stressed through movement. Redness of skin is noted. A skin pressure point is considered to be 1st degree if the red mark has not faded 100% in 30 minutes.
Second Degree, Grade 2	Moderate pain that increases significantly during palpation or movement. The pain is significant enough to cause most patients to stop activity. If ligaments are involved in the injured sections, the patient may experience a decrease in stability because of torn ligaments that cause an increase in joint mobility. Blistering or torn skin is evident in the case of skin pressure points.
Third Degree, Grade 3	Over 50% of the tissue involved is torn or avulsed. Severe pain is experienced even without movement; movement of affected part does not significantly increase pain. Significant joint instability may be noted if tendons or ligaments are involved.

ders, stereotypical behavior.

tightness a mild *contracture* of a group of muscles and tendons usually caused by inactivity and easily resolved through gentle, frequent enjoyable activities that promote range of motion of the involved area.

tilt table a firm stretcher that has a platform for the patient's feet. The tilt table works on the same principle as a teeter-totter — the head end raises and the feet go down. Since the elasticity of the blood vessels requires regular exposure to the vertical pull of gravity, a patient who has been on bed rest will have physically weakened vessel walls. If a patient with this condition stands up, the blood vessel walls will not be able to contain the blood causing the blood to pool in the lowest parts of the body. This causes a lack of oxygen (with subsequent fainting). A tilt table is used to help "exercise" the blood vessel walls to reduce the risk of fainting. See *conditioning.*

time management skills skills that allow the individual to schedule his/her day in such a manner as to get done what s/he needs to get done (in time) and to get where s/he wants to go (on time). Some skills related to time management are 1. ability to read a clock, 2. ability to develop a reasonable schedule, 3. ability to follow a schedule, 4. ability to *problem solve* and prioritize using good *judgment* when conflicts arise in scheduling, and 5. ability to notify appropriate others when the schedule changes. See *goal setting and time management, relaxation techniques.*

tissue injury, degree of Health care professionals usually divide injury to tissue into three levels or degrees. It is important for the professional to be aware of the three degrees and to be able to make a reasonable determination of the degree of injury received during an activity. Frequently an incident report will need to be written for any second- or third-degree tissue damage and a continuous quality improvement program will be required to reduce the likelihood of a repeat incident. A summary table of tissue injury is shown above.

titer the concentration of a substance in a solution, or the strength of such a substance detected by titration.

titrate to experiment with dosages to determine how much of a treatment is needed to produce an effect. While commonly used in chemistry and the study of the impact of doses of medicine on a patient's condition, therapists can also titrate treatments such as muscle strengthening programs, endurance, and tolerance.

T lymphocyte immune cells produced by bone marrow that mature in the thymus gland. T lymphocytes are critical to the functioning of the cellular immune response. (CDC) The most common type of lymphocyte, itself divided into at least three subpopulations on the basis of function: cytotoxic or killer T lymphocytes, helper T lymphocytes, and suppressor T lymphocytes. T cells play a cardinal role in regulating the immune system.

TNM See *cancer staging and grading.*

toilet hygiene For a patient to be able to be considered independent in toilet hygiene s/he would need to be able to complete the following tasks without cueing or other assistance:

1. ability to know the supplies needed and where to obtain them
2. ability to use supplies and ability to perform toileting tasks to achieve cleanliness
3. ability to transfer to; maintain body position; and then transfer back from a bedpan, toilet, commode, or other similar equipment.

While the patient's initial training in these skills will most likely come from an occupational therapist, other therapists will need to supervise, assist, and evaluate the patient in his/her skills related to toilet hygiene while on community integration outings.

tolerance 1. the ability to ignore irritating stimuli. 2. related to *substance dependence*, tolerance is the need for greatly increased amounts of the drug to obtain the desired effects and/or intoxication. The amount of tolerance an individual can develop depends on the substance being abused. After extended use of opioids and stimulants, the user can develop a tolerance so high that s/he needs ten or more times the amount to achieve the level of intoxication that s/he originally desired. In fact, opioids and stimulant users may develop a tolerance so high that the dose would normally be fatal to less seasoned users. The two key symptoms of substance tolerance are the need for increased amounts to achieve the same "high," and/or a significantly reduced "high" using the same amount over a period of time.

tone the degree to which the muscles display strength and the ability to recover from normal stretching and contracting. See *efficiency, flaccid, neuro-developmental techniques.*

tonus the normal state of balance achieved by the body through the partial contraction or alternate contraction and relaxation of muscle tissues that are in close proximity to each other.

toxic shock syndrome (TSS) an acute disease that manifests by sudden onset of fever, chills, vomiting, diarrhea, muscle pains, and rash. Hypotension and mucous membrane, multi-system involvement, and later desquamation are features of the disease. Staphylococcus aureus, a bacterium, is the etiologic agent. In the United States, annual incidence is 1-2/100,000 women 15-44 years of age (last active surveillance done in 1987). S. aureus commonly colonizes skin and mucous membranes in humans. TSS has been associated with use of tampons and intravaginal contraceptive devices in women and occurs as a complication of skin abscesses or surgery. 5% of all cases are fatal. Menstruating women, women using barrier contraceptive devices, and per-

sons who have undergone nasal surgery are especially at risk.

tracheostomy an opening through the skin into the trachea made so a tracheostomy tube can be inserted. A tracheotomy tube (usually made out of plastic or Silastic material) becomes flexible at body temperature to be able to move with the trachea. Depending on the patient's ability to breath, a ventilator may or may not be hooked up to the cuff of the tube. See *artificial airway, endotracheal airway.* Compare with *tracheotomy.*

tracheotomy an opening through the skin and between the second and fourth tracheal rings into the trachea (windpipe). The opening is made to allow air to reach the lungs and is either closed or converted into a tracheostomy. Compare with *tracheostomy.*

traction a treatment that uses equipment to provide pull and counter-pull on the skeletal system. The "pull" aspect of traction is achieved through the use of weights or springs to apply outward (stretching) force on a specific part of the skeletal system. The "counter-pull" aspect of traction is usually achieved by using the patient's own body. Using the patient's body as the counter-pull of the traction may increase skin integrity problems at the sight of the counter-pull. There are three primary categories of traction: 1. manual, 2. skin, and 3. skeletal. *Manual traction* is the use of one's hands and muscles to provide the "pull." This type of traction is usually used in first aid or emergency care (e.g., reducing a fracture or relocating a joint). *Skin traction* is the use of equipment to provide a pulling force on the skin surface indirectly causing a pull on the skeletal system itself. Because the counter-pull is frequently achieved by the patient's weight on the mattress, activities that involve rolling or other movement may reduce the effectiveness of the treatment and are therefore contraindicated. *Skeletal* traction is the use of pins surgically inserted into one or more bones. A weight or other means of pull is then attached to these pins to achieve traction. Some of the concerns for therapy related to traction are shown below. Specific types of traction are shown on the next page.

Traction, Concerns for Therapy

Concern	Action
Incorrect positioning	Instruct patient in correct positions to take for each activity.
Sheet burn to elbows and heels (friction and sheer)	Provide elbow and heel protection (bed pillows are actually good protection if sheering action is reduced).
Loss of muscle tone and range of motion	Provide activities which do not compromise traction but which promote range of motion activities and isometric exercise.

Types of Traction

Traction	Description
Bryant's	A type of traction used only on infants to treat a femur fracture or to correct congenital dislocation of the hip. This traction immobilizes the infant's lower extremities in a vertical position while the rest of the body is supine on the bed. The rope, weight, and pulley system is connected to footplates on the bottom of the infant's feet.
Buck's	A common type of traction that uses ropes, weights, and pulleys connected to a metal bar extending from the foot of the bed and applied to the patient's body through the use of a cast or splint over the affected body part. Traction is applied to one or both legs to treat contractures or disorders of the knees or hips. The patient is placed in a relatively horizontal position on the bed.
Crutchfield Skeletal	Crutchfield tongs are inserted into the skull to allow traction to be placed on the cervical vertebrae. The traction applied to the cervical vertebrae is usually 10 to 20 pounds, which is connected by a rope that travels through a pulley and connects to a freely hanging weight at the head of the bed. Patient care is staff intensive during the time an individual is in a Crutchfield skeletal traction, including deep-breathing exercises usually every two hours, massages to reduce decubiti, and passive range of motion to all extremities. Body alignment must be maintained during the weeks that the patient is in traction.
Halo	A traction device/splint that immobilizes the neck and head to promote the healing of cervical injuries. The halo splint sits on the trunk with four poles extending up to and connecting to a "halo" band around the skull.
Russell's	A traction for the lower extremities that includes both traction and suspension. Traction is applied to immobilize, position, and align the lower extremities (one or both sides). Additional immobilization is often applied using a jacket restraint to keep the patient from sliding downward on the bed. Suspension is used for positioning, such as a sling to support the weight of the lower extremity that is in traction.

trait an attribute that is relatively stable. A trait tends to remain consistent regardless of situational or environmental factors. An individual who has blue eyes (eye color = trait) will have blue eyes all of his/her life. An individual who is slow of thought (speed of cognitive processing = trait) will likely hold that trait throughout his/her life span. Traits are acquired through two primary vectors: genetic characteristics (e.g., blue eyes) or through learning (e.g., well spoken). An individual who was an extrovert prior to most injuries or illnesses will retain that trait through treatment and beyond. See *state*.

tram (ADA) refers to several types of motor vehicles consisting of a tractor unit, with or without passenger accommodations and one or more passenger trailer units, including but not limited to vehicles providing shuttle service to remote parking area, between hotels and other public accommodations, and between and within amusement parks and other recreation areas. The ADA accessibility guidelines for trams may be found in the **Trams, Similar Vehicles, and Systems Technical Assistance Manual** (US Architectural and Transportation Barriers Compliance Board).

trans fats (HHS) substances occurring naturally in beef, butter, milk, and lamb fats and in commercially prepared, partially hydrogenated margarines and solid cooking fats. The main sources of trans fats in the American diet today are margarine, shortening, commercial frying fats, and high-fat baked goods. Partially hydrogenated vegetable oils were developed in part to help displace highly saturated animal and vegetable fats used in frying, baking, and spreads. However, trans fats, like saturated fats, may raise blood LDL cholesterol levels (the so-called "bad" cholesterol) but not as much as the saturates do. At high consumption levels, it may also reduce the HDL or "good" cholesterol levels.

transference 1. attribution of thoughts and feelings, which were originally experienced with important people in a patient's life, to other people currently interacting with the patient. 2. the feelings a psychiatric patient has for the analyst, which were originally felt towards others who were significant in the patient's life. 3. shifting symptoms from one part of the body or producing physical symptoms because of emotional upset as in a conversion disorder. See *countertransference*.

transient ischemic attack (TIA) temporary symptoms of a *cerebrovascular accident*. Complete recovery usually results within 24 hours. A clot may have occluded the blood vessel and then released.

People having TIAs are advised to seek medical attention immediately because TIAs are predictors of future cerebrovascular accidents. People who have had a cerebrovascular accident may also have TIAs. Always alert a doctor to these "mini-strokes." See *cerebrovascular accident.*

transient lodging (ADA) a building, facility, or portion thereof, excluding inpatient medical care facilities, that contains one or more dwelling units or sleeping accommodations. Transient lodging may include, but is not limited to, resorts, group homes, hotels, motels, and dormitories.

transmission control protocol (HCO) a communications protocol governing data exchanged on the Internet. Also known as an Internet protocol.

transtheoretical model a model that posits that individuals can be classified into one of four stages that reflect their propensity to change specific behaviors. The four categories are 1. precontemplators/contemplators, 2. preparation, 3. action, and 4. maintenance. There are specific behaviors related to each category that need to be addressed for progression to occur and continue. For instance, precontemplators and contemplators, who tend to be sedentary, need to alter their thinking if they are to progress to the preparation and action stages. At the same time, those in the preparation and action stages want to change, thus skill development to create positive habits and ensure success is required. Finally, those in the maintenance stage need to develop cognitive/behavioral strategies to help them avoid relapse or begin again after relapse (Sallis & Owen, 1999). The model is a useful research and clinical tool.

transverse deficiency a weakness or other disabling condition which affects the entire width of a limb. Compare with *paraxial deficiency.*

traumatic brain injury (TBI) injury to the brain as a result of a traumatic event. There are two major classes of brain injuries: open head and closed head. An open head injury is one which penetrates the scalp or skull such as a gun shot wound. A closed head injury results in brain damage without penetration of the scalp or skull and may be due to an impact (e.g., being hit on the head by a baseball) or acceleration/deceleration (e.g., being hit from behind in your car while wearing your seatbelt). The skull may or may not be fractured in a closed head injury. The types of disabilities seen as a result of a TBI depend on the location that the brain was injured and the class of head injury. Open head injuries tend to produce discreet and focal lesions. Closed head injuries tend to produce generalized or diffused brain injury. (CDC) Of all types of injury, those to the brain are among the most likely to result in death or permanent disability. Estimates of traumatic brain injury incidence, severity, and cost reflect the enormous losses to individuals, their families, and society from these injuries. These data demonstrate a critical need for more effective ways to prevent brain injuries and care for those who are injured. Using national data for 1995-1996, the CDC estimates that TBIs have this impact in the United States each year: 1 million people are treated and released from hospital emergency departments. 230,000 people are hospitalized and survive, 50,000 people die. Using preliminary hospitalization and mortality data col-

Potential Impairments as a Result of Combining a Positive Blood Alcohol Level and TBI (Gill & Sparadeo, 1989)

Etiology	Findings
Metabolic changes that occur with ingestion of alcohol	• Increased potential for developing hematomas. In particular, alcoholics with cerebral atrophy are at risk due to increased capillary fragility and decreased brain counter-pressure to deal with low-pressure leaks. • Decreased tolerance of blood loss and decreased blood pressure on admission. • Fluid electrolyte abnormalities that could exacerbate cerebral edema. • The possibility of respiratory depression, which would increase the risk of hypoxia. • Increased vulnerability to infection. • Increased hemorrhaging. For example, cats administered alcohol and then subjected to an experimental brain lesion had a greater extent of hemorrhage than cats without alcohol.
Apart from the acute effects of alcohol, a second possible etiology is the long-term effects of alcohol abuse or dependency	• Well-documented cognitive deficits, particularly in visual spatial abilities, memory, psychomotor speed/coordination, and abstraction. • Cerebral atrophy on CT scans. • Increased risk of other medical conditions (e.g., liver damage).

lected from 12 states (Alaska, Arizona, Sacramento County [California], Colorado, Louisiana, Maryland, Missouri, New York, Oklahoma, Rhode Island, South Carolina, and Utah) during 1995-1996, CDC finds the following: The average TBI incidence rate (combined hospitalization and mortality rate) is 95 per 100,000 population. Twenty-two percent of people who have a TBI die from their injuries. The risk of having a TBI is especially high among adolescents, young adults, and people older than 75 years of age. For persons of all ages, the risk of TBI among males is twice the risk among females. The leading causes of TBI are motor vehicle crashes, violence, and falls.

Nearly two-thirds of firearm-related TBIs are classified as suicidal in intent. The leading causes of TBI vary by age: *falls* are the leading cause of TBI among persons aged 65 years and older, whereas transportation leads among persons aged 5 to 64 years. The outcome of these injuries varies greatly depending on the cause: 91% of firearm-related TBIs resulted in death, but only 11% of fall-related TBIs are fatal. Based on national TBI incidence data and preliminary data from the Colorado Traumatic Brain Injury Registry that describe TBI-related disability in 1996-1997, CDC estimates the following: Each year more than 80,000 Americans survive a hospitalization for traumatic brain injury but are dis-

Bicycle Related Head Injuries (CDC)

Topic	Discussion
Scope of Problem in the United States	In 1997, 813 bicyclists were killed in crashes with motor vehicles, an increase of 7% over the previous year. Of these, 31% were riders younger than 16 years old and 97% were not wearing helmets. In 1997, an estimated 567,000 Americans sustained a bicycle-related injury that required emergency department care. Approximately two-thirds of these cyclists were children or adolescents. An estimated 140,000 children are treated each year in emergency departments for head injuries sustained while bicycling. In 1991, societal costs associated with bicycle-related head injury or death were estimated to exceed $3 billion.
Prevention Strategies	Riders should wear bicycle helmets every time they ride. In the event of a crash, wearing a bicycle helmet reduces the risk of serious head injury by as much as 85% and the risk for brain injury by as much as 88%. Helmets have also been shown to reduce the risk of injury to the upper and mid-face by 65%. In fact, if each rider wore a helmet, an estimated 500 bicycle-related fatalities and 151,000 nonfatal head injuries would be prevented each year—that's one death per day and one injury every four minutes. Unfortunately, estimates on helmet usage suggest that only 25% of children ages 5-14 years wear a helmet when riding. The percentage is close to zero when looking at teen riders. Children and adolescents' most common complaints are that helmets are not fashionable, or "cool," their friends don't wear them, and/or they are uncomfortable (usually too hot). Riders also convey that they do not think about the importance of bike helmets, nor about the need to protect themselves from injury, particularly if they are not riding in traffic. Accordingly, the national health goal for 2010 is for 50% of teenage bicyclists in 9th-12th grade to wear helmets.
What strategies are available to get bicyclists to wear helmets?	The primary strategies to increase bike helmet use include education, legislation, and helmet-distribution programs. Educational programs have been conducted in different communities and schools around the nation, with generally positive results. The most successful programs are multifaceted and often multi-site campaigns that combine education with helmet giveaways or discount programs and state or local legislation requiring helmet use. Some evidence suggests that legislative efforts are more cost-effective than school- or community-based programs.
How many states have bicycle helmet laws?	By early 1999, 15 states and more than 65 local governments had enacted some form of bicycle helmet legislation. Most of these laws pertain to children and adolescents.
What standards exist to ensure that helmets are truly protective?	The US Consumer Product Safety Commission issued a new safety standard for bike helmets in 1999. The new standard ensures that bike helmets will adequately protect the head and that chinstraps will be strong enough to prevent the helmet from coming off in a crash, collision, or fall. In addition, helmets intended for children up to age five must cover a larger surface of the head than before. All bike helmets made or imported into the United States must meet the CPSC standard.

Treatment Plan

problem/need	treatment	outcome	date
⇓ ability to find room	1. provide large lettered name on door (service)	⇑ ability to identify room due to label	3/2/02
	2. develop memory book with pictures and directions from activity room to bedroom (service)	ownership of prosthetic device to assist with ⇓ pathfinding ability	3/5/02
	3. practice with memory book five days a week, two times a day (therapy)	⇑ ability/skill in using memory book and residual memory to pathfind to room.	5/6/02

charged with TBI-related disabilities. 5.3 million Americans are living today with a TBI-related disability. There are several published epidemiological studies of TBI-related hospitalizations and deaths in the US. Kraus has reviewed some of these studies in detail. Recent data suggest a decline in rates of hospitalization for less severe TBI, possibly due to changes in hospital admission criteria. The lower TBI incidence rate seen today may be due in part to a real decline in brain injuries but also appears to be an artifact of counting methods, which capture only hospitalized and fatal cases. There was a 22% decline in the TBI-related death rate from 24.6/100,000 US residents in 1979 to 19.3/100,000 in 1992. Firearm-related rates increased 13% from 1984 through 1992, undermining a 25% decline in motor vehicle-related rates for the same period. Firearms surpassed motor vehicles as the largest single cause of death associated with traumatic brain injury in the United States in 1990. These data highlight the success of efforts to prevent traumatic brain injury due to motor vehicles and failure to prevent such injuries due to firearms. The increasing importance of penetrating injury has important implications for research, treatment, and prevention of traumatic brain injury in the United States. A number of studies have shown that males are about twice as likely to incur TBI as females. Most studies indicate that the highest rates of these injuries are found in persons 15-24 years of age. Persons under the age of five or over the age of 75 are also at high risk. There is no way to describe fully the human costs of traumatic brain injury: the burdens borne by those who are injured and their families. Only a few analyses of the monetary costs of these injuries are available, including the following estimate (lifetime cost of all brain injuries occurring in the United States in 1985): direct annual expenditures are $4.5 billion, indirect annual costs are $33.3 billion and total costs are $37.8 billion. The use of alcohol immediately prior to sustaining a head injury may exacerbate the short-term neurological and behavioral effects, which are different than what would be experienced

simply by withdrawal symptoms. Gill and Sparadeo (1989) reported the short-term neurobehavioral effects of a positive blood alcohol level combined with a traumatic brain injury in the table at the beginning of TBI. The table on the previous page shows information about bicycle-related head injuries. See *acceleration factors, brain plasticity, contrecoup lesions, coup, diabetes, echolalia, executive function, generalization, graphic input, neuropsychologist, secondary brain injury, second impact syndrome.*

treatment the use of identified methods of *intervention* to manage the patient's care. This management consists of assessment, specific interventions, and reassessment. See *critical pathway, current procedural terminology, day treatment program, diversional program, documentation, focused review, frame of reference, Functional Assessment of Characteristics of Therapeutic Recreation — Revised, functional treatment, holistic approach, hypothesis, indications, medical play, modality, patient satisfaction, progress notes, protocol, psychiatric hospital, remotivation, sensory integration, sign, visual impairment.*

treatment plan the formally outlined set of treatment interventions and services for a patient to ameliorate an illness or injury. A treatment plan is based on a formal assessment to determine need and clinical opinion/judgment and pre-established treatment interventions to anticipate an outcome. An example of a treatment plan is shown above. See *appropriateness, care plan, clinical privileging.*

tremor the rhythmic and quivering movements caused by the alternating contraction then relaxation of opposing muscle groups. Tremors are purposeless movements and may be due to advancing age, a medication side effect, or a degenerative neurological disorder. See a list of types of tremors on the next page.

trichotillomania the impulsive behavior of pulling one's hair out to relieve tension, for pleasure, or self-gratification. The behavior is prevalent enough to cause noticeable hair thinning and loss.

Type of Tremors

Type	Description
action tremor	Involuntary oscillating and rhythmic movements of the outstretched upper limb during activity.
coarse tremor	Slow, rhythmic movements.
essential tremor	Inherited tendency to develop a fine tremor, usually after the age of fifty. Also known as a familial tremor.
fine tremor	Fast, rhythmic movements.
intention tremor	Increase in intensity when the individual attempts a voluntary movement that requires coordination.
intermittent tremor	Occurs when voluntary movement is attempted or occurs in hemiplegia.
motofacient tremor	In muscle groups of the face.
passive tremor	Only seen when the patient is at rest.
persistent tremor	Present whether the patient is resting or attempting activity.
resting tremor	Present when the limb is supported and the patient is at rest, as in Parkinsonism.
volitional tremor	Seen throughout the entire body during voluntary movement, as in multiple sclerosis.

Trichotillomania is a recognized psychiatric diagnosis found in the **DSM-IV** under the category of impulse control disorders not elsewhere classified.

trigger something that causes action. In the case of long-term care facilities in the US, a "trigger" means that a patient has scored in an unacceptable range on one or more sections of the MDS. This identifies a patient who needs further evaluation using assessment protocols designated either by the state or the federal government. See *minimum data set.*

triglycerides serum laboratory test Dietary fat is absorbed through the small intestine and resynthesized by mucosal cells. An increase in triglyceride serum can indicate hypothyroidism, chronic alcoholism, stress, viral hepatitis, anorexia nervosa, diabetes mellitus, or nephrotic syndrome. A decrease can indicate malnutrition or malabsorption.

triple X syndrome See *chromosomal aberrations.*

trisomy 13 syndrome See *chromosomal aberrations.*

trisomy 18 syndrome See *chromosomal aberrations.*

trisomy 21 syndrome See *chromosomal aberrations, Down syndrome.*

trust a belief system that has three parts: 1. the belief in one's own ability to act in a trustworthy manner, 2. the belief in the potential of another person to respond in mutually respectful ways, and 3. the belief in one's own capability to assess the trustworthiness of another person accurately. By the time an individual is six months old s/he will have formed the basis for his/her level of trust and spend the rest of his/her life adjusting that level up or down. Traumatic events in an individual's life, such as rape or the burglary of one's home, can dramatically decrease the patient's ability to trust anyone, not just the individual(s) who harmed him/her. The ability to be able to be independent in the community requires at least a moderate degree of trust. A patient whose ability to trust others is low may have a difficult time integrating back into the community.

tubbing See *debridement.*

tuberculosis (TB) a chronic infection caused by the TB bacteria — Mycobacterium tuberculosis. While TB is a chronic lung infection, individuals with AIDS may experience a spread of the infection to multiple organs. *Fatigue,* chest pain, weight loss, and fever are early signs of TB. TB requires long-term antibiotic treatment. See *AFB isolation.*

tumor (HHS/NMDP) any abnormal mass resulting from the excessive multiplication of cells. Tumors can be cancerous or non-cancerous. (HHS) An abnormal mass of tissue that grows more rapidly than normal, and continues to grow after the stimuli that initiated the new growth cease.

Turner syndrome See *chromosomal aberrations.*

Twelve-Step program See *Alcoholics Anonymous.*

two-point discrimination test a test that measures the degree of sensation that a patient has on specific parts of his/her skin. The therapist or physician measures the patient's ability to perceive the difference between one or two points (measured in centimeters or millimeters). If a patient has been assessed to have poor two point discrimination, the therapist will need to ensure that appropriate safety measures are taken during activities, as the patient will have a decreased ability to sense that his/her skin is being injured.

type and cross match laboratory test a series of laboratory experiments on a person's blood to help determine blood type groups (ABO and Rh) and antibody screen and cross match. This test is used prior to surgery when it is considered likely that blood transfusions will be needed.

Type I diabetes See *diabetes*.

Type II diabetes See *diabetes*.

U

UE the abbreviation used for u̲pper e̲xtremity.

ulcer tissue death in the skin or mucous membrane that causes an open sore to form. *See autogenics, dyspepsia, pressure sore.*

umami (HHS) In addition to the four main taste components (sweet, sour, salty, and bitter), there is the additional taste characteristic called "umami" or savory. One of the food components responsible for the umami flavor in foods is glutamate, an amino acid. See *glutamate* and *MSG*.

umbrella legislation a consolidation of regulatory boards to reduce impact on state governments. Umbrella legislation may place the state credentialing of physical therapy, occupational therapy, speech therapy, and recreational therapy all under one review board. While each profession would maintain its own separate credential and scope of practice, the administrative tasks of each would be handled by a single board.

uncompensated care (FB) care for which a provider or health care facility does to expect to receive payment.

underlying cause the processes, policies, or procedures that allow an event to happen. The underlying cause may be due to a common-cause *variation*, a special-cause variation, or both.

underutilization not using services available. A provider who doesn't get bus passes for a patient who could use them is allowing or causing the patient to underutilized the transportation services available. Appropriate levels of service are based on what would be expected and required when measured against standards and coverage.

Unified Medical Language System (UMLS) (HCO) a computer-based system for translating among disparate clinical nomenclatures, maintained by the National Library of Medicine (NLM).

Unified Nursing Language System (UNLS) (HCO) a system similar to the United Medical Language System that focuses on nursing services.

Uniform Data System for Medical Rehabilitation (UDSmr) a system for documenting both the severity of patient disability and his/her response to rehabilitation intervention. Developed by C. V. Granger, MD and B. B. Hamilton, MD, PhD in 1987, this nationally used system helps keep track of national and regional trends in rehabilitation medicine. The data kept by the UDSmr includes information on patient demographics, medical diagnoses, disability groups, the length of stay (inpatient), and the cost of the rehabilitation services provided. The screening tool used to gather this information is called the Uniform Data Set Forms and employs either the FIM Scale for patients over 8 years of age or the WeeFIM (FIM for children) as the basis of the assessment. Facilities who use the UDSmr must subscribe to the service. In return they get management tools which provide information on trends in rehabilitation medicine, on how their facility compares to other facilities, data on which to base treatment, a basis for quality assurance programs, and a basis for the justification of services and billing. See *documentation.*

unilateral neglect lack of awareness of one side of the body. See *neglect.*

United States Association for Blind Athletes (USABA) a national organization that promotes opportunities for individuals who are visually impaired to compete on a regional, national, and international level. The national sports offered through USABA are goalball, gymnastics, judo, power lifting, tandem cycling, track and field, wrestling, alpine skiing, Nordic skiing, speed skating, and marathon running. Competitors are divided into three classifications for competition: "B1" (totally blind, may posses light perception but unable to recognize hand shapes at any distance), "B2" (recognize hand shapes up to and including 20/600 or field limited to less than 5 degrees), and "B3" (visual acuity greater than 20/600 up to 20/200, field limitation from 5 to 20 degrees). The address for USABA is 33 N. Institute St., Colorado Springs, CO 80903, 719-630-0422 voice, 719-630-0616 fax, 719-632-8180 bulletin board.

United States Department of Agriculture (USDA) (HHS) The United States Department of Agriculture is comprised of many agencies charged with different tasks related to agriculture and our food supply. Among these is ensuring a safe, affordable, nutritious, and accessible food supply. The USDA also enhances the quality of life for the American population by supporting production of agricultural products; caring for agricultural, forest, and range lands; supporting sound development of our rural communities; providing economic opportunities for farm and rural residents; expanding global markets for agricultural and forest products and services; and working to reduce hunger in America and throughout the world.

update a written report of the patient's response to placement and treatment placed in the medical record based on a reassessment, at least quarterly, of the patient. Updates are to reflect, but are not limited to: health status, psychosocial needs, change in ability to participate in activities, and new or improved or increased behavior problems with a related program of behavioral interventions.

upper respiratory infection an infection located in the nose, throat, sinuses, ear, and/or larynx. See *lower respiratory infection.*

urea the chief end product of nitrogen metabolism in mammals, excreted in the urine; carbonyl diamide, $CO(NH_2)_2$.

uremia an increased level of urea in the blood; a sign of kidney failure.

ureter a tube that carries urine from the kidneys to the bladder.

uric acid, serum laboratory test Uric acid is an end product excreted by the kidney. An increase in uric acid serum can indicate renal failure, gout, leukemia, lymphoma, myeloma, psoriasis, or lead nephropathy. A decrease in uric acid serum can indicate low-purine diets, neoplastic disease, or liver disease. Normal range in males is 2.4 - 7.4 and females 1.4 - 5.8 mg/dL. Serum levels can be affected by age and sex and tend to be higher in some racial groups, such as Filipinos.

urinary tract infection (UTI) (CDC) an infection of the urinary tract. Ranges from painful urination in uncomplicated urethritis or cystitis to severe systemic illness associated with abdominal or back pain, fever, sepsis, and decreased kidney function in some cases of pyelonephritis. Usually caused by Escherichia coli, but other Enterobacteriaceae are also important causes of infection. In the United States, urinary tract infections account for about 4 million ambulatory-care visits each year, representing about 1% of all outpatient visits. Severe infections associated with sepsis can be fatal. It is usually contracted through fecal contamination of the urinary tract.

utility systems management See *environment of care.*

utilization management the evaluation process, and subsequent change in procedures based on the results of the evaluation, to promote the best use of available resources. Utilization management has five main components: *prior review, concurrent review, retrospective review, discharge planning,* and *case management.*

utilization review (UR) the review of services furnished by a facility to individuals entitled to benefits under the Medicare and Medicaid programs or other third party payers. These services are then compared to standards of practice. UR, which is conducted either by the facility itself or by a PRO (*Peer Review Organization*), is directed at evaluating the admissions to the facility, the durations of stay, the professional services furnished with respect to the medical necessity of the services and the most efficient use of available health facilities and services. The impact that UR has on each practitioner is significant. UR requires that 1. each practice group conform to the appropriate *standards* of practice and 2. the practice group provide services based on diagnosis and functional need with very little variation given to patients with similar clinical conditions. Practitioners must use testing tools, protocols, and other standard outcome measurements to be able to demonstrate their ability to comply with good utilization review expectations. There are six indicators that may trigger a negative UR and a denial of claims (Foto and Swanson, 1993):

1.   misuse of procedure or service codes
2.   use of inappropriate treatment methods
3.   lengthy stays
4.   lack of change in treatment, with little or no results
5.   lack of appropriate cost alternatives
6.   spotty documentation

See *concurrent review, medical management systems, pharmacy management, peer review, retrospective review.*

VA Veteran's Affairs (Medical Centers).

vaginal photoplethysmograph a test used to measure sexual arousal in women. This test, similar to the penile *plethysmograph* for men, measures vaginal blood flow, vaginal pulse rate and amplitude, and the duration of the response.

valgus the outward twisting or bending of a body part causing a malformation and/or loss of functional ability. Opposite of *varus*.

validation in senior care, the acceptance of memories of the past without attempting to check them for correctness. For individuals who are very disoriented, the validation of the memories and feelings that they have is an important aspect of humane treatment. Validation activities do not focus on *orientation*; they focus on the patient's perception of what happened in the past (correct or incorrect — it doesn't matter).

validation survey of an accredited hospital a survey of Joint Commission on Accreditation of Healthcare Organizations/American Osteopathic Association accredited hospitals to validate the presumed compliance through the hospital's "deemed" status and the Joint Commission/AOA survey process. These surveys are selected on a random sample basis or are conducted in response to an allegation of a significant deficiency.

validity how well an assessment is able to measure what it states it is measuring. There are three factors which reduce the validity of testing tools: factors relating to the testing tool itself, factors relating to the administration of the testing tool, and factors relating to the designation of subjects. Dunn (1990) states, "The instrument itself might have unclear directions, unclear or ambiguous items, items at an in-

appropriate level of difficulty for the designated subjects, items not related to the construct being measured, too few items, or items with an identifiable pattern of response. (p. 68)" If the testing tool states that it is measuring the skills necessary to ride the city bus, has the tool actually "captured" all of the functional skills necessary to do so, or has it left some out? The BUS (Bus Utilization Scale by burlingame, 1989) is a case in point. The clients of a set of group homes had passed all of the bus riding functional assessments the staff could find, and yet, most of the clients were refused access to the bus due to their behavior. The bus riding assessments the staff were using did not capture all of the skills (i.e., social skills) necessary to be able to ride the bus. So, with input from the city transportation staff, staff in charge of training clients, and the clients themselves, the BUS was developed. This test appeared to have better content validity because it "captured" the actual functional abilities required to ride the city bus. Clients (and the control group) who received a passing score were, in fact, able to (and allowed to) ride the city bus, while clients who did not have a passing score could not (and were asked to leave the bus), demonstrating an inability to ride the bus. This type of validity is be content validity. The **Community Integration Program** (Armstrong and Lauzen, 1994) used at Harborview Medical Center in Seattle helped staff predict the risk of re-admittance due to *pressure sores* in patients with spinal cord injuries. Patients who successfully completed five modules had a significantly decreased risk of re-admission due to *pressure sores* (criterion-related validity). In 1990 Julie Dunn presented a workshop on client assessment validation procedures. The table below is

Three Types of Validity

Type	Meaning	Procedure
content validity	How well the test measures subject matter content and behavior under consideration.	Compare test content to the universe of content and behaviors to be measured.
criterion-related validity	How well test performance predicts future performance or estimates current performance on some valued measure other than the test itself.	Compare test scores with another measure of performance obtained at a later date (for prediction) or with another measurement of performance obtained concurrently (for estimating present status).
construct validity	How test performance can be described psychologically.	Experimentally determine what factors influence score on the test.

from that presentation.

Valsalva maneuver the action of holding one's breath while lifting. This action can cause a significant increase in one's blood pressure and increase the load on the heart.

value 1. a personal belief. 2. a numeric representation assigned to an object to help in its evaluation. See *ethics*.

value added network (VAN) (HCO) a data communication network that provides services beyond normal transmission, such as error correction or message storage and forwarding.

variable (HHS) any characteristic that may vary in study subjects, such as gender, age, body weight, diet, behavior, attitude, or other attribute. In an experiment, the treatment is called the independent variable; it is the factor being investigated. The variable that is influenced by the treatment is the dependent variable; it may change as a result of the effect of the independent variable.

variance the amount of difference or variability one would expect in a set of scores. In other words, if you knew what the "average" or "mean" score was, the variance would be differences from that score that would still be considered to be within a normal range. (An example would be the "average" IQ score is 100 but the expected variance is between 90 and 110.) *Standard deviation* is obtained by taking the square root of the variance.

variation the differences found in measuring the same phenomenon more than once. The Joint Commission on Accreditation of Health Care Organizations recognizes two types of variations found when measuring processes: common-cause variation and special-cause variation. The ability to identify and correct excessive variations in processes is important for managing health care costs and treatment outcomes, as large variations tend to increase costs and decrease beneficial outcomes. Common-cause variances (also known as endogenous cause variation or systemic cause variation) are normal fluctuations in a process and its outcomes. The variation is due to the process itself and, because of this, the variation cannot be eliminated without some basic changes being made in the process. An example is getting a treatment group started on an arts and crafts project that allows fine motor range of motion of the hands. The therapist has run this group every other week for the last three years. S/he knows that explaining to a group how to do the activity takes an average of ten minutes (with a normal range of eight to twelve minutes). The typical events that are anticipated and which create a normal range of eight to twelve minutes include reminding patients to put

the brakes on their wheelchairs, making sure that everyone can reach the glue and other supplies, repeating the instructions for patients who have trouble with three-step commands, and listening to quick comments from other staff as they help patients into the room. These "normal" and anticipated events are common-cause variations. Special-cause variations would be events that are outside of what is normally expected and that negatively impact (i.e., increase) the time it takes to explain the activity. Some examples of these special-cause variations would be a fire drill, a patient having a grand mal seizure during the explanation, or finding that someone has replaced all of the glue in the bottles with milk.

varus the inward twisting or bending of a body part causing a malformation and/or loss of functional ability. Opposite of *valgus.*

vascular pertaining to the blood vessels.

vascular dementia a type of *dementia* that is similar to late onset dementia in the types of cognitive losses demonstrated by the patient, only that the damage to the brain is in measurable step-downs due to cerebrovascular accidents and not systematically progressive in a downward flowing manner. (Formerly called multi-infarct dementia.) See *cerebrovascular accident.*

vascular sensation awareness of a change in the tone of the surface capillaries (e.g., blushing). See *sensation.*

vasospasm transient, abnormal constriction of a blood vessel.

vegetarian (HHS) According to the Vegetarian Resource Group, less than 1% of Americans are true vegetarians. Such people never eat meat, fish, or poultry, although they may eat foods derived from animals such as dairy products and eggs (lacto-ovo vegetarians). There are even fewer vegans, strict vegetarians who avoid all animal-derived foods, even honey.

vehicle the transmission of the infectious agent without direct person-to-person transmission. An example would be transmission through tainted food or through arthropods (such as mosquitoes). See *infection, infection control.*

vehicle lift (ADA) the ADA outlines minimum size, function, and weight-bearing ability of vehicle lifts used to help individual's access the vehicle.

vehicular way (ADA) a route intended for vehicular traffic, such as a street, driveway, or parking lot.

venereal disease a dated term now referred to as *sexually transmitted disease* or STD.

ventilator a variety of machines that assist in the breathing process by filling (or causing the lungs to fill) with air. See *bronchopulmonary dysplasia.*

ventral suspension holding an infant, face down, and horizontal across the inside of the professional's lower arm, providing trunk support. This is used as a test to measure the degree of head, leg, back, and hip control the child is able to demonstrate.

verbalize using words to express thoughts.

vertebral artery a branch of the subclavian artery that supplies blood to the brain.

vertigo a feeling of being faint; dizziness.

vestibular pertaining to a *vestibule.*

vestibular board a platform placed on rockers that may be tilted in different directions. The patient is placed on the vestibular board (sitting or lying down) and the platform is rocked so that the orientation of the patient changes as the platform is moved. This allows assessment of the patient's ability to right himself/herself and adjust neuro-muscularly to position changes and provides practice opportunities to improve that ability.

vestibular stimulation activities that help exercise the person's awareness of body position and balance. Swinging, rocking, and dancing are examples of vestibular stimulation.

vestibular system the nerves and bony structures of the ears that are responsible for being able to discern which way is up (equilibrium).

vestibule any of several openings or cavities in the body, especially ones that appear to be an entrance to another cavity. Examples include the structure of the inner ear and the part of the left ventricle below the aortic opening.

vibration a technique used in addition to *percussion* to facilitate drainage of secretions from the airway. The therapist uses both of his/her hands (either side-by-side or on top of one another) and applies slight pressure and rapid vibration on the chest as the patient exhales.

victim thinking the point at which an individual feels that s/he is not able to control the specific situation, current events, or his/her whole life. During traumatic events, it is normal and reasonable for an individual to feel this way. However, if the patient continues to view himself/herself as a "victim," his/her ability to function independently significantly decreases. Matsakis (1994) suggests that the therapist use the checklist below to gauge whether a patient is engaging in "victim thinking." If the patient checks 10 or more of the following 22 statements, Matsakis suggests that this indicates victim thinking. Please note that this checklist is to be used

Victim Thinking

To begin, check the boxes beside those statements that sound like something you find yourself thinking or feeling.

☐ I have to accept bad situations because they are part of life and I can do nothing to make them better.

☐ I don't expect much good to happen in my life.

☐ Nobody could ever love me.

☐ I am always going to feel sad, angry, depressed, and confused.

☐ There are situations at work and at home that I could do something about, but I don't have the motivation to do so.

☐ Life overwhelms me, so I prefer to be alone whenever possible.

☐ You can't trust anyone except a very few people.

☐ I feel I have to be extra good, competent, and attractive in order to compensate for my many defects.

☐ I feel guilty for many things, even things that I know are not my fault.

☐ I feel I have to explain myself to people so that they will understand me. But sometimes I get tired of explaining, conclude it's not worth the effort, and stay alone.

☐ I'm often afraid to do something new for fear I will make a mistake.

☐ I can't afford to be wrong.

☐ I feel that when people look at me, they know right away that I'm different.

☐ Sometimes I think that those who died during the traumatic event I experienced were better off than me. At least they don't have to live with the memories.

☐ I am afraid of the future.

☐ Most times I think things will never get better. There is not much I can do to make my life better.

☐ I can be either a perfectionist or a total slob depending on my mood.

☐ I tend to see people as either for me or against me.

☐ I feel pressure to go along with others, even when I don't want to. To avoid such pressure, I avoid people.

☐ I am never going to get over what happened to me.

☐ I find myself apologizing for myself to others.

☐ I have very few choices in life.

as a gauge and should not be used as a standardized assessment.

Vineland Adaptive Behavior Scales a standardized testing tool which uses a parent interview to measure a client's communication skills, daily living skills, socialization skills, fine, and gross motor skills. The Vineland may be used by the therapist as a beginning point to determine which testing tools to use to obtain a clearer idea of the client's actual functional ability.

violence in the workplace The workplace can be a violent place for staff. The booklet **Healthcare Violence** (Coastal Health Train Publication #V1002H) states that as many as one-third of all nurses are assaulted each year on the job. While most attacks on staff occur on psychiatric units, other units are also experiencing an increase in the frequency of violence against staff. Staff can decrease the chance of violence by taking three preventative steps: 1. Be a good listener. Respond to the patient and their families in a sensitive manner. Be realistic by not promising the unachievable in response to requests. 2. Wear clothing and jewelry which cannot be used against you, e.g., necklaces, tight clothing which limit your physical ability, etc., and 3. Keep physically fit so that you can respond with stamina and strength when you need it. Each unit should have at least two different ways to reach security. This may mean having phone lines in two different places, having an intercom and a phone line, or any other dual means of calling for help. By being ready for violence in the workplace and understanding the *assault cycle*, staff will be able to maintain a safe workplace.

visual acuity the measurement of how clearly a person can perceive objects at different distances. Visual acuity is measured by stating "20/____," with the value placed in the blank space representing how far/close a person must be to an object to perceive it as clearly as a person with normal vision would at 20 feet. In other words, if a patient had a visual acuity of 20/200, the patient could see clearly at 20 feet what most people can see clearly at 200 feet.

visual arts When used as a treatment modality, visual arts is either a process or product which creates a form that can be seen or touched. There is a continuum of visual arts experiences — from fine arts (focus on beauty, art for art's sake) to crafts (art which also has utilitarian purposes) to therapeutic art (art processes to serve a therapeutic purpose).

visual cues the objects in the environment which, when seen, help an individual interpret his/her world. Parking signs, restroom signs, and familiar restaurant signs are different type of visual cues which we use every day. A staff person may use a hand gesture as a visual cue to help a patient remember which way to go back to his/her room. See *cueing*.

Visual Disability Rating Levels a scale containing six levels that describe the degree to which an individual is visually impaired. (no disability to slight = reduced reading distance; moderate = vision correctable with magnifiers; severe = reduced reading speed and/or endurance; profound = inability to manage detailed visual tasks, increased reliance on other senses, and/or difficulty with gross visual tasks such as mobility; near total visual disability = unreliable vision, relies mainly on other senses; total visual disability = no vision, relies on other senses altogether).

visual field the total area the patient is able to see without moving his/her eyes or head.

visual function (RAP) the aging process leads to a gradual decline in visual acuity; a decreased ability to focus on close objects or to see small print, a reduced capacity to adjust to changes in light and dark and diminished ability to discriminate color. The aged eye requires about 3-4 times more light than the young eye in order to see well. The leading causes of visual impairment in the elderly are macular degeneration, cataracts, glaucoma, and diabetic retinopathy. In addition, visual perceptual deficits (impaired perceptions of the relationship of objects in the environment) are common in the nursing home population. Such deficits are a common consequence of *cerebrovascular accidents* and are often seen in the late stages of *Alzheimer's disease* and other *dementias*. The incidence of all these problems increases with age. In 1974, 49% of all nursing home patients were described as being unable to see well enough to read a newspaper with or without glasses. In 1985, over 100,000 nursing home patients were estimated to have visual impairment or no vision at all. Thus, vision loss is one of the most prevalent losses of patients in nursing facilities. A significant number of patients in any facility may be expected to have difficulty performing tasks depending on vision as well as problems adjusting to vision loss.

visual impairment the ability to see is a seven step process. If there is an interruption or malfunction in any of the seven steps, the individual will experience a visual impairment. The degree of impairment, even after treatment, depends on which step is impaired and to what degree. Since information that we receive visually is one of our greatest learning and survival tools, any loss of function changes the way we interact with the world around us.

1. The cornea is a protective covering over the surface of the eye. If this covering is damaged, it distorts the image. A cornea transplant is one means of correction, especially with elderly populations.
2. The anterior chamber is filled with a clear fluid to help the cornea maintain its proper shape.
3. The iris regulates the amount of light allowed into the eye. This regulation of light helps to protect the retina from being "burned" by too much light and helps control the amount of light to allow the best interpretation of objects.
4. The lens adjusts focus to allow better interpretation of images. If the lens becomes cloudy (*cataracts*), everything appears to be blurred and dimmed.
5. The vitreous body contains a clear jell which helps maintain the correct distance between the lens and the retina. It also helps maintain the correct curvature of the retina, allowing better vision. *Glaucoma* is a condition where there is an increased fluid build up in the vitreous body. This buildup stretches the outer perimeter of the eye, stretching the optic nerves to the point of failure. This stretching usually impacts the outer optic nerves first (peripheral vision). Untreated, it progressively stretches the optic nerves toward the center. The end result is tunnel vision or total blindness.
6. The retina's function is to change images into electronic signal that can be interpreted by the brain. There are various causes for deterioration or malformation of the retina, but the professional will most frequently see individuals with damage caused by diabetes and/or aging. *Diabetes* may cause multiple hemorrhages in the retina. These hemorrhages cause dark spots to appear in the individual's vision.
7. The optic nerves transmit the signals from the retina to the vision center of the brain. Youth who have sustained a severe *traumatic brain injury* are at increased risk of damage to these nerves.

Damage to the parts of the brain that interpret vision, may make vision impossible, even if all seven of these steps/body parts are not damaged. The occurrence of severe visual impairment is approximately one in four thousand (Blackman, 1990) for the "normal" population. However, that occurrence rate increases to almost one in three for individuals with multiple disorders. Too frequently, the professional will overlook the importance of training the individual with *developmental disabilities*, dementia, or severe cognitive impairment to wear his/her glasses. The pressure of the glasses on the bridge of the nose or over the ears is difficult to tolerate if you do not understand the reason for the irritation. However, not wearing glasses significantly increases sensory deprivation due to the lack of visual input. The long-term prognosis from this deprivation is a greater degree of disability. Staff sometimes become confused about the issue of an individual's right to refuse to wear glasses. An individual, even one with significant cognitive impairment, cannot give an "informed" refusal for treatment (wearing glasses) if the staff have not first informed the individual about the benefits vs. risks. Since few of these individuals learn well via verbal communication, a training program which 1. promotes the wearing of the glasses to allow the individual to experience improved vision and 2. promotes praise, a positive atmosphere and experiences of success resulting from the improved vision should be implemented.

visualization a type of relaxation technique. Visualization is the process of guiding and controlling your thoughts (like daydreams) to promote a positive mental environment. There are three different types of visualization techniques: guided visualization, programmed visualization, and receptive visualization. Guided visualization is the process of creating a scenario that makes you feel good and then letting your mind "float" as it makes the scene clearer and more enjoyable (e.g., skiing your favorite ski run but with light powder up to your waist which brushes past your face in a sensual manner as you ski perfectly down the slope). Programmed visualization is the process of creating a positive scenario of something that you really want to have happen but question your ability to do (e.g., you want to create a spectacular quilt and slowly "walk" through the design and construction process until you have the whole thing mentally completed). Receptive visualization is the process of emptying your mind except for asking yourself a question and waiting until an answer "floats" into your consciousness (e.g., "Why can't I get up enough courage to ask Chris out?"). See *relaxation techniques*.

visual neglect See *visuospatial neglect, neglect*.

visuospatial neglect lack of awareness of one side of the body. See *neglect*.

vital capacity the largest amount of air that a person can expel from his/her lungs after the person has breathed in as much air as s/he feels his/her lungs can handle. Patients with obstructive airway diseases or severe obesity will have impaired vital capacities. Patients with spinal cord injuries that affect their intercostals and abdominal muscles may lose half of their vital capacity.

vital signs the four basic measurable functions of health are called vital signs: 1. *blood pressure*, 2. *pulse*, 3. respiration, and 4. temperature. See *fever.*

vitamin (HHS) an organic compound that is nutritionally essential in small amounts to control metabolic processes and cannot be synthesized by the body. Vitamins are usually classified by their solubility, which to some degree determines their stability, occurrence in foodstuffs, distribution in body fluids, and tissue storage capacity. Each of the fat-soluble vitamins (A, D, E, and K) has a distinct and separate physiologic role. Several have antioxidant properties to depress the effects of metabolic byproducts called free radicals, which are thought to cause degenerative changes related to aging. Most of the water-soluble vitamins are components of essential enzyme systems. Many are involved in the reactions supporting energy metabolism. These vitamins are not normally stored in the body in appreciable amounts and are normally excreted in the urine. Thus, a daily supply is desirable to avoid depletion and interruption of normal physiologic functions.

vitamin D deficiency (HHS) (causes rickets and osteomalacia) In children, the condition prevents normal bone development; in adults, a lack of vitamin D causes demineralization of bone, particularly in the spine, pelvis, and lower extremities.

vitamin D intoxication (HHS) an overdose of vitamin D; a disorder marked by weight loss, nausea, vomiting, and impaired renal function.

vocational activities functional ability related to the work (vocational) environment including vocational exploration, acquisition of a job, and timely and effective vocational performance. Different from *work activities.*

volition the act of voluntarily and purposely selecting an action to take.

volitional tremor See *tremor.*

volt the International System of Units unit of potential difference and electromotive force, equal to the difference of electric potential between two points of a conductor carrying a constant current of one ampere, when the power dissipated between these points is equal to one watt.

volume indicators a term used in *quality assurance* programs. Volume indicators are measurements which provide the professional with scope (types of interventions required by patients with a C1-C4 complete spinal cord injury), frequency (number of times patients utilize public transportation systems for leisure activities after completing the transportation protocol), and incidence (number of patients who receive medications more than 30 minutes late due to being on a community integration outing). The type of information gathered with volume indicators provides the department with key information to fine-tune strategic planning, develop a realistic budget, and allocate resources better.

voluntary admission admissions where the patient admits himself/herself to a treatment program and is free to leave at any time. See *psychiatric admissions.*

voucher (FB) a form of check indicating a credit against future purchases or expenditures.

WAID See *What Am I Doing.*

walk (ADA) an exterior pathway with a prepared surface intended for pedestrian use, including general pedestrian areas such as plazas and courts.

walker a category of devices that assist with ambulation. Walkers are lightweight devices that usually have four legs and allow the patient to place some or much of his/her weight onto the device to help with balance and movement. They provide more support for the patient than canes do. The patient is usually best positioned for safe ambulation with his/her hands on the handgrips at the side of the walker with his/her elbows bent at a 30° angle. The patient's should place his/her feet approximately 6" to 8" apart, stand up straight, and look forward. Looking down may increase the patient's risk of falling or running into objects. Walkers may have wheels or caps (or a combination of the two) on the ends of the legs. Walkers without wheels are usually used by patients who have at least moderate reciprocal leg action for walking but need added balance support. The patient with this type of walker picks up the walker by holding on to the horizontal side bars, lifting up and forward to place the walker further in front. The patient then takes a few steps up to the walker and repeats the movement. A walker with wheels on all four legs is referred to as a rollator. Rollators are used by patients who need to conserve energy and balance is not as great of an issue (if the patient has poor balance and leans too far forward, holding onto the walker, the patient will fall forward as the walker scoots ahead).

water (HHS) a chemical compound with two hydrogen atoms and one oxygen atom (H_2O). Although deficiencies of energy or nutrients can be sustained for months or even years, a person can survive only a few days without water. Experts rank water second only to oxygen as essential for life. In addition to offering true refreshment for the thirsty, water plays a vital role in all bodily processes. It supplies the medium in which various chemical changes of the body occur, aiding in digestion, absorption, circulation, and lubrication of body joints. For example, as a major component of blood, water helps deliver nutrients to body cells and removes waste to the kidneys for excretion.

water loading the process of drinking excessive amounts of fluids to temporarily increase one's body weight. This is a technique used by patients with eating disorders who are not complying with eating the prescribed number of calories or who are engaging in excessive exercise, and thus have not gained the anticipated weight. To appear to be in compliance with the treatment program, the patient will drink excessive amounts of water right before being weighed.

water mattress bed See *bed.*

watt the International System of Units unit of power, equivalent to one joule per second and equal to the power in a circuit in which the current of one ampere flows across a potential difference of one volt.

Wechsler Preschool and Primary Scale of Intelligence-Revised (WPPSI-R) a standardized test which measures the verbal and performance skills of children between the ages of two and six and a half years.

weight bearing refers to the degree of one's own weight that can be supported by one or more body parts. The abbreviations for different levels of weight bearing are
- Non-weight bearing (NWB)
- Partial weight bearing (PWB)
- Full weight bearing (FWB)

WEST an acronym for <u>w</u>ork <u>e</u>valuation <u>s</u>ystems <u>t</u>echnology, equipment to help the therapist measure the patient's work tolerance for upper extremity and/or total body work. WEST measurements include lifting capabilities and also the torque strength of the hands.

wet-to-dry dressing a type of treatment used with open wounds. The *dressing* is impregnated with normal saline and allowed to dry.

What Am I Doing? (WAID) The WAID was developed by John Neulinger based on his belief that leisure is not a matter of free time but a matter of attitude. The important elements of this attitude are threefold: 1. Perceived Freedom (Choice), 2. Intrinsic Motivation (Reason), and 3. Feeling Tone (Feeling). The WAID Manual and the WAID form were intended to be more than just an assessment tool. The patient was to fill out the form daily, as a kind of journal. Following the rather detailed instructions in the manual, the patient was then to score the assessment himself/herself as an educational/enlightening experience meant to make the patient evaluate his/her own priorities toward leisure. There are two problems associated with using the WAID with patients. The primary one is that the copyright on the forms is still in effect but no additional forms have been available for purchase since the death of Dr. Neulinger in 1992. Only facilities that still have some left over can use the assessment. The second problem associated with using the assessment with patients is that the form requires the patient to use a lot of insight and cognitive energy to complete the form — attributes that are already stressed when an individual is dealing with the effects of an illness or disability. While of historical value, for all intents and purposes, this assessment is not appropriate or available for use with patients.

WIC See *women, infant, and children program.*

Wide Range Achievement Test 3 (WRAT3) The WRAT3 is an IQ/achievement test administered to patients from age 5 through 75. The WRAT3 is usually administered by a psychologist to help identify *learning disabilities* in the areas of reading (recognizing and naming letters, pronouncing printed words), spelling (writing names, writing letters and words from dictation), and arithmetic (counting, reading number symbols, oral problem computations). The results from the WRAT3 are helpful in determining the types of intervention the patient may need from the therapist when combined with the results from specific ability and functional assessments. For example, the therapist can anticipate potential problems related to independent leisure functioning (e.g., being able to read a menu) and be able to identify the patient's problem solving skills related to that deficit (e.g., the patient can use pictures on the menu to order).

willingness-to-pay approach (HCO) a valuation approach used in *cost-benefit analysis* that assigns monetary value to human life by considering how much individuals are willing to pay for a reduction in the risk of death or illness.

Wiscott-Aldrich syndrome (HHS/NMDP) an inherited disease affecting the immune system. Chronic skin problems and frequent infections are characteristics of the disease.

withdrawal related to *substance dependence,* the negative behavioral, cognitive, and physiological changes that are a direct result of the reduction of a substance (drug of abuse) in one's body. Different substances have different withdrawal symptoms, but all generally lead the user to begin using the substance again to avoid withdrawal symptoms. Withdrawal symptoms can be unpleasant, even leading to death. Patients who are incarcerated or on a substance abuse unit are usually "detoxed" on the unit under close medical supervision. During the first

three to seven days of withdrawal the patient will probably not be able to tolerate activities. The two key symptoms of withdrawal are 1. the typical physiological and behavioral symptoms associated with withdrawal for the specific drug and/or 2. the taking of another, similar drug to reduce or avoid the withdrawal symptoms. See *alcohol dependence.*

Woman, Infants, and Children Program (WIC) a federally funded endowment program that provides food vouchers, nutritional counseling and health care referrals to participants who qualify. Established in 1972, the WIC program provides food and nutrition education to improve the nutritional status of medically high-risk pregnant and lactating women and children up to 5 years of age from low-income families. The program is administered by the US Department of Agriculture.

word salad a speech disorder where the patient seems to randomly toss together words without any meaning or sense. Word salad is sometimes seen in patients with *aphasia* or with *schizophrenia.*

work activities activities related to home management skills (preparing meals, cleaning the house, taking care of clothing, maintaining the house), care of others, and safety awareness and skills. See *ergonomics, vocational activities.*

work hardening an interdisciplinary approach to prepare an injured worker for return to the workplace. This includes education in appropriate body mechanics, strengthening of appropriate muscles, and acquisition of appropriate safety equipment (e.g., wrist brace). See *ergonomics, physical activities.*

World Health Organization (WHO) the public health care agency which is part of the United Nations. WHO is best known as the publisher of the *International Classification of Impairments, Disabilities, and Handicaps; A Manual of Classification Relating to the Consequences of Disease* (ICIDH). The ICIDH is the only internationally recognized system of standardized terminology that is used by all health care professionals (clinicians as well as researchers).

WPPSI-R See *Wechsler Preschool and Primary Scale of Intelligence-Revised.*

WRAT3 See *Wide Range Achievement Test 3.*

wrist disarticulation an amputation through the wrist joint. Special wrist disarticulation prosthesis are designed to help retain as normal as possible *range of motion* in the wrist joint. The socket edge of the prosthetic device is usually cut back anteriorly to allow maximum flexion. The prosthesis for a wrist disarticulation has four parts:

1.   figure 8 harness control

2. flexible elbow hinges
3. wrist unit
4. a terminal device

This prosthesis greatly enhances the patient's functional ability. But, the extensive "hardware" which extends from the wrist, up the back of the arm, and crisscrosses the back and the chest, poses a challenge for normalization. The wrist disarticulation is abbreviated "WD."

X Y Z

xenobiotics (HHS) synthetic chemicals believed to be resistant to environmental degradation. A branch of biotechnology called bioremediation is seeking to develop biological methods to degrade such compounds.

xenophobia an abnormal fear of strangers or of strange places.

X-linked dominant disorder any disorder that is transferred via the dominant gene on the X chromosome.

X-linked recessive disorder any disorder that is transferred via the recessive gene on the X chromosome.

X-value the value of the score on the x-axis.

XYY syndrome See *chromosomal aberrations*.

YAVIS syndrome an acronym for y̲oung, a̲ttractive, v̲erbal, i̲ntelligent, s̲uccessful. A tongue-in-check term which describes a group of people who tend to seek professional help (counseling) for "problems" usually resolvable through cognitive therapy. YAVIS patients help balance the practitioner's load, giving some relief from patients who have very complex problems. While YAVIS patients want to seek help to be more "mentally healthy," there is some discussion about the ethical use of insurance funds to pay for such services, draining resources from companies who also have patients with more severe, organic mental disorders.

zooerasty sexual intercourse with an animal.

zoomatology the study of diseases and parasites which can be transmitted between animals and humans.

Analytical List

A

a(n)	absence, without
ab-	away from
abdomin-	abdomen
acid	sour
acou-	hear
acre-	extremity
act-	do, act
actin-	radius, ray
ad-	toward
aden-	gland
adip(o)-	fat
-aemia	blood
aer-	air
aesthe-	perceive, feel
-agogue	inducing, leading
-agra	catching, seizure
alb-	white
alg-	pain
all-	different, other
alve-	channel, cavity
ambi-	on both sides
an	negative
ana-	positive, up
andr-	man
angi-	vessel
anis(o)-	unequal
ankyl-	looped, crooked
ante-	before
anti-	against, counter to
antr-	cavern
-aph	touch
apo-	away from, detached
arch-	beginning, origin
arter(i)-	artery, windpipe
arthr(o)-	joint
articul-	joint
-ase	enzyme
aur-	ear
aut(o)-	self

B

ba-	walk, stand, go
ball-	throw
bar-	weight
bi-	life, two
bil-	bile

bio-	pertaining to life
-biosis	life
blast-	bud, early stages
blep-	see, look
blephar-	eyelid
bol-	ball
brachi-	arm
brachy-	short
brady-	slow
brom-	stench
bronch-	windpipe
bucc-	cheek

C

cac-	abnormal, bad
calc-	heel
calor-	heat
cancr-	cancer
capit-	head
caps-	container
carcin-	cancer
cardi-	heart
cat-	down
cata-	negative
caud-	tail
cav-	hollow
cec-	blind
-cele	tumor, hernia
cell-	room, cell
cen-	common
cent-	hundred
cente-	to puncture
centre-	point, center
cephal-	head
cept-	receive
cerebr-	cerebrum
cervic(i)(o)-	neck
cheil-	lip
cheir-	hand
chem-	chemical
chlor-	green
chol-	bile
chondr-	cartilage
chord-	string, cord
chro-	color
chron-	time

chy-	pour
-cid(e)	kill, cut
cili-	eyelid
circum-	around
-cis	cut, kill
clas-	break
clin-	bend, incline
clus-	shut
co-, com-	together
cocc-	seed, pill
coel-	hollow
col-	colon
colon-	lower intestine
colp-	hollow, vagina
con-	with, together
contra-	against
corpor-	body
cost-	rib
crani-	skull
creat-	meat, flesh
-crescent	grow
cret-	separate off, different
crur-	shin, leg
cry-	cold
crypt-	conceal
cult-	tend
cune-	wedge
cut-	skin
cyan-	blue
cycl-	circle
cyst-	bladder
cyt-	cell

D

dacry-	tears
dactyl(o)-	finger, toe
de-	down from
dec-	ten
demi-	half
dent-	tooth
derm-	skin
-derm	skin
desm-	band, ligament
dextr-	right, hand
di-	two
dia-	apart, through, across

didym-	twin	fract-	break	hypo-	below
digit-	finger, toe	front-	front, forehead	**I**	
diplo-	double	-fug(e)	avoid		
dis-	away from, negative, absence of	funct-	perform, function	-iasis	pathological state, condition
disc-	disk	fund-	pour	iatr-	physician
dors-	back	**G**		idi-	separate, self
-dorsal	back			ile-	ileum
drom-	course	galact-	milk	ili-	lower abdomen
-ducent	lead, conduct	gam-	union	im-	in, on
dur-	hard	gangli-	swelling	in-	fiber *also* in, on, *also* negative
dynam(i)-	power	gastr-	stomach		
dys-	improper, bad, painful, out from	gelat-	congeal, freeze	infra-	beneath
		gemin-	twin, double	inter-	among, between
E		gen-	become, originate	intra-	inside
				is-	equal
ec-	out of	ger(o)	aging	ischi-	hip
-ech-	have, hold	germ-	bud, growth	-ism	condition, theory
ect-	outside	gest-	carry	iso-	equal
-ectomy	surgical removal	gli-	glue like	-itis	inflammation
ede-	swell	gloss-	tongue	-ize	to use special method
-elc-	sore, ulcer	glott-	tongue, language		
-em	blood			**J**	
-emesis	vomiting	gluc(o)	sweet		
en-	in, on, inside	glyc(y)-	sweet	jact-	throw
end-	inside	gnath-	jaw	-ject	throw
enter-	intestine	gno-	know	jejun-	jejunum
ento-	within	gon(o)-	semen, seed	jug-	yoke
epi-	upon, after, additionally	grad-	walk, take steps	junct-	join, yoke
		-gram	letter, drawing	juxta-	near
erg-	work	gran-	particle, grain	**K**	
eso-	inside	-graph	write, record		
esthe-	perceive, feel	grav-	heavy	kary-	nucleus
eu-	good, normal	gyn-	woman	kil-	one thousand
ex-	out of	**H**		kine-	move
exo-	outside			-kinesis	motion
extra-	beyond, outside	hapt-	touch	**L**	
F		hect-	hundred		
		helc-	sore, ulcer	labi-	lip
faci-	face	hem(at)-	blood	lact-	milk
-facient	make	hemi-	half	lal-	babble
fasci-	band, bundle	hen-	one	lapar-	flank
febr-	fever	hepat-	liver	laryng-	windpipe
-ferent	carry, bear	hered-	heir	lat-	carry
ferr-	iron	hetero-	other, different	later-	side
feto-	fetus	hidr-	sweat	lep-	take, seize
fibr-	fiber	hist-	web, tissue	leuk-	white
fil-	thread	hod-	path	lien-	spleen
fiss-	split	hom-	common, same	lig-	bind
-flect-	divert, bend	horm-	impulse	lingu-	tongue
flu-	flow	hydat-	water	lip-	fat
for-	opening	hydr-	water	loc-	place
fore-	in front of	hyper-	above	log-	speak
-form	shape	hypn-	sleep	-logia	science of

lumb- loin
lute- yellow
ly- loose
lymph- water, lymph
lyo- dissolved
-lysis setting free: disintegration

M

macr- long, large
mal- abnormal, bad
malac- soft
mamm- breast
man- hand
mani- mental aberration
mast- breast
medi- middle
mega- large
megal- great
mel- limb, member
melan- black
men- month
mening- membrane
meno- menses
ment- mind
mer- part
mes- middle
meta- after
mill- one thousand
mio- less
-mittent send
mne- remember
mon- one, only
morph- form
mot- move
multi- many
my- muscle
myc- fungus
myel- marrow, spinal cord
myx- mucus

N

narc- numbness, stupor
nas- nose
ne- new, young
necr- corpse
neo- new
nephr- kidney
neur- nerve
nom- custom
non- no
nos- disease
nutri- nourish

O

ob- against, toward
ocul- eye
-ode path, road
odont- tooth
-odyn pain, distress
-oid form, resemblance
ole- oil
olig- few, small
-oma tumor
omo- shoulder
onc- mass
onych- nail, claw
op- see
ophthamal- eye
or- mouth
orb- circle
orchi- testicle
orth- straight, normal
-osis condition, disease, intensive
-osm smell
oss- bone
ost(e)- bone
ot- ear
ox- oxygenation

P

pachy(n)- thicken
pag- fix, make
pan- all, entire
par- bear
para- beside, beyond
part- give birth to
path- sickness, disease
pec- fix, make fast
ped- child
pell- skin
-pellent drive
pen- need, lack
pend- hang down
peps- digest
pept- digest
per- through
peri- around
pet- seek
pex- make fast
pha- say, speak
phac- lens

phag- eat
pharmac- drug
pharyng- throat
phen- show, be seen
pher- support
phil- have affinity for
phleb- vein
phleg- burn
phob- fear, dread
phon- sound
phot- light
phren- mind
phthi- waste away, decay
phy- produce
phyl- kind, tribe
phylac- guard
phys(a) blow
pil- hair
plas- mold, shape
-plasia growth
platy- broad, flat
pleg- strike
-plegia paralysis
pleur- rib, side
plex- strike
plur- more
pne- breathing
pneumo(n) lungs
pod- foot
poie- make, produce
pol- axis of a sphere
poly- many
pont- bridge
-por passageway
posit- place, put
post- after
-praxia movement
pro- before
proct- anus
prosop- face
proto- first
pseud- false
psych- soul, mind
pub- adult
pulmo(n)- lung
puls- drive
punct- pierce
pur- pus
pyel- pelvis, kidney
pyl- orifice
pyr- fire

Q

quadr- four

R

rachi-	spine
radi-	ray
re-	again, contrary
ren-	kidneys
retro-	backwards
rhag-	break
-rhage	hemorrhage
rhaph-	suture
rhe-	flow
rhex-	break
rhin-	nose
rot-	wheel
-rrhea	fluid discharge
rub-	red

S

sacro-	sacrum
sanguin-	blood
sarc-	flesh
schis-	split
scler-	hard, dry
scolio-	crooked
scop-	look at, observe
sect-	cut
semi-	half
sens-	perceive, feel
sep-	rot, decay
sial-	saliva
sin-	fold
sit-	food
solut-	loose, set free
somat-	body
spas-	draw
spectr-	appearance
spers-	scatter
sphen-	wedge
spher-	ball
sphygm-	pulsation
spin-	spine
spirat-	breathe
splen-	spleen
sta-	make stand, stop
stal-	send
stear-	fat
sten-	narrow
ster-	solid
-stol	send
stom(a)	orifice
-stomy	opening
strep(h)	twist
-strict	draw tight, cause pain

sub-	under, below
super-	beyond, above
syn-	with, together

T

tachy-	swift, rapid
tack-	order
tact-	touch
tax-	order
-taxis	movement
teg-	cover
tel-	end
tele-	at a distance
tempor-	timely
ten-	tightly stretched band
tens-	stretch
tetra-	four
the-	put
therap-	treatment
therm-	heat
thorac-	chest
thromb-	lump, clot
thym-	spirit
thyr-	shield
tom-	cut
ton-	stretch, put under tension
top-	place
tors-	twist
tox-	poison
trache-	windpipe
trachel-	neck
tract-	draw, drag
trans-	across
traumat-	wound
tri-	three
trich-	hair
trip-	rub
trop-	turn, react
troph-	nurture
tuber-	swelling
typ-	type
typhl-	blind

U

ultra-	beyond
un-	one
ur-	urine
-uria	urine

V

vagin-	sheath
vas-	vessel

ven(o)	vein
ventr(o)-	belly, front
vert-	turn
vertebr(o)	vertebra
vesic(o)	bladder
vit-	life
vuls-	pull, twitch

Y

-yl-	substance

Z

zo-	life

Units of Measure

Le Système Internationale d'Unités is an international set of rules which govern the way medical and scientific units of measure are reported. Below are some of the rules for using abbreviations and other scientific symbols.
1. Do not use periods in abbreviations e.g., kg, not k.g.
2. Do not use an "s" to indicate plurals e.g., 25 mm not 25 mms
3. Avoid using commas as a spacer in larger numbers, as some countries use commas to mean decimal points.
4. Do not use the degree sign (°) when using the Kelvin temperatures e.g., 310k not 310° k

Temperature
$0°C = 32°F$
$100°C = 212°F$
$273k = 0°C = 32°F$
$°C = (°F - 32) \times 5/9$
$°F = (9/5 \ °C) + 32$

Distance
1 inch = 2.54 centimeters (cm) = 25.4 millimeters (mm) = 0.0254 meters (m)
1 foot = 30.48 cm = 304.8 mm = 0.305 m
1 mile = 5280 feet = 1760 yards = 1609.35 meters = 1.61 kilometers (km)
1 cm = 0.3937 inch
1 m = 39.37 inches = 3.28 feet = 1.09 yards
1 km = 0.62 mile

Oxygen
1 liter of oxygen consumed = 5.05 kcal = 15,575 foot pounds = 2153 kg-m = 1.057 quarts
1 quart = 0.946 liter

Energy and Work
Work = energy = application of a force over a distance
1 kilocalorie (kcal) = amount of energy required to heat 1 kilogram (kg) of water 1 degree centigrade
1 foot-pound (ft-lb) = the amount of work required to move 1 lb by 1 foot
1 kilogram-meter (kg-m) = the amount of work required to move 1 kg by 1 meter
1 kcal = 3086 foot-pounds = 426.4 kg-m
1 foot pound = 0.1383 kg-m
1 kg-m = 723 foot pounds

Weights
1 ounce (oz) = 0.0625 pounds = 28.35 grams (g) = 0.028 kg
1 pound (lb) = 16 oz = 454 g = 0.454 kg
1 g = 0.035 oz = 0.0022 pounds = 0.001 kg
1 kg = 35.27 oz = 2.2 pounds = 1000 grams

Velocity
1 foot per second (ft/sec) = 0.3048 m/sec = 18.3 m/min = 1.1 km per hour (km/hr) = 0.68 mile/hr (mph)
1 mph = 88 ft/min = 1.47 ft/sec = 0.45 m/sec = 26.8 m/min = 1.61 km/hr
1 km/hr = 16.7 m/min = 0.28 m/sec = 0.91 ft/sec = 0.62 mph

Medical Abbreviations

Introduction

In today's health care arena, professionals are expected to have acquired a working knowledge of medical abbreviations and terminology. There seems to be, however, confusion on exact usage and meaning for many abbreviations and terms. This primer is designed to offer a "ready reference" for many of the terms therapists may encounter in the delivery of services within clinical and non-clinical settings.

It is important to note that this primer should not be interpreted as the final word but does integrate abbreviations and terminology from multiple authorities. Frequently, however, the practitioner and pre-professional may find exceptions that are agency specific. In such situations, the practitioner should defer to the agency's accepted abbreviations or terminology.

Medical Abbreviations

Abbreviations are listed in alphabetical order, using Roman letter ordering. The absence of a letter precedes the letter A. For instance L precedes LA. Furthermore, abbreviations using numbers are alphabetized by letter first then by number. The abbreviation qh precedes q2h which precedes q hor and qid. Likewise, numbers may also be ignored in the ordering of abbreviations. Therefore, 3-D is listed in the D section but follows D and 2-D. Punctuation, such as a dash, and spaces are ignored in deciding the order. For example:

D	date, daughter, day…
d	diarrhea, divorced, doctor, …
1-D	one-dimensional
2-D	two-dimensional
3-D	three-dimensional
D1…D12	dorsal vertebrae 1 through 12

Greek letters and non-alphabetical symbols are listed in separate sections. The Greek alphabet is listed in alphabetical order. However, symbols are listed by categorical use.

Again, it is important to recognize that many abbreviations have multiple usages and should be interpreted in context of use. The user should also acknowledge the diversity of interpretation for medical abbreviations and terminology.

Terminology

It is not the intent of this primer to provide a comprehensive listing of medical terminology. It is the intent to this primer to offer terminology that enhances a working knowledge of frequently encountered terms for the practice of therapy.

A

A ....abnormal; absolute (also abs); absorbency; adrenaline; adult; age; allergy; alternate; assistance; atomic weight; axial; water (aqua); year (annum); accommodation; area; alveolar (gas)

a ....absent; accommodation; acid; ampere; anterior; artery; arterial; asymmetric; prefix meaning no, not, without (i.e. atypical); anode; before/prior to (ante)

Å ....Ångstrom unit

A2 ....aortic second sound (heart)

AA ....achievement age; active assistance; acetic acid; adjuvant arthritis; Administration on Aging; affirmative action; Alcoholics Anonymous; atomic absorption; African-American

aa........................of each (ana); arteries (arteriae)

AAA....................abdominal aortic aneurysm; acquired aplastic anemia; acute anxiety attack; androgenic anabolic agent; American Academy of Allergy

aaa......................amalgam (amalgama)

A&A ....aid and attendance; awake and aware

AADL ....advanced activities of daily living

AAEM................American Academy of Emergency Medicine

AAF ....acetylaminoflourene; acetic acid-alcohol-formalin mixture; ascorbic acid factor

AAHPERD ....American Alliance for Health, Physical Education, Recreation, and Dance

AAL ....anterior axillary line

AALR ....American Association for Leisure and Recreation

AAM..................amino acid mixture

AAP ....air at atmospheric pressure; American Academy of Periodontology; American Association of Physicians

AAPCC..............average adjusted per capita cost

AAPS.................American Association of Physician Specialists

AAR....................antigen-antiglobulin reaction; Australian antigen radioimmunoassay

AAROM ....active assistive range of motion

AARP.................American Association of Retired Persons

AASA ....American Association of School Administrators

AAT ....acute abdominal tympani

AB......................able-bodied; blood type; abnormal; asthmatic bronchitis

Ab ....abortion; antibody

ab ....about; prefix meaning away from (Latin); abortion

ABA....................antibacterial activity; Architectural Barriers Act

abbr ....abbreviations

abd ....abduction; abdominal

ABDA.................American Board of Disability Analysts

ABE ....acute bacterial endocarditis; adult basic education

ABEM................American Board of Emergency Medicine

ABG...................arterial blood gases

ABL ....antigen-binding lymphocytes

abnl ....abnormal

ABO...................absent bed occupant/occupancy

ABP ....arterial blood pressure

ABR...................absolute bed rest

abras..................abrasions

abs......................absent; absolute; absorb

ABS ....acute brain syndrome

absc ....abscissa

ABS-RC:2..........adaptive behavior scale — residential and community: 2nd edition

AC......................acetylcholine; acromioclavicular; adaptive control; adherent cell; adrenal cortex; air conduction; alternating current; ambulatory care; anticoagulant; aortic closure; ascending colon; atriocarotid; axiocervical; acid; antiphlogistic corticoid

ac........................acid; acute; before meals (ante cibum)

ACA....................acute cerebellar ataxia; adenocarcinoma; anterior cerebral artery; American College of Allergist; American College of Anesthesiologist; American Counseling Association

acad....................academy

ACB ....aortocoronary (saphenous vein) bypass; arterialized capillary blood

acc......................according to; accident; accommodation

ACC ....adenoid cystic carcinoma; alveolar cell carcinoma; ambulatory care center; American College of Cardiology; activity coordinator, certified

accel.....................acceleration

ACCH ....Association for the Care of Children's Health

accid....................accident

accom..................accommodation (eye)

accum..................accumulation

accur....................accurately (accuratissime)

ACD.....................absolute cardiac dullness; acid, citrate, dextrose; allergic contact dermatitis

ACE ....adrenal cortical extract; angiotensin converting enzyme

ACEP ....American College of Emergency Physicians

ACF ....accessory clinical finding; advanced communications function; anterior cervical fusion

AC-G...................accelerator globulin

ACGIH................American Conference of Governmental Industrial Hygienists

ACHi....................arm girth, chest depth, hip width index

ACL ....anterior cruciate ligament

ACLD ....Association for Children with Learning Disabilities

ACLF ....adult congregate living facility

ACLS ....advanced cardiac life support training course

ACO.....................acute coronary occlusion

ACOA ....Adult Children of Alcoholics

acous ....acoustics

ACP ....aspirin, caffeine, and phenacetin; American College of Physicians

ACR ....abnormal contracting regions; anticonstipation regime; America College of Radiology

acr ....acrylic

ACROS ....Automated Cross Referencing Occupational System

ACS ....acute confusional state; ambulatory care services

ACT ....anticoagulant therapy; activated coagulation (clotting) time; anxiety control training; American College Testing

act ....activity

ACTH ....adrenocorticotropic hormone

activ ....activity

ACTS..................advanced communication and technology satellite

ACU.....................acute care unit; ambulatory care

unit

ACV.....................arterial, carotid, ventricular; atherosclerotic cardiovascular

ACVD.................acute cardiovascular disease

Ac/W...................acetone/water

AD ....activity director; active disease; achievement drive; adenoidal degeneration; admitting diagnosis; Alzheimer's disease; average deviation; axis deviation; right atrium (atrium dexter); right ear (auras dextra)

ad ....add; to (Latin)

A&D ....ascending and descending

ADA...................Americans with Disabilities Act; American Dental Association; American Diabetes Association; American Dietetic Association; American Dermatological Association

ad aur ....to the ear (ad aur em)

ADC....................Aid to Dependent Children

ADD....................attention deficit disorder

add ....let there be added (adde); adduction

ADE....................acute disseminated encephalitis

ad def an..............to the point of fainting (ad defectionem animi)

ad deliq ....to faint (ad deliquium)

ad effect ....until effective (ad effectum)

ADEM ....acute disseminated encephalomyelitis

ADH....................anti-diuretic hormone

ADHD................attention-deficit hyperactivity disorder

adhib ....to be administered; apply; take (adhibendus)

ADHR................anti-diuretic-hormone-resistant diabetes

ad int ....in the meantime (ad interim)

adj ....adjoining; adjunct; adjutant

ADL ....activities of daily living

ad lib ....as desired (ad libitum)

adm ....administrator; admission; admit

ADM..................average daily membership

ad man med........deliver to the physician (ad manus medici)

admin ....administration

admov ....let it be applied (ad move)

ADMR ....average daily metabolic rate

ad naus ....producing nausea (ad nauseum)

ad neut...............to neutralize (ad neutralizandum)

ADP ....alternative disposition plan

ad part dol ....to the painful parts (ad partes dolentes)

ADPL...................average daily patient load

ad pond om ....to the weight of the whole (ad pondus omnium)

adq ....adequate

ADR....................accepted dental remedies; adverse drug reaction; alternative dispute resolution; appropriate dispute resolution

Adr ....adrenaline

ADS ....antibody deficiency syndrome; anti-diuretic substance

ad sat...................at saturation (ad saturandum)

adst feb................while fever is present (adstante febre)

ADT....................any desired thing (any damn thing); placebo labeling; automated dithionate test

ad us ext..............for external use (ad usum externum)

ad us....................according to custom (ad usum)

adv ....advanced; advertisement; against (adversum)

ad 2 vic................for two doses (ad duas vices)

ADVOC-NET .....Adult Vocational Network

AE......................above elbow; accurate empathy; acro-dermatitis enteropathica; adaptive equipment; age equivalent

AEC ....at earliest convenience

AECG ....abnormal electrocardiograph

AED....................automatic external defibrillator

AEE ....Association for Experiential Education

AEG ....air encephalogram

aeg......................patient (aeger, aegra)

AEM ....ambulatory EKG monitor

AEP....................auditory evoked potential; average evoked potential

AEq....................age equivalent

aeq......................equal (aequales)

AER ....Association for Education and Rehabilitation of the Blind and Visually Impaired

AERA ....American Educational Research Association

aet ....at the age of (aetas); aged

AF ....acid fast; antibody forming; atrial fibrillation or flutter; auricular fibrillation

AFB ....acid-fast bacillus; a type of isolation procedure for TB

AFDC.................Aid to Families with Dependent Children

AFG ....auditory figure ground

AFIB ....atrial fibrillation

AFl......................atrial flutter

AFO ....ankle-foot orthosis

AFRD.................acute febrile respiratory disease

AFRI ....acute febrile respiratory illness

AFS(D) ....Adult and Family Services Division

AFT....................American Federation of Teachers

Ag ....antigen; silver

AG ....antiglobulin; atrial gallop

A/G ....albumin/globulin ratio

AGA...................accelerated growth area; appropriate for gestational age

AGE ....angle of greatest extension

AGF ....angle of greatest flexion

ag fed ....while the fever increases (aggrediente febre)

agit ante sum ....shake before taking (agita ante sumendum)

agit vas................shake the vile (agitato vase)

AGL ....acute granulocytic leukemia

agt ....agent

AGT ....antiglobulin test; automated guideway transit

AGTT ....abnormal glucose tolerance test

AH ....auditory hallucination

A&H ....accident and health

AHA...................American Heart Association; American Hospital Association

AHCA ....American Health Care Association

AHCPR..............Agency for Health Care Policy and Research

AHPB.................adjusted historical payment base

AHSD ....adult high school diploma

AHTA ....American Horticultural Therapy Association

AI.......................aortic insufficiency

AIDS..................acquired immune deficiency syndrome

AIMS ....Academic Instrumental Measurement System

AIR ....American Institute for Research

AIT ....Agency for Instructional Technology; auditory integrated training

AITN..................Arizona International Telemedicine Network

AIVR ....accelerated idioventricular rhythm

AJ.......................ankle jerk

AK ....above knee

AKA...................above knee amputation; also known as

ALB ....albumin; white

ALJ ....administrative law judge

alk p'tase.............alkaline phosphatase

ALL....................acute lymphoblastic leukemia

ALO...................alternative learning options

ALS....................amyotrophic lateral sclerosis; advanced life support

alt dieb. ....every other day

alt hor.................every other hour

AMA..................against medical advice; American Medical Association

AMAC ....adults molested as children

AMB ....ambulate

AMC ....arthrogryposis multiplex congenita

AMD..................age-related macular degeneration

AMI ....acute myocardial infarction; Alliance for the Mentally Ill

AML ....acute myeloblastic leukemia

AMOL.................acute monoblastic leukemia

amp ....ampule

amt ....amount

ANA..................antinuclear antibodies; American Nurses Association; American Neurological Association

anat....................anatomy

anes ....anesthesiology

ANLL..................acute non-lymphocytic leukemia

ANOVA ....analysis of variance

ANSI..................American National Standards Institute

ant ....anterior; antenna

ante....................before

AO ....ankle orthosis

AOA...................American Osteopathic Association

AODM ....adult onset diabetes mellitus

AOPA.................American Orthotic and Prosthetic Association

AOTA ....American Occupational Therapy Association

AOTCB...............American Occupational Therapy Certification Board

AP ....anterior-posterior; appendix; atrial pressure; alum precipitated; action potential; Academy of Periodontology; apical pulse

A/P.....................anterior-posterior

APA....................American Psychiatric Association; American Psychological Association

APCOR...............advanced portable coronary observation radio

APE....................acute pulmonary edema; adapted physical education

AP&L.................anterior, posterior, and lateral

APLS ....advanced pediatric life support

approx ....approximately

APTA ....American Physical Therapy Association

aq ....water

AR-177 ....an anti-HIV drug

ARC...................American Red Cross

Arc ....formerly Association for Retarded Citizens

arch ....architectural

ARDS.................adult respiratory distress syndrome

ARF ....acute renal failure

AROM ....active range of motion

AS ....aortic stenosis; androsterone sulfate; ankylosing spondylitis; arteriosclerosis; atrial stenosis; left ear

ASA ....aspirin (acetylsalicylic acid); America Standards Association; Autism Society of America

ASAP ....as soon as possible

ASC ....accredited standards committee; ambulatory surgical center; Advanced Study Center

ASCD.................Association for Supervision and Curriculum Development; American Society for Curriculum Development

ASCVD...............arteriosclerotic cardiovascular disease

ASD ....atrial septal defect

ASHA ....American Speech, Language, and Hearing Association

ASHD ....arteriosclerotic heart disease

ASIA ....American Spinal Injury Association

ASL....................American Sign Language

ASOHI ....Association for Severely Other Health Impaired

ASTM ....American Society for Testing and Materials

AT ....assistive technology

ATA....................Alliance for Technology Access

ATBCB ....Architecture and Transportation Barriers Compliance Board

ATC....................area technical center

ATLS..................advanced trauma life support training course

ATM...................asynchronous transfer mode; automated teller machine

ATP....................advanced technology program; adenosine triphosphate

ATRA.................American Therapeutic Recreation Association

ATSDR...............Agency for Toxic Substances and Disease Registry

AU ....both ears

Au ....gold

AV ....arteriovenous; atrioventricular

AVA.....................American Vocational Association
AVEA..................Adult Vocational Education Association
AVEPDA.............American Vocational Education Personnel Development Association
AVERA ....American Vocational Education Research Association
AVPU..................alert, verbal, pain, unresponsive (trauma alertness scale)
AVTI ....area vocational technical institute
ax ....axillary; axis

B

B ....bilateral
BA......................bachelor of arts
Ba......................barium
BAC...................blood alcohol concentration
BaEn ....barium enema
BAEP.................brainstem auditory evoked potential
BAER.................brainstem auditory evoked response
BAL ....blood alcohol level
BASIS................Basic Adult Skills Inventory System
b/c ....because
BCEM................Board of Certification in Emergency Medicine
BCP....................biochemical profile; bromcresol purple; Blue Cross Plan
BD.....................behavior disorder; brain damaged
BE ....below elbow; base excess; bacterial endocarditis; barium enema
BEA ....below elbow amputation
BEE....................basal energy expenditure
BEH ....behaviorally/emotionally handicapped
BES....................balanced electrolyte solution
BEST ....basic education study team
BH.....................behaviorally handicapped
BHT ....blunt head trauma
BI ....bodily injury; brain injury
BIA ....Brain Injury Association; Bureau of Indian Affairs
BIBA..................brought in by ambulance
bid......................twice a day (bis in die)
bil.......................bilateral; bilirubin
BK......................below knee
BKA...................below knee amputation
bl cult.................blood culture
BLE....................bilateral lower extremities
BLRS ....Brief Leisure Rating Scale
BLS.....................basic life support

BM.....................bowel movement; bone marrow; basal metabolism
BMP...................behavior modification program
BMR ....basal metabolic rate
BNL ....below normal limits
BP ....blood pressure; birthplace; bed pan; British pharmacopoeia
BPD ....bronchopulmonary dysplasia
BPH ....benign prostatic hypertrophy
bpm ....beats per minute
BR......................bed rest
BRAT ....bananas, rice (cereal), applesauce, and toast
BRBPR ....bright red blood per rectum
BRFSS ....Behavioral Risk Factor Surveillance System
BRP....................bathroom privileges
BRT....................Business Round Table
BS ....bowel sounds; breath sounds; bachelor of science
bs........................breath sounds
BSE....................bovine spongiform encephalopathy
BSN ....bachelor degree in nursing; bowel sounds normal
BSP ....bromsulphalein
BSW ....bachelor degree in social work
BTW ....by the way
BUN...................blood urea nitrogen
BUO...................bilateral ureteral obstruction
B/V ....bivalve
BVM ....bag-valve mask (ventilation)
BW.....................body weight; biological warfare; birth weight; blood Wassermann
Bx ....biopsy

C

C ....content; contraction; cortex; coulomb; coefficient; color sense; complement; compound; carbohydrate; carbon; cathode; Catholic; Caucasian; cerebrospinal fluid; certified; cervical; chest; cholesterol; clearance; clonus; closure; centigrade; Celsius; calorie; canine; capacitance; capillary; contact; curie; cycle; hundred
c̄ ....with
°C......................degrees Celsius or centigrade
C1 to C7.............cervical vertebrae or nerves
Ca......................cancer; carcinoma; cathode; calcium
CA......................chronological age
CAAM ....complimentary and alternate medicine

CAAS.................Commission on Accreditation of Ambulance Services

CABG ....coronary artery bypass graft

CAD..................coronary artery disease

CALS ....Canadian Association for Leisure Studies

CAM ....certificate of advanced mastery

CAMH ....Comprehensive Accreditation Manual for Hospitals

cap(s) ....capsules; capacity; let him take

CAPD................central auditory processing disorder

CAP-MR/DD ......community alternatives program for people who are severely mentally retarded/developmentally disabled

cardio ....cardiology; cardiac surgery

CARF................CARF: the Rehabilitation Accreditation Commission.

CASA................court appointed special advocate

CAT..................computerized axial tomography; Committee on Accessible Transportation

cath..................catheter; cathartic; cathode

CBA..................cost-benefit analysis

CBC..................complete blood count

CBS..................chronic brain syndrome

CC....................chief complaint; coronary collateral; critical condition; cord compression; correlation; clean catch; commission certified as in CCC - Audiology

cc......................cubic centimeter(s)

CCC-A ....Certificate of Clinical Competence - Audiology

CCC-SLP ....Certificate of Clinical Competence - Speech, Language Pathology

CCS..................Children's Coma Scale

CCU..................coronary care unit

CDC..................Centers for Disease Control

CDH..................congenital dislocation (or dysplasia) of hip

CDRC ....Child Development and Rehabilitation Center

CD-ROM ....compact disk, read-only memory

CDS ....child development specialist; controlled dangerous substance

CDSS ....clinical decision support system

CEA ....cost-effectiveness analysis

ceph..................cephalic

CERT ....Comprehensive Evaluation in Recreational Therapy

CF ....cystic fibrosis

CFIDS...............chronic fatigue and immune dysfunction syndrome

CFR...................Code of Federal Regulations; certified first responder

CFS ....chronic fatigue syndrome

CFSEI ....Culture Free Self-Esteem Inventories

CG....................contact guard; center of gravity; chorionic gonadotropin

CH....................cholesterol

CHADD ....Children & Adults with Attention Deficit Disorder

CHAP................Child Health Assurance Program

CHB ....complete heart block

CHD..................congenital heart disease; congenital hip dysplasia

CHESS...............comprehensive health enhancement support system

CHF ....congestive heart failure

CHI ....consumer health informatics; closed head injury

CHMIS...............community health management information system

cho ....carbohydrates

chol ....cholesterol

CHRIE ....Commission for Hotel & Restaurant Industry Educators

CIL...................center for independent living

CIM..................certificate of initial mastery

CIP..................Community Integration Program

CIRF ....cocaine-induced respiratory failure

Cl ....chlorine (Cl ion)

CLC ....Child Life Council

CLEIRS..............Comprehensive Leisure Rating Scale

CLL..................chronic lymphocytic leukemia

cm ....centimeter(s); costal margin; tomorrow morning

CME..................continuing medical education

CMHC ....community mental health center

CMHP................community mental health program

CML..................chronic myelogenous leukemia

CMML...............chronic myelomonocytic leukemia

CMP..................civil monetary penalty

CMV ....cytomegalovirus

cm^2 ....square centimeter(s)

cm^3 ....cubic centimeter(s)

CNA..................certified nursing assistant

CNC..................confirmed negativity condition

CNS ....central nervous system; clinical nurse specialist

CN (2-12)...........cranial nerves 2-12

CO....................carbon monoxide; cardiac output; cervical orthosis

c/o ....complains of

CO_2 ....carbon dioxide

COA ....children of alcoholic parents
cog ....cognition; cognitive
cog rem ....cognitive remediation
comp ....compress
CON ....certificate of need
conf ....conference
cont ....continue
COPD...............chronic obstructive pulmonary disease
COPE...............Committee on Prosthetic-Orthotic Education
cor ....heart
CORF................comprehensive outpatient rehabilitation facility
COTA................certified occupational therapy assistant
CP ....cerebral palsy; capillary pressure; cerebellopontine; constant pressure; cor pulmonate; creatine phosphate; cold pack; chest pain
CPC...................clinicopathological conference; chronic passive congestion
CPK ....creatine phosphokinase
CPM..................continuous passive motion
CPP ....cerebral perfusion pressure
CPR...................cardiopulmonary resuscitation; cardiac and pulmonary rehabilitation
CPS ....current population survey; Child Protective Services
CPT ....chest physiotherapy; combining power test; Current Procedural Terminology
CQI ....continuous quality improvement
CRIPA...............Civil Rights of Institutionalized Persons Act
CR Ph................consultant registered pharmacist
CRTT ....certified respiratory therapy technician
C+S ....culture and sensitivity
CSF ....cerebrospinal fluid
CSFII ....Continuing Survey of Food Intake of Individuals
CSLP.................certified speech-language pathologist
CSN ....community services network
CSPD ....comprehensive system of personnel development
CT ....CAT scan (computer tomography); confirmatory typing
CTA...................clear to auscultation
CTLSO..............cervicothoracolumbosacral orthosis
CTRS ....certified therapeutic recreation specialist
CTS...................carpal tunnel syndrome

CV ....cardiovascular; closing volume; coefficient of variation; cardiovascular accident; costovertebral angle; concentrated volume; conduction volume; curriculum vitae
CVA ....cerebrovascular accident (stroke)
CVC..................central venous catheter
CVP ....central venous pressure
CVS ....cardiovascular system
CXR...................chest x-ray

D

D ....dependent; date; daughter; day; dead space; deciduous; density; dermatology; deuterium; diameter; diopter; distal; diverticulum; divorced; dorsal; duration; right (dexter); vitamin D unit
DC.....................discharge from hospital; dental corps; direct current; discontinue
d/c or dc ....discharge; discontinue; diarrhea/constipation
DD ....developmental delay; developmental disability
DDE...................direct data entry
DDST.................Denver Developmental Screening Tool
DDx ....differential diagnosis
DE.....................Department of Education
D&E..................diagnosis and evaluation
DEA ....Drug Enforcement Administration
DEMPAQ...........Developing and Evaluating Methods to Promote Ambulatory Care Quality
derm ....dermatology
DG ....diagnosis
DH ....developmentally handicapped
DHHS ....Department of Health and Human Services
DHR...................Department of Human Resources
DICOM..............digital imaging and communications in medicine
dieb alt ....on alternate days
dieb tert...............on every third day
diff ....differential
dim....................one-half (dimidius)
DIMOAD...........(syndrome) diabetes insipidus, diabetes mellitus, optic atrophy, and deafness
div ....divide
DJD...................degenerative joint disease
DKA..................diabetic ketoacidosis
DM....................diabetes mellitus
DNR...................do not resuscitate

DNS .... director of nursing services
D5 0.3NS .... dextrose in 1/3 normal saline
D5 0.45NS .... dextrose in 1/2 normal saline
D5 0.9NS .... dextrose in normal saline
DO .... doctor of osteopathy; diamine oxidase
DOA .... dead on arrival
DOB .... date of birth
DOC .... Department of Commerce
DOE .... dyspnea on exertion; depending on experience
DOH .... Department of Health
DOJ .... Department of Justice
DOL .... Department of Labor
dp .... depression
DP .... distal pulses
dr .... dram; dressing
Dr. .... doctor
DRG .... diagnostic related group
D5 RL .... dextrose in Ringer's lactate
DRS .... Dementia Rating Scale
DRSP .... drug-resistant Streptococcus pneumoniae
DS .... Down syndrome
DSD .... dry sterile dressing
DSG .... dressing
DSM III-R .... Diagnostic and Statistical Manual of Mental Disorders, Third Edition, Revised
DSM IV .... Diagnostic and Statistical Manual of Mental Disorders, Fourth Edition
DS-0, DS-1, D3 ... digital telecommunication channels
DT .... delirium tremens; distance test; doubling time; duration of tetany; diet technician
DTLA .... Detroit Tests of Learning Aptitude
DTR .... deep tendon reflex
DUB .... dysfunctional uterine bleeding
DUI .... driving under the influence
DVT .... deep vein thrombosis
D/W .... dextrose in water
D5/W .... dextrose (5%) in water
DWI .... driving while impaired
dx .... diagnosis

E

EBD .... emotional/behavioral disorder
EBV .... Epstein-Barr virus
EC .... early childhood
ECE .... early childhood education
ECF .... extended care facility; extracellular fluid
ECG .... electrocardiogram; electrocardio-graph
ECSE .... early childhood special education
ECT .... electroconvulsive treatment
ED .... elbow disarticulation; emergency department; emotionally disturbed
EDGAR .... Education Department General Administrative Regulations
EDI .... electronic data interchange
EEG .... electroencephalogram
EENT .... eye, ear, nose, and throat
EEOC .... Equal Employment Opportunity Commission
e.g. .... for example
EGTA .... esophageal gastric tube airway
EHA .... Education of Handicapped Children Act (later called IDEA)
EI .... early intervention
EIB .... exercise-induced bronchospasms
EKG .... electrocardiogram; electrocardio-graph
elb .... elbow
elix .... elixir
ELL .... English language learner
EMD .... emergency medical doctor
EMG .... electromyogram; exophthalmos-macroglossia-gigantism
EMH .... educable mentally handicapped
EMR .... educable mentally retarded
EMS .... electrical muscle stimulation; emergency medical service; eosinophilia myalgia syndrome
EMT .... emergency medical technician
EMV .... (Glasgow Coma Scale grading) eyes, motor, voice. Written: $E_3M_4V_3$
ENT .... ear, nose, and throat
EO .... elbow orthosis
EOM .... extraocular movement
EP .... ectopic pregnancy; emergency physician; evoked potentials
EPA .... Environmental Protection Agency
epith .... epithelium; epithelial
EPS .... extrapyramidal symptoms
EPSDT .... early periodic screening, diagnosis, and treatment
equip .... equipment
ER .... emergency room; endoplasmic reticulum; estradiol receptor; external receptor
ERISA .... Employee Retirement Income Security Act
ERT .... estrogen replacement therapy
es .... electrical stimulation
ESL .... English as a second language

ESLD ....end stage liver disease

esp.......................extrasensory perception; especially

ESR..................erythrocyte sedimentation rate; electron spin resonance

ESRD ....end stage renal disease

ESY....................extended school year (K-12)

ET ....education therapy; endotracheal

ETA...................estimated time of arrival

et al ....and the rest

ETHOL ....ethanol

ETOH.................ethyl alcohol

ETT....................exercise tolerance test; endotracheal tube

EUA ....examination under anesthesia

EUD ....etiology undetermined

eval....................evaluation

EWHO ....elbow-wrist-hand orthosis

ex ....exercise, examination

exam..................examination

exp ....expiration or expiratory; exponent; example

EXT ....extensor; extension

ext ....extremities; exterior; external; extract spread

F

F ....female; farad; father; fecal; fellow; field; formula; fractional concentration; French; fair

°F ....degrees Fahrenheit

FACTR/R...........Functional Assessment of Characteristics in Therapeutic Recreation/Revised

FAE....................fetal alcohol effect

FAPE.................free and appropriate public education

FAS ....fetal alcohol syndrome

FB ....foreign body

FBLA ....Future Business Leaders of America

FBS ....fasting blood sugar

FC ....foster care; facilitated communication

FDA ....Food and Drug Administration

Fe ....iron

FEAT..................Families for Early Autism Treatment

FERPA ....Family Educational Rights and Privacy Act

FES ....functional electrical stimulation

FeSO₄.................ferrous sulfate

FF.......................forced feeding; forced fluids; fat free; foster father; filtration fraction; fixing fluid

FFA ....Future Farmers of America

FFP ....Federal Financial Participation, section 1905(d)

FH ....family history

FHA ....Future Homemakers of America

FIM ....Functional Independence Measure

FIO₂ ....fractional inspiration oxygen

fl.........................fluid

flex ....flexion; flexor

FLSA.................Fair Labor Standards Act

FMC...................fine motor coordination

FMLA ....Family Medical Leave Act

FNS....................functional neuromuscular stimulation

FO ....foot orthosis

FOB ....foot of bed

FR ....Federal Register

freq....................frequent

FRG ....function related groups

FSA...................Family Support Act

FSP ....family support plan

ft..........................feet; foot

FTA ....fluorescent treponemal antibody test

FTE....................full-time equivalent

F to N ....finger to nose test

FTT ....failure to thrive

F/U ....follow-up

(5-) FU ....fluorouracil

FUO ....fever of unknown origin

FWB ....full weight bearing

Fx.......................fracture

FY ....fiscal year

FYI.....................for your information

G

G ....good; gastric; gauss; giga; gingival; Greek

g ....gram(s); Newtonian constant of gravitation

GAF ....Global Assessment of Functioning

gal ....gallon(s); galactose

GALF.................Global Assessment of Leisure Functioning

GAO...................General Accounting Office

GAS ....general adaptation syndrome

GB.....................gallbladder; Guillain-Barré

GBS ....gallbladder series

gc ....gonococcus; gas chromatography

GCS ....Glasgow Coma Scale

GED...................general educational development

gen ....general

GER ....gastroesophageal reflux

GERD ....gastroesophageal reflux disease

GFR ....glomerular filtration rate
GI ....gastrointestinal; glomerular index; globin insulin
gm ....gram(s)
GMC ....gross motor coordination
Gold sol...............colloidal gold curve
GPO ....Government Printing Office
gr......................grain
GRAS.................generally recognized as safe
grav ....gravity
grm......................grooming
GRST ....General Recreation Screening Tool
GRT ....graduate respiratory therapist
GRTT.................graduate respiratory therapist technician
GSA ....General Services Administration
GSI......................genuine stress incontinence
GSR ....galvanic skin response
GSW ....gunshot wound
GT......................gait training
gt......................gait; drop (of a liquid)
GT/LD ....gifted and talented and learning disabled
GTT ....glucose tolerance test
gtt......................drops
GU ....genitourinary; gastric ulcer
GVH..................graft vs. host disease
gyn ....gynecologist; gynecology

H

H ....height; high; horizontal; hypermetropia; hypodermic
h ....hour; Planck's constant
HA ....headache(s); hemaglutination; heated aerosol
HAA..................hepatitis associated antigen
HACCP.............hazard analysis and critical control points
HAL ....handicapped assistance loans
HAP ....Human Activity Profile
HAV ....hepatitis A virus
Hb ....hemoglobin
HBD..................hydroxybutyrate dehydrogenase
HBIG ....hepatitis B immune globulin
HBOC...............hyperbaric oxygen chamber
HBP ....high blood pressure
HBV..................hepatitis B virus
HC..................hydro collator packs; head compress; high calorie; home care; hospital corps; house calls; hydrocephalus; hydrocortisone
HCFA.................Health Care Financing Administration
HCL ....hairy cell leukemia

HCl..................hydrochloric acid
HCO..................Health Care Online
HCO$_3$ ....bicarbonate
HCPCS...............Health Care Financing Administration's Common Procedure Coding System
hct ....hematocrit
HCV..................hepatitis C virus
HCVD.............hypertensive cardiovascular disease
HD..................hip disarticulation
HDV.............hepatitis D virus
HEENT ....head, eyes, ears, nose, and throat
HELP ....health evaluation through logical processing
hemi ....hemiplegia
hep lock...............heparin lock
HERO ....Home Economics Related Occupations
HFA..................high functioning autism
HFCS ....high-fructose corn syrup
Hg ....mercury
Hgb ....hemoglobin
HH ....hard of hearing
HHA..................home health agency
HHC..................home health care
HHV-4 ....human herpesvirus 4
HI..................homicidal ideation; hearing impaired; health impaired
HIB ....*Haemophilus influenzae*, type B
HISPP ....Healthcare Information Standards Planning Panel
HIV ....human immunodeficiency virus
HKAFO.............hip-knee-ankle-foot orthosis
HLA ....human leukocyte antigens
HLHS.................hypoplastic left heart syndrome
HL7..................health level 7
HM..................home management; hand movement
HMO..................health maintenance organization
HNP ....herniated nucleus polposus
HO ....heterotopic ossification; house officer; hand orthosis; hip orthosis
h/o ....history of
H$_2$O ....water
H$_2$O$_2$ ....hydrogen peroxide
HOH..................hard of hearing
HOSA ....Health Occupations Students of America
HOST.................Healthcare Open System and Trials Consortium
HP ....hot pack
H&P ....history and physical
H+P ....history and physical
HPCC..................high performance computing and

communications
HPI.....................history of present illness
HR......................heart rate
hr.......................hour
HRmax...............maximum heart rate
HRRR ....heart regular rate and rhythm
HRS ....health and rehabilitative services
hs.......................bedtime; hour of sleep (hora somni)
HS ....Head Start; high school
HSC ....high school completion
HSQB................Health Standards and Quality Bureau
ht.......................height
HT.....................Hubbard tank; hyper-dermic tablet; hydroxytryptamine
HTN..................hypertension
HTR ....horticultural therapist, registered
HTU ....head trauma unit
HUD..................Housing and Urban Development
HUM..................heat, ultrasound, and massage
HUS ....hemolytic uremic syndrome
Hx ....history
hyg ....hygiene
hypo ....hypodermic injection (subcutaneous)
HZV ....herpes zoster virus

I

I..........................independence; independent
IBD ....inflammatory bowel diseases
IBW ....ideal body weight
ICD ....implanted cardiac defibrillator
ICD-9-CM..........International Classification of Disease, Ninth Revision, Clinical Modification
ICF-MR..............Intermediate Care Facility for the Mentally Retarded
ICP.....................intracranial pressure
ICS.....................intercostal space
ICU ....intensive care unit
I+D.....................incision and drainage
IDDM.................insulin dependent diabetes mellitus
IDEA..................Individuals with Disabilities Education Act
IDELR ....Individuals With Disabilities Education Law Report
IDS.....................integrated delivery system
i.e. ....that is
I/E ....inspiratory/expiratory ratio
IED ....intermittent explosive disorder
IEE.....................independent educational evaluation
IEEE ....Institute of Electrical and Electronics Engineers
IEP ....individualized education program

IEU ....intermediate educational unit
IFEA ....International Festivals and Events Association
IFSP ....individualized family service plan
IHE ....institutions of higher education
IHP.....................individualized habilitation program or plan
IHTP ....individualized habilitation and treatment plan
IITF....................Information Infrastructure Task Force
ILC.....................independent living center
ILP ....independent living plan
IM ....intramuscular; infectious mononucleosis; internal medicine; intra medullary
imp.....................impression; improved
IMV ....intermittent mandatory ventilation
in ....inch(es)
incont ....incontinent
ind ....independence
indep ....independent
inf......................inferior
INH ....inhalation; isoniazid (isonicotinic acid hydrazide)
inj......................injection; injury
insp.....................inspiration; inspection
invol ....involuntary
I&O....................intake and output
I+O.....................intake and output
IOM ....Institute of Medicine
IOP.....................improving organizational performance; intraocular pressure
IPA ....independent practice association
IPC ....Industry Planning Council
IPL ....initial program load
IPM ....integrated pest management
IPP ....individualized program plan
IPPB...................intermittent positive pressure breathing
IPPV ....intermittent positive pressure ventilation
IQ.......................intelligence quotient
IR ....internal rotation
IRB ....internal review board (research approval board)
IRCA..................Immigration Reform and Control Act
IS........................intercostal space
ISDN..................integrated services digital network
ISP ....individualized service plan
ITEA ....International Technology Education Association
ITIP...................instructional theory into practice

ITP ....individualized treatment plan
IU ....international unit
IV ....intravenous; inter-ventricular; in-
                          tervertebral
IVP ....intravenous polygram; intraven-
                          tricular pressure; intravenous
                          pyelography

J

JAMA ....Journal of the American Medical
                          Association
JAN ....Job Accommodation Network
JCAHO ....Joint Commission on Accreditation
                          of Healthcare Organizations
JOBS ....job opportunities and basic skills
JPEG ....Joint Photographic Experts Group
JRA ....juvenile rheumatoid arthritis
jt ....joint
JTPA ....Job Training Partnership Act

K

K ....potassium; cathode; equilibrium
                          constant; electrostatic capacity
k ....Kelvin
KAFO ....knee-ankle-foot orthosis
K/B ....knee bearing (disarticulation)
kcal ....kilocalorie
KCl ....potassium chloride
kg ....kilogram
kHz ....kilohertz
KJ ....knee jerk
KO ....knee orthosis
KS ....Kaposi's sarcoma
KTW ....Klippel-Trenaunay-Weber syn-
                          drome
KUB ....kidney-ureter-bladder (x-ray)
KVO IV ....keep vein open IV

L

L ....left; coefficient of induction; lacto-
                          bacillus; lambert; Latin; left;
                          length; lethal; lowest; licensed;
                          light sense; liter; lumbar; limitation
l ....liter
L1 to L5 ....lumbar vertebrae or nerves
L+A ....light and accommodation
LAAM................L-alpha-acetyl-methadol
lab ....laboratory
lac ....lactation
LAN ....local area network
LAS ....Leisure Attitude Scale
lat ....lateral; latitude
LATA ....local access transport area
LB ....lower body

lb ....pound
LBI ....Leisure Barriers Inventory
LBPH ....Library for the Blind and Physi-
                          cally Handicapped
lcm ....left costal margin; lymphocytic
                          choriomeningitis
LCM ....Leisure Competency Measure
LCSW ....licensed clinical social worker
LD ....learning disability; learning differ-
                          ence; learning disabled; Legion-
                          naire's disease
LDA ....Learning Disabilities Association
LDB ....Leisure Diagnostic Battery
LDH ....lactose dehydrogenate
LE ....lower extremity; left eye
LEA ....local education agency (school dis-
                          trict)
LEDS ....Law Enforcement Data System
lei ....leisure
LENI ....lower extremity noninvasive
LEO ....law enforcement officer
LEP ....limited English proficient
LFA ....low functioning autism
LFT ....liver function test
lg ....large
LGIB ....lower gastrointestinal bleeding
LIM ....Leisure Interest Measure
liq ....liquid
LKS ....Landau-Kleffler syndrome
LL ....lumbar laminectomy
LLB ....long lower brace
LLE ....lower left extremity
LLL ....lower left lobe (limb)
LLQ ....lower left quadrant
l/m ....liters per minute
LMN ....lower motor neuron
LMP ....last menstrual period; left mento-
                          posterior
LMS ....Leisure Motivation Scale
LOC ....loss of consciousness; laxative of
                          choice; level of consciousness; lo-
                          cus of control
LOINC ....laboratory observation identifier
                          names and codes
LOM ....limitation of motion; loss of motion
LOS ....length of stay
LP ....lumbar puncture; latent period;
                          light perception; low pressure; lym-
                          phoid predominance; little person,
                          little people (dwarfism)
LPM ....liters per minute
LPN ....licensed practical nurse
LPTA..................licensed physical therapy assistant
LRE ....least restrictive environment

LRI .... Leisure and Recreation Involvement Measurement
LS .... lumbosacral spine
LSA .... Leisure Studies Association, Britain; list of CFR sections affected
LSC .... Life Safety Code
LSD .... lysergic acid diethylamide
LSK .... liver, spleen, kidney
LSM .... Leisure Satisfaction Measure
LSS .... Life Satisfaction Scale
lt .... left
LT .... long term; lymphocyte transformation; lymphotoxin
L/T .... light touch
LTC .... long-term care
LTCF .... long-term care facility
LTCT .... long-term care and treatment
LTD .... long-term disability
LT/M .... long-term memory
LUE .... left upper extremity
LUL .... left upper lobe (limb)
LUQ .... left upper quadrant
LV .... left ventricle
LVH .... left ventricle hypertrophy
L+W .... living and well
LWCT .... Lee-White clotting time
LWV .... League of Women Voters
lyphs .... lymphocytes
lytes .... electrolytes

M

M .... male; handful; macerate; malignant; massage; mature; mean; media; median; medical; medium; membrane; metabolite; meter; micrococcus; mixture; molar; Monday; mother; muscle; myopia; moon; thousand; mammillaria nucleus; memory; mictoporum; morning; morphine; mouth; murmur; mycobacterium; mycoplasma; married
m .... meter; minimum; minute; murmur
M/ED .... mental or emotional disturbance
M1 .... mitral first sound
M2 .... heart sound at apex; mitral second sound
MA .... master of arts; mental age
mA .... milliampere(s)
MAL .... mid-axillary line
mand .... mandible
mass. .... massage
max .... maximum; maximal assist
MBA .... master's in business administration

MBD .... minimal brain dysfunction
MBO .... management by objective
mcg .... microgram
MCH .... maternal and child health; mean corpuscular hemoglobin
MCHC .... mean corpuscular hemoglobin concentration
MCL .... mid-clavicular line
MCO .... managed care organization
MCP .... metacarpal phalangeal
MCS .... multiple chemical sensitivities
MCV .... mean corpuscular volume
MD .... doctor of medicine; medical doctor; manic depressive; mean deviation; medical department; mentally deficient; muscular dystrophy; maternal deprivation
MDS .... Minimum Data Set
MDT .... multidisciplinary team
ME .... medical examiner
med .... medicine
MEDTEP .... AHCPR's Medical Treatment Effectiveness Program
mEq .... milliequivalent
MET .... metabolic equivalent
MFR .... myofascial release
Mg .... magnesium
mg .... milligram(s)
MGRAD .... Minimum Guidelines and Requirements for Accessible Design
MgSO₄ .... magnesium sulfate
MH .... multiply handicapped; mental health
MHA .... master's in health administration
MHC .... mental hygiene clinic
MI .... myocardial infarction; mitral insufficiency; mental illness
MIB .... medical information bus; men in black
MICU .... medical intensive care unit
MID .... multi-infarct dementia
min .... minute; minimum
MIS .... management information systems
ML .... midline; middle lobe
ml .... milliliter(s)
MLC .... mixed lymphocyte culture
MLM .... medical logic module
MM .... manual muscle; mucous membrane; multiple myeloma
mm .... millimeter
MMACS .... Medicare/Medicaid Automated Certification System
MMH .... mild-moderate mentally handicapped

MMPI-2 ....Minnesota Multiphasic Personality Inventory
MMS.................Mini-Mental State Exam
MMT................manual muscle test
mod ....moderate
Mod A...............moderate assist
Mod I ....moderate independence
MODS...............multiple organ dysfunction syndrome
MODY ....maturity onset diabetes of youth
MOF.................multiple organ failure
MOM ....milk of magnesia
mono ....monocyte
MP ....mercaptopurine; metacarpophalangeal; metatarsalphangeal; mucopolysaccharide; muscle power
MPA ....main pulmonary artery; medroxyprogesterone acetate; master's in public administration
MPC.................multidisciplinary pain center
MPEG ....Motion Picture Experts Group
MPH ....master's in public health; miles per hour
MR...................mental retardation; mitral regurgitation
MR/DD ....mentally retarded/developmentally disabled
MRI..................magnetic resonance imaging
MRM ....modified radical mastectomy
MR/MED ....mentally retarded and mentally or emotionally disturbed
MS ....mass spectrometer; master of surgery; mitral stenosis; morphine sulfate; multiple sclerosis; muscle strength; mental state; master of science
ms.....................muscle
MSBP ....Munchausen syndrome by proxy
MSDD...............multi-sensory developmental delays
MSDS ....material safety data sheet
msec ....millisecond(s)
MSG.................monosodium glutamate
MSL..................mid-sternal line
MSN..................master's in nursing
MSO_4 ....morphine sulfate
MSW.................master's in social work
mV ....millivolt(s)
MVA ....motor vehicle accident
MVO_2................myocardial oxygen consumption
MVP ....mitral valve prolapse
mvt...................movement

N

N ....normal; nasal; negative; Negro (Black); *Neisseria*; nerve; neurology; nonmalignant; normal; nitrogen
NA ....nursing assistant; *Nomina Anatomica*; noradrenaline; not applicable; not available; numeric aperture; nurse anesthetist; nurse's aide
Na ....sodium
N/A ....not applicable
NAAP ....National Association of Activity Professionals
NAB..................National Alliance of Business
NABS................normoactive bowel sounds
NaCl..................sodium chloride (table salt)
NAD..................no appreciable disease; no acute distress
NADS ....National Association for Down Syndrome
NAEMSP ....National Association of Emergency Medical Service Physicians
NAEO ....National Activity Education Organization
NAEP................National Assessment of Educational Progress
NAEYC.............National Association for the Education of Young Children
NAGB ....National Assessment Governing Board
$NaHCO_2$.............sodium bicarbonate
NAIS.................National Association of Independent Schools
NALQO ....National Assisted Living Quality Organization
NAPPA..............National Association of Prevention Professionals and Advocates
NARIC..............National Rehabilitation Information Center
NARRP ....National Association of Recreation Resource Planners
NAS ....National Academy of Sciences; neonatal abstinence syndrome; no added salt
NASASPS..........National Association of State Administrators and Supervisors of Private Schools
NASBE ....National Association of State Boards of Education
NASDSE............National Association of State Directors of Special Education
NASP ....National Association of School

Principals

NASSP................National Association of Secondary School Principals

NAVE.................National Academy for Vocational Educators

NB.......................newborn

nb ....note well

NBPTS................National Board for Professional Teaching Standards

N/C.....................nasal cannula; no complaints

NC/AT................normocephalic/atraumatic (no head injury)

NCCAP ....National Certification Council for Activity Professionals

NCD...................National Council on Disability

NCDD................National Council on Developmental Disabilities

NCES ....National Center for Education Statistics

NCEST...............National Council for Evaluation, Standards, and Testing

NCHS.................National Center for Health Statistics

NCHSR ....National Center for Health Services Research

NCI ....National Cancer Institute

NCME................National Council on Measurement in Education

NCOVE ....National Council on Vocational Education

NCP ....nursing care plan

NCQA ....National Committee for Quality Assurance

NCRVE ....National Center for Research in Vocational Education

NCSESA ....National Committee on Science Education Standards and Assessment

NCTRC ....National Council for Therapeutic Recreation Certification

NCVHS ....National Committee on Vital and Health Statistics

ND ....non-distended

NDA...................no diagnosis of anything

NDSC.................National Down Syndrome Congress

NDSS ....National DS Society

NDT...................neuro-developmental treatment

NEA ....National Education Association

NEC ....not elsewhere classified

NECTAS ....National Early Childhood Technical Assistance System

neg ....negative

NEJM.................New England Journal of Medicine

neonat.................neonatology

NERRC ....New England Regional Resource Center

NESRA ....National Employee Services & Recreation Association

neuro ....neurology; neurosurgery

NF ....National Formulary; non-function

NFB ....National Federation of the Blind

N/G ....nasogastric

NGA...................National Governors Association

NGT ....nasogastric tube

NH ....nursing home

NH_4Cl ....ammonium chloride

NHE...................national health expenditures

N/I......................not indicated

NICEM ....National Information Center for Educational Media

NICHCY ....National Information Center for Children and Youth with Disabilities

NICU ....neonatal intensive care unit

NIDDM...............non-insulin dependent diabetes mellitus

NIDRR...............National Institute on Disability and Rehabilitation Research

NIE ....National Institutes of Education

NIH ....National Institutes of Health

NII......................National Information Infrastructure

NIRSA ....National Intramural Recreational Sports Association

NIST ....National Institute for Standards and Technology

NKA...................no known allergies

NL......................normal limits

NLD...................nonverbal learning disability

NLM ....National Library of Medicine

NLS....................National Library Service for the Blind and Physically Handicapped

NMS...................neuromuscular stimulation

No. (#)................number

N_2O ....nitrous oxide

noct ....nocturnal; at night

NOK...................next of kin

NORD................National Organization for Rare Disorders

NOS ....not otherwise specified

NP ....neuropsychiatric; neuropsychology; nucleoplasmic index; nucleoprotein; nursing procedure; neck pain

NPC ....nonproductive cough; nasopharyngeal cancer; nasopharyngeal carcinoma; near point of convergence

NPIN..................National Parent Information Network

NPND ....National Parent Network on Disabilities

NPO ....nothing by mouth (nil per os)

NPPSIS ....National Parent to Parent Support & Information Systems, Inc.

NPRM ....notice of proposed rulemaking

NPTA ....National Parents and Teachers Association

NR.....................do not repeat; no refill; no response; non-reactive; normal range; non-rebreathing; nodal rhythm

NRC ....National Research Council

NRPA ....National Recreation and Parks Association

NS ....normal saline

N/S ....no show

NSAID ....non-steroidal anti-inflammatory drug

NSBA.................National School Boards Association

NSF ....National Science Foundation

nsg.....................nursing

NSR ....normal sinus rhythm; non-systemic reaction

NSVD ....normal spontaneous vaginal delivery

NT......................non-tender

NTD ....neural tube defect

NTG ....nitroglycerin

NTIA..................National Telecommunications and Information Administration

NTRS.................National Therapeutic Recreation Society

NUBC ....National Uniform Billing Committee

N&V ....nausea and vomiting

NVD...................normal vaginal delivery

NWB...................non-weight bearing

NYD...................not yet diagnosed

O

O ....oriented; eye; female

O_2......................oxygen

OA ....osteoarthritis; old age; oxalic acid; occiput anterior

OB......................obstetrics

OBRA ....Omnibus Budget Reconciliation Act

OBS ....organic brain syndrome

OC......................oral contraceptive

occ......................occasional

OCD...................obsessive-compulsive disorder

OCR...................optical character recognition; Office for Civil Rights

OD ....right eye (oculus dexter); outside diameter; optical density; doctor of optometry; overdose; officer of the day

ODAS ....Occupational Data Analysis System

ODD...................oppositional defiant disorder

OFCCP...............Office of Federal Contract Compliance Programs

OHI ....other health impairments

OI ....osteogenesis imperfecta

OIG ....US Department of Health and Human Services Office of the Inspector General

OJ......................orange juice

OJT ....on the job training

OLAP.................on-line analytical processing

OM....................oral motor; occupational medicine; otitis media

om ....every morning

OMB ....Office of Management and Budget

on ....every night

oncol ....oncology

op ....operation

O&P ....ova and parasites

OPA....................oropharyngeal airway

OPD ....outpatient department; optical path difference

oph ....ophthalmology

OPIM ....other potentially infectious material

OPM ....Office of Personal Management

OPT...................out-patient; out-patient physical therapy

OPTH.................ophthalmology

OR......................operating room; oxidation reduction

ORIF ....open reduction internal fixation

ortho..................orthopedics

OS ....left eye (oculus sinister)

os.........................mouth; left eye

OSEP ....Office of Special Education Programs, US Department of Education

OSERS...............Office of Special Education and Rehabilitative Services, US Department of Education

OSHA ....Occupational Safety and Health Act; Occupational Safety and Health Administration

OSPI ....Office of the Superintendent of Public Instruction

OT......................occupational therapy; objective test; old tuberculin; otolaryngology; over time

OTA ....occupational therapy assistant
OTC ....over the counter (medication)
OTR/L.............occupational therapist regis-
tered/licensed
OU ....both eyes; each eye
Ox3 ....oriented to person, place, and time
oz ....ounce

P

P......................poor; by weight; handful; near;
pharmacopoeia; phenolphthalein;
pico; plasma; pole; population;
position; posterior; post partum;
protein; psychiatry; pulse; pupil
p̄........................after or post
p2 ....pulmonic second heart sound
PA ....posterior-anterior; physician's
assistant; procainamide; pernicious
anemia
pa ....pulmonary artery
P&A ....protection and advocacy
P+A ....percussion and auscultation
PAC..................premature atrial contraction; phenacetin, aspirin, and caffeine; political
action committee
PACS................Picture Archiving and Communica-
tions System
PAL..................posterior axillary line
P and A ....protection and advocacy
Pap ....Papanicolaou test
para ....multipara; primapara
PAS ....para amino salicylic acid
pas...................passive
PAT ....paroxysmal atrial tachycardia
path ....pathology; pathologist
PAVE................Parents Advocating for Vocational
Education
PBI...................protein-bound iodine
PBM.................pharmacy benefit management
PBSC ....peripheral blood stem cell
PBX ....private branch exchange
pc ....after meals; after food; percent
PC ....personal computer
PCA ....patient controlled analgesic; per-
sonal care attendant
PCD ....pacing cardioverter/defibrillator
PCEPD..............President's Commission on the Em-
ployment of People with Disability
PCMR...............Presidents Committee on Mental
Retardation
PCN ....penicillin
pCO$_2$ ....partial pressure carbon dioxide
PCP ....phencyclidine (angel dust);
pneumocystis carinii pneumonia;

primary care physician
PD ....postural drainage; doctor of pharmacy; pulmonary disease; interpu-
pillary distance
PDA ....personal digital assistant; patent
ductus arteriosus
PDD ....pervasive developmental disorder
PDD/NOS ....pervasive developmental disorder,
not otherwise specified
PDQ ....Physician Data Query; pretty damn
quick
PDR ....Physician's Desk Reference
PE ....pulmonary embolus; pulmonary
edema; probable error; physical ex-
amination, physical education
peds.................pediatrics
PEEP................positive end expiratory pressure
per ....perceptual; through; by
PERL ....pupils equal, react to light
PERRLA...........pupils equal, round, react to light,
accommodation
PERS................Public Employees Retirement Sys-
tem
PFT ....pulmonary function test
PG ....pregnant
PH ....past history; personal history
pH ....hydrogen ion concentration,
acid/base
PHN ....public health nurse
PI......................present illness; pressure on inspira-
tion; performance improvement;
personal injury; physically im-
paired
PID...................pelvic inflammatory disease
PIE ....problem, intervention, evaluation
(form of charting)
PIP ....parent information packet
PJC..................premature junctional tachycardia
PKU ....phenylketonuria
pl......................plural
PL ....public law
PL 89-97 ....Social Security Act of 1965
PL 90-480 ....Architectural Barriers Act of 1968
PL 91-517 ....Developmental Disabilities and Fa-
cilities Construction Act of 1970
PL 92-603 ....Social Security Amendments of
1972.
PL 93-112 ....Rehabilitation Act of 1973
PL 93-516 ....Rehabilitation Act Amendment of
1974.
PL 94-103 ....The Developmental Disabilities
Assistance Bill of Rights Act of
1975
PL 94-142 ....Education of Handicapped Chil-

dren Act of 1975 (now PL 101-476)

PL 95-602 ....Rehabilitation Act Amendments of 1978

PL 96-247 ....The Civil Rights of Institutionalized Persons Act (CRIPA).

PL 97-248 ....Tax Equity and Fiscal Responsibility Act (TEFRA)

PL 98-21 ....Social Security Amendments of 1983

PL 99-319 ....Protection and Advocacy for the Mentally Ill Individual Act of 1986.

PL 99-457 ....Education of the Handicapped Amendments of 1986.

PL 99-506 ....Rehabilitation Act (reauthorization).

PL 100-203 ....Omnibus Budget Reconciliation Act (OBRA)

PL 101-336 ....Americans with Disabilities Act

PL 101-476 ....1991 Amendments (IDEA)

PL 105-15 ....Individuals with Disabilities Education Act of 1997 (formerly PL 101-476)

PL 105-17 ....1997 Amendments (IDEA)

PL 105-476 ....Individuals with Disabilities Education Act of 1990 (formerly PL 94-142 and 99-457)

PLATO ....Programmed Logic Automatic Teaching Operations

PLT ....platelets

pm ....afternoon or evening (post meridiem)

PM ....participative management; post mortem

PMEALS.............after meals

PMH ....past medical history

PMN ....polymorphonuclear

PM&R................physical medicine and rehabilitation

PMS ....premenstrual syndrome (premenstrual dysphoric disorder)

PNB ....pulseless non-breathing

PND ....paroxysmal nocturnal dyspnea

PNF...................proprioceptive neuromuscular facilitation

PNI....................psychoneuroimmunology

PNP...................pediatric nurse practitioner

po ....by mouth; orally (per os)

PO ....phoned order; postoperative

pO$_2$.....................partial pressure oxygen

pod ....podiatric surgery

POR ....problem oriented record

PORT ....patient outcomes research team

pos.....................positive

post op ....postoperative

post ....posterior or after; post mortem

PPBS.................postprandial blood sugar

PPD...................purified protein derivative

PPE ....personal protective equipment

PPO...................preferred provider organization

PPS ....prospective payment system; post polio syndrome; pupil personnel services

PRE...................progressive resistive exercise

pre ....before

pre-op................before operation

prep ....preparation

prn.....................as needed or desired (pro re nata)

PRO ....peer review organization

pro.....................protein; pronation

PROM................passive range of motion; prolonged range of motion

PROMISE..........Providence Regional Outreach for Medically Impaired Students Education

prox...................proximal

PS......................pulmonary stenosis

PSA...................prostate-specific antigen

PSF ....posterior spine fusion

psi ....pounds per square inch

psig...................pounds per square inch by gauge

PSVT ....paroxysmal supraventricular tachycardia

psych.................psychology

PT ....physical therapy; posterior tibial; prothrombin time

pt........................pint, patient

PTA...................prior to admission; post-traumatic amnesia; physical therapy assistant; peroxidase labeled antibodies; Parent Teacher Association

PTAC ....Professional and Technical Advisory Committee

PTB...................patellar tendon-bearing prosthesis

PTCA ....percutaneous transluminal coronary angioplasty

PTG...................parent teacher group

PTSD ....post-traumatic stress disorder

PTT...................partial thromboplastin time; prothrombin time

PTX...................pneumothorax

PUD ....peptic ulcer disease

pulm ....pulmonary medicine

PVC ....premature ventricular contraction; polyvinyl chloride

PVD ....peripheral vascular disease

PVS...................persistent vegetative state; private vocational schools

PWA...................person with AIDS
PWB ....partial weight bearing
PWS..................Prader-Willi Syndrome
PWV ....pulse wave velocity
Px......................prognosis
PY ....project year
PZI ....protamine zinc insulin

Q

q ....every; four
QA ....quality assurance; quality assessment
qam ....every morning
QC.....................quality circle; quad cane
qd ....every day
qh ....every hour
q2h ....every two hours
q3h ....every three hours
q4h ....every four hours
q hor..................every hour
QHS ....every night at bedtime
QI......................quality indicator
qid ....four times a day (quarter in die)
QIDM.................four times daily with meals and at bedtime
ql ....as much as you please
QMRP................qualified mental retardation specialist
qn ....every night
qns.....................quantity not sufficient
qod ....every other day
qoh ....every other hour
qp ....at will
qpm ....every night
qs.......................quantity sufficient; as much as required
qt ....quart
quad ....quadriplegia

R

R ....respiration; right; far; reference file; radiology; rectal; regression coefficient; resistance; respiration; response; review; Rickettsia; Rennes test
RA......................rheumatoid arthritis; rennin activity; repeat action; residual air; right arm; right atrium
RAI ....Resident Assessment Instrument
RAID ....redundant array of independent disks
RAM ....rapid alternating movement; random access memory
RAP ....Resident Assessment Protocol

RBBB ....right bundle branch block
RBC ....red blood cell; erythrocyte count
rBST ....bovine somatotropin
RC......................respiratory therapy care; red cell; respiration ceases; respiratory center; Roman Catholic
RCA ....rehabilitation center for alcoholics; red blood cell agglutinations; right coronary artery
RCF....................residential care facility
RCH ....residential care home
RCM ....right costal margin; red cell mass
RCRA ....Resort & Commercial Recreation Association
RD......................registered dietitian
R&D...................research and development
RDS ....respiratory distress syndrome
RDT ....registered diet technician
re:......................regarding
rec ....recommended
REDS.................Recreation Early Development Screening Tool
Reg No...............register number
Rehab.................rehabilitation
REM...................rapid eye movement; right eye movement
resp ....respiration
RF ....rheumatoid factor; relative flow
RFP ....request for proposal
RHC ....rural health clinic
RHD...................rheumatic heart disease
RICE ....rest, ice, compression, and elevation
RIND ....reversible ischemic neurologic deficit
RLE....................right lower extremity
RLL....................right lower limb; right lower lobe
RLQ ....right lower quadrant
RML...................right middle lobe
RMRS ....Regenstrief medical record system
RMS...................rehabilitation medicine service; root mean square
RMT ....regional management team
RN......................registered nurse
R/O....................rule out
RODEO NET......Rural Options for Development and Educational Opportunities Network
ROM ....range of motion; read only memory
ROP ....retinpathy of prematurity
ROS ....review of systems
RPD ....Recreation Participation Data Sheet
RPE....................rating of perceived exertion
RPh ....registered pharmacist
RPR....................rapid plasma reagent

RPT....................registered physical therapist
RR....................respiratory rate; rate and rhythm
RR&E ....round, regular, and equal
RRI....................recurrent respiratory infections
RRR ....regular rate and rhythm
RRT ....registered respiratory therapist
RSA ....Regional Service Agency;
                     Rehabilitation Services Administra-
                     tion
RSD ....reflex sympathetic dystrophy
RSR....................regular sinus rhythm
RT ....recreational therapy; radiotherapy;
                     reaction time; reading test; regis-
                     tered technician; respiratory ther-
                     apy
rt......................right
R&T ....research and training
RTA....................recreational therapy assistant;
                     Roundtable Associates, Inc.
RTC....................return to clinic
RTH ....residential training home
Rt lab..................routine laboratory work
RUE ....right upper extremity
rupt....................ruptured
RUQ..................right upper quadrant
RVR ....rapid ventricular response
RWQC ....regional workforce quality commit-
                     tee
Rx......................therapy; treatment; prescription

S

S........................supervise; supervision; supervised;
                     half; left; mark; percentage of satu-
                     ration; sacral; second; sedimenta-
                     tion coefficient; sensation; sensi-
                     tive; serum; single; soluble; spheri-
                     cal; stimulus; subjects
s̄........................without
S1 to S5..............sacral vertebra or nerves
S+A....................sugar and acetone
SAN ....side arm nebulizer
SAS....................sleep apnea syndrome
SAT ....Scholastic Aptitude Test
SBA ....Small Business Administration;
                     standby assist
SBE....................state board of education
SBP....................systolic blood pressure
sc......................subcutaneously
SCI....................spinal cord injury
SD ....shoulder disarticulation; standard
                     deviation
SDA....................service delivery area
SE ....signed English
SEA....................state education act; state education

agency
SEC....................special education child
SECC..................special education child count
Section 503/504 ..Sections of the Rehabilitation Act
                     of 1973
SED....................seriously emotionally disabled
sed rate..............sedimentation rate
SEE....................signing exact English
SERVE..............Secondary Education Reporting of
                     Vocational Enrollment
SET ....student effectiveness team
SEWHO.............shoulder-elbow-wrist-hand orthosis
SFA....................safety awareness; serum folate
SGA ....small for gestational age
SGOT..................serum glutamic-oxaloacetic transa-
                     minase
SGPT ....serum glutamic-pyruvic transami-
                     nase
sh......................shoulder
SH ....social history; somatotropic hor-
                     mone
shd....................shoulder
SHHH ....self-help for hard of hearing
SHI....................Specialized Housing, Inc.
SI......................sensory integration; suicidal idea-
                     tion
SIB....................self-injurious behavior
SICU ....surgical intensive care unit
SIDS..................sudden infant death syndrome
sig......................to write; to label; signal; signifi-
                     cant; signature
SILP..................semi-independent living program
SIO....................sacroiliac orthosis
SIS ....shared information systems; shaken
                     infant syndrome
SIT-R ....Slosson Intelligence Test — Re-
                     vised
SLB....................short leg brace
SLC....................structured learning center
SLD....................specific learning disability
SLE....................systematic lupus erthematosis
SLP ....speech language pathologist
SLR....................straight leg raise; state liaison
                     representative
SLT ....speech language therapist
sm......................small
SMA..................sequential multiple analyzer;
                     smooth muscle antibodies; superior
                     mesenteric artery; spinal muscular
                     atrophy
SN ....special needs
SNOMED ....Systematic Nomenclature of Medi-
                     cine
SO ....shoulder orthosis

SOAP .... subjective, objective, assessment, plan (form of charting)

SOB .... shortness of breath; side of bed

sol .... solution

SOS .... one dose only

S/P .... status post

spec. .... specimen

SPED .... special education or special education teacher

sp gr .... specific gravity

Sp. Path .... speech pathology

sq .... subcutaneously (into fat layer)

SROM .... self range of motion

ss .... one half

SS .... social security

SSA .... Social Security Act

SSD .... Social Security Disability

SSDI .... Social Security Disability Income; segmental sequential irradiation

ss e .... soapsuds enema

SSI .... Supplemental Security Income

SSKI .... saturated solution of potassium iodide

SSN .... social security number

SST .... sensory stimulation; student study team

st .... short term; let it stand; straight

ST/M .... short-term memory

Staph .... staphylococcus

stat .... immediately; at once

STD .... sexually transmitted disease; standard

Stim .... stimulation

Strep .... streptococcus

STSG .... split thickness skin graft

STSS .... Streptococcal toxic shock syndrome

STTE .... Society of Travel & Tourism Educators

subcu .... subcutaneously (into fat layer)

subq .... subcutaneously (into fat layer)

sup .... superior

supp .... suppository

sur .... surgery

susp .... suspension

SVC .... superior vena cava

SVT .... supraventricular tachycardia

SW .... social work

SWS .... Sturge-Weber syndrome

Sx .... symptoms or systems; signs

T

T .... temperature; trace; tension; thoracic; tidal; transverse; *Treponema*; total

T1 to T12 .... thoracic vertebrae or nerves

T 3 .... triiodothyronine

T 4 .... thyroxin level

T&A .... tonsillectomy and adenoidectomy

tab(s) .... tablets

TAG .... talented and gifted

TAH .... total abdominal hysterectomy

T and C .... Tylenol and codeine

TASH .... The Association for Persons with Severe Disabilities

TB .... tuberculosis; total body; thymol blue

T bar .... trapeze bar

TBI .... traumatic brain injury

TBSA .... total body surface area

Tbsp .... tablespoon

TCA .... tricyclic antidepressant

TDBW .... touch down bearing weight

TDD .... telecommunications device for the deaf

TEE .... transesophageal echocardiogram

temp .... temperature

TENS .... transcutaneous electrical nerve (neuromuscular) stimulation

TFC .... Together for Children

THA .... total hip arthroplasty; tetrahydroaminacrine

Ther/Ex .... therapeutic exercises

Thor Surg .... thoracic surgery

Thpy .... therapy; counseling

THR .... total hip replacement

TIA .... transient ischemic attack

tid .... three times daily

TIDM .... three times daily with meals

tinc .... tincture

TIP .... teacher improvement process

TIW .... three times weekly

TKA .... total knee arthroplasty

TKR .... total knee replacement

TLC .... tender loving care; thin layer chromatography; therapeutic learning center

TLSO .... thoracolumbosacral orthosis

TMH .... trainable mentally handicapped

TMJ .... temporomandibular joint

TMR .... trainable mentally retarded

TNM .... tumor size, nodal involvement, metastatic process (method of describing cancers)

TO .... telephone order

TOF .... tetralogy of Fallot

TP .... total protein; toilet paper; *Treponema pallidum*

TPM....................total passive motion
TPN....................total parenteral nutrition; triphos-
phopyridine nucleotide
TPR....................temperature, pulse, respiration
TPR, BP.............temperature, pulse, respiration,
blood pressure
TQI ....total quality improvement
TQM ....total quality management
TR.....................therapeutic recreation
trach ....tracheostomy
TRAIDS.............transfusion related AIDS
trp.....................transportation
TS ....thoracic surgeon; Tourette syn-
drome
tsp ....teaspoon
TSPC.................Teacher Standards and Practices
Commission
TSS ....toxic shock syndrome
TT ....tilt table; tetanus toxoid; thrombin
time; thymol turbidity; transit time;
text telephone
TTRA.................Travel & Tourism Research Asso-
ciation
TTWA.................toe touch weight bearing
TTY ....teletypewriter
TUR ....transurethral resection
TVH...................transvaginal hysterectomy
Tx......................treatment
TxP ....treatment plan

U

U ....unit
UA ....urinalysis
UAF ....university affiliated facility
UAP ....university affiliated program
UB......................upper body
UBW...................usual weight bearing
U/C.....................unit clerk
UCG...................urine chorionic gonadotropin
UCHD.................usual childhood diseases
UCP ....United Cerebral Palsy
ud ....as directed
UE......................upper extremity
UGI....................upper gastrointestinal series
UGIB ....upper gastrointestinal bleeding
UHF ....ultra-high frequency
UL......................upper lobe
UMLS ....unified medical language system
UMN..................upper motor neuron
ung ....ointment (unguentum)
UNLS.................unified nursing language system
UO ....undetermined origin
UR......................utilization review
URI.....................upper respiratory infection

US......................ultrasound
USC ....United States Code
USDE.................United States Department of
Education
USDmr...............Uniform Data System for Mental
Retardation
USED.................United States Education Depart-
ment
USN ....ultrasonic nebulizer
USP....................US Pharmacopoeia
UTI ....urinary tract infection
UV ....ultraviolet

V

V ....volt; unipolar chest lead; velocity;
ventilation; verbal; vibrio; viral; vi-
sion; visual acuity; volume
vag ....vaginal
VAMC................Veteran's Affairs Medical Center
VAN ....value-added network
VCFS ....velo-cardio-facial-syndrome
VD ....venereal disease
VE......................vocational education
VEDS.................vocational education data systems
VF......................ventricular fibrillation
VFIB ....ventricular fibrillation
VH......................visual hallucination
VI.......................visual impairment
via ....by way of
vis......................visibility
viz......................namely
VLCD ....very low calorie diet
VO ....verbal order
VO$_2$max ....maximum oxygen consumption
rate
vol......................volume
VPB ....ventricular premature beats
VR......................vocational rehabilitation
VRD...................vocational rehabilitation division
VS ....vital signs
VSA ....very special arts
VSD ....ventricular septal defect
VT......................ventricular tachycardia

W

W ....watt(s); water; weight; white; white
cell; widow; word fluency
w̄ ....with
w/ ....with
W/A ....while awake
WAC ....work activity center
WAID.................What Am I Doing
WAIS ....Wechsler Adult Intelligence Scale
WBAT................weight bearing as tolerated

WBC ....white blood cell; leukocyte count
WBS ....weight bearing status
WC.......................worker's compensation
w/c ....wheelchair
WCST ....Wisconsin Card Sorting Test
WD, w/d..............well developed; wet dressing; Wilson's disease
WDWN...............well developed, well nourished
WEST ....work evaluation systems technology
WFL....................within functional limits
WHO...................World Health Organization
WIC ....Women, Infant, and Children Program
WISC-R ....Wechsler Intelligence Scale for Children –Revised
WLRA.................World Leisure & Recreation Association
WNL ....within normal limits
w/o ....without
wp ....whirlpool
WPPSI-R ....Wechsler Preschool and Primary Scale of Intelligence — Revised
WQC...................Workplace Quality Council
WRAT3 ....Wide Range Achievement Test 3
WRRC ....Western Regional Resource Center
WS ....waivered services
wt ....weight

X Y Z

x ....times
y/o ....year old
YPLL ....years of potential life lost
yr..........................year
YTP....................youth transition program
ZPP ....zone of partial paralysis

Miscellaneous Symbols

@	at
−	no change; minus; negative; absent
″	inch; second
′	foot
24 A	24-hour assistance
>	more than/ greater than
<	less than
3	tertiary/ third-degree; dram
2	secondary
1	primary
↓	low; decreased; worsening
↑	high; increased; improvement
‖	parallel bars
♀	female
♂	male
+1 or +2	requiring one or two people to assist
~	approximately
→	to/ from
Δ	change
/ |	flexion/ extension
°	degree (s)
%	percent
−	minus
+	plus
μg	microgram
§	Section
2 + 2	two years in HS, two years CC

Greek Alphabet

A	α	alpha
B	β	beta
Γ	γ	gamma
Δ	δ	delta
E	ϵ	epsilon
Z	ζ	zeta
H	η	eta
Θ	θ	theta
I	ι	iota
K	κ	kappa
Λ	λ	lambda
M	μ	mu
N	ν	nu
Ξ	ξ	xi
O	o	omicron
Π	π	pi
P	ρ	rho
Σ	σ	sigma
T	τ	tau
Υ	υ	upsilon
Φ	ϕ	phi
X	χ	chi
Ψ	ψ	psi
Ω	ω	omega

Growth and Development

Developmental Age: Birth to 12 Months

Psychosocial Stage of Development (Erikson)	*Stage One: Infancy*	Trust vs. Mistrust	Ability to trust others and a sense of one's own trustworthiness; a sense of hope. Withdrawal and estrangement. Emotional dissatisfaction if needs have not been consistently met.
Moral Judgment (Kohlberg)	Kohlberg does not recognize a moral judgment awareness at this level.		
Radius of Significant Relationships (Sullivan)	*Maternal person* may be either uni-polar or bipolar. Given the extent of child care used today, this distinction is slipping.		
Cognitive Stage (Piaget)	Piaget calls this stage the *sensorimotor stage* and extends the chronological age of this stage to two years.		
Psychosexual Stage (Freud)	*Oral-Sensory* One of the major sources of pleasure from this age comes from exploring the world through oral activities such as vocalizing, sucking, chewing.		
Play Behaviors	Engages in playful activity alone and independently. Will engage in play with someone who is older but play behavior is centered on what interests him/her. Explores world visually by random movement. As ability to grasp and ability to put things in his/her mouth develops, explores the world this way also.		
Basic Physiological Events	Develops basic control of body through space (hand to mouth, sitting up, pulls self to standing, crawling, roll from back to abdomen when lying down). Develops basic fine motor control (palmer grasp, radial-digital grasp, scissor grasp, 3-jaw chuck grasp, and pincer grasp).		
Common Fears	Loss of care/support from trusted adults, strangers, animals, loud noises, sudden movements, and bright lights.		
Medical Preparation Concerns	Patients who are functionally under one year of age rely heavily on the support of a parent or familiar staff to survive unknown and scary situations. Explain the procedure to a parent or staff person who has a trusting relationship with the patient and is willing to stay with the patient through the procedure. Patients, lacking the general ability to control their environment, are soothed by the physical presence of a parent or staff person that they can trust. These patients are also extremely limited in their ability to adjust quickly to new environments. Provide the patient with familiar objects from his/her room along with the company of the parent or familiar staff person while the procedure is being performed.		

Developmental Age: 1 Year to 3 Years

Psychosocial Stage of Development (Erikson)	*Stage Two: Late infancy and early childhood*	Autonomy vs. Shame and Doubt	Self-control without loss of self-esteem; ability to cooperate and to express oneself. Compulsive self-restraint or compliance; defiance, willfulness. Shame. Doubt: feelings that nothing one does is any good.
Moral Judgment (Kohlberg)	*Pre-conventional* (pre-moral). External morality, directed and imposed by authoritarian figures. There are two levels associated with pre-conventional stage. The first one, punishment-and-obedience orientation (where actions are labeled as "good/bad" based on the consequences received), falls into this age group.		
Radius of Significant Relationships (Sullivan)	*Parental Persons* (tri-polar)		
Play Behavior	Plays alone and independently. Others may be playing nearby but their actions have little to moderate influence on the child's play.		
Psychosexual Stage (Freud)	*Anal Stage.* Individuals learn to withhold or expel fecal material at will. Future personality traits such as stinginess, stubbornness, expansiveness, over-generosity, and orderliness or messiness are developed and fine-tuned.		
Basic Physiological Events	Turns pages in books, can build a tower of blocks up to 9 blocks tall, walks up and down stairs, stands on one foot for a few seconds, in artwork is able to copy circles and crosses.		
Common Fears	Separation from parent/primary care takers, injury, certain persons or locations (e.g., doctor, dentist office), loud or sudden noises, dark places, large machines.		
Medical Preparation Concerns	Patients rely heavily on the gross and fine motor ability that they have. Restricted movement may increase the patient's level of stress. Simple procedures like a blood pressure check may produce anxiety. For painless procedures, showing the equipment, performing the procedure on an anatomically correct doll or "teaching" the patient how to imitate the procedure on the doll may reduce fear. Play may need to be done a few times prior to the actual appointment. This group does not have an understanding of what is inside the body. Avoid lengthy discussions about what is going to be "fixed" or "examined." Concentrate on how the treatment/procedure will feel. Intense emotional upset and physical resistance is developmentally normal. A procedure should be done as quickly and gently as possible with a trusted staff person or parent physically close. After a painful procedure, numerous opportunities to "work out" fear and misunderstanding are appropriate. Frequently this group equates pain directly with punishment. If the patient is verbal and talks about the doll being "bad" or needing a time out prior to having the procedure, the staff can direct the patient's play to reflect a truer picture of what happened.		

Developmental Age: 3 to 6 Years

Psychosocial Stage of Development (Erikson)	*Stage Three: Early Childhood*	Initiative vs. Guilt	The courage to try to achieve desired goals tempered by a sense of conscience. Self-denial and self-restriction.
Moral Judgment (Kohlberg)	*Pre-conventional* (pre-moral). Morality is external, being directed and imposed by authoritarian figures. There are two levels associated with pre-conventional stage. The second one, the instrumental-relativist orientation (where behaviors are considered to be "right" if they brings pleasure), falls into this age group.			
Radius of Significant Relationships (Sullivan)	*Basic Family*			
Play Behavior	Child plays with toys; engages in activities similar to the others nearby, but plays next to, instead of with, others. Engages in make-believe and dramatic play.			
Psychosexual Stage (Freud)	*Phallic Stage.* Freud noted that it is during this developmental period that children begin to recognize that there are differences between the sexes. They also discover that their genitals are interesting and sensitive. He speculated that penis envy and castration anxiety were important concerns for children in this age group. Freud associated such personality traits as shyness/brashness, blind courage/timidity, and stylishness/plainness as developing during this stage.			
Basic Physiological Events	Skips and hops on one foot, throws and catches balls well, walks backward, ties shoelaces, uses seven to nine parts when drawing a stickman, constantly active.			
Common Fears	Monsters, ghosts or other supernatural beings, injury, death, "bad" people, the dark.			
Medical Preparation Concerns (Material in this section is based on the developmental needs of patients between the ages of three years and seven years. Around the age of seven children are more able to understand medical and health issues.)	(Ages 3 to 7 years.) Patients tend to think egocentrically and explain unknowns through magical thinking. Without adequate preparation, their minds can become quite active with imagination, making the procedure more exaggerated, bizarre, and frightening than it actually is. Explain the procedure to them using dolls, puppets, and other visual aids. Allow them to take the part of the practitioner prior to the procedure until they feel more relaxed. This reduces the need for both physical and chemical restraints. Children of this age tend to have concerns about mutilation, especially fears of castration. While some adults who function at this developmental age don't exhibit this behavior, many patients will still experience this fear. Be very explicit about the part of the body that the procedure will be done on. Frequently patients want to act like "grown men and women." To them this means that they are not allowed to express their fears, cry, or even to scream. With the use of the puppets or dolls, staff can help the patient learn appropriate ways in which to express feelings.			

Developmental Age: 6 to 12 Years

Psychosocial Stage of Development (Erikson)	*Stage Four: Middle Child-hood*	Industry vs. Inferiority	Realization of competence, perseverance. Feeling that one will never be "any good," withdrawal from school and peers.
Moral Judgment (Kohlberg)	*Conventional Stage* where conformity, loyalty, and maintenance of social order is paramount. This stage, closely corresponds to the child's operational level of cognitive function. The two levels of this stage (stages 3 and 4, building upon earlier stages) are 3. the interpersonal concordance (one earns approval by following "norms" and being a good girl/good boy) and 4. the "law and order" orientation where following the rules set out by authority equals "correct" behavior.		
Radius of Significant Relationships (Sullivan)	*Neighborhood and School.*		
Play Behaviors	Plays with others in an organized manner for a purpose (e.g., sports teams, to make something). Feelings of belonging to the group. The youth plays a role (leader/follower) and the others support that role to some degree.		
Psychosexual Stage (Freud)	*Latency Period.* Freud identified this time of maturation to be one of polishing previously acquired personality traits and using one's energy to acquire knowledge.		
Basic Physiological Events	Can follow three step commands, repeats performances to improve skill, prefers to play with members of own sex, dresses self completely, generally likes competition, pubescent changes may begin to develop.		
Common Fears	Storms, the dark, staying alone, failure in school and tests, supernatural beings (esp. seen on TV or in movies), death.		
Medical Preparation Concerns (Material in this section is based on the developmental needs of patients between the ages of seven years and thirteen years. Around the age of thirteen adolescents are confused with the physiological changes and also want to have a say in what happens.)	Patients who are able to function in this developmental category are at least somewhat aware of different illnesses and how people cannot live without certain body organs. When preparing this group for invasive procedures, explain the procedure in a non-hurried manner first. Some of the patients will ask many, many questions to gain a sense of control. Please be patient. Understanding what is going to happen will reduce the need for restraints. Use scientific terminology for body parts and medical procedures. Unlike patients functioning below seven years or above 13 years, this group of patients may be embarrassed by having other people know that dolls were used to explain the procedure. If they don't want to use dolls or similar training props, explain the procedure with pictures.		

Developmental Age: 12 to 19 Years

Psychosocial Stage of Development (Erikson)	*Stage Five: Adolescence & Post Adoles-cence. "Identity Crisis."*	Identity vs. Role Diffusion	Sexual maturation/individuation. Coherent sense of self; plans to actualize one's abilities. Feelings of confusion, indecisiveness, and antisocial behavior.
Moral Judgment (Kohlberg)	*Postconventional.* Social contract, legalistic orientation. Moral judgment tends to reflect generally accepted social standards and follow community laws. Individuals tend to believe that they can influence change of standards if changes need to be made to increase fairness and rights of the community in general.		
Radius of Significant Relationships (Sullivan)	*Outgroups.* Relationships during this time period tend to be an outgrowth of previously developed close friendships, first with individuals of the same sex, then branching out to members of the opposite sex.		
Play Behaviors	Generally both sexes engage in activities that involve their peers; females tend to spend more time talking about "things" than the males. Sports, hobbies, and entertainment (computer games, videos, and music) tend to make up much of the adolescents' "play behavior."		
Psychosexual Stage (Freud)	*Genital Stage.* This stage begins at the onset of puberty and the production of sexual hormones. While interactions tend to move toward developing a significant relationship, a major source of pleasure comes from sexual pleasures and tensions.		
Basic Physiological Events	Top age group for participation in sports, developmentally a need for independence and freedom from authority, likely to take risks, very strong need for approval from peers, girls generally two years ahead of boys developmentally.		
Common Fears	Social isolation, physical changes in body and own sexuality, divorce of parents, gossip, speaking in public, making mistakes in public.		
Medical Preparation Concerns	Use visual aids to provide visualization of the procedures. Include a description of the expected external appearance after the procedure if the patient's normal appearance will change (e.g., cast, stitches). Patients functioning at this developmental level prefer not to have any familiar staff or a parent with them as the procedures are being explained. Respect their wish for privacy. Additional feelings of control, which should reduce the need for restraints, can be gained by having the patients make their own appointments.		

Developmental Age: 18 to 25 Years

Psychosocial Stage of Development (Erikson)	Stage Six: Early Adulthood	Intimacy vs. Isolation	Capacity for love as mutual devotion; commitment to work and relationships without loss of self. Impersonal relationships, prejudice.

Developmental Age: 25 to 65 Years

Psychosocial Stage of Development (Erikson)	Stage Seven: Adulthood. 40 mid-life crisis; 42 - 65 middle age.	Generativity vs. Stagnation	Creativity, productivity, concern for others and the next generation. Self-indulgence, impoverishment of self.

Developmental Age: 65 Years Plus

Psychosocial Stage of Development (Erikson)	Stage Eight: Old Age. Possible loss of social and economic status, diminishing physical stamina, institutionalization, disengagement from commercial and professional activities; relative, family, and friends may become more important.	Ego Integrity vs. Despair	Acceptance of the worth and uniqueness of one's life. Emotional integration. That enables one to honor the past while preparing to relinquish leadership to younger people. Sense of loss, contempt for others. Life has been too short to achieve one's desires and that it is too late to begin again.

References

Accardo, P. J. & B. Y. Whitman. (1996). *Dictionary of developmental disabilities terminology*. Baltimore, MD: Paul H. Brookes Publishing Company.

Accu-Med Services. (1998). What and why of three-tier architecture. Software solutions: Special advertising section of *Contemporary Long Term Care, 21*(6), 2-3.

Adams, R. & J. McCubbin. (1991). *Games, sports, and exercises for the physically disabled, fourth edition*. Philadelphia, PA: Lea & Febiger.

Ader, R., Felten, D. & Cohen, N. (1991). *Psychoneuroimmunology*. New York: Academic Press.

American Conference of Governmental Industrial Hygienists, (1995). Threshold limits for chemical substances and physical agents and biological exposure indices. Cincinnati, OH: ACGIH.

American Occupational Therapy Association. (1989). *Uniform terminology for reporting occupational therapy, 2nd ed*. Bethesda, MD: AOTA.

American Psychiatric Association. (1987). *Diagnostic and statistical manual of mental disorders, third edition — revised*. Washington, DC.

American Psychiatric Association. (1994). *Diagnostic and statistical manual of mental disorders, fourth edition*. Washington, DC.

Anderson, K., L. Anderson & W. Glanze. (1994). *Mosby's medical, nursing & allied health dictionary, fourth edition*. St. Louis, MO: C. V. Mosby.

Armstrong, M. & S. Lauzen. (1994). *Community integration program, second edition*. Ravensdale, WA: Idyll Arbor, Inc.

Association of Operating Room Nurses, Inc. 1996. PEW Health Professions Commission taskforce on health care workforce regulation. http://www.aom.org/NSGTODAY/GOV/pew.htm (12-03-96 01:19:13 P.M.).

Austin, D. R. (1994). *Comprehensive glossary of recreational therapy*. Bloomington, IN: D. R. Austin.

Austin, D. R. (1997). *Therapeutic recreation: Processes and techniques (third edition)*. Champaign, IL: Sagamore Publishing.

Battle, J. (1992). *Culture-free self-esteem inventories, second edition*. Austin, TX: PRO-Ed.

Baum, A & Grunberg, N. (1995). Measurement of stress hormones. In Cohen, S., Kessler, R. C. & Gordon, L. U. (Eds.). *Measuring stress*. New York: Oxford.

Benson, H. & Stuart, E. M. (1992). *The wellness book*. New York: Simon & Schuster.

Benson, H. (1993). The relaxation response. In Goleman, D. & Gurin, J. (Eds.). *Mind body medicine* (pp. 233-257). New York: Consumer Reports Publishing.

Best Martini, E., M. Weeks & P. Wirth. (1996). *Long term care, second edition*. Ravensdale, WA: Idyll Arbor, Inc.

Best Martini, E., M. Weeks & P. Wirth. (2001). *Long term care, third edition*. Ravensdale, WA: Idyll Arbor, Inc.

Blackman, J. A. (1990). *Medical aspects of developmental disabilities in children birth to three*. Gaithersburg, MD: Aspen Publications.

Blauvelt, C. & F. Nelson. (1990). *A manual of orthopaedic terminology, fourth edition*. St. Louis, MO: C. V. Mosby.

Blauvelt, C. & F. Nelson. (1994). *A manual of orthopaedic terminology, fifth edition*. St. Louis, MO: C. V. Mosby.

Blumenthal, S. J. (1994). Introductory remarks: New frontiers in behavioral medicine research. In Blumenthal, S. J., Matthews, K., & Weiss, S. P. (Eds.). *New frontiers in behavioral medicine: Proceedings of the national conference* (pp. 9-15). Washington, DC: US Government Printing Office.

Blumenthal, S. J., Matthews, K., & Weiss, S. P. (1994). *New frontiers in behavioral medicine: Proceedings of the national conference*. Washington, DC: US Government Printing Office, #94-3772.

Borden, P., S. Fatherly, K. Ford & G. Vanderheiden. (1993). *Trace resourcebook: Assistive technologies for communication, control and computer access*. Madison, WI: Trace R&D Center.

Bourne, E. J. (1995). *The anxiety and phobia workbook, revised second edition*. Oakland, CA: New Harbinger Publications, Inc.

Bradford, L. P. (1976). *Making meetings work: A guide for leaders and group members*. La Jolla, CA: University Associates.

Brookfield, S. D. (1986). *Understanding and facilitating adult learning*. San Francisco, CA: Jossey-Bass.

Buchanan, L. & D. Nawoczenski. (1987). *Spinal cord injury: Concepts and management approaches*. Baltimore, MD: Williams & Wilkins.

Bunting, C.J., Tolson, H., Kuhn, C, Suarez, E., & Williams, R. B. (2000). Physiological stress response of the neuroendocrine system during outdoor adventure tasks. *Journal of Leisure Research, 32*(2), 197-207.

Burdge, R. (1961). The development of a leisure orientation scale. Unpublished master's thesis, Ohio State University.

Burisch, M. (1984). Approaches to personality inventory construction: A comparison of merits. *American Psychologist, 39*, 214-227.

burlingame, j. (1989). *Bus utilization skills assessment manual (BUS)*. Ravensdale, WA: Idyll Arbor, Inc.

burlingame, j. (1990). *burlingame software scale*. Ravensdale, WA: Idyll Arbor, Inc.

burlingame, j. (1996a). Quality assurance, safety, and risk management In E. Best Martini, M. Weeks and P. Wirth. *Long term care for activity and social services professionals, second edition*. Ravensdale, WA: Idyll Arbor, Inc.

burlingame, j. (1996b). Overview of evaluation. In A. D'Antonio-Nocera, N. DeBolt, & N. Touhey. *The professional activity manager and consultant*. Ravensdale, WA: Idyll Arbor, Inc.

burlingame, j. (1998a) Customer service. In F. Brasile, T. Skalko & j. burlingame (Eds.). *Perspectives in recreational therapy: Issues of a dynamic profession*. Ravensdale, WA: Idyll Arbor, Inc.

burlingame, j. (1998b) The role of information technologies. In F. Brasile, T. Skalko & j. burlingame (Eds.). *Perspectives in recreational therapy: Issues of a dynamic profession*. Ravensdale, WA: Idyll Arbor, Inc.

burlingame, j. & T. M. Blaschko. (1991). *Therapy in intermediate care facilities for the mentally retarded*. Seaside, OR: Frontier Publishing.

burlingame, j. & T. M. Blaschko. (1997). *Assessment tools for recreational therapy, second edition*. Ravensdale, WA: Idyll Arbor, Inc.

burlingame, j. & J. Peterson. (1987). *Recreation participation data sheet*. Ravensdale, WA: Idyll Arbor, Inc.

Card, J., D. Compton & G. Ellis. (1996.) *The comprehensive leisure rating scale*. Letter from J. Card to author.

Carruthers, C. (1993). Leisure and alcohol expectancies. *Journal of Leisure Research 25*(3), 229-244.

Caruso, Joseph J. (1982). Eight practices of good supervisors. *Children's Health Care 11*(1), 29-32.

Caudill, M. (1993). The biopsychosocial model of health: The mind body connection. In Wells, C. L. (Ed.). *Clinical training in behavioral medicine provider's manual*. Boston: Mind Body Medical Institute.

Caudill, M. (1995). *Managing pain before it manages you*. New York: Guilford Press.

Chrousos, G. P. & Gold, P. W. (1992). The concepts of stress and stress system disorders: Overview of physical and behavioral homeostasis. *Journal of the American Medical Association, 267*(9), 1244-1252.

Clark, W. A. (1920). System of joint measurement. *J. of Orthopedic Surgery. 2*:687. Reported in Rothstein, Roy & Wolf, *The rehabilitation specialist's handbook*. Philadelphia, PA: F. A. Davis Company.

Coastal Health Train. (1996). *Healthcare violence: Be part of the cure*. Virginia Beach, VA: Coastal Health Train.

Cohen, S., Kessler, R. C. & Gordon, L. U. (1995). *Measuring stress*. New York: Oxford.

Cohen, S., Tyrell, D., & Smith, A. (1991). Psychological stress and susceptibility to the common cold. *New England Journal of Medicine, 325*(9), 606-612.

Coile, R. C. Jr. (1994). Forecasting the future, part two. *Rehab Management 7*(2), 59-63.

Coleman, J. (1993). *The early intervention dictionary: a multidisciplinary guide to terminology*. Bethesda, MD: Woodbine House.

Congressional Record, 100 Stat. 478. Public Law 99-319. May 23, 1986. Protection and Advocacy for Mentally Ill Individuals Act 1986.

Connolly, P. (1997). Credentialing. In F. Brasile, T. Skalko & j. burlingame (Eds.). *Perspectives in recreational therapy: Issues of a dynamic profession*. Ravensdale, WA: Idyll Arbor, Inc.

Cunninghis, R. (1995). *Reality activities: A how to manual for increasing orientation, second edition*. Ravensdale, WA: Idyll Arbor, Inc.

Cunninghis, R. & E. Best Martini. (1996). *Quality assurance for activity programs, second edition*. Ravensdale, WA: Idyll Arbor, Inc.

D'Antonio-Nocera, A., N. DeBolt & N. Touhey. Editors. (1996). *The professional activity manager and consultant*. Ravensdale, WA: Idyll Arbor, Inc.

Daniels, L. & C. Worthingham. (1972). Muscle testing techniques of manual. In *Evaluation by comparison, third edition*. Philadelphia: W B Saunders Company.

Davidow, W. & Uttal, B. (1989). *Total customer service: The ultimate weapon*. New York: HarperPerennial.

Davis, J. E. (1952). *Clinical applications of recreational therapy*. Springfield: Charles C. Thomas.

Davis, M., E. Robbins-Eshelman & M. McKay. (1995). *The relaxation and stress reduction workbook, fourth edition*. Oakland, CA: New Harbinger Press.

Dehn, D. (1995). *Leisure step up*. Ravensdale, WA: Idyll Arbor, Inc.

Deutsch, A. & H. Fishman., Editors. (1970). *The encyclopedia of mental health*. Metuchen, NJ: Mini-Print Corporation.

Devine, Mary Ann. (2000). Constructing social acceptance in inclusive leisure contexts. Presentation at the National Parks and Recreation Congress, Phoenix, AZ.

DiGregorio, V. (1984). The burn problem, the burn team, and the physical therapist. In DiGregorio, V. (Ed.). *Rehabilitation of the burn patient*. New York: Churchill Livingstone.

Dorland, W. (1988). *Dorland's illustrated medical dictionary, 27th edition*. Philadelphia, PA: W. B. Saunders Co.

Dunn, J. (1990). Client assessment validation procedures. Handout from Class, University of North Texas.

Engel, G. L. (1977). The need for a new medical model: A challenge for biomedicine. *Science, 196*, 129-136.

Equal Employment Opportunity Commission & the US Department of Justice. (1991). *Americans with disabilities act handbook*. Washington, DC: US Government Printing Office.

Folkow, B. (1993). Physiological organization of neurohormonal responses to prolonged psychosocial stimuli: Implications for health and disease. *Annals of Behavioral Medicine, 15*(4), 236-244.

Folstein, M. F., S. Folstein, & P. R. McHugh. (1975). Mini-mental state: A practical method for grading the cognitive state of patients for the clinician. *Journal of Psychiatric Research 12*, 189-198.

Foto, M & G. Swanson (1993). Utilization review and managed care. *Rehab Management. 6*(5), 123-125.

Frankel, H. L., D. O. Hancock & G. Hyslop. (1969). The value of postural reduction in the initial management of closed injuries of the spine with paraplegia and tetraplegis. *Paraplegia 7*(3):179-92.

Friedman, M. & Ulmer, D. (1984). *Treating type A behavior and your heart*. New York: Fawcett Crest.

Garb, S., E. Krakauer, & C. Justice. (1976). *Abbreviations and acronyms in medicine and nursing*. New York: Springfield Publishing, Inc.

Gerhardt, J. J. & O. A. Russe. (1975). International SFTR method of measuring and recording joint motion. In Rothstein, J. S. Roy & S. Wolf (1991). *The rehabilitation specialist's handbook*. Philadelphia, PA: F. A. Davis Company.

Gill D. & Sparadeo F. (1989). Focus on clinical research: Effects of prior alcohol use on head injury recovery. *Journal of Head Trauma Rehabilitation 4*(1), 75-82.

Glanze, W., K. Anderson & L. Anderson. (1996). *The Signet Mosby medical encyclopedia, revised edition*. St. Louis, MO: C. V. Mosby.

Godfried, M. R. (1973). Reduction of generalized anxiety through a variant of systematic desensitization. In M. R. Godfried and M. Merbaum (Eds.). *Behavior change through self-control*. New York: Holt, Rinehart, and Winston.

Goldenson, R., J. Dunham, and C. Dunham. (1978). *Disability and rehabilitation handbook*. New York: McGraw-Hill, Inc.

Goldstein, T. (1995). *Functional rehabilitation in orthopaedics*. Gaithersburg, MD: Aspen Publishers.

Goleman, D. & Gurin, J. (1993). *Mind body medicine*. New York: Consumer Reports Publishing.

Goleman, D. (1995). *Emotional Intelligence*. New York: Bantam.

Gordon, N. F. (1993). *Breathing disorders: Your complete exercise guide*. Champaign, IL: Human Kinetics Publishers.

Graham Scott, G. (1990). *Resolving conflict with others and within yourself*. Oakland, CA: New Harbinger Publications, Inc.

Grosvenor, B. J. (1997). Unpublished manuscript. Ravensdale, WA: Idyll Arbor, Inc.

Hafen, B. Q., Frandsen, K. J., Karren, K. J., Hooker, K. R. (1992). *The health effects of attitudes emotions relationships*. Provo: EMS Associates.

Hamilton, B., & Guidos, B. (Eds.). (1984). *Medical acronyms, symbols, and abbreviations*. New York: Neal-Schuman Publishing, Inc.

Harnest, J. (1988). *Teach-a-bodies: An effective resource for sex education, investigation, therapy, and courtroom testimony*. Forth Worth, TX: Teach-A-Bodies.

Hartshorne, H. and May, M. A. (1928). *Studies in deceit*. New York: MacMillian.

Head, A. A. (1993). Let the record show. *Rehab Management, 6*(6), 110-111.

Health Care Financing Administration. (1989). *Health facility surveyor training basic course manual*. Baltimore: MD.

Health Care Financing Administration. (1990). *Patient assessment system for long-term care facilities*. US Department of Commerce National Technical Information Service. Springfield, VA.

Health Care Financing Administration. (1992). *State operations manual provider certification*. US Department of Commerce National Technical Information Service. Springfield, VA.

Hewitt, P. (1999). Psychological treatment works for perfectionism. www.cpa.ca/factsheets/perfectionism.htm. Canadian Psychological Association.

Hopkins, H. L. & H. D. Smith. (1983). *Willard and Spackman's occupational therapy, sixth edition*. New York: J. B. Lippincott Company.

Hughes, H. K. (1977). *Dictionary of abbreviations in medicine and the health sciences*. Lexington, MA: Lexington Books.

Inlander, C. & The Staff of the People's Medical Society. (1995). *The People's Medical Society health desk reference*. New York: Hyperion.

Institute of Medicine. (1989). *Prevention and treatment of alcohol problems: Research opportunities*. Washington DC: National Academy Press.

Jackson E. (1993). Recognizing patterns of leisure constraints: Results from alternative analyses." *Journal of Leisure Research,* *25*(2), 129-149.

Jay, R. (1997). Other considerations in selecting a support surface. *Advances in Wound Care, 10*(7), 37-42.

Joint Commission on Accreditation of Healthcare Organizations. (1995). *1996 comprehensive accreditation manual for hospitals.* Oakbrook Terrace: IL: Joint Commission.

Julien, R. (1992). *A primer of drug action, sixth edition.* New York: W. H. Freeman and Company.

Kane, R. A. & Kane, R. L. (1981). *Assessing the elderly: A practical guide to measurement.* Lexington, MA: Lexington Books.

Kaplan, H., B. Sadock & J. Grebb. (1994). *Kaplan and Sadock's synopsis of psychiatry, seventh edition.* Baltimore, MD: Williams & Wilkins.

Karam, C. (1989). *A practical guide to cardiac rehabilitation.* Gaithersburg, MD: Aspen Publications.

Kaufman, G. & L. Raphael. (1990). *Stick up for yourself: Every kid's guide to personal power and positive self-esteem.* Minneapolis, MN: Free Spirit Publishing.

Kaye, P. (1990). *Notes on symptom control in hospice & palliative care, revised first edition.* Essex, CT: Hospice Education Institute.

Kemp, B., K. Brummel-Smith & J. W. Ramsdell. (1990). *Geriatric rehabilitation.* Boston, MA: College Hill Publications.

Kiecolt-Glaser, J. K. & Glaser, R. (1995). Measurement of the immune response. In Cohen, S., Kessler, R. C. & Gordon, L. U. *Measuring stress.* New York: Oxford University Press.

Kiehnel, T. G., R. P. Liberman, D. Storzbach, & G. Rose. (1990). *A resource book for psychiatric rehabilitation — elements of service for the mentally ill.* Baltimore, MD: Williams and Wilkins.

Kisner, C. and L. A. Colby. (1990). *Therapeutic exercise: Foundations and techniques, second edition.* Philadelphia. F. A. Davis.

Klapp, O. (1986). *Overload and boredom: Essays on the quality of life in the information society.* Westport, CT: Greenwood Press, Inc.

Klein, J. B. 1994. Managed care contracting. *Rehab Management, 7*(5), 85-87.

Knaus, D. L. & J. B. Davis. (1993). *Medicare rules and regulations: A survival guide to policies, procedures, and payment reform.* Los Angeles: PMIC.

Knight-Ridders Newspapers, *The News Tribune* (Tacoma, WA, January 7, 1998). Confirmed negativity condition

Knowles, M. (1978). *The adult learner: A neglected species.* Houston, TX. Gulf Publishing Company.

Knowles, M. (1984). *Andragogy in action: Applying modern principles of adult learning.* San Francisco, CA: Jossey Bass.

Kreitner, C, A. J. Hartz, and R. D. Pflum. (1994). Patient-Centered Care. *Rehab Management, 7*(3.), 25-30, 119

Kübler-Ross, E. (1969). *On death and dying.* New York: Macmillan Publishing Co., Inc.

Kurtzke, P. (1983). Expanded Disability Status Scale. *Neurology, 33,* 1444-52.

Lamers-Winhelman, F. (1988). Recognition of child sexual abuse in young children. In Harnest, J. *Teach-a-bodies: An effective resource for sex education, investigation, therapy, and courtroom testimony.* Fort Worth, TX: Teach-A Bodies.

Lewis, C. B. (1989). *Improving mobility in older persons: A manual for geriatric specialists.* Gaithersburg, MD: Aspen Publication.

Locke, S. (1992). Introduction. In G. F. Von Bozzay (Ed.). *Behavioral medicine, stress management and biofeedback: A clinician's desk reference.* San Francisco: Biofeedback Press.

Locke, S. & Colligan, D. (1986). *The healer within.* New York: Mentor.

Lohmann, N. (1976). *Life Satisfaction Scale.* Morgantown, WV: West Virginia University.

Lopez, M. (1998). Musculoskeletal ergonomics: An introduction. in V. B. Rice (Ed.) *Ergonomics in health care and rehabilitation.* Boston: Butterworth-Heinemann.

Luborsky, L. (1962). Clinician's judgment of mental health. *Archives of General Psychiatry, 7*:407-417.

Luckasson, R. A. (1992). *Mental retardation: Definition, classification, and systems of support, ninth edition.* American Association on Mental Retardation.

Mackay, H. (1996). *Swim with the sharks without being eaten alive: Outsell, outmanage, outmotivate, and outnegotiate your competition.* New York: Ballantine.

Malkin, M. and C. Howe. (1993). *Research in therapeutic recreation: Concepts and methods.* State College, PA: Venture Publishing.

Matsakis, A. (1994). *Post-traumatic stress disorder: A complete treatment guide.* Oakland, CA: New Harbinger.

McKay, M., M. Davis & P. Fanning. (1983). *Messages: The communication skills book.* Oakland. New Harbinger Publications.

McKay, M, M. Davis & P Fanning. (1995). *Messages: The communication skills book, second edition.* Oakland, CA: New Harbinger Publications.

Merla, J. L and S. J. Spaulding. (1997). The balance system: Implications for occupational therapy intervention. *Physical and Occupational Therapy in Geriatrics, 15*:1, 21-36.

Miller, E. E. (1997). *Deep healing.* Carlsbad, CA: Hay House, Inc.

Moyers, B. D. (1993). *Healing and the mind.* New York; Bantam Doubleday, Inc.

Nash, T. B. (1953). *Philosophy of recreation and leisure.* Dubuque, IA: Wm. C. Brown Company.

Nathan, A. & S. Mirviss. (1997). *Therapy techniques using the creative arts.* Ravensdale, WA: Idyll Arbor, Inc.

National Adult Learning and Literacy Center. (1990). *Teaching adults who have learning disabilities.* Washington, DC: The Adult Learning and Literacy Clearinghouse, US Department of Education.

National Archives and Records Administration. (1990). *Code of federal regulations 42: part 430 to end.* Washington, DC: U. S. Government Printing Office.

National Committee for Quality Assurance. (1996). *1996 reviewer guidelines: Standards for accreditation.* Washington, DC: National Committee for Quality Assurance.

Navar, N. & C. A. Peterson. (1990). *State Technical Institute leisure activities project.* Ravensdale, WA: Idyll Arbor, Inc.

Niemeyer, L. O. & burlingame, j. (1998). Outcomes. In F. Brasile, T. Skalko & j. burlingame (Eds.). *Perspectives in recreational therapy: Issues of a dynamic profession.* Ravensdale: Idyll Arbor, Inc.

O'Morrow, G. & Reynolds, R. P. (1989). *Therapeutic recreation.* Englewood Cliffs, NJ: Prentice Hall.

Occupational Safety and Health Administration, (1995). *Ergonomic protection standard* (Draft). Washington, DC: Government Printing Office.

Ornstein, R. & Sobel, D. (1989). *Healthy pleasures.* Reading, Mass: Addison Wesley.

Pearsall, P. (1996). *The pleasure prescription.* Alameda CA: Hunter House, Inc.

Pelletier, K. R. (1994) *Sound mind, sound body.* New York: Simon & Schuster.

Pert, C. B. (1997). *Molecules of emotion.* New York: Scribner.

Peters, E. (1979). Notes toward an archaeology of boredom. *Social Research, 42*:493-511.

Peterson, C. A., J. Dunn & C. Carruthers. (1983). *Functional assessment of characteristics of therapeutic recreation.* Ravensdale, WA: Idyll Arbor, Inc.

Peterson, C. A., J. Dunn & C. Carruthers. (1996). *Functional assessment of characteristics of therapeutic recreation, revised.* Ravensdale, WA: Idyll Arbor, Inc.

Peterson, C.A. and S. L. Gunn. (1984). *Therapeutic recreation program design, second edition.* Englewood Cliffs, NJ: Prentice-Hall.

Peterson, C. A. & Stumbo, N. (2000). *Therapeutic recreation program design.* Boston: Allyn and Bacon.

Pollock, M. L. & Wilmore, J. H. (1990). *Exercise in health and disease.* Philadelphia: W. B. Saunders.

Pool, J. L. (1991). Age related changes in sensory system dynamics related to balance. *Physical & Occupational Therapy in Geriatrics, 10*:55-66).

Pozgar, G. (1996). *Legal aspects of health care administration.* Gaithersburg, MD: Aspen Publications.

Pyle, V. (1996). *Current medical terminology, sixth edition.* Modesto, CA: Health Professions Institute.

Ragheb, M. (1996). Measuring leisure and recreation involvement. Presentation at the National Congress for the National Recreation and Park Association. Kansas City.

Ragheb, M. (1997). *Leisure and recreation involvement measurement.* Ravensdale, WA: Idyll Arbor, Inc.

Ragheb, M. G. & J. G. Beard. (1990). *Leisure motivation scale.* Ravensdale, WA: Idyll Arbor, Inc.

Ragheb, M. G. & J. G. Beard. (1991a). *Leisure attitude measurement.* Ravensdale, WA: Idyll Arbor, Inc.

Ragheb, M. G. & J. G. Beard. (1991b). *Leisure interest measure.* Ravensdale, WA: Idyll Arbor, Inc.

Ragheb, M. G. & J. G. Beard. (1991c). *Leisure satisfaction measure.* Ravensdale, WA: Idyll Arbor, Inc.

Ragheb, M. G. & S. P. Merydith (1995). *Free time boredom.* Ravensdale, WA: Idyll Arbor, Inc.

Rakowski, W. (1996). The transtheoretical model of behavioral change: Application to clinical practice. *Mind/Body Medicine, 1*(4), 207-220.

Randall-David, E. (1989). *Strategies for working with culturally diverse communities and patients.* Bethesda, MD: Association for the Care of Children's Health.

Reber, A. S. (1985). *Dictionary of psychology.* New York: Penguin Books.

Roat, C. (1996). Letter to author. Seattle, WA: The Cross Cultural Health Care Program.

Robbins, J. (2000). *Symphony in the brain.* New York: Atlantic Monthly Press.

Rodman, G. P., C. McEwen & S. L. Wallace. (1973). Primer on the rheumatic diseases. Reprinted from *The Journal of the American Medical Association 224*(5) (Supplement).

Rogers, R. (Ed.) (1997). *Clinical Assessment of Malingering and Deception.* New York: Guilford.

Rook, J.L. (1995). Geriatric pain management. *Rehab Management 8*(1), 25-26, 30-32.

Rossi, E. L. (1993). *The psychobiology of mind-body healing.* New York: W. W. Norton.

Rothstein, J., S. Roy & S. Wolf. (1991). *The rehabilitation specialist's handbook.* Philadelphia, PA: F. A. Davis.

Russoniello, C. V. (1994). An exploratory study of physiological and psychological changes in patients after recreational therapy treatments. Annals of Behavioral Medicine: Fourth International Congress Proceedings, 228.

Russoniello, C.V. (1997). Behavioral medicine: A model for therapeutic recreation. In Compton, D. M. (Ed.). *Issues in therapeutic recreation.* (pp. 461-488). Champaign: Sagamore.

Sainsbury, R. (1993). Life satisfaction as it relates to recreational therapy. Presentation at the Third International TR Conference, August 1993, Richmond Hill, Ontario.

Sallis, J. F. & Owen, N. (1999). *Physical activity and behavioral medicine.* Thousand Oaks, CA: Sage.

Sanderson, C. (1995). *Counseling adult survivors of child sexual abuse.* Bristol, PA: Jessica Kingsley Publishers, Ltd.

Sapolsky, R. M. (1994). *Why zebras don't get ulcers.* New York: W. H. Freeman and Company.

Schenk, C. (1995). *Leisurescope plus.* Tallahassee, FL: Leisure Dynamics.

Scotece, G. (1993). The pain team. *Rehab Management, 6*(6): 290-293.

Searight, H. R. (1999). *Behavioral medicine: A primary care approach.* Philadelphia: Brunner/Mazel.

Seattle-King County Department of Public Health. (1994). *Questions & answers about HIV and AIDS.* Seattle, WA.

Seligman, M. E. P. (1994). *What you can change & what you can't.* New York: Knopf.

Seligman, M. E. P. (1995). The effectiveness of psychotherapy. The Consumer Reports study. *American Psychologist, 50*(12), 965-974.

Selye, H. (1978). *The stress of life.* New York: McGraw-Hill.

Shank, J. W., Kinney, W. B. & Coyle, C. (1993). Efficacy studies in therapeutic recreation research: The need, the state of the art, and future implications. In Malkin, M. J. & Howe, C. Z. *Research in therapeutic recreation.* State College, PA: Venture.

Shannon, M. L. (1984). Five famous fallacies about pressure sores. *Nursing 84*(14):34-41.

Shelton, S. B. (1999). The doctor-patient relationship. In Stoudemire, A. (Ed.). *Human behavior.* Philadelphia: Lippincott-Rave.

Skalko, T., R. Mitchell., A. Kaye, & M. Dalton. (1994). *Basic guide to physical and psychiatric medication for recreational therapy.* Hattiesburg, MS: American Therapeutic Recreation Association.

Slivkin, K. & R. Crandell. (1978). A new leisure ethic scale. Unpublished Paper, AAHPER Convention, Kansas City, KS.

Smilkstein, G. 1978. The family APGAR: A proposal for a family function test and its use by physicians. *Journal of Family Practice 6*:1231-1239.

Smith, R. (1994). Trends in medical rehab. *Rehab Management, 7*(6), 33-38.

Sobel, D. S. (1994). Mind matter, money matter: The cost-effectiveness of clinical behavioral medicine. In Blumenthal, S. J., Matthews, K., & Weiss, S. P. (Eds.). *New Frontiers in behavioral medicine: Proceedings of the national conference.* Washington, DC: US Government Printing Office, #94-3772.

Springhouse Corporation. (1997). *Diseases, second edition.* Springhouse, PA: Springhouse Corporation.

Stedman, T. L. (1995). *Stedman's medical dictionary: Illustrated in color, 26th edition.* Baltimore, MD: Williams & Wilkins.

Stolov, W. C. (1992). New ASIA standards for neurological and functional classification of spinal cord injury. *Rehabilitation Spinal Cord Injury Update 2*(4), 1-2.

Suinn, R. M. & F. Richardson. (1971). Anxiety management training: A non-specific behavior therapy program for anxiety control. *Behavior Therapy 2*:498-510.

Timby, B. and L. Lewis. (1992). *Fundamental skills and concepts in patient care, fifth edition.* Philadelphia, PA: J. B. Lippincott.

Towell, J. E. & H. E. Sheppard. (Eds.). (1987). *Acronyms, initialisms & abbreviations dictionary, eleventh edition.* Detroit, MI: Gale Research Company.

United States Congressional Office of Technology Assessment. (1990). *The use of integrity tests for pre-employment screening.* Report No. OTA-SET-442. Washington DC: US Government Printing Office.

University of Texas at Austin Counseling and Mental Health Center (1999). www.utexas.edu/student/cmhc/perfect.html.

US Architectural and Transportation Barriers Compliance Board. (1991). *Americans with Disabilities Act accessibility guidelines checklist for buildings and facilities.* Washington, DC: US Government Printing Office.

US Department of Health and Human Services. (1981). *Lead poisoning.* Washington, DC: US Government Printing Office.

US Department of Health and Human Services. (1983). *CDC guidelines for isolation precautions in hospitals and CDC guidelines for infection control in hospital personnel.* Atlanta: Centers for Disease Control.

US Department of Health and Human Services. (1990). *International classification of diseases, ninth edition, clinical modification.* Washington, DC: US Government Printing Office.

Voelkl, J. E. (1988). *Risk management in therapeutic recreation: A component of quality assurance.* State College, PA: Venture Publishing.

Washington State Department of Social and Health Services. (1988). *Facts about hepatitis.* Olympia, WA.

Waters, R. L., R. H. Adkins, & J. S. Yakura (1991). Definition of complete spinal cord injury. *Paraplegia 29*(9):573-81.

Webster's collegiate dictionary, fifth edition. (1946). Springfield, MA: G. & C. Merriam Co., Publishers.

Werner, A., R. J. Campbell, S. H. Frazier, E. M. Stone, J. Edgerton & APA Staff. (1984). *The American Psychiatric Association's psychiatric glossary.* Washington DC: American Psychiatric Press, Inc.

West, C. C. (1945). Measurement of Joint Motion. *Arch. Physical Medicine* 26:414. In Rothstein, Roy & Wolf. *The rehabilitation specialist's handbook.* Philadelphia, PA: F. A. Davis Company.

Whaley, L. & D. Wong. (1985). *Essentials of pediatric nursing, second edition.* St. Louis, MO: C. V. Mosby.

Whaley, L and D. Wong. (1991). *Nursing care of infants and children, fourth edition.* St. Louis, MO: Mosby.

White and Wooten. (1986). *Professional ethics and practice of organizational development.* NY: Praeger Publishers.

Whitehead, W. (1994). Assessing the effects of stress on physical symptoms. *Health Psychology, 13*(2), 99-102.

Wieder-Singer, D. (1994). Putting muscle in referral relationships. *Rehab Management, 7*(6), 115-116.

Witt, P. & G. Ellis. (1990). *Leisure diagnostic battery.* State College, PA: Venture Publishing.

Wolfe, G. (1993). Case management and managed care. *Rehab Management, 6*(6), 114-115.

Ylvisaker, M. (Ed.). (1985). *Head injury rehabilitation: Children and adolescents.* Boston, MA: College-Hill Press.

Zane, L. (1984). Evaluation of the acutely ill burn patient. In DiGregorio, V. R. (Ed.). *Rehabilitation of the burn patient.* New York, NY: Churchill Livingstone.

Zuckerman, E. L. (1994). *The clinician's thesaurus third edition.* Pittsburgh, PA: The Clinician's ToolBox.